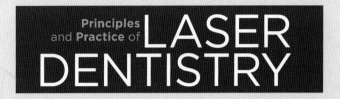

6/11/05

To Pete

Happy Layering !!

signature

2nd Edition

Principles and Practice of LASER DENTISTRY

Robert A. Convissar, DDS, FAGD

Director, Laser Dentistry
New York Hospital Queens
Master, Academy of Laser Dentistry
Private Practice
New York, New York

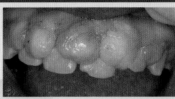
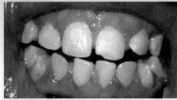
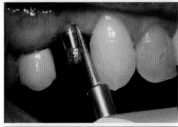
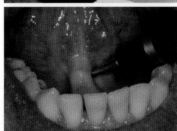
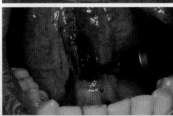

ELSEVIER

3251 Riverport Lane
St. Louis, Missouri 63043

PRINCIPLES AND PRACTICE OF LASER DENTISTRY, SECOND EDITION   ISBN: 978-0-323-29762-2
Copyright © 2016 by Elsevier, Inc. All rights reserved.

Notices

Previous edition copyrighted 2010.

International Standard Book Number: 978-0-323-29762-2

Executive Content Strategist: Kathy Falk
Content Development Manager: Jolynn Gower
Senior Content Development Specialist: Brian Loehr
Publishing Services Manager: Julie Eddy
Project Manager: Sara Alsup
Design Direction: Amy Buxton

Printed in China

Last digit is the print number: 9 8 7 6 5 4 3 2 1

Working together to grow libraries in developing countries

www.elsevier.com • www.bookaid.org

*To my wife, partner, and source of inspiration
not just in dentistry, but in life:*

Dr. Ellen Goldstein Convissar

Contributors

Eugenia Anagnostaki, DDS, FALD, SOLA Master
Private Practice
Rethymno, Greece

Ana Cecilia Corrêa Aranha, DDS, MSc, PhD
Special Laboratory of Lasers in Dentistry (LELO)
School of Dentistry, University of São Paulo
São Paulo, Brazil

Per Hugo Beck-Kristensen, DDS
Board Member, Nordic Laser Dental Society
Main Lecturer, SOLA Academy
Vienna, Austria;
Staff Dental Surgeon
Frederiksberggårdens Tandklinik/Dental Clinic
Frederiksberg, Denmark

Marina Stella Bello-Silva, DDS
School of Dentistry, University Nove de Julho (UNINOVE)
São Paulo, Brazil

Louis G. Chmura, DDS, MS
Owner and Director, Laser Training–Egghead Ortho
Private Practice
Marshall, Michigan

Michael Coleman, DDS
Private Practice, Oral and Maxillofacial Surgery
Cornelius, North Carolina

Donald J. Coluzzi, DDS, FACD
Associate Clinical Professor
University of California, San Francisco School of Dentistry
San Francisco, California

Robert A. Convissar, DDS, FAGD
Director, Laser Dentistry
New York Hospital Queens
Master, Academy of Laser Dentistry
Private Practice
New York, New York

George R. Deeb, DDS, MD
Associate Professor
Department of Oral and Maxillofacial Surgery
Virginia Commonwealth University
Richmond, Virginia

James C. Downs, DMD
Clinical Director, Cosmetic and Restorative Dentistry
Dr. Dick Barnes Group
Sandy, Utah
Private Practice
Denver, Colorado

Carlos de Paula Eduardo, DDS, MSc, PhD
Full Professor, Department of Restorative Dentistry
Chairman, Special Laboratory of Lasers in Dentistry (LELO)
School of Dentistry, University of São Paulo
São Paulo, Brazil

John D.B. Featherstone, MSc, PhD
Dean and Professor
School of Dentistry
University of California San Francisco
San Francisco, California

Patricia Moreira de Freitas, DDS, MSc, PhD
Special Laboratory of Lasers in Dentistry (LELO)
School of Dentistry, University of São Paulo
São Paulo, Brazil

Charles R. Hoopingarner, DDS, FAGD
Associate Professor
University of Texas Dental School-Houston
Master Academy of Laser Dentistry
Private Practice
Houston, Texas

Jon Julian, DDS
Private Practice
CEO, North Star Dental Education
Travelers Rest, South Carolina

Lawrence Kotlow, DDS
Board-Certified Specialist in Pediatric Dentistry
Private Practice
Albany, New York

Samuel B. Low, DDS, MS, MEd
Professor Emeritus
University of Florida College of Dentistry
Gainesville, Florida

Erica Krohn Jany Migliorati, DDS
Assistant Professor, Department of Periodontics
University of Tennessee Health Science Center
College of Dentistry
Memphis, Tennessee

Joshua Moshonov, DMD
Clinical Associate Professor and Acting Chair
Department of Endodontics
Hebrew University–Hadassah School of Dental Medicine
Jerusalem, Israel

Angie Mott, RDH
Certified Dental Laser Educator
Master, Academy of Laser Dentistry
Clinical Private Practice
Tulsa, Oklahoma

Steven Parker, BDS, LDS RCS, MFGDP
Past President, Academy of Laser Dentistry
Associate Editor, *Journal of Lasers in Medical Science*
Visiting Professor, Faculty of Medicine and Dentistry
University of Genoa
Genoa, Italy;
Private Practice
Harrogate, United Kingdom

Karen Muller Ramalho, DDS, MSc
Biodentistry Master Program
School of Dentistry, Ibirapuera University (UNIB)
São Paulo, Brazil

Daniel Simões de Almeida Rosa, DDS
Laboratório Experimental de Laser em Odontologia
Special Laboratory of Lasers in Dentistry (LELO)
School of Dentistry, University of São Paulo
São Paulo, Brazil

David M. Roshkind, DMD, MBA, FAGD
Former Adjunct Professor
College of Dental Medicine, Nova Southeastern University
Certified Dental Laser Educator
Master, Academy of Laser Dentistry
Private Practice
West Palm Beach, Florida

Alana Ross, BScH
Medical Device Marketing and Education
Toronto, Ontario

Gerald Ross, DDS
College of Dental Surgeons of Ontario
Private Practice
Tottenham, Ontario

Sharonit Sahar-Helft, DMD
Clinical Instructor, Department of Endodontics
Hebrew University–Hadassah School of Dental Medicine
Jerusalem, Israel

Todd J. Sawisch, DDS
Diplomate, American Board of Oral and Maxillofacial Surgery
Voluntary Associate Professor of Surgery
University of Miami School of Medicine
Miami, Florida;
Private Practice
Fort Lauderdale, Florida

Mary Lynn Smith, RDH, BM, AAS
McPherson Dental Care
McPherson, Kansas

Adam Stabholz, DMD
Former Dean
Faculty of Dental Medicine
Professor and Former Chairman
Department of Endodontics
Hebrew University–Hadassah School of Dental Medicine
Jerusalem, Israel

Robert A. Strauss, DDS, MD
Professor of Surgery
Director, Residency Training Program
Department of Oral and Maxillofacial Surgery
Virginia Commonwealth University School of Medicine
Richmond, Virginia

John G. Sulewski, MA
Director of Education and Training
The Institute for Advanced Dental Technologies
Bloomfield Hills, Michigan

Grace Sun, DDS
Accredited Fellow, American Academy of Cosmetic Dentistry
Master, Academy of General Dentistry
Master and Educator, Academy of Laser Dentistry
Fellow, International Congress of Implantologists
Director, Sun Dental Group
West Hollywood, California

Jan Tunér, DDS
Former Secretary, World Association for Laser Therapy
Former Vice President, Swedish Laser Medical Society
Former Chair, Department of Prosthodontics
Former Lecturer, European Master Degree Program on Oral Laser Applications
Grangesberg, Sweden

Foreword

When the first dental laser came on the market in the late 1980s, there was great excitement in the world of dentistry. Unfortunately, the laser wavelength for that first device was chosen because it was available, not because it was the best one for the purpose desired. Laser dentistry has come a long way since then, with accumulation of an extensive science base on laser interactions with both soft and hard tissues. In recent years, lasers have been developed for medicine and dentistry based on the best evidence to date, including the optimal conditions for these clinical applications. A whole new energy has emerged regarding the use of lasers in dentistry and much of it is captured in this second edition of Dr. Robert Convissar's *Principles and Practice of Laser Dentistry*.

Dr. Convissar is one of the pioneers of the clinical use of lasers in dentistry, with almost 25 years of experience with carbon dioxide, neodymium-doped yttrium-aluminum-garnet (Nd:YAG), diode, and erbium wavelengths. He has presented more than 300 laser seminars on five continents. For this revised edition, he has brought together a team of authors whose knowledge base and skills are state of the art, for preparation of a treatise worth reading.

In these days of electronic communication and indeed electronic books, journals, media, music, and much more, it is hard to imagine that yet another textbook could be useful.

On the contrary, this is a great read for anyone who wants a comprehensive review of the world of lasers and their use in dentistry. The attentive reader will gain an understanding of how lasers work, how they interact with the tissues, and thus how best to apply this knowledge in clinical practice.

I started my research into the possibilities of using lasers in dentistry in 1980, well before there was even much use of these devices for surgery and treatments in the rest of the human body. Things were very primitive at that time, with much unknown. My team has worked for more than 30 years on laser interactions with hard tissues. Together with other groups across the world, we were able to contribute to an in-depth understanding of how to use lasers for teeth and bone applications. Only recently was all of this work brought together by a company to build and then market a new laser that takes advantage of this science and the clinical research that followed. This new technology has helped to set the stage for the next big move forward in the everyday adoption of lasers in dental practice.

Other big steps forward have been achieved in recent years, as detailed in the following pages. There is definitely more to come in the future, as a dream of more than 25 years ago for some of us is realized.

John D.B. Featherstone, MSc, PhD

Preface

In the five years since the publication of the first edition of this book, the field of laser dentistry has made great strides in delivering superior patient care. Manufacturers new to the industry have entered the field with state-of-the-art devices. Well-established companies have come out with new models that offer significant improvements over previous versions. A new wavelength on the market, a 9300-nm carbon dioxide laser with both hard- and soft-tissue applications, may revolutionize dentistry—or may fall by the wayside, as did the argon and holmium wavelengths in the context of general dentistry. As usual, the clinical experience will determine this outcome.

Clinicians are finding ever more procedures that have a positive impact on the lives of their patients. Five years ago, just a handful of pediatric laser dentistry pioneers were performing lingual tongue-tie and maxillary frenectomy procedures on newborn babies to help them latch onto their mothers' nipples and nurse. It was rare for dentists to receive referrals from other health care professionals for this type of procedure. Today, laser dentists are receiving referrals from pediatricians, neonatologists, pediatric otolaryngologists, lactation specialists, and many more to help babies nurse more successfully. For treating teenagers and older patients, dentists are receiving referrals on a regular basis from speech therapists, orofacial myologists, specialists in osteopathic manipulative medicine, and many more. For drug-induced gingival hyperplasia treatment, dentists are working with transplant surgeons and primary care physicians of organ transplant recipients. The list keeps growing.

As with the first edition, this book is written both for the clinician who wants to learn how to use a laser and for the established laser user who wants to expand the range of procedures for the practice's instrument or to add a device with different capabilities. For each procedure described, the peer-reviewed literature that validates its use also is presented. Procedures that are neither supported by the peer-reviewed literature nor based on sound biologic foundations are not included in this book. Each of the chapters is written by a "wet-fingered" practitioner with extensive laser experience—and, in most cases, with specialty board certification in his or her field of expertise. Virtually every procedure is fully documented with preoperative, intraoperative, and postoperative photographs. Suggestions and "Clinical Tips" are highlighted throughout, making the most pertinent clinical information for the practitioner readily available.

A textbook of any scope and depth cannot be written without the dedication of a number of people. Thanks are due to each and every contributing author, who gave up months of valuable time away from their practices and families to work on this most worthwhile project. Thanks also to the best team in dental textbook publishing: Brian Loehr, Jaime Pendill, Sara Alsup, and Kathy Falk. Finally, this book would never have been possible without the love, encouragement, and support of my wife and partner, Dr. Ellen Goldstein, and our children Craig, Alex, and Dana.

Contents

1

Einstein's "Splendid Light": Origins and Dental Applications

JOHN G. SULEWSKI

Humankind's fascination with the properties of light and its applications in medicine can be traced to ancient times. Developments in physics at the beginning of the twentieth century laid the foundation for laser theory postulated by Albert Einstein, culminating in the invention of this special form of light in 1960. Soon thereafter, researchers began to explore possible applications of laser technology in medical and dental treatment.

The medicinal use of light for diagnostic and therapeutic purposes dates from antiquity. Light allowed early physicians to observe skin color, inspect wounds, and choose a suitable therapeutic course of action. Heat from sunlight or campfires was used for therapy. Greeks and Romans took daily sunbaths, and the solarium was a feature of many Roman houses.[1] Ancient Egyptians, Chinese, and Indians used light to treat rickets, psoriasis, skin cancer, and even psychosis.[2]

The ancient Egyptians, Indians, and Greeks also used natural sunlight to repigment affected skin in patients with vitiligo by activating the naturally occurring photosensitizer *psoralen,* found in parsley and other plants.[3-5] In the eighteenth and nineteenth centuries, European physicians used sunlight and artificial light to treat cutaneous tuberculosis, psoriasis, eczema, and mycosis fungoides.[3] These and other applications of light were precursors to the invention and subsequent use of optical amplifier devices that generate a special form of light—*lasers*—in the medical field over the past several decades.

This chapter examines the efforts of select laser pioneers in dentistry and summarizes current intraoral clinical applications of lasers.

Early Published Theories of Light

Philosophers and scientists long pondered the nature of light: Was it composed of particles, waves, pressure, or some other substance or force?

In his *Book of Optics,* published in 1021, Persian mathematician, scientist, and philosopher Ibn al-Haytham described light as being composed of a stream of tiny particles that travel in straight lines and bounce off objects that they strike.[6] Pierre Gassendi, a French philosopher, scientist, astronomer, and mathematician, described his particle theory of light (published posthumously in 1658 in Lyon, France, as part of the six volumes of his collected works, the *Opera Omnia*), in effect introducing to European scholars the atomism view of the universe identified by the ancient Greek philosopher Epicurus (341-270 BCE)[7] (Figure 1-1).

Gassendi's work influenced English physicist Sir Isaac Newton (1642-1727), who described light as "corpuscles" or particles of matter that "were emitted in all directions from a source"[8,9] (Figure 1-2). Newton proposed the theory of particle dynamics, which later would be developed to describe the behavior of particles reacting to the influence of arbitrary forces.[10] The particle view of light differed from that of French philosopher and scientist René Descartes, who in his 1637 *Discourse* saw light as a type of "pressure," which foreshadowed the postulation of the wave theory of light[11] (Figure 1-3).

In 1665, English scientist Robert Hooke suggested his wave theory of light, likening the spread of light vibrations

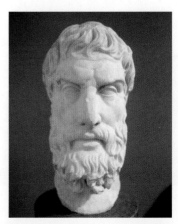

• **Figure 1-1** Greek philosopher Epicurus (341-270 BCE).

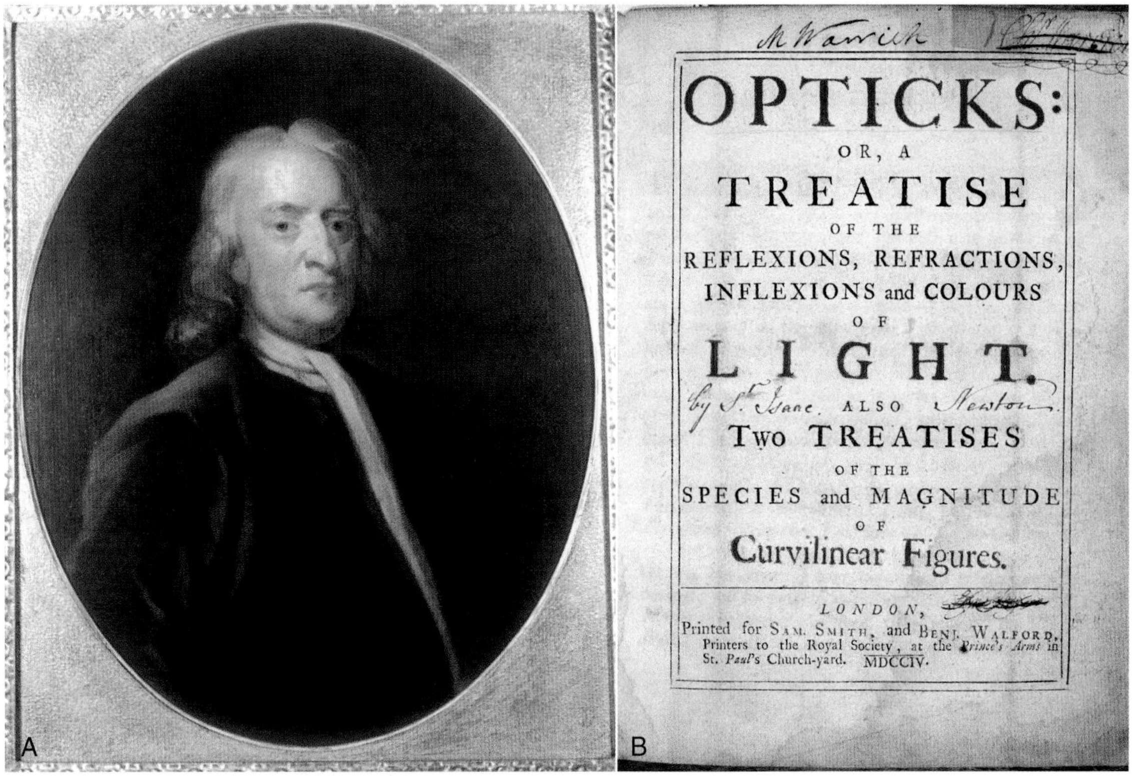

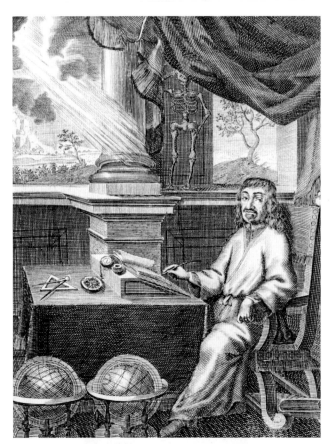

• **Figure 1-2 A,** Sir Isaac Newton (1642-1727). **B,** Title page from Newton's work *Opticks*, 1704.

• **Figure 1-3** René Descartes (1596-1650).

to that of waves in water: "every pulse or vitration of the luminous body will generate a sphere, which will continually increase, and grow bigger, just after the same manner (though infinitely swifter) as the waves or rings on the surface of the water do swell into bigger and bigger circles about a point."[12] The wave concept subsequently was proved experimentally by Scottish physicist James Clerk Maxwell, who in 1865 proposed an electromagnetic wave theory of light and demonstrated that electromagnetic waves traveled at precisely the speed of light.[13]

Development of Quantum Theory

The previous theories, useful as they might have been before 1900, did not entirely or satisfactorily describe the characteristics of light observed by the scientific community: Light behaved as particles in some cases and as waves in others. This context of inquiry led to the field of *quantum theory.*

On December 14, 1900, German physicist Max Planck delivered a lecture before the German Physical Society (Deutsche Physikalische Gesellschaft) in which he theorized that light consisted of discrete and indivisible packets of radiant energy that he named *quanta.* He described what eventually became known as the elemental unit of energy *(E)*, as $E = hv$, where h is a constant of nature with the dimension of action (= energy × time, with a value of 6.626×10^{-34} joule-second), subsequently called Planck's constant, and v is the frequency of radiation. Planck's theory was published late in 1900.[14-16] Eleven years later, British physicist Ernest Rutherford contributed to quantum theory when he postulated a planetary model of the atom based on his experimental observations of the scattering of alpha particles by atoms. In his view an atom comprises a central charge surrounded by a distribution of electrons orbiting within a sphere.[17]

Danish physicist Niels Bohr synthesized Rutherford's atom model with Planck's quantum hypothesis (Figure 1-4). In a series of papers published in 1913, Bohr proposed a theory in which electrons revolve in specific orbits around a nucleus without emitting radiant energy. He described the stable, "ground state" of an atom, when all of its electrons are at their lowest energy level. Bohr also theorized that an electron may suddenly jump from one specific orbital level to a higher level; to do so, an electron must gain energy. Conversely, an electron must lose energy to move from a higher energy level to a lower energy level. Thus an electron can move from one energy level to another by either absorbing or emitting radiant energy or light.[18,19]

It was in this burgeoning milieu of nascent quantum theory that Albert Einstein made three significant contributions. First, in 1905, Einstein developed his light quantum theory: "In the propagation of a light ray emitted from a point source, the energy is not distributed continuously over ever-increasing volumes of space, but consists of a finite number of energy quanta localized at points of space that move without dividing, and can be absorbed or generated as complete units."[20] Singh[21] points out that this

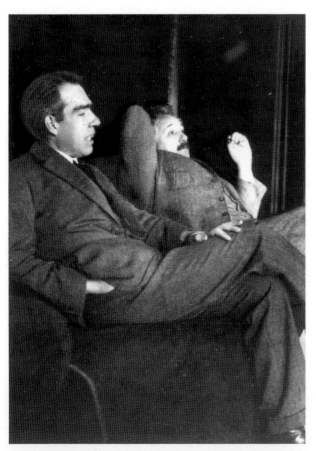

• **Figure 1-4** Niels Bohr and Albert Einstein in 1925.

paper on photoelectric effect was the first that Einstein published during his *annus mirabilis* ("extraordinary year"), in the scientific journal *Annalen der Physik* in 1905; his other papers that year treated Brownian motion, special theory of relativity, and matter and energy equivalence ($E = mc^2$). Notably, Einstein himself regarded his light quantum paper as the "most revolutionary" of those that he had published in 1905. He was awarded the 1921 Nobel Prize in physics for this paper. Hallmark and Horn[22] stated that Einstein's light quantum theory was so radical in comparison with other contemporary theories of light that it was not generally accepted until American physicist Robert A. Millikan performed additional experiments in 1916 to support the theory.

Einstein's 1905 paper made the case for the particle nature of light. In 1909, Einstein made his second significant contribution to laser theory by publishing the first reference in physics to the *wave-particle duality* of light radiation, using Planck's radiation law. Einstein stated: "It is my opinion that the next phase in the development of theoretical physics will bring us a theory of light which can be interpreted as a kind of fusion of the wave and emission theory. ... Wave structure and quantum structure ... are not to be considered as mutually incompatible. ... We will have to modify our current theories, not to abandon them completely."[21,23] British mathematician and physicist Banesh Hoffmann fancifully characterized the quandary for many early twentieth-century physicists regarding the apparent wave-particle duality of light: "They could but make the best of it, and went around with woebegone faces sadly complaining that on Mondays, Wednesdays, and Fridays they must look on light as a wave; on Tuesdays, Thursdays, and Saturdays, as a particle. On Sundays they simply prayed."[24]

In 1916-1917, Einstein made his third important contribution to laser theory by providing a new derivation of Planck's radiation law,[25-27] with vast implications. As he wrote to his friend Michele Angelo Besso in 1916, "A splendid light has dawned on me about the absorption and emission of radiation."[21] Indeed, his new idea provided the basis for subsequent laser development.

Based on quantum theory, two fundamental radiation processes associated with light and matter were known before Einstein's new derivation: (1) *stimulated absorption,* a process in which an atom can be excited to a higher energy state through such means as heating, light interaction, or particle interaction; and (2) *spontaneous emission,* the process of an excited atom decaying to a lower energy state spontaneously, by itself. Einstein's breakthrough was the addition of a third alternative: *stimulated emission,* the reverse of the stimulated absorption process. In the presence of other incoming radiation of the same frequency, excited atoms are stimulated to make a transition to the lower energy state— more quickly than in spontaneous emission—and in the process release light energy identical to the incoming form of light. The emitted light has the same frequency and is *in phase* (i.e., coherent) with the stimulating radiation wave. Stimulated emission occurs when there are more excited atoms than atoms that are not excited (i.e., more atoms in upper of two energy levels than in lower level), a condition called *population inversion*. Einstein also showed that the process of stimulated emission occurs with the same probability as for absorption from the lower state.[28-31] Hey et al.[32] summarized the significance of Einstein's insight as follows:

> For over 35 years this stimulated emission process gained hardly more than a cursory comment in quantum mechanics textbooks, since it seemed to have no practical application. What had been overlooked, however, was the special nature of the light that is emitted in this way. The photons that are emitted have exactly the same phase as the photons that induce the transition. This is because the varying electric fields of the applied light wave cause the charge distribution of the excited atom to oscillate in phase with this radiation. The emitted photons are all in phase—they are coherent—and, furthermore, they travel in the same direction as the inducing photon.

At this point, it should be clarified that the term *photon* was not used by Planck, Bohr, or Einstein up to the time of Einstein's 1916-1917 papers. American chemist Gilbert Lewis[33] apparently was the first to use the term when he argued, in a letter to the editor of *Nature* magazine in 1926, for the need for new nomenclature to describe discrete units of radiant energy:

> It would seem inappropriate to speak of one of these hypothetical entities as a particle of light, a corpuscle of light, a light quantum, or a light quant, if we are to assume that it spends only a minute fraction of its existence as a carrier of radiant energy, while the rest of the time it remains as an important structural element within the atom. It would also cause confusion to call it merely a quantum, for later it will be necessary to distinguish between the number of these entities present in an atom and the so-called quantum number. I therefore take the liberty of proposing for this hypothetical new atom, which is not light, but plays an essential part in every process of radiation, the name *photon*.

The following accepted definition appears in the *American Heritage Dictionary*[34]:

> **photon** n. *Physics.* The quantum of electromagnetic energy, regarded as a discrete particle having zero mass, no electric charge, and an indefinitely long lifetime.

Decades followed Einstein's 1916-1917 articles on stimulated emission before significant progress was made in laser development, both theoretically and practically, in the 1950s and 1960s, partly because of the outlook and training of physicists at that time, as suggested by American physicist Arthur L. Schawlow and later observers. Schooled in the idea that "thermodynamic equilibrium," a state of energy balance, was the normal condition of matter throughout the universe, these scientists tended to believe that population inversion was merely an unusual event or brief permutation, not something particularly significant.[35,36]

However, the 1920s and 1930s were not entirely bereft of discovery and insight. In 1928, German physicist Rudolf Ladenburg indirectly observed stimulated emission while studying the optical properties of neon gas at wavelengths near a transition where the gas absorbed and emitted light. This was the first evidence that stimulated emission existed.[35,37] In his 1939 doctoral dissertation, Soviet physicist Valentin A. Fabrikant had envisioned a way to produce a population inversion, writing that "such a ratio of populations is in principle attainable. … Under such conditions we would obtain a radiation output greater than the incident radiation."[35,36,38]

Nevertheless, the works of Ladenburg and that of Fabrikant were isolated incidents. Another impediment to laser development after Einstein was two world wars, although World War II then actually accelerated research toward laser development. Efforts of physicists were diverted from performing fundamental research to helping propel technology that would help win the war. Afterward, the sophisticated equipment developed for the war effort became military surplus, and physicists accustomed to low budgets received some of this equipment as they resumed their research.

Masers and Lasers

The impact of the wartime research focus on laser development is exemplified by the work of American physicist Charles H. Townes at Bell Telephone Laboratories in Manhattan and later at Columbia University, which he joined in 1948 (Figure 1-5). In 1941, Townes was assigned to work on a military radar project. Modern radar, a system of using transmitted and reflected radio waves for detecting a reflected object to determine its direction, distance, height, or speed, was developed in the 1930s, when systems used radio waves about a meter long and could not discern much detail. During the war, the military was interested in developing a radar system that used much higher radio frequencies to attain greater sensitivity, tighter radio beams, and transmitting antennas small enough to fit on an airplane. Townes began working on microwave frequencies of 3, 10, and 24 gigahertz (GHz).[35] Although none of these systems was used in battle, Townes' experience with the 24-GHz system, interest in microwave spectroscopy, and use of surplus equipment guided him toward subsequent development.

In 1951, at the spring meeting of the American Physical Society in Washington, D.C., Townes proposed the concept of a *maser*, an acronym he and his students coined for *m*icrowave *a*mplification by *s*timulated *e*mission of *r*adiation. He indicated that the "primary object of the work that led to the maser was to get shorter wavelengths so we could do better spectroscopy in a new spectral region."[39] Townes elaborated on April 26, 1951: "I sketched out and calculated requirements for a molecular-beam system to separate high-energy molecules from lower [-energy] ones and send them through a cavity which would contain the electromagnetic radiation [photons] to stimulate further emission from the molecules, thus providing feedback and continuous oscillation."[40] On May 11, Townes sketched the idea in his laboratory notebook, dated it, and signed it "Chas. H. Townes." In February 1952, his colleague and brother-in-law Arthur L. Schawlow also signed the page.[35,36]

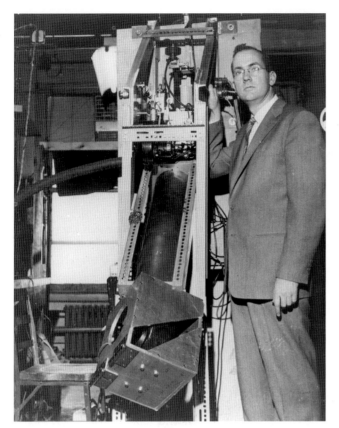

• **Figure 1-5** Charles H. Townes with a ruby microwave maser amplifier developed for radio astronomy in 1957. (Courtesy Alcatel-Lucent USA.)

On his return to Columbia University after the April 1951 conference, Townes and postdoctoral fellow Herbert J. Zeiger and doctoral student James P. Gordon commenced work on building a maser. They began to experiment with a beam of ammonia molecules, a compound familiar to Townes from his work on the 24-GHz radar system. It was known that ammonia molecules absorb microwaves at a frequency of 24 GHz, causing the nitrogen atom of that molecule to vibrate. Initial success was achieved in late 1953, when Gordon saw evidence of stimulated emission and amplification from their device; then, in early April 1954, they achieved the desired oscillation.[35] They reported their success in a late paper presented at a meeting of the American Physical Society on May 1 and then in a short paper published in the journal *Physical Review*.[41]

While on sabbatical from Columbia University in 1955, Townes worked with French physicist Alfred Kastler at the École Normale Supérieure in Paris. Kastler developed the technique of "optical pumping," a process by which light is used to raise (or pump) electrons from a lower to a higher energy level, as a new way to excite materials for microwave spectroscopy.[35] Townes recognized that optical pumping might excite the optical energy levels necessary for an optical maser. In fall 1957, Townes and Schawlow, a postdoctoral fellow under Townes at Columbia until he joined Bell Labs in 1951, proposed extending maser principles to the infrared and visible regions of the electromagnetic spectrum.[36,39]

They subsequently published their influential paper in *Physical Review* in 1958.[42]

Meanwhile, another American physicist, Gordon Gould, a Columbia graduate student in 1957, asked whether optical pumping could excite light emission. He recorded his ideas in nine handwritten pages of a laboratory notebook, with the first page titled "Some rough calculations on the feasibility of a LASER: Light Amplification by Stimulated Emission of Radiation"—the first time the term *laser* was used. Gould had his notes notarized on November 13, 1957, which he saw as a necessary step in applying for a patent. His patent defense efforts were finally recognized after 30 years of delays, challenges, and litigation.[35,39,43]

The Schawlow and Townes paper stirred a number of organizations to conduct additional research into optical masers as follows[35]:

- In September 1958, Townes and Columbia University received funding from the U.S. Air Force Office of Scientific Research to pursue investigation of a potassium-vapor laser.
- Schawlow began to work with crystals (including synthetic pink ruby, composed of aluminum oxide doped with chromium atoms) at Bell Labs, which was interested in developing the technology to expand the transmission capacity of Bell's communications network.
- Ali Javan and William R. Bennett, Jr., also at Bell, worked on employing an electrical discharge tube filled with helium and neon gas.
- Gould had joined the Technical Research Group (TRG) in Manhattan, a military contractor that secured funding from the Pentagon to research the potential military applications of a laser, including communications, marking targets for weapons, and measuring the range to targets. Gould's group explored the potential of a laser using alkali metal vapors.
- Westinghouse Research Laboratories in Pittsburgh had an Air Force contract to examine solid-state microwave masers. Irwin Wieder and Bruce McAvoy explored the characteristics of ruby using bright tungsten lamps and (unsuccessfully) pulsed light sources.
- IBM entered the laser race with Peter Sorokin and Mirek Stevenson at the T.J. Watson Research Center in Yorktown Heights, N.Y.

Numerous other companies also had joined the quest for building the first laser, including aerospace company Hughes Research Laboratories in California, which was under a maser development contract with the U.S. Army Signal Corps. The Corps became interested in developing a more practical version of a previously developed ruby solid-state microwave maser, one that could serve as a low-noise microwave amplifier aboard an airplane. American physicist Theodore H. Maiman, who joined Hughes in 1956, and his assistant, Irnee D'Haenens, were assigned to the project. Their task was daunting; the existing desk-size device weighed 2.5 tons. They succeeded in developing a 4-pound version, but the continuing need to incorporate cryogenic cooling of the device limited its practicality.

Nevertheless, Maiman used this experience with ruby in his later work on the laser. Some investigators, including Wieder at Westinghouse as well as Schawlow and others at Bell Labs, had dismissed ruby as an unsuitably inefficient laser material, but their calculations were based on inadequate data. Maiman conducted his own investigation and found that ruby could indeed be suitable, provided that it could be optically pumped with an intensely bright light source. His calculations showed that a pulsed flashlamp would provide enough light to excite a ruby laser. His experimental laser design ultimately was elegant, incorporated in a device that could fit in the palm of the hand: a ruby rod 1 cm in diameter and 2 cm long placed within the coils of a small flashlamp, and an aluminum cylinder with reflective interior surface that slipped around the lamp to reflect light toward the ruby rod. The ends of the rod were polished flat, perpendicular to the length of the rod and parallel to each other. Maiman applied a reflective silver coating to both ends and then removed the silver from the center of one end, to allow a transparent opening for the laser beam to escape and subsequently be detected. The apparatus was connected to a separate power supply.[35]

On May 16, 1960, Maiman and D'Haenens aimed the laser cylinder toward a white poster board. They started firing the flashlamp with pulses of 500 volts (V), gradually increasing the voltage to produce progressively more intense light flashes, and measured the laser's output tracing on an oscilloscope. Finally, with the power supply set above 950 V, the oscilloscope's trace surged, a red glow filled the room, and a brilliant red spot appeared on the poster board. After 9 months of intense effort, Maiman accomplished his goal, and the laser was born. In so doing, he beat out Bell Labs, TRG, Westinghouse, IBM, Siemens, RCA Labs, Massachusetts Institute of Technology's Lincoln Laboratory, General Electric, and all others in contention.[35,36,39,44] Maiman submitted a paper reporting his evidence for a ruby laser to *Physical Review Letters,* the leading U.S. journal for publishing new physics research. Its editor, Samuel Goudsmit, rejected the manuscript, apparently not appreciating the breakthrough Maiman had achieved, perhaps mistakenly believing it was just a follow-up to previously published work on masers. Maiman then submitted his report to the British weekly journal *Nature,* which accepted it immediately and published it on August 6, 1960.[45,46]

Other laser types followed[36,39,46]:

- Sorokin and Stevenson demonstrated the solid-state uranium laser in November 1960.[47]
- Javan, Bennett, and Herriott demonstrated the first gas laser, a helium-neon (HeNe) laser emitting at 1.15 μm, in December 1960 at Bell's Murray Hill, New Jersey, laboratory.[48]
- In 1961, Johnson and Nassau at Bell Labs demonstrated a 1.06-μm laser from neodymium (Nd) ions in a host crystal of calcium tungstate.[49]
- Also in 1961, Snitzer of American Optical (Southbridge, Massachusetts) built an Nd laser in optical glass.[50]

- White and Rigden developed the 632.8-nm-wavelength HeNe laser at Bell Labs in 1962.[51]
- Also in 1962, Rabinowitz, Jacobs, and Gould demonstrated the optically pumped cesium laser at TRG.[52]
- Further in 1962, Hall and colleagues of the General Electric Research Center (Schenectady, NY) developed a cryogenically cooled gallium-arsenide (GaAs) semiconductor laser.[53]
- The year 1964 marked the demonstration of the neodymium-doped yttrium-aluminum-garnet (Nd:YAG) laser by Geusic, Marcos, and van Uitert at Bell Labs.[54]
- Patel developed the carbon dioxide (CO_2) laser at Bell Labs in 1964.[55]
- Also in 1964, Bridges of Hughes Research Laboratories developed the argon ion laser.[56]
- Silfvast and colleagues at the University of Utah conducted extensive research with metal-vapor lasers in the mid-1960s.[57]
- Sorokin and Lankard developed the dye laser in the mid-1960s.[58,59]
- Ewing and Brau of the Avco Everett Research Laboratory (Everett, Massachusetts) were the first to demonstrate three excimer lasers: krypton fluoride, xenon fluoride, and xenon chloride lasers.[60]
- Madey of Stanford University demonstrated the free electron laser on January 7, 1975.[61]
- Schawlow and one of his students even concocted a Jello-O laser by firing a ruby laser into a bowl of Jell-O doped with the organic dye rhodamine 6G.[35,39]

During a July 7, 1960, press conference announcing his accomplishment, Maiman identified five potential uses for the laser:

1. The first true amplification of light
2. A tool to probe matter for basic research
3. High-power beams for space communications
4. Increasing the number of available communication channels
5. Concentrating light for industry, chemistry, and medicine

The accuracy of his insight was affirmed in subsequent discoveries and applications; only his third prediction has not been put into regular use.[35] A few years later, when commenting on the outlook for medical applications of the laser, Maiman foresaw the use of the device as a "bloodless" surgical tool, in the treatment of malignancies, and as a dentist's drill.[62] He cited the interconnection of blood vessels to relieve arterial blockage as one example of successful experimentation. He also discussed microsurgical laser equipment capable of destroying individual red blood cells, as well as a laser destroying single genes and other tiny masses, with practically no effect on surrounding tissue.[63]

Lasers In Dentistry and Oral Surgery

Soon after his invention was demonstrated, researchers began to examine Maiman's vision of the laser as a useful instrument for medicine. Their efforts laid the foundation for the present clinical use of lasers in ophthalmology, neurosurgery, urology, gynecology, gastroenterology, general surgery, cardiovascular surgery, orthopedics, esthetic/dermatologic/plastic surgery, otorhinolaryngology, oral surgery and dentistry, and veterinary medicine. This section briefly outlines select pioneering efforts in the application of laser technology to dentistry and oral surgery and then summarizes the types of lasers and current range of intraoral clinical applications. (See also Chapter 2.)

To find new and effective methods of removing caries, pioneering examinations into the interactions of ruby laser energy with tooth structure were reported in the mid-1960s.[64-72] Investigators discovered that the ruby laser could vaporize caries, but that the high energy densities caused irreversible necrotic changes in pulpal tissues. Years later, the development of erbium (Er) laser wavelengths and CO_2 lasers operating at 9300 and 9600 nm, better suited to the clinical requirements for cavity preparation without the detrimental effects on pulp, led to further investigations.[73-84]

Early intraoral soft tissue investigations were conducted using the ruby laser.[71,85,86] The development of the CO_2 laser with its ability to ablate soft tissue with minimal hemorrhage led to studies in oral surgery.[87-99] Other groups of workers followed up with soft tissue studies involving the Nd:YAG laser.[100-103]

Other researchers examined the photopolymerization of dental composites[104-109] with the argon laser, the possible use of Nd:YAG lasers in the welding of prosthetic devices and gold alloys,[107-110] and the application of various lasers in endodontics.[111-113] An extensive survey of the published scientific research and clinical reports on the use of lasers in dentistry discusses the first experimental uses in 1964 through the numerous clinical applications into 2000.[114]

Otolaryngologists, oral surgeons, and periodontists were among the first practitioners to use medical lasers intraorally to perform a variety of soft tissue surgical applications. On May 3, 1990, the first laser designed specifically for general dentistry, the dLase 300 Nd:YAG laser, developed by Myers and Myers, was introduced in the United States.[115] This event marked the beginning of the clinical use of lasers by dentists—a development anticipated by a pioneer in laser surgery, Leon Goldman (1905-1997).

Goldman had been reporting on the biomedical aspects of the laser since 1963 and had published findings on the effect of the laser on dental caries, teeth, and other tissues as part of his early research. Concerning the prospects of laser applications in dentistry, Goldman[116] wrote in 1967:

> Although the possibilities of the development of laser dentistry appear to us to be excellent, there has been too little interest in the clinical and applied phases of laser dentistry by dentists and dental research groups. … These studies at present then indicate that a significant portion of the laser laboratory should be devoted to the field of laser dentistry. Unlike many dentists, we feel that this is a profitable area for research, especially in the treatment of caries and perhaps even of calculus. The dentist and especially dental histopathologist and electron microscopist must work with the biologists and the physicians and the engineers engaged in laser research. The purpose of this cooperative study is to develop flexible, effective and safe laser instrumentation needed for laser dentistry. Dentists should be active in this program, not wait until other disciplines do the work for them.

Almost 2 decades later, a dental practitioner heeded Dr. Goldman's call to develop what became the first laser designed specifically for general dentistry. Michigan dentist Dr. Terry D. Myers joined with his ophthalmologist brother Dr. William D. Myers, himself among the first to incorporate a laser into his ophthalmic practice, in exploring the advances in lasers, electronics, and optics to produce a device appropriate for the dental operatory. In contrast with a medical laser adapted for dental use, their instrument would be designed for the specific needs of the dental practitioner. It would feature an easy-to-use control panel that selected safe and effective operational parameters for the lasers' numerous clinical indications. It would be portable, with a self-contained cooling system, requiring no special electrical hookups, and would be simple to set up and maintain. It would have built-in self-diagnostics, autoclavable or disposable components, and a flexible fiberoptic delivery system to facilitate intraoral access and provide the necessary tactile feedback to which dental professionals are accustomed.

Currently, a number of laser wavelengths are used in oral surgery and dentistry, including two CO_2 wavelengths, Nd:YAG, argon, various diode wavelengths, two Er wavelengths, and potassium titanyl phosphate (KTP). Applications include the following[117-121]:

- Soft tissue procedures: gingivectomy/gingivoplasty, uvulopalatoplasty, excision of tumors and other lesions, incision/excision biopsies, frenectomy, removal of hyperplastic/granulation tissue, second-stage recovery of implants, guided tissue regeneration, and treatment of periodontal disease, aphthous ulcers, herpetic lesions, leukoplakia, and verrucous carcinoma
- Control of bleeding in vascular lesions
- Arthroscopic temporomandibular joint surgery
- Caries diagnosis and removal
- Curing of composites
- Activation of tooth-bleaching solutions
- Caries diagnosis and removal
- Root canal debridement and preparation
- Osteotomy and osseous crown lengthening
- Detection of subgingival dental calculus

Many professional societies are dedicated to the use of lasers in medicine and dentistry (Table 1-1). All have international representation, and some have links to their component societies or country representatives. Affiliated selected journals of interest to dentists who use lasers in their practice include the following and are listed in Table 1-2.

TABLE 1-1 Professional Societies Dedicated to the Use of Lasers in Medicine and Dentistry

Organization	Web Address	Year Formed
Academy of Laser Dentistry	www.laserdentistry.org	1993
American Society for Laser Medicine and Surgery	www.aslms.org	1981
Deutsche Gesellschaft für Laserzahnheilkunde	www.dgl-online.de	1991
Japanese Society for Laser Dentistry	http://jsld.jp	1989
Society for Oral Laser Applications	www.sola-int.org	ca. 2000
Laser Institute of America	www.laserinstitute.org	1968
SPIE* (an international society for optics and photonics)	www.spie.org	1955
World Association for Laser Therapy	www.walt.nu	1994
World Federation for Laser Dentistry	www.wfld-org.infolaser.com	1988

*Originally founded as the "Society of Photographic Instrumentation Engineers."

TABLE 1-2 Selected Journals of Interest to Dental Laser Practitioners

Journal	Web Address	Years of Publication
International Journal of Laser Dentistry	www.jaypeejournals.com/eJournals	2011-present
Journal of Biomedical Optics	www.spie.org/x866.xml	1996-present
Journal of Dental Lasers	www.jdentlasers.org	2007-present
Journal of Laser Applications	www.lia.org/subscriptions/jla	1988-present
Journal of Laser Dentistry	www.laserdentistry.org	1992-present
Journal of Oral Laser Applications	www.quintpub.com/journals/jola/gp.php?journal_name=jola	2001-2010
Journal of the Japanese Society for Laser Dentistry	www.jstage.jst.go.jp/browse/jjpnsoclaserdent	1990-present
Journal of the Laser and Health Academy	www.laserandhealthacademy.com/en/journal	2007-present
Laser International	www.dental-tribune.com/epaper/issues/product/33	2010-present
Laser Journal	http://www.zwp-online-info/de/publikationen/laser-journal	2003-present
Lasers in Medical Science	http://link.springer.com/journal/10103	1986-present
Lasers in Surgery and Medicine	http://onlinelibrary.wiley.com/journal/10.1002/(ISSN)1096-9101	1980-present
Optical Engineering	http://spie.org/x867.xml	1962-present
Photochemistry and Photobiology	http://onlinelibrary.wiley.com/journal/10.1111/(ISSN)1751-1097	1962-present
Photomedicine and Laser Surgery	http://www.libertpub.com/overview/photomedicine-and-laser-surgery/128	1983-present
Zeitschrift für Laser Zahnheilkunde	http://lzhk.quintessenz.de	2004-2008

Conclusions

Fifty years after their initial experimental use in dentistry, and almost 25 years after their practical introduction into the dental operatory, lasers are becoming more commonplace and even routine, either as adjunctive treatment methodologies or as stand-alone additions to the dental armamentarium. Researchers continue to investigate new laser wavelengths and clinical applications as they apply to dentistry, extending the vision of Maiman and other pioneers. The growing number of dental laser practitioners, propelled by the increasing body of evidence concerning the safe, effective, and appropriate use of lasers in dentistry, will continue to advance the application of Einstein's "splendid light" in their operatories, to the benefit of patient and practitioner alike.

If laser clinicians find themselves simultaneously awed over the multifaceted capabilities of laser light and confounded in their attempts to fully explain it, they might find consolation in the knowledge that others have expressed similar fascination. Einstein himself wrote to Besso on December 12, 1951: "All the fifty years of conscious brooding have brought me no closer to the answer to the question, 'What are light quanta?' Of course today every rascal thinks he knows the answer, but he is deluding himself."[122] Rascals or not, laser clinicians are in good company in their sense of wonder!

References

1. Katzir A: *Lasers and optical fibers in medicine*, San Diego, 1993, Academic Press.

2. Daniell MD, Hill JS: A history of photodynamic therapy, *Aust NZ J Surg* 61(5):340–348, 1991.

3. Wheeland RG: History of lasers in dermatology, *Clin Dermatol* 13(1):3–10, 1995.

4. Fitzpatrick TB, Pathak MA: Historical aspects of methoxsalen and other furocoumarins, *J Invest Dermatol* 32(2, pt 2):229–231, 1959.

5. Kalka K, Merk H, Mukhtar H: Photodynamic therapy in dermatology, *J Am Acad Dermatol* 42(3):389–413, 414–416 (quiz), 2000, errata, 43(4):609, 2000, and 44(1):150, 2001.

6. Gribbin JR: *Q is for quantum: an encyclopedia of particle physics*, New York, 2000, Touchstone.

7. *Opera omnia … haetenus edita auctor ante obitum recensuit … posthuma vero, totius naturae explicationem complectentia, in lucem nunc primum proderunt ex bibliotheca … Henrici-Ludovici-Haberti Mon-Morii … [Accesit Samuelis Sorberii praefatio, in qua de vita et moribus Petri Gassendi disseritur]*, Lyon, 1658, Laurent Anisson and Jean Baptiste Devenet, I, pp 422a–432b.

8. Newton I: Correspondence: Isaac Newton to Henry Oldenburg, Cambridge, Dec 7, 1675. In Turnbull HW, Scott JP, Hall AR, Tilling L, editors: *The correspondence of Isaac Newton* (5 vols, continuing), Cambridge, UK, 1959, Royal Society at the University Press, vol I, pp 362–389.

9. Newton I: *Opticks: or, a treatise of the reflexions, refractions, inflexions and colours of light. Also two treatises of the species and magnitude of curvilinear figures*, London, 1704, Smith and Walford, Printers to the Royal Society.

10. Mehra J, Rechenberg H: *The historical development of quantum theory*, vol 5, Erwin Schrödinger and the rise of wave mechanics: Part 1. Schrodinger in Vienna and Zurich 1887–1925, New York, 1987, Springer-Verlag.

11. Descartes R: Discours de la méthode pour bien conduir sa raison et chercher la vérité dans les sciences plus la dioptrique, les meteores, et la geometrie, qui sont des essais de cete methode [Discourse on the method for properly conducting reason and searching for truth in the sciences, as well as the dioptrics, the meteors, and the geometry, which are essays in this method], 1637. In Cottingham J, Stoothoff R, Murdoch D, translators-editors: *The philosophical writings of Descartes*, vol 1, Cambridge, UK, 1985, Cambridge University Press.

12. Hooke R: *Micrographia; or, some physiological descriptions of minute bodies made by magnifying glasses with observations and inquiries thereupon*, London, 1665, Martyn & Allestry.

13. Maxwell JC: A dynamical theory of the electromagnetic field, *Philos Trans R Soc Lond* 155:459–512, 1865.

14. Planck M: Zur theorie des gesetzes der energieverteilung im normalspektrum, *Verh Dtsch Phys Ges* 2:237–245, 1900.

15. Van der Waerden BL, editor: *Sources of quantum mechanics*, Amsterdam, 1967, North-Holland Publishing.

16. Torretti R: *The philosophy of physics*, Cambridge, UK, 1999, Cambridge University Press.

17. Rutherford E: The scattering of α and β particles by matter and the structure of the atom, *Philos Mag*, Series 6 21:669–688, 1911.

18. Bohr N: On the constitution of atoms and molecules. Parts I–III, *Lond Edinb Dublin Philos Mag J Sci, Sixth Series* 26(151):1–25, (153):476–501, (155):857–875, 1913.

19. Billings CW: *Lasers: the new technology of light*, New York, 1992, Facts on File.

20. Einstein A: Über einen die erzeugung und verwandlung des lichtes betreffenden heuristichen geischtpunkt [On a heuristic point of view concerning the generalization and transformation of light], *Ann Phys* 17:132–148, 1905.

21. Singh V: Einstein and the quantum. In Wadia SR, editor: *The legacy of Albert Einstein: a collection of essays in celebration of the year of physics*, Singapore, 2007, World Scientific Publishing.

22. Hallmark CL, Horn DT: *Lasers: the light fantastic*, ed 2, Blue Ridge Summit, Pa, 1987, TAB Books.

23. Einstein A: Über die Entwickelung unserer Anschauungen über das Wesen und die Konstitution der Strahlung [On the evolution of our vision on the nature and constitution of radiation], *Phys Z* 10(22):817–826, 1909.

24. Hoffmann B: *The strange story of the quantum*, ed 2, New York, 1959, Dover Publications, p 42.

25. Einstein A: Strahlungs-emission und -absorption nach der quantentheorie, *Verh Dtsch Phys Ges* 18(13–14):318–323, 1916.

26. Einstein A: Zur quantentheorie der strahlung [On the quantum theory of radiation], *Mitt Phys Ges Zurich* 18:47–62, 1916.

27. Einstein A: Zur quantentheorie der strahlung [On the quantum theory of radiation], *Phys Z* 18:121–128, 1917. (identical to 1916 paper of the same name, with a minor correction).

28. Schilling BW: Lasers. In Driggers RG, editor: *Encyclopedia of optical engineering*, vol 2, New York, 2003, Marcel Dekker.

29. Institute for Advanced Dental Technologies: *The laser course. Laser dentistry: a clinical training seminar*, Southfield, Mich, 1999, The Institute, III.6.

30. *The photonics dictionary, int'l ed 46, Pittsfield, Mass, 2000, Laurin Publishing, D-111.*

31. Carruth JA, McKenzie AL: *Medical lasers: science and clinical practice*, Bristol, UK, 1986, Adam Hilger.

32. Hey AJ, Hey T, Walters P: Quantum co-operation and superfluids. In *The new quantum universe*, Cambridge, UK, 2003, Cambridge University Press.

33. Lewis GN: The conservation of photons, *Nature* 118(2):874–875, 1926.

34. *American Heritage dictionary of the English language*, ed 5, Boston, 2012, Houghton Mifflin.

35. Hecht J: *Beam: the race to make the laser*, New York, 2005, Oxford University Press.

36. Hecht J: *Laser pioneers*, rev ed, Boston, 1992, Academic Press.

37. Ladenburg R: Untersuchungen über die anomale Dispersion angeregter Gase. I. Teil. Zur Prüfung der quantentheoretischen Dispersionsformel [Research on the anomalous dispersion of gases], *Z Phys A* 48(1–2):15–25, 1928.

38. Bertolotti M: *Masers and lasers: an historical approach*, Bristol, UK, 1983, Adam Hilger.

39. *Laser pioneer interviews with an introduction to laser history by Jeff Hecht*, Torrance Calif, 1985, High Tech Publications.

40. Townes CH: The laser's roots: Townes recalls the early days, *Laser Focus* 14(8):52, 1978.

41. Gordon JP, Zeiger HJ, Townes CH: Molecular microwave oscillator and new hyperfine structure in the microwave spectrum of NH₃, *Phys Rev* 95(1):282–284, 1954.

42. Schawlow AL, Townes CH: Infrared and optical masers, *Phys Rev* 112(6):1940–1949, 1958.

43. Bromberg JL: Amazing light, *Invent Technol Mag* 7(4)[~118 pp], 1992 [online serial] http://www.americanheritage.com/articles/magazine/it/1992/4/1992_4_18.shtmlinnovationgateway.org/content/amazing-light-1. Accessed March 2014.

44. Friedman G: Inventing the light fantastic: Ted Maiman and the world's first laser, *OE Rep* (200):5–6, August 2000. Also available as: *Lasers & sources. Inventing … laser*, Greg Friedman [website]. DOI: 10.1117/2.6200705.0001. SPIE. c200914. [~45 pp]; http://spie.org/x13999.xml. Accessed March 2014.

45. Maiman TH: Stimulated optical radiation in ruby, *Nature* 187(4736):493–494, 1960.

46. Townes CH: *How the laser happened: adventures of a scientist*, New York, 1999, Oxford University Press.

47. Sorokin PP, Stevenson MJ: Stimulated infrared emission from trivalent uranium, *Phys Rev Lett* 5(12):557–559, 1960.

48. Javan A, Bennett Jr WR, Herriott DR: Population inversion and continuous optical maser oscillation in a gas discharge containing a He-Ne mixture, *Phys Rev Lett* 6(3):106–110, 1961.

49. Johnson LF, Nassau K: Infrared fluorescence and stimulated emission of Nd3+ in CaWO, *Proc Inst Radio Eng* 49(12):1704, 1961.

50. Snitzer E: Optical maser action of Nd3+ in a barium crown glass, *Phys Rev Lett* 7(12):444–446, 1961.

51. White AD, Rigden JD: Continuous gas maser operation in the visible, *Proc Inst Radio Eng* 50(7):1697, 1962.

52. Rabinowitz P, Jacobs S, Gould G: Continuous optically pumped Cs laser, *Appl Opt* 1(4):513–516, 1962.

53. Hall RN, Fenner GE, Kingsley JD, et al.: Coherent light emission from GaAs junctions, *Phys Rev Lett* 9(9):366–368, 1962.

54. Geusic JE, Marcos HM, Van Uitert LG: Laser oscillations in Nd-doped yttrium aluminum, yttrium gallium, and gadolinium garnets, *Appl Phys Lett* 4(10):182–184, 1954.

55. Patel CKN: Continuous-wave laser action on vibrational-rotational transitions of CO_2, *Phys Rev A* 136(5):1187–1193, 1964.

56. Bridges WB: Laser oscillation in singly ionized argon in the visible spectrum, *Appl Phys Lett* 4(7):128–130, 1964, erratum 5(2):39.

57. Silfvast WT, Fowles GR, Hopkins BD: Laser action in singly ionized Ge, Sn, Pb, In, Cd and Zn, *Appl Phys Lett* 8(12):318–319, 1966.

58. Sorokin PP, Lankard JR: Stimulated emission observed from an organic dye, chloro-aluminum phthalocyanine, *IBM J Res Dev* 10(2):162–163, 1966.

59. Sorokin PP, Lankard JR: Flashlamp excitation of organic dye lasers: a short communication, *IBM J Res Dev* 11(2):148, 1967.

60. Ewing JJ, Brau CA: Laser action on the $^2\Sigma^+_{1/2} \rightarrow {}^2\Sigma^+_{1/2}$ bands of KrF and XeCl, *Appl Phys Lett* 27(6):350–352, 1975.

61. Madey JM: Stimulated emission of bremsstrahlung in a periodic magnetic field, *J Appl Phys* 42(5):1906–1913, 1971.

62. Maiman comments on his precocious five-year-old [editorial], *Laser Focus* 1(9):2–4, 1965.

63. Maiman TH: A look at things to come: biomedical lasers evolve toward clinical applications, *Hosp Manage* 101(4):39–41, 1966.

64. Stern RH, Sognnaes RF: Laser beam effect on dental hard tissues, *J Dent Res* 43(5):873, 1964. [abstract 307].

65. Kinersly T, Jarabak JP, Phatak NM, Dement J: Laser effects on tissue and materials related to dentistry, *J Am Dent Assoc* 70(3):593–600, 1965.

66. Goldman L, Gray J, Goldman J, et al.: Effect of the laser beam impacts on teeth, *J Am Dent Assoc* 70(3):601–606, 1965.

67. Goldman L, Hornby P, Meyer R, Goldman B: Impact of the laser on dental caries, *Nature* 203(4943):417, 1964.

68. Gordon Jr TE: Laser interactions with extracted human teeth: a preliminary report, *Dent Digest* 72(4):154–158, 1966.

69. Gordon TE: Some effects of laser impacts on extracted teeth, *J Dent Res* 45(2):372–375, 1966.

70. Lobene RR, Fine S: Interaction of laser radiation with oral hard tissues, *J Prosthet Dent* 16(3):589–597, 1966.

71. Taylor R, Shklar G, Roeber F: The effects of laser radiation on teeth, dental pulp, and oral mucosa of experimental animals, *Oral Surg Oral Med Oral Pathol* 19(6):786–795, 1965.

72. Adrian JC, Bernier JL, Sprague WG: Laser and the dental pulp, *J Am Dent Assoc* 83(1):113–117, 1971.

73. Paghdiwala AF: Application of the erbium:YAG laser on hard dental tissues: measurement of the temperature changes and depths of cut. In Profio AE, editor: *Laser research in medicine, dentistry and surgery* vol 64, 1988. ICALEO Santa Clara, Calif, Proceedings, Toledo, Ohio, 1988, Laser Institute of America, pp 192–201.

74. Dostálová T, Jelínková H, Kucerová H, et al.: Clinical evaluation of Er-YAG laser caries treatment. In Wigdor HA, Featherstone JD, Rechman P, editors: *Lasers in dentistry III*, 1997. San Jose, Calif Proc SPIE 2973, Bellingham, Wash, 1997, International Society for Optical Engineering, pp 85–91.

75. Matsumoto K, Nakamura Y, Mazeki K, Kimura Y: Clinical dental application of Er:YAG laser class V cavity preparation, *J Clin Laser Med Surg* 14(3):123–127, 1996.

76. Sonntag KD, Klitzman B, Burkes EJ, et al.: Pulpal response to cavity preparation with the Er:YAG and Mark III free electron lasers, *Oral Surg Oral Med Oral Pathol Oral Radiol Endod* 81(6):695–702, 1996.

77. Eversole LR, Rizoiu I, Kimmel AI: Pulpal response to cavity preparation by an erbium, chromium:YSGG laser-powered hydrokinetic system, *J Am Dent Assoc* 128(8):1099–1106, 1997.

78. Pellagalli J, Gimbel CB, Hansen RT, et al.: Investigational study of the use of Er:YAG laser versus dental drill for caries removal and cavity preparation—phase I, *J Clin Laser Med Surg* 15(3):109–115, 1997.

79. Wigdor HA, Walsh Jr JT, Featherstone JD, et al.: Lasers in dentistry, *Lasers Surg Med* 16(2):103–133, 1995.

80. Fried D, Seka W, Glena RE, et al.: Thermal response of hard dental tissues to 9- through 11-μm CO_2 laser irradiation, *Opt Eng* 35(7):1976–1984, 1996.

81. Featherstone JDB, Fried D: Fundamental interactions of lasers with dental hard tissues, *Med Laser Appl* 16(3):181–194, 2001.

82. Fan K, Bell P, Fried D: Rapid and conservative ablation and modification of enamel, dentin, and alveolar bone using a high repetition rate transverse excited atmospheric pressure CO_2 laser operating at λ = 9.3 μm, *J Biomed Opt* 11(6), 2006. 064008-1–064008-11.

83. Staninec M, Darling CL, Goodis HE, et al.: Pulpal effects of enamel ablation with a microsecond pulsed λ = 9.3-μm CO_2 laser, *Lasers Surg Med* 41(4):256–263, 2009.

84. Nguyen D, Chang K, Hedayatollahnajafi S, et al.: High-speed scanning ablation of dental hard tissues with a λ = 9.3 μm CO_2 laser: adhesion, mechanical strength, heat accumulation, and peripheral thermal damage, *J Biomed Opt* 16(7), 2011. 071410-1–071410-9.

85. Yamamoto H, Okabe H, Ooya K, et al.: Laser effect on vital oral tissues: a preliminary investigation, *J Oral Pathol* 1(5):256–264, 1972.

86. Tanaka H: Effect of ruby-laser irradiation on gingiva, *Shigaku [Odontol]* 63(4):355–364, 1975.

87. Schafir R, Slutzki S, Bornstein LA: Excision of buccal hemangioma by carbon dioxide laser beam, *Oral Surg Oral Med Oral Pathol* 44(3):347–350, 1977.

88. Adrian JC: Effects of carbon dioxide laser radiation on oral soft tissues: an initial report, *Mil Med* 144(2):83–89, 1979.

89. Strong MS, Vaughan CW, Jako GJ, Polanyi T: Transoral resection of cancer of the oral cavity: the role of the CO_2 laser, *Otolaryngol Clin North Am* 12(1):207–218, 1979.

90. Tuffin JR, Carruth JA: The carbon dioxide surgical laser, *Br Dent J* 149(9):255–258, 1980.

91. Horch HH, Gerlach KL: CO_2 laser treatment of oral dysplastic precancerous lesions: a preliminary report, *Lasers Surg Med* 2(2):179–185, 1982.

92. Horch HH, Gerlach KL, Schaefer HE: CO_2 laser surgery of oral premalignant lesions, *Int J Oral Maxillofac Surg* 15(1):19–24, 1986.

93. Frame JW: Carbon dioxide laser surgery for benign oral lesions, *Br Dent J* 158(4):125–128, 1985.

94. Frame JW: Removal of oral soft tissue pathology with the CO_2 laser, *J Oral Maxillofac Surg* 43(11):850–855, 1985.

95. Frame JW, Das Gupta AR, Dalton GA: Rhys Evans PH: Use of the carbon dioxide laser in the management of premalignant lesions of the oral mucosa, *J Laryngol Otol* 98(12):1251–1260, 1984.

96. Kamami YV: Outpatient treatment of sleep apnea syndrome with CO_2 laser, LAUP: laser-assisted UPPP results on 46 patients, *J Clin Laser Med Surg* 12(4):215–219, 1994.

97. Wilder-Smith P, Arrastia A-MA, Liaw L-H, et al.: Incision properties and thermal effects of three CO_2 lasers in soft tissue, *Oral Surg Oral Med Oral Pathol Oral Radiol Endod* 79(6):685–691, 1995.

98. Wilder-Smith P, Dang J, Kurosaki T: Investigating the range of surgical effects on soft tissue produced by a carbon dioxide laser, *J Am Dent Assoc* 128(5):583–588, 1997.

99. Payne BP, Nishioka NS, Mikic BB, et al.: Comparison of pulsed CO_2 laser ablation at 10.6 μm and 9.5 μm, *Lasers Surg Med* 23(1):1–6, 1998.

100. Myers TD, Myers WD, Stone RM: First soft tissue study utilizing a pulsed Nd:YAG dental laser, *Northwest Dent* 68(2):14–17, 1989.

101. White JM, Goodis HE, Rose CL: Use of the pulsed Nd:YAG laser for intraoral soft tissue surgery, *Lasers Surg Med* 11(5):455–461, 1991.

102. Neill MF, Mellonig JT: Clinical efficacy of the Nd:YAG laser for combination periodontitis therapy, *Pract Periodont Aesthet Dent* 9(Suppl 6):1–5, 1997.

103. Yukna RA, Carr RL, Evans GH: Histologic evaluation of an Nd:YAG laser-assisted new attachment procedure in humans, *Int J Periodont Restorative Dent* 27(6):577–587, 2007.

104. Benedicenti A, Daneo M, Verrando M, et al.: Valutazione dell'assorbimento d'acqua di un composito, il Durafill, polimerizzato in luce laser argon rispetto alla normale polimeriizzazione [Evaluation of water absorption by a composite, Durafill, polymerized with argon laser light, in relation to normal polymerization], *Parodontol Stomatol (Nuova)* 23(3):27–29, 1984.

105. Séverin C: Apport du rayonnement laser-argon à la polymerization des photocomposites: collage des verrous orthodontiques [The effect of argon laser radiation on the polymerization of photocomposites: bonding of orthodontic brackets], *J Biomater Dent* 1(2):111–112, 1985. 161–165.

106. Séverin C, Maquin M: Argon ion laser beam as composite resin light curing agent. In Yamamoto H, Atsumi K, Kusakari H, editors: *Lasers in dentistry: proceedings of the International Congress of Laser in Dentistry, Tokyo, 1988*, Amsterdam, 1989, Excerpta Medica, pp 241–246.

107. Gordon TE, Smith DL: Laser welding of prostheses: an initial report, *J Prosthet Dent* 24(4):472–476, 1970.

108. Smith DL, Burnett AP, Gordon Jr TE: Laser welding of gold alloys, *J Dent Res* 51(1):161–167, 1972.

109. Huling JS, Clark RE: Comparative distortion in three-unit fixed prostheses joined by laser welding, conventional soldering, or casting in one piece, *J Dent Res* 56(2):128–134, 1977.

110. Apotheker H, Nishimura I, Seerattan C: Laser-welded vs soldered nonprecious alloy dental bridges: a comparative study, *Lasers Surg Med* 4(2):207–213, 1984.

111. Weichman JA, Johnson FM: Laser use in endodontics: a preliminary investigation, *Oral Surg Oral Med Oral Pathol* 31(3):416–420, 1971.

112. Dederich DN, Zakariasen KL, Tulip J: Scanning electron microscopic analysis of canal wall dentin following neodymium-aluminum-garnet laser irradiation, *J Endod* 10(9):428–431, 1984.

113. Yamazaki R, Goya C, Yu DG, et al.: Effects of erbium, chromium:YSGG laser irradiation on root canal walls: a scanning electron microscopic and thermographic study, *J Endod* 27(1):9–12, 2001.

114. Sulewski JG: Historical survey of laser dentistry, *Dent Clin North Am* 44(4):717–752, 2000.

115. Myers TD: The future of lasers in dentistry, *Dent Clin North Am* 44(4):971–980, 2000.

116. Goldman L: Dental applications of the laser. In Goldman L, editor: *Biomedical aspects of the laser: the introduction of laser applications into biology and medicine*, New York, 1967, Springer-Verlag.

117. Ball KA: *Lasers: the perioperative challenge*, ed 3, Denver, 2004, AORN.

118. Catone GA, Alling III CC: *Laser applications in oral and maxillofacial surgery*, Philadelphia, 1997, Saunders.

119. Clayman L: *Oral Maxillofac Surg Clin North Am* 9(1):1–131, 1997.

120. Joffe SN: Lasers in medicine. In Driggers RG, editor: *Encyclopedia of optical engineering*, vol 2, New York, 2003, Marcel Dekker.

121. Sulewski JG: *Selected US FDA marketing clearances*, San Diego, 2014, Academy of Laser Dentistry 21st Annual Conference and Exhibition. 08.

122. Klein MJ: The first phase of the Bohr-Einstein dialogue. In McCormmach R, editor: *Historical studies in the physical sciences*, vol 2, Philadelphia, 1970, University of Pennsylvania Press, pp 1–39.

2

Laser Fundamentals

DONALD J. COLUZZI, ROBERT A. CONVISSAR, AND DAVID M. ROSHKIND

The word *laser* is an acronym for *light* *a*mplification by *s*timulated *e*mission of *r*adiation. In this chapter, brief descriptions of these five terms, within the context of the unique qualities of a laser instrument, are presented as background for a subsequent overview of the uses of lasers in dentistry.

Light

Light is a form of electromagnetic energy that exists as a particle and that travels in waves at a constant velocity. The basic unit of this radiant energy is called a *photon*.[1] The waves of photons travel at the speed of light and can be defined by two basic properties: amplitude and wavelength (Figure 2-1). *Amplitude* is defined as the vertical height of the wave from the zero axis to its peak as it moves around that axis. This correlates with the amount of intensity in the wave: The larger the amplitude, the greater the amount of potential work that could be performed. For a sound wave, amplitude correlates with *loudness*. For a wave emitting light, amplitude correlates with *brightness*. A joule (J) is a unit of energy; a useful quantity in laser dentistry is a *millijoule* (mJ), or one thousandth (10^{-3}) of a joule (0.001 J).

The second property of a wave is *wavelength* (λ), the horizontal distance between any two corresponding points on the wave. This measurement is important to both how the laser light is delivered to the surgical site and how it reacts with tissue. Wavelength is measured in meters (m). Dental lasers have wavelengths on the order of much smaller units, using terminology of either *nanometer* (nm), equal to one billionth (10^{-9}) of a meter, or *micrometer* (μm), one millionth (10^{-6}) of a meter (replaces the micron [μ] unit, still occasionally seen in laser science).

As waves travel, they rise and fall about the zero axis a certain number of times per second; this is called *oscillation*. The number of oscillations per unit time is defined as *frequency*. Frequency is measured in hertz (Hz); 1 Hz equals one oscillation per second. Frequency is inversely proportional to wavelength: The shorter the wavelength, the higher the frequency, and vice versa. Although the hertz as just defined is a basic unit in physics, it also is used more specifically to describe the number of pulses per second of emitted laser energy.

Ordinary light, such as that produced by a table lamp, usually is a warm, white color. "White" as seen by the human eye is really the sum of the many colors of the visible spectrum: red, orange, yellow, green, blue, and violet. The light usually is diffuse—that is, not focused. Laser light is distinguished from ordinary light by two properties. Laser light is *monochromatic*: It is generated as a beam of a single color, which is invisible if its wavelength is outside of the visible part of the spectrum. In addition, the waves of laser light are *coherent*, or identical in physical size and shape. Thus the amplitude and frequency of all of the waves of photons are identical. This coherence results in the production of a specific form of focused electromagnetic energy.

The beams emitted from laser instruments are *collimated* (produced with all waves parallel to each other) over a long distance, but once the laser beam enters certain delivery systems such as optical fibers or tips (e.g., in neodymium-doped yttrium-aluminum-garnet [Nd:YAG], erbium, and diode lasers), it diverges at the fiber tip. This monochromatic, coherent beam of light energy can be used to accomplish the treatment objective.

Using a household fixture as an example, a 100-watt (W) lamp will produce a moderate amount of light for a room area, with some heat. On the other hand, 2 W of laser light can be used for precise excision of a fibroma while providing adequate hemostasis at the surgical site, without disturbing the surrounding tissue.[2] The difference between the 100 W of an ordinary light bulb able to light up a room and the 2 W of a laser able to perform a surgical procedure lies in the property of coherence. As an apt analogy, imagine a crew race on a river. The boat that comes in first is the boat in which all of the members of the crew team are working together. At any given moment, they are all at the same stage of the stroke cycle, so that all of their energies are working together to propel the boat. All of the members of the crew team place their oars in the water at the same instant. They all remove their oars from the water at the same instant. They are working together in perfect unison. In similar fashion, all of the light waves in a laser work together in a beam of coherent energy. By contrast, in the boat that comes in last, the crew members may be seen to be at different stages of the stroke cycle. Some have their oars going

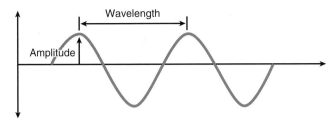

• **Figure 2-1** Properties of electromagnetic waves. Amplitude is the height of the wave from the zero axis to the peak. Wavelength is the horizontal distance between two adjacent parts of a wave.

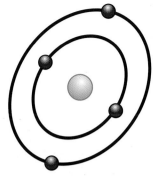

• **Figure 2-2** An atom of an active medium in ground state.

into the water, and some have their oars coming out of the water; some are at the top of the stroke cycle, and some are at the bottom of the stroke cycle. The team members are not working together as one. The work expended by this disorganized crew, which cannot propel their boat forward with any effective speed, would be analogous to the energy from an ordinary light bulb, which is insufficient for excision of soft tissue.

Amplification

Amplification is the part of this process that occurs inside the laser. In this section, the components of a laser instrument are identified to show how laser light is produced.

The center of the laser is called the *laser cavity*. The following three components make up the laser cavity:

- Active medium
- Pumping mechanism
- Optical resonator

The *active medium* is composed of chemical elements, molecules, or compounds. Lasers are generically named for the material of the active medium, which can be (1) a container of gas, such as a canister of carbon dioxide (CO_2) gas in a CO_2 laser; (2) a solid crystal, such as that in an erbium-doped YAG (Er:YAG) laser; (3) a solid-state semiconductor, such as the semiconductors found in diode lasers; or (4) a liquid, such as that used in some medical laser devices.

Surrounding this active medium is an excitation source, such as a flash lamp strobe device, electrical circuit, electrical coil, or similar source of energy that pumps energy into the active medium. When this *pumping mechanism* drives energy into the active medium, the electrons in the outermost shell of the active medium's atoms absorb the energy. These electrons have absorbed a specific amount of energy to reach the next shell farther from the nucleus, which is at a higher energy level. A "population inversion" occurs when more of the electrons from the active medium are in the higher energy level shell farther from the nucleus than are in the ground state (Figure 2-2). The electrons in this excited state then return to their resting state and emit that energy in a form known as a photon (Figure 2-3). This is called *spontaneous (not stimulated) emission* (Figure 2-4).

Completing the laser cavity are two mirrors, one at each end of the optical cavity, placed parallel to each other; or in the case of a semiconductor diode laser, two polished

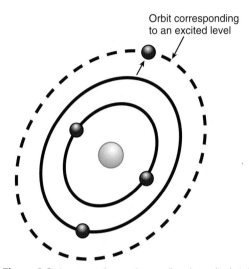

• **Figure 2-3** An atom of an active medium in excited state.

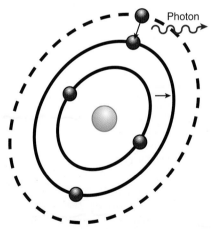

• **Figure 2-4** An atom of an active medium spontaneously emits a photon and returns to a stable orbit, giving off the energy that it had just absorbed, according to the principle of conservation of energy.

surfaces at each end. These mirrors or polished surfaces act as *optical resonators,* reflecting the waves back and forth, and help to collimate and amplify the developing beam. A cooling system, focusing lenses, and other controlling mechanisms complete the mechanical components. Figure 2-5 shows a schematic of a gas or solid active-medium laser (e.g., CO_2, Nd:YAG). Figure 2-6 shows a schematic of a semiconductor diode device.

Laser components, e.g., CO_2 or Nd:YAG

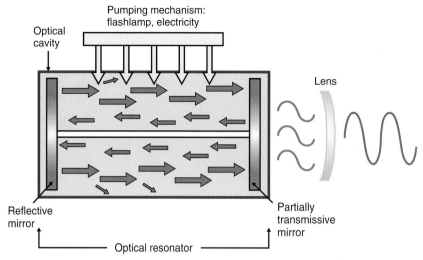

• **Figure 2-5** A gas or solid active-medium laser, such as CO_2 or Nd:YAG laser.

Semiconductor diode laser components

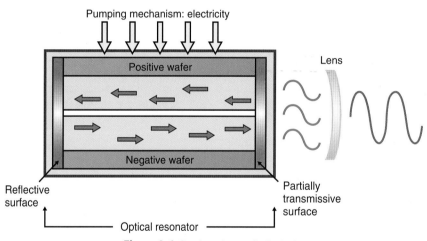

• **Figure 2-6** Semiconductor diode device.

Stimulated Emission

Stimulated emission is the process by which laser beams are produced inside the laser cavity. The theory of stimulated emission was postulated by Albert Einstein in 1916.[3] He based his work on some earlier work by physicists from Germany (Max Planck) and Denmark (Niels Bohr), who theorized a model of the atom as well as the quantum theory of physics, which defined a *quantum* as the smallest unit of energy emitted from an atom.[4,5] Einstein, using this concept, further theorized that an additional quantum of energy may be absorbed by the already-energized atom, resulting in a release of two quanta (Figure 2-7). This energy is emitted, or *radiated,* as identical photons, traveling as a coherent wave. These photons in turn are then able to energize more atoms in a geometric progression, which further causes the emission of additional identical photons, resulting in an amplification of the light energy—thereby producing a laser beam (Figure 2-8).

Radiation

The light waves produced by the laser are a specific form of electromagnetic energy.[6] The *electromagnetic spectrum* is the entire collection of wave energy, ranging from gamma rays, with wavelengths of 1×10^{-12} m, to radio waves, with wavelengths of thousands of meters. All currently available dental laser devices have emission wavelengths of approximately 500 to 10,600 nm, which places them in either the visible or the invisible (infrared) nonionizing portion of the electromagnetic spectrum, as shown in Figure 2-9. Of note, the dividing line between the ionizing, cellular DNA–mutagenic portion of the spectrum and the nonionizing portion is at the junction of ultraviolet and visible-violet light. Thus all current dental lasers emit either a visible-light wavelength or an invisible, infrared-light wavelength in the portion of the nonionizing spectrum called *thermal radiation*.[7] The word radiation in this context does not imply radioactive or carcinogenic but simply means the *emission of electromagnetic energy*.

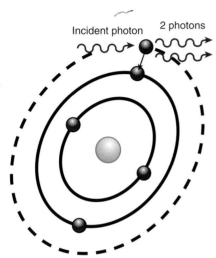

• **Figure 2-7** An atom of an active medium showing stimulated emission, releasing two identical photons before returning to a stable state.

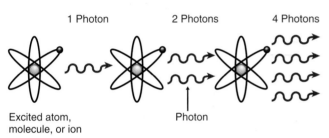

• **Figure 2-8** Light amplification by stimulated emission of radiation.

The following four dental laser instruments emit visible light:
• Argon laser: blue wavelength of 488 nm
• Argon laser: blue-green wavelength of 514 nm
• Frequency-doubled Nd:YAG laser, also called a potassium titanyl phosphate (KTP) laser: green wavelength of 532 nm
• Low-level lasers: red nonsurgical wavelengths of 600 to 635 nm (for photobiomodulation) and 655 nm (for caries detection)

Argon lasers are no longer manufactured as dental surgical instruments, although they are still used for medical procedures.

Other dental lasers emit invisible laser light in the near, middle, and far infrared portion of the electromagnetic spectrum. These include photobiomodulation devices with wavelengths between 800 and 900 nm, as well as surgical instruments, as follows:
• Diode lasers: various wavelengths between 800 and 1064 nm, using a semiconductor active medium of gallium and arsenide, with the addition of either aluminum or indium in some devices
• Nd:YAG laser: 1064 nm
• Erbium-chromium–doped yttrium-scandium-gallium-garnet (Er,Cr:YSGG) laser: 2780 nm
• Er:YAG laser: 2940 nm
• CO_2 laser: 9300 nm and 10,600 nm

Laser Delivery Systems

Laser energy should be delivered to the surgical site by a method that is ergonomic and precise.[8] Shorter-wavelength instruments, such as KTP, diode, and Nd:Y-AG lasers, have

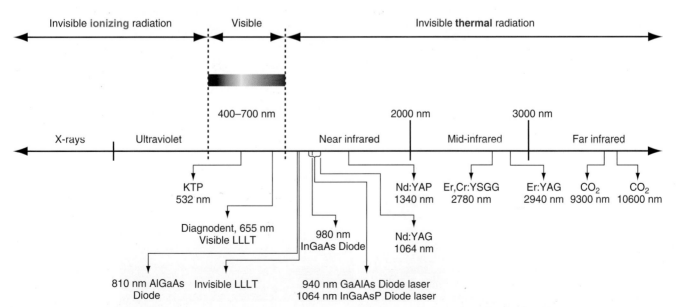

• **Figure 2-9** Part of electromagnetic spectrum showing division into ionizing, visible portion, and nonionizing portion.

small, flexible fiberoptic systems with bare glass fibers that deliver the laser energy to the target tissue (Figure 2-10). Because the erbium and CO_2 laser wavelengths are absorbed by water, which is a major component of conventional glass fibers, these wavelengths cannot pass through these fibers. Erbium and CO_2 devices are therefore constructed with special fibers capable of transmitting the wavelengths, with semiflexible hollow waveguides, or with articulated arms (Figure 2-11). Some of these systems employ small quartz or sapphire tips that attach to the laser device for contact with target tissue; others employ noncontact tips (Figure 2-12). In addition, the erbium lasers incorporate a water spray for cooling hard tissues. Lasers may have different fiber diameters, handpieces, and tips (Figure 2-13). Each of these elements plays a significant role in the delivery of energy (Figure 2-14).

All conventional dental instrumentation, either hand or rotary, must physically touch the tissue being treated, which gives the operator instant feedback. As mentioned, dental lasers can be used either in contact or out of contact. The fiber tip can easily be inserted into a periodontal pocket to remove small amounts of granulomatous tissue or treat an aphthous ulcer (Figures 2-15 to 2-17). In non-contact use, the beam is aimed at the target some distance away (Figure 2-18). This modality is useful for following various tissue contours, but with the loss of tactile sensation, the surgeon must pay close attention to the tissue interaction with the laser energy. All of the invisible-light dental lasers—Nd:YAG, CO_2, diode, and erbium—are equipped with a separate aiming beam, which can be either a laser or a conventional light. The aiming beam is delivered coaxially along the fiber or waveguide and shows the operator the exact spot at which the laser energy will strike the tissue.

Spot Size

Lenses focus the active beam. With hollow-waveguide or articulated-arm delivery systems, there is a precise spot at the point where the amount of energy is the greatest.

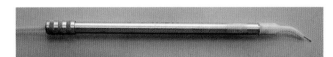

• **Figure 2-10** An assembled fiberoptic delivery system consisting of the bare fiber, a handpiece, and a disposable tip.

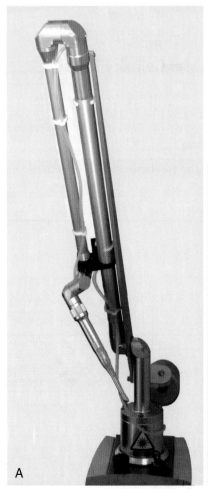
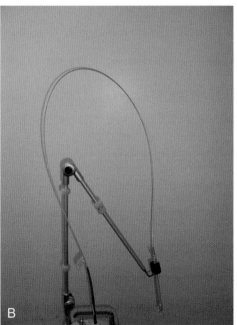

A   B

• **Figure 2-11** A, Articulated-arm delivery system, typical of CO_2 lasers and some erbium devices. B, Hollow waveguide delivery system of a CO_2 laser.

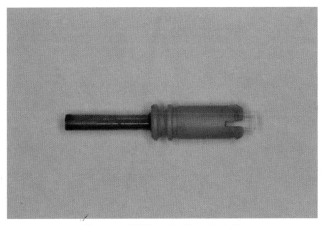

• **Figure 2-12** Typical erbium laser tip.

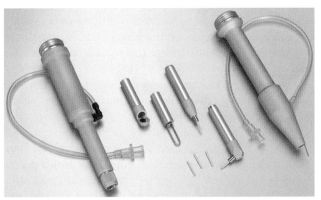

• **Figure 2-13** A variety of handpieces available with most CO_2 laser systems offer a variety of spot sizes and focal distances.

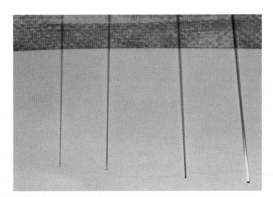

• **Figure 2-14** Fiber diameters for Nd:YAG and diode lasers, yielding different spot sizes.

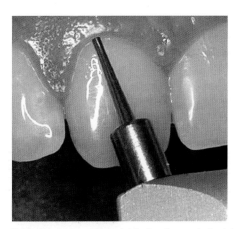

• **Figure 2-15** CO_2 laser periodontal tip treating periodontal pocket.

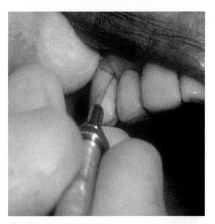

• **Figure 2-16** Nd:YAG laser fiber entering periodontal pocket.

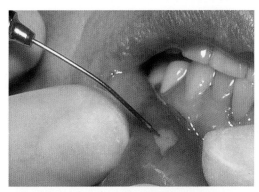

• **Figure 2-17** Nd:YAG laser fiber contacting aphthous ulcer.

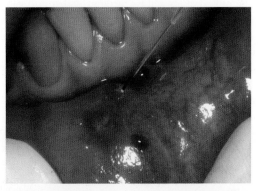

• **Figure 2-18** Nd:YAG laser fiber out of contact treating aphthous ulcer.

This *focal point* is used for incision and excision surgery. For fiberoptic contact delivery systems, the focal point is at or near the tip of the fiber, which again has the greatest amount of energy. For CO_2 lasers, which are used out of contact, the focal point may be anywhere from 1 to 12 mm from the tissue surface, depending on the handpiece being used (Figure 2-19). When the handpiece is moved away from the tissue and away from the focal point, the beam is *defocused* (out of focus) and becomes more divergent and therefore delivers less energy to the surgical site (Figure 2-20). At a small

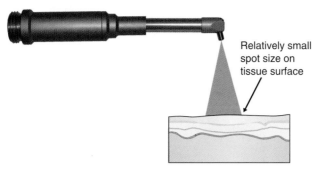

• **Figure 2-19** A handpiece at the correct distance from the tissue for maximal effect is "in focus."

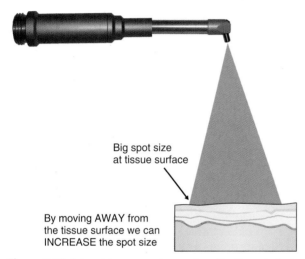

Big spot size
at tissue surface

By moving AWAY from
the tissue surface we can
INCREASE the spot size

• **Figure 2-20** A handpiece moved away from the tissue is "out of focus," resulting in a larger spot size and less fluence. Out-of-focus mode is excellent for hemostasis.

divergent distance, the beam can cover a wider area, which would be useful in achieving a wide yet shallow ablation of tissue or, at a more divergent distance, hemostasis. At a greater distance, the beam will lose its effectiveness because the energy will dissipate.

Emission Modes

Dental laser devices can emit light energy in two modalities as a function of time: (1) constant on or (2) pulsed on and off.[8] The pulsed lasers can be further divided into gated and free-running modes for delivering energy to the target tissue. Thus three different emission modes are described, as follows:

1. **Continuous-wave mode,** in which the beam is emitted at only one power level for as long as the operator depresses the foot switch.
2. **Gated-pulse mode,** characterized by periodic alternations of the laser energy, similar to a blinking light. This mode is achieved by the opening and closing of a mechanical shutter in front of the beam path of a continuous-wave emission. All surgical devices that operate in continuous-wave mode have this gated-pulse feature. Some instruments can produce pulses as short as

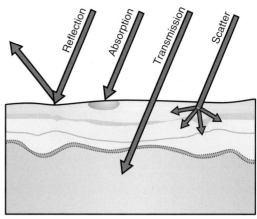

• **Figure 2-21** Four potential laser-tissue interactions.

microseconds (μsec) or milliseconds (msec). Peak powers of approximately 10 to 50 times that of continuous-wave power measurements are produced, and charring of the tissue can be reduced. The more advanced units have computer-controlled shutters that allow for these very short pulses. Manufacturers have coined many terms to describe these short pulse durations, including "super pulse" and "ultra speed."

3. **Free-running pulsed mode,** sometimes referred to as *true pulsed* mode. This emission is unique in that large peak energies of laser light are emitted usually for microseconds, followed by a relatively long time in which the laser is off. For example, with a free-running pulsed laser with pulse duration of 100 μsec and pulses delivered at 10 per second (10 Hz), the energy at the surgical site is present for 0.01% of a second and absent for the remaining 99.99% of that second. Free-running pulsed devices have a rapidly strobing flash lamp that pumps the active medium. With each pulse, high peak powers in hundreds or thousands of watts are generated. Because the pulse duration is short, however, the average power that the tissue incurs is small. Free-running pulsed devices cannot have a continuous-wave or gated-pulse output.

True pulsed lasers are driven by the action of the pumping mechanism within the laser cavity. Gated-pulse lasers are pulsed as a result of a shutter outside the laser cavity. Medical and scientific laser instruments are available with pulse durations in the nanosecond (one billionth of a second), picosecond (one trillionth of a second), or smaller range. These can generate tremendous peak powers, but the calculated average pulse energies are small, allowing increased surgical precision. Some instruments can be controlled to emit a single pulse.

Laser Effects on Tissue

Depending on the optical properties of the tissue, the light energy from a laser may have four different interactions with the target tissue (Figure 2-21), as follows[9]:

• Reflection
• Absorption

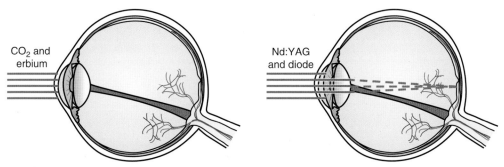

• **Figure 2-22** Diagram of the eye showing the effects of different wavelengths on various tissue types. In general, CO_2 and erbium lasers interact with the cornea and lens, whereas Nd:YAG and diode lasers penetrate to the retina.

- Transmission
- Scattering

A good way to remember these four types of laser-tissue interactions is with the mnemonic device RATS.

Reflection is simply the beam being redirected off the surface, with no effect on the target tissue. The reflected light may maintain its collimation in a narrow beam, or it may become more diffuse. As stated previously, the laser beam generally becomes more divergent as the distance from the handpiece increases. With some lasers, however, the beam can still have adequate energy at distances greater than 3 m. In any event, this reflection can be dangerous because the energy could be redirected to an unintentional target, such as the eyes. This potential mistargeting is a major safety concern in laser operation and the reason that every person in the dental treatment room must wear wavelength-specific safety glasses with appropriate side shields. An example of reflection would be the interaction between a CO_2 laser and a patient's titanium implants. CO_2 laser energy reflected off the implants could be redirected to the dentist's eyes.

The second interaction with tissue is *absorption*. Absorption of the laser energy by the intended target tissue usually is the most desirable effect. The amount of energy absorbed by the tissue depends on that tissue's characteristics, such as pigmentation and water content, and on the laser wavelength. The primary and beneficial goal of laser energy is therefore absorption of the laser light by the intended biologic tissue.

The third effect is *transmission* of the laser energy directly through the tissue, with no effect on the target tissue (Figure 2-22). This effect also is highly dependent on the wavelength of laser light. Water, for example, is relatively "transparent" to (does not absorb) the diode and Nd:YAG wavelengths, whereas the water component of tissue fluids readily absorbs erbium and CO_2 wavelengths at the surface, so minimal energy is transmitted to adjacent tissues. The diode and Nd:YAG wavelengths are transmitted through the sclera, lens, iris, cornea, vitreous humor, and aqueous humor of the eye before being absorbed on the retina.

The fourth tissue interaction is *scattering* of the laser light, which weakens the intended energy. Scattering is the predominant event with use of the near-infrared lasers in healthy soft tissue. Scattering causes the photons to change directions, leading to increased absorption, with

correspondingly increased chances of interacting with the predominant chromophore of those wavelengths. Scattering of the laser beam also could cause heat transfer to the tissue adjacent to the surgical site, with the potential for injury from unwanted laser effects. However, a beam that is scattered, or deflected in different directions, would be useful in facilitating laser curing of composite resin.

The following photobiologic effects are possible with use of a dental laser[10]:

- The principal laser-tissue interaction is *photothermal,* which means the laser energy is transformed into heat. The three primary photothermal laser-tissue interactions are *incision/excision, ablation/vaporization,* and *hemostasis/coagulation.* By varying the various laser parameters of beam diameter (called *spot size*), energy, and time, lasers can be made to perform any of the three photothermal interactions:
  1. A laser beam in focus with a small spot size is used for incision/excision procedures (Figure 2-23).
  2. A laser beam with a wider spot size will interact with the tissue over a wider area, but more superficially, producing a surface ablation (Figure 2-24).
  3. A laser beam out of focus will produce hemostasis/coagulation (Figure 2-25).
- *Photochemical* effects occur when the laser is used to stimulate chemical reactions, such as the curing of composite resin by an argon laser. The breaking of chemical bonds, such as using photosensitive compounds exposed to laser energy, can produce singlet oxygen radical for disinfection of periodontal pockets and endodontic canals.
- Certain biologic pigments, when absorbing laser light of a specific wavelength, can *fluoresce;* this property can be used for caries detection on occlusal surfaces of teeth. More information on the use of laser fluorescence for caries detection may be found in the chapter on the use of lasers in operative dentistry.
- A laser can be used in a nonsurgical mode for *biostimulation* for more rapid wound healing, pain relief, increased collagen growth, and a general antiinflammatory effect. More information on this application can be found in Chapter 15, on low-level laser therapy (photobiomodulation) in dentistry.
- The pulse of laser energy on hard dentinal and osseous tissues can produce a shock wave, which is an example of

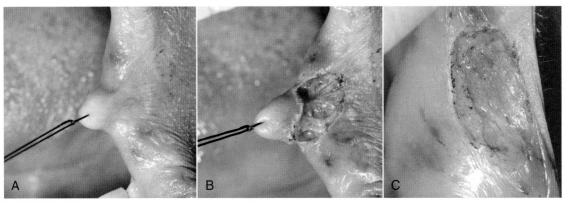

• **Figure 2-23** Laser excisional biopsy. **A,** Traction suture in place immediately preoperatively. **B,** Beginning laser excision of lesion. **C,** Immediate postoperative view of excision site. Note the complete absence of bleeding at the surgical site, one of the many advantages of laser surgery over conventional techniques.

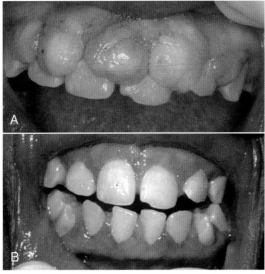

• **Figure 2-24** Laser ablation of excess tissue for treatment of cyclosporine-induced gingival hyperplasia. The patient was an adolescent kidney transplant recipient. **A,** Immediate preoperative view. **B,** One-week postoperative view of laser-ablated area.

the *photoacoustic* effect of laser light. This process often is called *spallation.*

More information on spallation is presented in Chapter 10, on operative dentistry. As discussed next, the main photothermal effect of dental lasers is tissue water vaporization; accordingly, the primary treatment goal is surgical, that is, the removal of tissue, as opposed to fluorescence or biostimulation.

Tissue Temperature

The thermal effect of laser energy on tissue primarily involves the water content of tissue and change in the temperature of the tissue. As Table 2-1 shows, when target tissue containing water is heated to a temperature of 100° C, vaporization of the water within the tissue occurs; this process is called *ablation.*[11] Because soft tissue is composed of a very high percentage of water, excision/incision of soft tissue commences at this temperature. At temperatures between approximately 60° and 100° C, proteins begin to denature, without any vaporization of the underlying tissue. This phenomenon is useful in surgically removing diseased granulomatous tissue without affecting the healthy tissue, so long as the tissue temperature can be controlled.[12] At 70° to 80° C, soft tissue edges can be welded back together without sutures.[13]

If the tissue temperature is raised to approximately 200° C, the tissue becomes dehydrated and then starts to burn, and carbon is the end product. Carbon is a strong absorber of all wavelengths, so it can become a "heat sink" as the laser procedure continues.[14] The heat conduction will then cause extensive collateral thermal trauma, referred to as *tissue charring.* Tissue charring occurs when improper laser parameters are used.

For dental hard tissue, the primary interaction occurs at 100° C, when the water within the hydroxyapatite crystal is converted to steam, whose increased volume causes an explosive expansion and removal of that tissue.[15]

Laser emission modes play an important role in increasing the tissue temperature. The important principle of any laser emission mode is that the light energy strikes the tissue for a certain length of time, producing a thermal interaction.[16] If the laser is used in a pulsed mode, the targeted tissue may have time to cool before the next pulse of laser energy is emitted. In continuous-wave mode, the operator must cease the laser emission manually so that thermal relaxation of the tissue may occur. Thin or fragile soft tissue, for example, should be treated in a pulsed mode so that the amount and rate of tissue removal are slower, but the chance of irreversible thermal damage to the target tissue and the adjacent nontarget tissue is minimal. Longer intervals between pulses also can help avoid the transfer of heat to the surrounding tissue. In addition, a gentle air stream or an air current from the high-volume suction will aid in keeping the area cooler. Similarly, with use of hard tissue lasers, a water spray will help prevent microfracturing of the crystalline structures and reduce the possibility of carbonization.

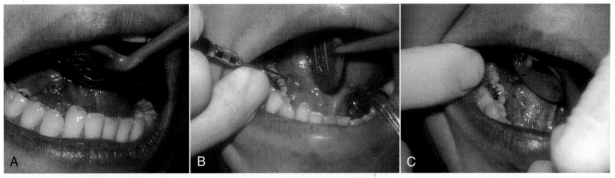

• **Figure 2-25** Laser coagulation of an aphthous ulcer on the floor of the mouth. **A,** Preoperative view. **B,** Applying laser energy to lesion. **C,** Immediate postoperative view of surgical site.

TABLE 2-1	Temperature Effects on Oral Soft Tissue	
Tissue Temperature (° C)	**Observed Effect(s)**	
37 C	normal body temperature	
>60 C	Coagulation and protein denaturation	
100 C	Vaporization of intra- and extra-cellular water	

Conversely, thick, dense, fibrous tissue requires more energy for removal. For the same reason, dental enamel, with its higher mineral content, requires more ablation power than softer, more aqueous carious tissue. In either case, if too much thermal energy is used, healing can be delayed, and postoperative discomfort may be greater than normal.

Lasers have wide-ranging variability in pulse parameters (Figure 2-26). To allow tissue cooling, some lasers permit the surgeon to change the amount of "on" time of the pulse, called the *pulse width*. Other lasers allow the surgeon to control the amount of "off" time between pulses. By varying the amount of time the laser pulses on and off, the surgeon is better able to treat different tissue types. The laser buyer should evaluate the amount of variability built into the unit. Some units have fixed pulse widths that cannot be changed. This limitation curtails the surgeon's ability to modify settings for optimal treatment of different tissues.

Duty cycle, also called *emission cycle,* is the term used to describe the amount of on and off time. A duty cycle of 10% means that the laser is on for 10% and off for 90% of the time. A duty cycle of 50% means that the laser is on for half the time and off for half. Thin, friable tissues should be treated with small duty cycles, whereas thicker tissue may be treated with larger duty cycles or with continuous-wave emission.

Absorption of Laser Energy by Dental Tissues

Different laser wavelengths have different absorption coefficients, with the primary oral tissue components of water,

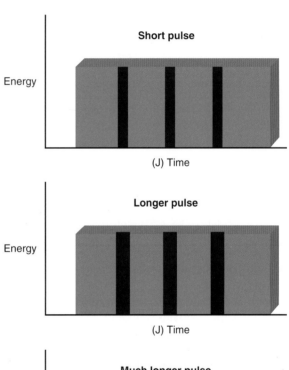
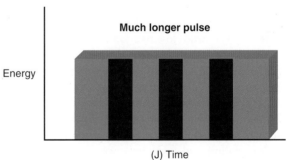

• **Figure 2-26** Various pulse parameters.

pigment, blood constituents, and minerals (Figure 2-27). Laser energy can therefore be reflected, absorbed, transmitted, or scattered, depending on the composition of the target tissue. The primary absorbers of specific laser energy are called *chromophores.*[7,17] Water, which is present in all biologic tissue, maximally absorbs the two erbium wavelengths, followed by the two CO_2 wavelengths. Conversely, water allows the transmission of the shorter-wavelength

Approximate net absorption curves of various tissue components

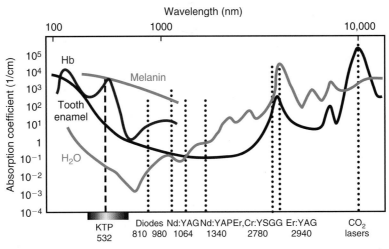

• **Figure 2-27** Approximate absorption curves of the prime oral chromophores.

lasers (e.g., diode, Nd:YAG). Tooth enamel is composed of carbonated hydroxyapatite and water. The apatite crystal readily absorbs the CO_2 wavelength and interacts to a lesser degree with the erbium wavelengths. It does not interact with the shorter wavelengths. Hemoglobin and other blood components and pigments such as melanin absorb diode and Nd:YAG laser wavelengths in variable amounts.

Human dental tissues are composed of a combination of compounds, so the clinician must choose the best laser for each treatment.[18] For soft tissue treatments, the practitioner can use any available wavelength, because all dental laser wavelengths are absorbed by one or more of the soft tissue components. For hard tissue, however, the erbium lasers and the 9.3-μm CO_2 laser with very short pulse durations easily ablate layers of calcified tissue with minimal thermal effects. Of interest, the short-wavelength lasers (e.g., diode, Nd:YAG) are essentially nonreactive with healthy tooth enamel. Recontouring gingival tissue close to a tooth can therefore proceed uneventfully with use of these wavelengths. Conversely, if soft tissue is impinging into a carious lesion, an erbium laser can remove the lesion and the soft tissue very efficiently, so long as appropriate settings are used for each tissue type.

In addition to unique absorptive optical properties, all wavelengths have different *penetration* depths through tissue. The erbium and CO_2 laser wavelengths are so well absorbed by tissue with a high water content (e.g., mucosa) that they penetrate only a few to several μm deep into the target tissue, whereas diode and Nd:YAG lasers can reach a few millimeters deeper. It is important to recognize that in keeping with the differences in penetration of the various wavelengths into mucosa, tissue interaction may continue at levels beyond the desired depth of the surgical field. This increased penetration could lead to deep thermal necrosis of underlying tissue and osteonecrosis of bone.

Extinction length is defined as the thickness of a substance in which 98% of the energy from the laser is absorbed.[19]

A small extinction length means that the laser energy is maximally absorbed by that tissue with no deep penetration and thus minimal possibility of deep thermal damage. A large extinction length means that the laser energy penetrates deep into that tissue. Because CO_2 and erbium lasers are the two wavelengths best absorbed by tissue with high water content, these wavelengths have the smallest extinction length in mucosa and are least likely to cause deep thermal damage, so long as proper operating parameters are used. The extinction length for CO_2 lasers in mucosa, for example, is 0.03 mm. Lasers with greater extinction lengths in mucosa, such as Nd:YAG (1 to 3 mm) and diode lasers, are safe to use provided that correct operating parameters are followed. Conversely, the use of these wavelengths by operators without adequate training carries the risk of thermal damage to the underlying tissue.

Laser-Tissue Summary

To determine the tissue interactions associated with a particular laser device, the following factors must be considered[20]:

1. Each laser wavelength will affect the interrelated components of the target tissue: water content, color of the tissue, vascularity, and chemical composition.
2. The diameter of the laser spot on the tissue, or spot size, whether delivered in contact or noncontact with the tissue, will create a certain amount of energy per square millimeter of tissue. This is called *energy density*, or *fluence*. An inverse relationship exists between spot size and fluence; the smaller the spot size, the greater the fluence (Figure 2-28). For example, a beam diameter of 200 μm, compared with a beam diameter of 300 μm at the same output setting, will have more than twice as much energy density. Use of the smaller spot size thus will result in greatly increased thermal transfer from the laser to the

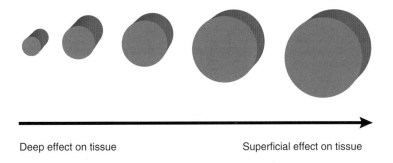

Deep effect on tissue   Superficial effect on tissue

Small spot size   **Large spot size**

5 W ← Same power → 5 W

Narrow, deep effect   Wide, shallow effect
(think incision)   (think ablation)

• **Figure 2-28** Graphic representation of the relationship between spot size and fluence. The same wavelength and power were used but the spot size was changed. On the *left*, the incision is narrow and deep with a smaller spot size; on the *right*, the incision is wide and shallow with a larger spot size.

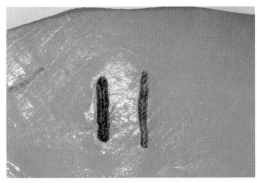

• **Figure 2-29** Effect of hand speed on incisions. Both incisions were made with the same handpiece and spot size. The incision on the *left* was performed with a very slow hand speed, whereas the incision on the *right* was performed with a faster hand speed.

tissue, with a corresponding increase in absorption of heat in that smaller area. If the beam has divergence, moving it away from the tissue will increase its diameter, thereby lessening the energy density.

3. The amount of time during which the beam is allowed to strike the target tissue will affect the rate of tissue temperature rise. Accordingly, two specific aspects of laser operation need to be addressed:

   a. *Repetition rate* of the pulsed-laser emission mode: the number of pulses per second. The repetition rate is measured in Hz.

   b. *Hand speed*: the speed of moving the laser through the tissue. A rapid movement of the laser through the surgical field may not permit adequate absorption of the energy by the tissue. Conversely, moving the laser through the surgical field too slowly may result in too much thermal damage to the tissue (Figure 2-29).

4. Using a water or air spray also can cool the tissue, which would affect the rate of vaporization.

The laser practitioner must be aware of these factors before beginning treatment. Selection of the appropriate wavelength, beam diameter (spot size), focused or defocused distance, Hz setting, and amount and type of tissue cooling can then be achieved. The correct combination of all of these parameters should ensure an efficient procedure and a beneficial outcome. Laser training is critically important in determining how to manipulate these parameters, as discussed in more detail in Chapter 16, on practice management considerations in laser dentistry.

Laser Safety

General Principles

All laser devices come with complete instructions on the safe use of the machine. Every laser practitioner should know certain fundamentals, but the primary responsibility for safe and effective operation of the laser is assigned to the laser safety officer for the clinical facility.[21,22] This person provides all necessary information, inspects and maintains the laser and its accessories, and ensures that all safety procedures are implemented. More information on the role of the laser safety officer may be found in Chapter 16.

The patient and all members of the surgical team must wear appropriate protective eyewear when the laser is operating, to prevent damage from any reflected or accidental direct energy exposure. The surgical environment must have a warning sign posted, with limited access to the treatment room. High-volume suction must be used to evacuate the plume formed by tissue ablation, and the normal infection protocol must be followed. The laser itself must be in good working order so that the manufacturer safeguards prevent accidental laser exposure. Masks must be of appropriate filtering capacity to prevent inhalation of laser plume. Most laser procedures should be performed with the surgeon wearing a 0.1-μm filtration mask. Regular cup-shaped dental masks are insufficient for filtering the laser plume and should not be worn during laser surgery. *Laser plume* results from the aerosol byproducts of laser-tissue interaction, which may contain particulate organic and inorganic matter (e.g., viruses, toxic gases, chemicals) and may be infectious and/or carcinogenic.

Laser Regulatory Agencies

In most countries, regulatory agencies control both the laser operator and the laser manufacturer, and standards are strictly enforced.

In the United States, the American National Standards Institute (ANSI) provides guidance for the safe use of laser systems by specifically defining control measures for lasers.[23] The Occupational Safety and Health Administration (OSHA) is primarily concerned with a safe workplace environment, and numerous requirements exist for laser protocols. The Center for Devices and Radiological Health (CDRH) is the bureau within the Food and Drug Administration (FDA) whose purpose is to standardize the manufacture of laser products and to enforce compliance with the medical devices legislation.[22] All laser manufacturers must obtain permission from the CDRH to make and distribute each device for a specific purpose; this *marketing clearance* means that the FDA is satisfied that the laser is both safe and effective to operate for that purpose. The owner's manual for the particular laser model instructs the operator on how to use the device for the particular CDRH-regulated procedure.

In countries and jurisdictions outside of the United States, the International Electrotechnical Commission (IEC), headquartered in Geneva, Switzerland, promulgates similar standards and regulations.

At present, approximately two dozen indications for use of specific dental lasers are recognized. All wavelengths and devices of adequate power may be used for every aspect of intraoral soft tissue surgery. The erbium lasers may be used for carious lesion removal, tooth preparation, endodontic, and osseous procedures. The 9300-nm CO_2 laser also may be used for some hard tissue procedures, with the possibility of more indications pending regulatory clearance. Some instruments have specific clearances for procedures such as sulcular debridement and tooth whitening. The dental practitioner may use the laser for procedures other than for the cleared indications because the FDA does not regulate dental practice; however, using a laser for a non–FDA-cleared procedure may have legal ramifications in the event of a malpractice claim.

Hospitals and institutions have their own credentialing programs for the use of lasers in their facilities, and a published curriculum guideline has established standards of dental laser education. The scope of practice—as defined by the dental practice act of each state or other jurisdiction—and the training and clinical experience of the dental laser operator are the primary factors that should determine how the device is used.

Benefits and Drawbacks of Dental Lasers

One of the main benefits of using dental lasers is the capability of selective and precise interaction with diseased tissues. Lasers also allow the clinician to reduce the amount of bacteria and other pathogens in the surgical field and, in the case of soft tissue procedures, achieve good hemostasis with reduced need for sutures.[24-27] Many researchers have shown that the ability of lasers to seal blood vessels and lymphatic channels results in reduced postoperative edema, which in turn results in less postoperative discomfort.[28]

The hard tissue laser devices can selectively remove diseased tooth structure because a carious lesion has much higher water content than healthy tissue, and water is the primary absorber of that wavelength of laser energy.[15,29-31] These same devices confer advantages over conventional high-speed handpieces as they interact with the tooth surface; for example, laser-treated dentin has no "smear layer," and the cavity preparation has been disinfected because of the bactericidal nature of laser energy.[32]

The disadvantages of the current dental laser instruments are the relatively high cost and the required training.[33] Most dental instruments are both side-cutting and end-cutting, so a modification of clinical technique is required in using lasers, which are almost exclusively end-cutting. The clinician must prevent overheating of the tissue and guard against air embolism caused by excessive pressure of air and water spray during laser procedures. Another drawback of erbium lasers is the inability to remove metallic restorations. In addition, despite laser manufacturers' claims to the contrary, no single wavelength will optimally treat all dental disease.[34]

Thus proper laser training is critical in deciding which wavelength to use and which model to purchase.[35] Some manufacturers provide excellent hands-on training both at seminars and in the office, whereas others give the buyer nothing more than a CD and training manual. This issue is discussed in more detail in Chapter 16.

Lasers in Dentistry: Now and in the Future

As mentioned, all dental surgical lasers currently available are designed for soft tissue procedures; only the two erbium and the 9.3-μm CO_2 wavelengths are safe and effective for use with teeth and bone. Therapeutic, or photobiomodulation, lasers show beneficial results for healing, although a majority of the reports are anecdotal. The initial clinical results with photoactivated disinfection also show promising applications for disease control. More information on photoactivated disinfection and low-level laser therapy is presented in Chapter 15.

The future holds the promise of additional laser applications. Optical coherence tomography using a laser to create a three-dimensional image will be a tremendous advance for dental diagnosis, and laser Doppler instruments will be able to measure blood flow rates to assess inflammation. Selective ablation of calculus and bacteria and enamel hardening for caries resistance are examples of new procedures under development.[36,37] Manufacturers continue to develop technologies, with clearance for other clinical applications and laser wavelengths pending. More information on what the future of lasers in dentistry may hold may be found in Chapter 17, on laser research.

Conclusions

The appropriate and effective use of dental lasers in clinical practice requires a firm grasp of their scientific basis and tissue effects, proper training in techniques and applications, and sufficient operative experience to achieve and maintain proficiency. The clinician can then choose the proper laser(s) for the intended application. Although the types of tissue interaction overlap somewhat, each wavelength has specific properties that can be used to accomplish a specific treatment objective. Laser energy requires some procedures to be performed much differently from those using conventional instrumentation, but the indications for laser use continue to expand, with further benefit for patient care.

References

1. *The photonics dictionary*, ed 43, Pittsfield, Mass, 1997, Laurin Publishing.
2. Myers TD: Lasers in dentistry: their application in clinical practice, *J Am Dent Assoc* 122:46–50, 1991.
3. Einstein A: Zur Quantum Theorie der Stralung, *Verk Deutsch Phys Ges* 18:318, 1916.
4. *Dictionary of scientific biography*, New York, 1971, Charles Scribner's Sons.
5. Bohr N: *The theory of spectra and atomic constitution*, ed 2, Cambridge, Mass, 1922, Cambridge University Press.
6. *The Columbia electronic encyclopedia*, New York, 2003, Columbia University Press. Available at http://www.encyclopedia.com Accessed July 30, 2008.
7. Manni JG: *Dental applications of advanced lasers*, Burlington, Mass, 2004, JGM Associates.
8. Coluzzi DJ, Convissar RA: *Atlas of laser applications in dentistry*, Hanover Park, Ill, 2007. Quintessence.
9. Miserendino LJ, Levy G, Miserendino CA: Laser interaction with biologic tissues. In Miserendino LJ, Pick RM, editors: *Lasers in dentistry*, Chicago, 1995, Quintessence.
10. Niemz MH: *Laser-tissue interaction: fundamentals and applications*, ed 3, (enlarged) Berlin, 2007, Springer.
11. McKenzie AL: Physics of thermal processes in laser-tissue interaction, *Phys Med Biol* 35(9):1175–1209, 1990.
12. Knappe V, Frank F, Rohde E: Principles of lasers and biophotonic effects, *Photomed Laser Surg* 22(5):411–417, 2004.
13. Springer TA, Welch AJ: Temperature control during tissue welding, *Appl Optics* 32(4):517–525, 1993.
14. Bornstein E: Near-infrared dental diode lasers: scientific and photo biologic principles and applications, *Dent Today* 23(3):102–104, 2004. 106–108.
15. Rechmann P, Goldin DS, Hennig T: Er:YAG lasers in dentistry: an overview. In Featherstone JD, Rechmann P, Fried DS, editors: *Lasers in dentistry IV*, January 25-26, 1998, San Jose, Calif, *Proc. SPIE 3248*, Bellingham, Wash, 1998, SPIE—The International Society for Optical Engineering.
16. White JM, Goodis HE, Kudler JJ, Tran KT: Photo thermal laser effects on intraoral soft tissue, teeth and bone in vitro. *Proceedings of the ISLD Third International Congress on Lasers in Dentistry*, Salt Lake City, 1992, University of Utah.
17. Goldman L: Chromophores in tissue for laser medicine and laser surgery, *Lasers Med Sci* 5(3):289–292, 1990.
18. Coluzzi DJ: Fundamentals of lasers in dentistry: basic science, tissue interaction, and instrumentation, *J Laser Dent* 16(spec. issue): 4–10, 2008.
19. Hale GM, Querry MR: Optical constants of water in the 200-nm to 200-μm wavelength region, *Appl Opt* 12(3):555–563, 1973.
20. Parker S: *Lasers in dentistry*, London, 2007, British Dental Association London.
21. Sliney DH, Trokel SL: *Medical lasers and their safe use*, New York, 1993, Springer-Verlag.
22. Piccione PJ: Dental laser safety, *Dent Clin North Am* 48:795–807, 2004.
23. American National Standards Institute: *American national standard for safe use of lasers in health care facilities*, Orlando, Florida, 1996, The Laser Institute of America.
24. Ando Y, Aoki A, Watanabe H, Ishikawa I: Bactericidal effect of erbium YAG laser on periodontopathic bacteria, *Lasers Surg Med* 19:190–200, 1996.
25. Moritz A, Gutknecht N, Doertbudak O, Goharkhay K, et al.: Bacterial reduction in periodontal pockets through irradiation with a diode laser, *J Clin Laser Med Surg* 15(1):33–37, 1997.
26. Raffetto N, Gutierrez T: Lasers in periodontal therapy, a five-year retrospective, *J Calif Dental Hyg Assoc* 16:17–20, 2001.
27. Coleton S: The use of lasers in periodontal therapy, *Gen Dent* 56(7):612–617, 2008.
28. White JM, Goodis HE, Rose CL: Use of the pulsed Nd:YAG laser for intraoral soft tissue surgery, *Lasers Surg Med* 11(5):455–461, 1991.

29. Dostalova T, Jelínkova H, Kucerova H, et al.: Noncontact Er:YAG laser ablation: clinical evaluation, *J Clin Laser Med Surg* 16(5):273–282, 1998.

30. Eversole LR, Rizoiu IM, Kimmel AI: Pulpal response to cavity preparation of an Erbium, Chromium:YSGG laser-powered hydrokinetic system, *J Am Dent Assoc* 128(8):1099–1106, 1997.

31. Hossain M, Nakamura Y, Yamada Y, et al.: Effects of Er, Cr:YSGG laser irradiation in human enamel and dentin: ablation and morphological studies, *J Clin Laser Med Surg* 17(4):155–159, 1999.

32. Aoki A, Ishikawa I, Yamada T, et al.: A comparison of conventional hand piece versus Erbium:YAG laser for caries in vitro, *J Dent Res* 77(6):1404–1414, 1998.

33. Weiner GP: Laser dentistry practice management, *Dent Clin North Am* 48:1105–1126, 2004.

34. Coluzzi DJ, Rice JH, Coleton S: The coming of age of lasers in dentistry, *Dent Today* 17(10):64–71, 1998.

35. Myers TD, Sulewski JG: Evaluating dental lasers: what the clinician should know, *Dent Clin North Am* 48:1127–1144, 2004.

36. Rechmann P: Dental laser research: selective ablation of caries, calculus, and microbial plaque: from the idea to the first in vivo investigation, *Dent Clin North Am* 48(4):1077–1104, 2004.

37. Featherstone JD, Fried D, McCormack S, Seka W: Effect of pulse duration and repetition rate on CO_2 laser inhibition of caries progression. In Wigdor H, Featherstone JD, White J, Neev J, editors: *Lasers in dentistry II*, January 28, 1996, San Jose, Calif, *Proc SPIE 2672*, Bellingham, Wash, 1996, SPIE—The International Society for Optical Engineering, pp 79–87.

3

Laser-Assisted Nonsurgical Periodontal Therapy

MARY LYNN SMITH AND ANGIE MOTT

Periodontal disease affects 80% of the adult population in the United States.[1] Recent research suggests that bacteria associated with periodontal disease have been linked to an increased risk of heart disease, diabetes, stroke, premature birth,[2,3] and respiratory infection in susceptible persons.[4,5] Although periodontal disease should be one of the most frequently treated conditions in dentistry, traditional therapies have been poorly received, even feared, and viewed by many patients as "bad experiences." Patients are reluctant to pursue initial periodontal treatment and are even more reluctant to have further treatment when disease progression occurs.

This chapter discusses the use and benefits of lasers in treatment planning and delivery of nonsurgical periodontal procedures, as well as the efficiency and efficacy of these laser-assisted procedures. The use of lasers is widely accepted and is the standard of care in ophthalmology, dermatology, plastic and vascular surgery, and many other medical specialties. Dentistry also should embrace laser technology as a proven method to treat patients safely and effectively, with excellent results.

In many states, hygienists are permitted to perform laser-assisted nonsurgical periodontal therapy. In other states, only dentists are permitted to use lasers. Some state dental practice acts require certification of dentists and hygienists through successful completion of an Academy of Laser Dentistry Standard Proficiency Certification Course or similar educational program before practicing laser-assisted procedures. Other states have no educational requirements for clinicians to perform laser treatments. Procedures provided by health care professionals, whether the dentist or the hygienist, must be within the clinician's scope of practice according to the dental practice laws of the particular state or country.

Periodontal Diseases

Periodontal diseases are biofilm-initiated inflammatory conditions that affect susceptible persons.[6] *Gingivitis,* the first stage of periodontal disease, is defined as "gingival inflammation without loss of connective tissue attachment."[7]

Periodontitis is defined as follows: "the presence of gingival inflammation at sites where there has been a pathological detachment of collagen fibers from cementum and the junctional epithelium has migrated apically."[7] In addition, inflammatory events associated with connective tissue attachment loss also lead to the resorption of coronal portions of tooth-supporting alveolar bone.

Similar definitions are recognized for periimplant mucositis and periimplantitis, respectively. The disease process is disrupted and controlled by host resistance through therapy or natural defenses.[8]

The organization and activity of biofilm are important because biofilm is the first component of periodontal disease–targeted in therapy. *Biofilm* is a complex community of microorganisms protected by a secreted extracellular polymeric substance. As it becomes more mature, the microbes use a molecular communication, *quorum sensing,* to create a highly organized and adaptable infrastructure. The various microbes within the biofilm behave so as to preserve the entire community, in essence becoming a discrete, living organism.[9]

As the biofilm responds to its environment, its adaptation provides resistance to such factors as ultraviolet (UV) light, bacteriophages, biocides, antibiotics, immune system responses, and environmental stresses.[10] Manor et al.[11] found that biofilm penetrates epithelium and underlying connective tissue, possibly to a depth of 500 μm. Biofilm has been observed penetrating tissues along the path of capillaries. Through various means, including stimulating the host's inflammatory pathways, biofilm may control transudate production to supply its nourishment.[12] These findings demonstrate the parasitic nature of biofilm in tissue.

As the body responds to biofilm invasion, proinflammatory cytokines, prostanoids, and proteolytic enzymes are synthesized and released. Fluids increase within the tissues, circulation becomes stagnant, swelling occurs, and metabolic products become backlogged. Enzymes such as collagenase, gelatinase, elastase, and fibrinolysin,[3] which are instrumental in the initial healing stage, remain at the site, destroying the developing strands of healing matrix needed to form connective tissue. The inflamed tissue is unable to progress from the granulation phase of healing into the remodeling phase because of the continued insult, with pathogenic processes and further biofilm proliferation.[13] The site is now a biofilm-infested chronic wound[14]; without treatment, progression to localized destruction is likely, with associated adverse effects on systemic health.

All of the following terms used throughout this chapter refer to treatment of the soft tissue wall of the periodontal pocket:

- Nonsurgical periodontal therapy
- Sulcular debridement
- Active phase I periodontal infection therapy
- *Laser decontamination*—refers specifically to reducing the biofilm of the pocket, usually meaning what is contained within diseased tissue
- *Laser coagulation*—refers specifically to sealing of capillaries and lymphatics after laser decontamination of the tissue

Benefits of Laser Therapy

Lasers have a direct deleterious effect on bacteria, which supports the body's healing response. Incorporating lasers into conventional therapies helps accomplish treatment objectives. Conventional nonsurgical periodontal therapy entails debriding the affected area of bacteria, endotoxins, and hard deposits from the tooth structure to restore gingival health.[8] Instrumentation is focused on the tooth structure, and debridement most often is accomplished by means of manual and power scaling. In the future, lasers also will be used for root debridement.

To date, the U.S. Food and Drug Administration (FDA) has not yet cleared the use of lasers for removal of deposits and biofilm from tooth structure. However, Aoki et al.[15] determined that deposits and biofilm are more thoroughly removed and that a more biocompatible surface is created for reattachment with use of an erbium laser than with conventional methods.[16] The alexandrite laser also has been in development for selective removal of calculus from the root structure.[17] The carbon dioxide (CO_2) laser has been shown to increase adherence of fibroblasts to root surfaces, and the fibroblast adherence is superior to conventional techniques both in quantity of fibroblasts attached and in the quality of the attachment.[18]

Regardless of the instrument used, it is essential that contaminants be thoroughly removed from the tooth structure in any periodontal therapy. Current laser-assisted methods focus on the biofilm of the pocket wall, supplementing conventional methods that debride the tooth structure itself. A critical point in this context is that laser treatment is an *addition* to, not a replacement for, conventional periodontal therapy.

Both in vitro and in vivo studies show that lasers are bactericidal.[19–22] Although not specific to certain bacteria, the argon (Ar), neodymium-doped yttrium-aluminum-garnet (Nd:YAG), and diode laser wavelengths show strong absorption in darkly pigmented bacteria, with a consequent direct, increased effect on the red and orange–complex bacteria associated with periodontitis.[23] The CO_2 laser also has excellent bactericidal properties.[24,25] Both CO_2 and erbium lasers act on pathogens by heating intracellular fluids, causing the microbes to collapse.[26,27] The absorption of laser energy by tissues produces a photothermal effect. With use of the appropriate settings, most nonsporulating bacteria, including anaerobes, are readily deactivated at 50° C.[28,29]

In laser-assisted *active phase I periodontal infection therapy,* the diseased biofilm-infested tissues of periodontal pockets are debrided. With laser techniques that involve working close to the recommended parameter of 60° C,[30] the healthy tissue beneath the nonhealing granulation layer is not affected by the low energy. As noted earlier, biofilm can penetrate soft tissues. Localized removal of "bioburden" has a significant beneficial effect on wound bed preparation and wound healing.[31] Steed et al.[32] showed that more frequent debridement resulted in better healing than that obtained with debridement performed less frequently. Moritz et al.[19] reported that the bleeding index improved in 96.9% of the patients treated with laser-assisted periodontal therapy after conventional therapy, compared with 66.7% of patients treated conventionally without laser. These investigators concluded that "the diode laser assisted periodontal therapy provided a bactericidal effect, reduced inflammation, and supported healing of periodontal pockets through elimination of bacteria."[19] Administering laser energy to the affected tissues at specific, repeated intervals is key in targeting biofilm during periodontal therapy.

Lasers also have the ability to seal capillaries and lymphatics, thereby reducing swelling at the treated site and minimizing postoperative discomfort.[33]

Another benefit of laser-assisted procedures is the healing stimulated at the cellular level.[34] Medrado et al.[35] found that low-level laser treatment depresses the exudative phase while enhancing the proliferative processes during acute and chronic inflammation. Laser *photobiomodulation* can activate the local blood circulation and stimulate proliferation of endothelial cells.[36,37] Wound healing is supported, with reduced edema and polymorphonuclear (leukocyte) neutrophil (PMN) infiltrate, increased fibroblasts, and more and better-organized collagen bundles.[38] Karu[39] suggested that these effects are caused by an increase in mitochondrial synthesis. The slight scattering that occurs with more deeply absorbed energy of certain lasers may have photobiomodulation effects beyond the direct application. The aiming beams of the lasers also may have a photobiomodulation effect (see Chapter 15). More research needs to be conducted in this area.

Laser Types

Laser wavelengths used to treat active phase I periodontal infection include the diodes, Nd:YAG, CO_2, and erbium lasers. Chapter 2, on laser fundamentals, provides further information on each wavelength.

Argon Laser

The argon laser, emitting a 514-nm wavelength, was FDA-cleared for sulcular debridement in 1991. The energy is delivered through a fiberoptic system in contact or noncontact mode, depending on the procedure. These wavelengths are highly absorbed in hemoglobin and melanin, and have demonstrated bactericidal properties, particularly for *Prevotella* and *Porphyromonas*.[23,40] However, argon lasers are no longer being marketed to dentists.

Diode Lasers

The semiconductor diode lasers are available in four different wavelengths, as follows:
- 810–830 nm
- 940 nm
- 980 nm
- 1064 nm

Both the 810- to 830-nm and the 980-nm wavelengths may be used for nonsurgical periodontal therapy, with good results well supported by the literature. As yet, few published studies have examined the use or advantages of the 940-mn wavelength or the 1064-nm diode wavelength.

Like argon lasers, diode lasers also use fiberoptics for energy delivery in contact or noncontact mode, depending on the procedure. With diodes in this wavelength range, energy is absorbed in hemoglobin and pigment (e.g., melanin). These *chromophores,* or organic compounds that absorb light at a specific wavelength, are present in high concentrations within the diseased periodontal pocket, making these wavelengths applicable for sulcular debridement.

The 980-nm wavelength exhibits greater absorption in water than for the other three diode wavelengths, which may be an added benefit to the laser interaction within the pocket. However, no definitive studies yet show that the increased absorption in water leads to clinical results superior to those obtained with use of other diode wavelengths. Diode lasers are bactericidal[19,41,42] and aid in coagulation.

Diode lasers may be operated in continuous-wave mode (with energy emitted as a constant beam), with low settings and short application time, or in gated-pulse mode (with energy emitted as a constant but interrupted beam, or pulsed at specific intervals), with higher settings and longer application time. Some diode lasers offer specific pulse duration on–off time controls, allowing higher power to be applied to the tissue for shorter periods of time, which allow the tissues to cool adequately before receiving another pulse of energy. This energy pattern limits accumulation of heat, which decreases thermal collateral damage. Less collateral damage means less postoperative discomfort for the patient.

Neodymium:Yttrium-Aluminum-Garnet Laser

The Nd:YAG is a free-running pulsed laser. The laser energy is produced in bursts of photonic energy, rather than as a continuous beam. This laser also uses a fiberoptic delivery system for contact or noncontact procedures. The 1064-nm wavelength is most highly absorbed in melanin, less absorbed in hemoglobin, and slightly absorbed in water. The Nd:YAG laser also is bactericidal[20] and provides good hemostasis. Because it is a free-running pulsed laser, the Nd:YAG emits high peak powers but allows for tissue cooling during the off time. In choosing settings for treatment, the combination of higher millijoules (mJ) with fewer repetitions per second (i.e., hertz [Hz]) aids in coagulation, whereas lower mJ with higher Hz typically is used for decontamination.

> **CLINICAL TIP**
>
> A joule (J) is a measurement of energy available to do work in dentistry; dental professionals work in millijoules (mJ).

Micropulsed CO$_2$ Lasers

The micropulsed 10,600-nm CO$_2$ lasers incorporate the newest technology available in producing CO$_2$ laser energy. Delivery by an articulated arm or waveguide in noncontact mode facilitates treatment. A 250-μm tip (the diameter of a #25 endodontic file) is used for administering laser energy into the periodontal pocket. This wavelength interacts with water and hydroxyapatite and has a depth of penetration on the order of micrometers. Inflamed tissue has an increased water content and is therefore preferentially affected by the laser energy, as are crevicular fluids and intracellular fluids. Fluids are photothermally heated and then vaporized, with consequent collapse of the cell membranes. The bacteria are inactivated,[24,25] and dehydration occurs as energy is applied.

Earlier CO$_2$ lasers emitted energy in continuous-wave mode and, with later improvements, also could be gated, but only with longer pulses and higher mJ. The less sophisticated technology of those units was associated with increased thermal damage in surrounding tissue, often resulting in charring, and they could not be used within the periodontal pocket. The newest micropulsed CO$_2$ lasers provide greater control of the energy, making application safe and effective within the periodontal pocket. These lasers allow higher peak power for ultrashort pulse durations, with longer off times. This improvement provides for maximum thermal relaxation, decreasing collateral damage and discomfort. The mJ settings are greatly reduced in sulcular debridement compared with previous gated-pulse CO$_2$ technologies. Technique requires the same care as for any other soft tissue laser application: The laser energy must be directed *away from* the tooth structure. A new-wavelength CO$_2$ laser, emitting at 9300 nm, has recently been FDA-cleared for clinical use. To date, there have been no published studies or reports of its use in periodontal pocket therapy.

Erbium Lasers

Erbium lasers are FDA-cleared for both hard and soft tissue applications, and some erbium lasers are FDA-cleared for sulcular debridement. It is important to check with the manufacturer of the specific laser device to ensure that it is FDA-cleared for its intended use. The erbium-doped YAG (Er:YAG) 2940-nm and erbium plus chromium–doped yttrium-scandium-gallium-garnet (Er,Cr:YSGG) 2780-nm instruments are free-running pulsed lasers with wavelengths that are most highly absorbed in water, followed by good absorption in hydroxyapatite and poor absorption in hemoglobin. Thermal rise in the superficial tissue layers is minimal and even less with concurrent water spray during the laser procedure. This effect limits achievement of hemostasis and coagulation within the pocket. Although some clinicians view the associated bleeding as a hindrance when working with these lasers, a benefit of this wavelength is almost complete absence of operative or postoperative discomfort. Quicker healing also is another advantage reported with these wavelengths.[16,43] Studies have demonstrated significant population reduction of the periodontal pathogens *Porphyromonas gingivalis* and *Actinobacillus (Aggregatibacter) actinomycetemcomitans,* as well as positive long-term clinical results in attachment gain.[16,21,26] With the 9300-nm CO_2 laser, recently cleared for hard tissue applications, the energy is absorbed by the carbonate of hard tissue, rather than the hydroxyapatite. To date, there have been no studies or peer-reviewed published reports of its effects or use in pocket therapy.

Fundamentals of Laser Physics

Understanding basic laser physics is important to make needed adjustments while administering laser treatment. In laser-assisted procedures, laser energy is absorbed by the chromophores within the pocket and transformed into photothermal energy. Observing laser–tissue interaction is critical. Tissues containing different concentrations of the wavelength-specific chromophore will require different parameters.

The patient's comfort also is important. Often a treatment area is fully anesthetized during the initial appointment for debridement and laser decontamination but may require only topical or no anesthetic for laser therapy at repeat visits. Making adjustments will improve the patient's comfort while accomplishing the treatment goal.

The treatment goal for nonsurgical periodontal therapy is decontamination and coagulation, rather than incising. Procedures are accomplished through control of tissue temperature. The factors that affect tissue temperature are the mJ and Hz settings, speed at which the laser beam moves over the target tissue (hand speed), and cooling factors such as pulse "off" time, high-volume evacuation, and water application.

Some lasers allow more control of these parameters than that provided by others. For a free-running pulsed laser such as the Nd:YAG, high mJ with low Hz means more energy per pulse *but* more thermal relaxation time between pulses.

Typically this combination of parameters will improve hemostasis. If lower mJ is selected with more Hz, there is less energy in each repetition but also less thermal relaxation time, because more pulses are emitted into the tissue every second. With these settings, more even thermal absorption may be achieved. Diode lasers are operated in either continuous or gated mode; continuous operation does not allow any thermal relaxation. Lower-power settings should be chosen to prevent temperature increase beyond the treatment goal of decontamination or coagulation. If gated (pulsed) mode is selected, a higher energy may be required to raise the tissue temperature with each pulse. The gated mode allows the tissue to cool before the succeeding pulse.

All tissues have an *absorption threshold;* tissue can absorb only so much energy before it is overloaded by the energy and becomes painful and is damaged. Think of sitting on a beach and getting a nice suntan. To achieve that look, your tissue (skin) absorbs a certain amount of energy (sunlight). Think again of sitting on a beach for many hours, with prolonged exposure to the sun's rays. Your skin will then be overloaded with too much energy (sunlight), and the result will be a sunburn, with pain and charring of the tissue. The pain occur when more energy reaches the target tissue than it can absorb.

When the patient feels discomfort during laser treatment, the following adjustments can be made without changing the mJ or Hz settings:

- Move the laser fiber more quickly (adjust hand speed), decreasing total energy exposure.
- Move the suction closer to the operative site so that the circulating air decreases the accumulating temperature.
- Add a light spray of water to dissipate heat.

These adjustments work well with all wavelengths. Of note, however, because the CO_2 wavelength is highly absorbed in water, a high tissue fluid content (too much water) will inhibit tissue interaction, whereas a lower fluid content (not enough water) will increase discomfort.

Conversely, if the tissue is not responding, alterations are needed. First, check the settings; then inspect the aiming beam, ensuring patency of the optics. If parameters are correct, test-fire the laser on an appropriate chromophore, moving the laser more slowly. If results are still negative, increase the settings incrementally until interaction occurs. If a large increase is necessary, a technical problem is likely, and the laser instrument should be serviced by a certified technician. The clinician must understand the properties of the selected wavelength to provide optimal, beneficial laser treatment.

Treatment Objectives with Soft Tissue Lasers

The objective of active phase I periodontal infection therapy is to remove biofilm and deposits found above the gumline and within the periodontal pocket, whether on the tooth structure, on the pocket wall, or in the crevicular fluids. Such therapy assists the body's healing response. This aspect of treatment is accomplished through conventional scaling and root debridement as well as laser-assisted sulcular debridement. Sulcular debridement addresses the pocket wall for profound decontamination and seals the capillaries and lymphatics through coagulation.

Sulcular Debridement with Fiberoptic Laser Delivery

Preprocedural Decontamination

Preprocedural decontamination is a laser application done before any instrumentation, even probing. The objectives are to eradicate the bacteria within the sulcus, thereby reducing the risk of bacteremia from instrumentation, and to lower the microcount in aerosols created during ultrasonic instrumentation.[44] The technique uses very low energy. The fiber is placed within the sulcus and is swept vertically and horizontally against the pocket wall, away from the tooth, with a smooth, flowing motion, for 7 to 8 seconds on the lingual aspect and then on the buccal surface of each tooth's tissue wall. The benefits of preprocedural decontamination are seen in the reduced microbial translocation through the circulatory system.

Decontamination

Just as conventional root debridement removes biofilm and accretions from the hard tooth surface, laser decontamination removes biofilm within the necrotic tissue of the pocket wall. The laser energy interacts strongly with inflamed tissue components (owing to preferential absorption by chromophores, which are more abundant in diseased tissues) and less strongly with healthy tissue. This nonsurgical therapy uses very low settings and decontaminates rather than cuts the tissue.[28]

The administration of laser decontamination requires an understanding of current periodontal pocket topography, proficiency in technique, and recognition of laser–tissue interaction to determine the end point of therapy. An updated periodontal chart is needed for reference throughout therapy. With conventional root debridement provided just before laser decontamination, the pocket depths may need to be reprobed for accuracy of laser treatment. Laser therapy should address sites manifesting with inflammation and/or pocket depths of 4 mm or greater. It is helpful to visualize the extent of surface area being treated. For example, the diseased pocket lining requiring treatment in a patient with 50% generalized bone loss has an estimated tissue surface area of 40 cm² (6.2 in²), and with 4 to 5 mm of generalized pocketing, this area is 20 cm² (3.1 in²).[45] Knowing the depth and shape of pockets and the area to be addressed enables the clinician to be thorough with decontamination technique.

With fiberoptic technique, the fiber tip engages every millimeter of the diseased tissue–wall that corresponds to the indicated sites marked on the periodontal chart. Before initiation of the laser treatment, calibrate the amount of fiber exposed to measure 1 mm less than the pocket depth (Figure 3-1). Begin the procedure with the fiber placed just inside the gingival margin, progressing apically, *or* place the fiber 1 mm short of the depth of the pocket, working

coronally (Figure 3-2). The edge of the cannula indicates the treatment depth of the pocket being reached. Use a gliding, multidirectional motion with the tip of the fiber in constant contact with the pocket wall. The strokes should address small sections and should be systematically overlapping. The motion is somewhat analogous to sweeping a floor with a broom. It is helpful to mentally divide the pocket into affected sections, such as interproximal to the line angle, the direct buccal or lingual surface, and the line angle to the interproximal area. Continually inspect the fiber tip and remove any accumulated debris (Figure 3-3) with water-moistened gauze.

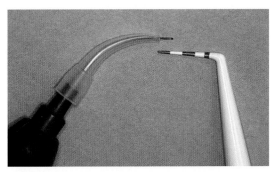

• **Figure 3-1** Calibrating optimal laser fiber length using a periodontal probe.

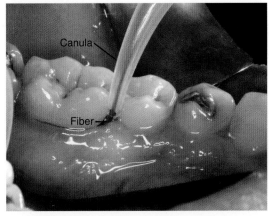

• **Figure 3-2** Laser fiber in periodontal pocket.

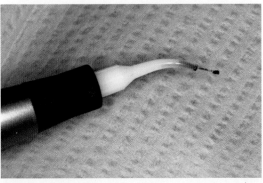

• **Figure 3-3** Small amount of granulomatous tissue debris on fiber tip.

When exiting the pocket, take care to inactivate the laser, preventing overexposure of the gingival margin's thin tissue. If the fiber tip becomes irreversibly coated (Figure 3-4), cleave the fiber, calibrate the length of the fiber, and continue the procedure.

Completion of laser decontamination is determined by laser parameters used, delivery time, and clinical signs. Decontamination is accomplished with less mJ and more Hz than for coagulation. A more inflamed pocket may require less average power because of increased concentration of the laser's preferred chromophores. With use of an initiated fiber and lower settings in continuous-wave mode, interaction is concentrated and will require less treatment time than with use of a noninitiated fiber with higher settings in pulsed mode. A deeper pocket will require longer treatment time because of increased surface area. As laser treatment progresses in an area, less and less debris should collect on the fiber. Fresh bleeding will occur, however, when the pocket wall is fully decontaminated and debrided (Figure 3-5). Keep in mind the laser parameters and application time. Observing tissue interaction is essential in determining the duration of laser exposure for the diseased site being treated.

> **EXERCISE:** To illustrate laser technique, try this simulation exercise. On paper, draw an area measuring 20 cm^2 (3 × 1–inch rectangle). Use a mechanical pencil with fine lead (0.5 mm) to color the area using flowing, methodical, overlapping, multidirectional strokes, leaving no areas uncolored. The laser fiber is actually only 0.4 or 0.3 mm, but this activity reflects the time and thoroughness needed for treatment within the pocket.

Coagulation

When biofilm has been removed, the second objective in active phase I periodontal infection therapy is coagulation, sealing the capillaries and lymphatics of the healthy tissue. As previously noted, biofilm tends to continue its invasion of the host tissue through the vessels. Coagulation may inhibit the biofilm's progression. It also counteracts the swelling that occurs with the inflammatory process. Coagulation is accomplished with increased mJ and decreased Hz compared with decontamination. Coagulation also requires less time within the pocket and does not address every millimeter of tissue.

For this procedure, a newly cleaved fiber is moved back and forth through the pocket, administering laser energy beyond the end of the fiber into the tissue. The application raises the temperature within the pocket slightly, to promote protein denaturation and sealing of the vessels. If continued hemorrhaging occurs on exiting the pocket, a freshly cleaved fiber may be used in noncontact mode to coagulate at the gingival margin, keeping the laser energy directed away from the tooth surface.

After coagulation, application of firm digital pressure to areas with deep pockets will support the re-adaptation of the tissue to the tooth and further enhance reattachment. Coagulation assists the first stages of healing after debridement.

Sulcular Debridement with Carbon Dioxide Laser

Whereas the argon, diode, and Nd:YAG lasers employ a contact technique for sulcular debridement, the micropulsed 10,600-nm CO_2 laser uses a defocused, noncontact technique. Marginal dehydration and pocket decontamination are two steps applied in CO_2 laser therapy. Because the CO_2 laser's wavelength is absorbed by the crevicular fluids and water content in the diseased tissue wall, it is important to direct the energy parallel to the tooth surface and toward the tissue.

Begin the debridement procedure by directing laser energy to the coronal edge of the marginal gingiva. Hold the tip perpendicular to the tissue crest at a distance of approximately 1 mm. Tissue interaction is observed as a slight "frosting" of the surface (Figure 3-6). Marginal dehydration will improve entry of the tip by drawing the tissue slightly away from the tooth structure. Epithelial growth will be inhibited by this application. This is the first step before pocket decontamination.

The technique for decontamination involves placement of the laser's defocusing tip 1 to 2 mm into the pocket (only 1 mm for pockets up to 6 mm in depth; only 2 mm for

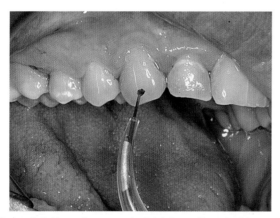

• **Figure 3-4** Excessive amount of debris on fiber. At this stage of treatment, the fiber should be cleaved and recalibrated.

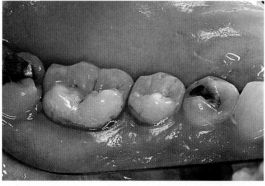

• **Figure 3-5** Gingiva immediately after fiber-based laser treatment, showing fresh bleeding from the pocket.

pockets greater than 6 mm in depth). Treatment should include the complete circumference of each tooth presenting with disease. Activate the laser as the tip is drawn through the crevicular space in an even, slow motion, working from the distal aspect to the mesial aspect on the buccal and again on the lingual side of the tooth. The laser tip is kept parallel to the long axis of the tooth (Figure 3-7).

Treatment time is a *maximum* of 16 seconds per buccal or lingual surface. The length of application time depends on the extent of disease and the surface area; larger teeth such as molars are treated longer than smaller teeth such as lower anteriors.[46] The tip must be kept open and free of coagulum for efficient energy flow. Keeping the tissue slightly moist

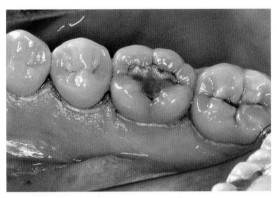

• **Figure 3-6** Laser marginal dehydration of gingival tissue immediately before pocket debridement and decontamination with CO_2 laser.

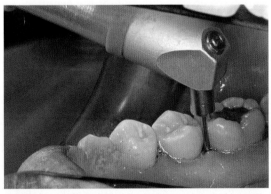

• **Figure 3-7** Tip of CO_2 laser in periodontal pocket. Note parallel orientation of tip to root surface.

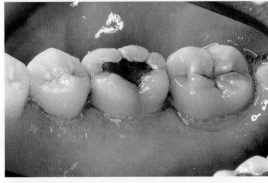

• **Figure 3-8** Gingiva immediately after CO_2 laser treatment.

and working in a single direction will enhance the laser's efficiency. Vertical, up-and-down movements or pushing the tip toward the tissue can cause the tip to clog. If the tip becomes occluded, both the tip and detritus inside will continue absorbing the energy, with consequent excessive heating of the tip. Coagulation occurs simultaneously with decontamination. No additional steps are necessary in using the CO_2 laser. Figure 3-8 shows the gingiva after laser treatment.

Postoperative Care

The therapeutic appointment concludes with several steps in professional postoperative care. After the laser treatment, allow the patient to rinse with water or with a non–alcohol-based rinse to freshen and moisten the mouth. A topical soothing agent such as vitamin E oil or aloe vera may be applied with a gloved finger or sterile cotton swab to the areas treated. Firm adaptation of tissue to the tooth with digital pressure may assist adhesion of fibrin between the tissue and tooth, particularly for deeper pockets.

Postlaser irrigation is a subject of debate. Although irrigation with chlorhexidine or other solutions is used in conventional treatment as a final step in disinfecting periodontal pockets, the authors believe that postlaser irrigation is unnecessary. In fact, Mariotti and Rumpf[47] found that solutions of chlorhexidine (0.12% or less) in contact with wound sites for even a short time could have serious toxic effects on gingival fibroblasts. Other studies report that subgingival irrigation has no significant additive effects on periodontal healing.[48–50]

When the laser procedure is completed, all the benefits of profound decontamination and coagulation are in place. Further manipulation of the tissues will reintroduce contaminated instruments into the pocket and disrupt the fibrin clot.

The final step in postoperative care is advising the patient on what to expect, addressing further concerns, and discussing continued self-care. Counsel the patient that mild discomfort is possible the first 24 to 48 hours. With laser-assisted nonsurgical periodontal therapy, discomfort is associated more often with root debridement than with the laser treatment. Excessive pain may indicate another issue and warrants investigation. The patient should avoid spicy, sharp, and crunchy foods for 24 hours to help prevent discomfort and trauma. Seeds and husks may become lodged between the gum and the tooth and should be avoided. The risk of impaired healing from presence of a foreign object is highest in the first few postoperative days, but risk may persist if the periodontal disease is more severe. Encourage the patient to be diligent in supporting the healing process by consistent and thorough daily cleaning. Patients appreciate instructions in written form for reference as well as in verbal form (Box 3-1).

Healing and Tissue Rehabilitation

Healing typically occurs without complications as the body responds to laser therapy. Through the first 24 to 72 hours, the patient may feel tenderness and experience light bleeding when eating or cleaning; after tooth debridement and tissue decontamination, epithelium begins to regenerate after 24 hours and then progresses 1 mm per day, protecting the pocket wall. Within 1 week, the wound surface is covered. Connective tissue begins proliferation by day 5. Because laser decontamination procedures are repeated at 10-day intervals, the epithelium is impaired during laser biofilm reduction. This allows the fibroblasts to continue organizing into a connective tissue attachment apparatus. The attachment will continue to mature for 12 months.[8] This attachment is easily disrupted, so only light-pressure probing is recommended after several months, with resumption of normal probing after 6 months of postoperative therapy.[51]

Classic signs of tissue rehabilitation include improved color, consistency, texture and stippling, and contour. These signs, as well as a decrease in or elimination of hemorrhaging during gentle tissue manipulation and a reduction of

pocket depth, all are desired indications of tissue healing. Figure 3-9 shows initial periodontal probing before treatment and periodontal probing 6 months after treatment. Figure 3-10 shows data for three sets of probings: initial probing, 8 weeks after treatment, and 5 months after treatment. Analysis of the probing results shows a resolution of 86% of the bleeding sites, a decrease in 86% of the pocketing sites, and a 58% decrease in the number of teeth exhibiting periodontal disease.

Complications and Adverse Reactions

Healing may be complicated by microbiologic, immunologic, and traumatic factors. Rapid pocket reinfection will occur with insufficient removal of subgingival biofilm, with inadequate supragingival biofilm control, or with uncorrected poor restorative conditions. Patients with a compromised immune system often exhibit a delayed or less optimal healing response; with the assistance of laser benefits, however, such patients could recover better than expected.

Traumatic injury, such as from excessive instrumentation or increased collateral damage from overexposure of laser energy, may result in prolonged tissue discomfort and soreness. Systemic diseases such as diabetes are associated with delayed healing. Evaluation for excessive occlusal stress, which may impair healing, also is important.

In states in which hygienists are allowed to perform laser therapy, it is incumbent on the hygienist to make certain that the dentist has performed a complete occlusal evaluation and correction/equilibration of the dentition. Occlusion is a risk factor for periodontal breakdown, so occlusal treatment needs to be considered as a part of the comprehensive treatment of periodontal disease.[52] Trauma from occlusal problems constitutes an additional risk factor for the progression and severity of periodontal disease. An understanding of the effect of trauma from occlusal loading on the periodontium is useful in the clinical management of periodontal problems.[53]

Adverse reactions are a result of inappropriate laser application: The wavelength is incorrect for the target site, the parameters are incorrect, or the duration of application is incorrect. Some lasers interact with metal, resulting in a

---

> • **BOX 3-1** **Patient Care Instructions after Laser-Assisted Periodontal Therapy**
>
> 1. Do not eat until numbness is gone.
> 2. *For patients who smoke*: Smoking compromises the healing processes; refrain from smoking for as long as possible (or preferably, take opportunity to stop smoking).
> 3. Avoid spicy, sharp, crunchy foods for 24 hours.
> 4. Avoid alcohol-containing products for 24 hours.
> 5. Avoid seeds or husks for 3 to 5 days (or as directed).
> 6. Rinse with salt water (1 tsp in 8 oz of warm water) three times daily until tissues are comfortable.
> 7. Any over-the-counter pain reliever may be taken as directed to manage mild discomfort.
> 8. More severe pain should be evaluated by the dentist.
> 9. Thorough but gentle cleaning is essential to the healing process. In treated areas, use an extra-soft toothbrush for 1 or 2 days, and floss gently. Regular brushing and flossing may be done in all other areas.
> 10. Oral irrigation may begin after 24 hours. Use a medium to low power setting, directing the water stream at a 90-degree angle to the tooth—*not* into the pocket. Subgingival irrigation is contraindicated until further evaluation.

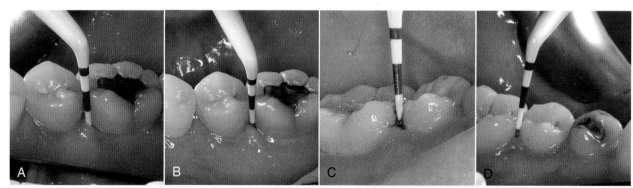

• **Figure 3-9** **A,** Periodontal pocket probing before CO_2 laser treatment. **B,** Periodontal pocket probing 6 months after CO_2 laser treatment. **C,** Periodontal pocket probing before fiber-based laser treatment. **D,** Periodontal pocket probing 6 months after fiber-based laser treatment.

percussive reaction and immediate heat generation. This heat could transfer to the nerve or surrounding tissue. Therefore the laser energy must not be directed toward metallic crown margins or metallic restorations at the gingival margins. Laser energy directed toward the tooth may cause irreversible damage to the tooth, such as cracking, pitting, melting, or charring. Excessive heat accumulation can cause damage to underlying bone. Intense overexposure of laser energy on tissue results in carbonized tissue.

Complications in healing and adverse reactions are minimized with adherence to appropriate treatment protocols. Understanding the laser settings and observing the laser–tissue interaction during application are crucial. The clinician must have adequate knowledge and proficiency whenever providing treatment with any instrument, whether ultrasonic, hand, or laser. All of these treatment modes are extremely beneficial when used properly.

Documentation

Documentation in the patient's chart serves to describe the conditions, diagnosis, and specific treatment rendered.

Written references concerning laser use should include the following:

- The wavelength and type of laser (e.g., 980-nm diode)
- The spot size (size of fiber, tip, or aperture of tip)
- The settings (e.g., mJ, Hz, W of average power)
- Mode of application (continuous or pulsed wave)
- Duration of application
- Application with or without water spray
- Type of anesthesia used (topical or injection, number of carpules)

Documentation also should (1) confirm that wavelength-specific laser safety glasses were worn, (2) describe any adverse reactions and how they were managed, and (3) state that postoperative instructions were given. Complete documentation should include content that serves to answer any question that a patient might ask about the treatment (Box 3-2).

Adjunctive Chemotherapeutics

The rationale for adding antibiotics in some cases is better biofilm suppression with concomitant therapies. If treatment

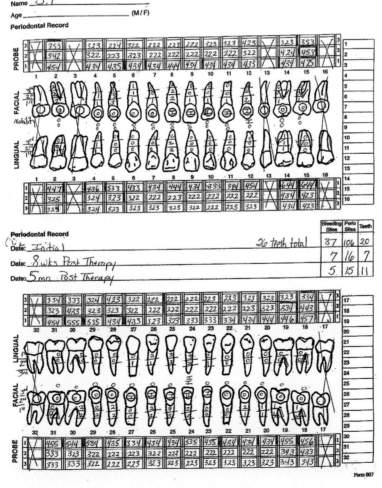

• **Figure 3-10** Periodontal charting showing pocket depths initially and at 8 weeks and then 5 months after laser treatment.

requires multiple strategies, chemotherapeutics may be used in conjunction with lasers and conventional treatment. Antibiotics such as doxycycline, tetracycline, and metronidazole are prescribed for systemic control of pathogens. Low-dose levels of oral doxycycline hyclate (Periostat) suppress the enzymatic activity of collagenase associated with the disease processes. Topical preparations of minocycline hydrochloride (Arestin), doxycycline hyclate (Atridox), and chlorhexidine gluconate (as the Periochip) may be placed to control localized growth of pathogens.

Biofilm is most susceptible to chemotherapeutics when it has been disrupted aggressively through debridement of both the tooth and the tissue. A systemic antibiotic should begin early in the treatment to assist the body as treatment progresses. A local antibiotic may be placed in an affected site *after* the last session of laser treatment; in this way, without disturbance, the effectiveness of the drug is maximized, because it works for several weeks. Locally administered antibiotics should *not* be used between lasing appointments.

It is prudent to assess the biofilm's composition and the susceptibility of pathogens before administration of chemotherapeutics. Many types of culturing do not test the antibiotic against the protective mechanisms in the biofilm and thus do not reflect the in vivo environment. Polymerase chain reaction (PCR) assay, 454 sequencing, and other molecular tests give a better view of what organisms are cohabitating within the biofilm. This information may determine which medication(s) would be most beneficial,

how long it should be administered, and whether a second phase with testing is needed. Chronic wounds should never be controlled merely with antibiotic therapy.

Laser Safety

The designated laser safety officer is responsible for educating the dental team in the safe use of the laser, as well as for enforcing safety practices, as follows:

1. Securing the operatory by limiting access to the room and posting "laser in use" signs
2. Using safety features of the laser, such as placing the laser in standby mode when not in use
3. Enforcing mandatory use of wavelength-specific protective eyewear within the treatment area
4. Evacuating with high-volume evacuation to remove aerosols and laser plume
5. Using a high-efficiency particulate filtration mask (particle filtration efficiency of 99.75% at 0.1 μm)

Test firing the laser before the patient's procedure is another important step in safety and procedure preparation. Test firing proves the laser energy is being delivered as expected. For this procedure, with safety measures in place, position the terminal end of the laser away from the patient. Select a suitable chromophore (for argon, Nd:YAG, and diode lasers: dark material; for CO_2 lasers: moist paper; and for erbium lasers: water) and activate the laser while holding it 1 to 2 mm from the material chosen. As energy is absorbed, an interaction will be observed, such as a mark and plume or water bubbling or evaporating. This test step is not the same as "initiating" the fiber but simply constitutes an assessment of interaction between the laser and an appropriate chromophore, to ensure the laser is working as anticipated.

Laser Plume

Although no set standard exists, strong recommendations (such as those from the Occupational Safety and Health Administration [OSHA], the Centers for Disease Control and Prevention [CDC], and the American National Standards Institute [ANSI]) address evacuation of the laser plume. High-volume evacuation is indicated for aerosol reduction during ultrasonic instrumentation,[54] as well as for plume removal during laser treatment. The plume is composed of 95% water and 5% particulate matter, organic and inorganic chemicals, and microorganisms.[55] Organic chemicals such as benzene, toluene, formaldehyde, and cyanide have been isolated within the plume; inorganic chemicals include carbon monoxide, sulfur, and nitrogen compounds.[56] The microorganism analysis shows bacteria, microbacteria, fungi, viruses, and DNA from intact viruses of human immunodeficiency virus (HIV), hepatitis B virus (HBV), and human papillomavirus (HPV).[57] Most particles are 0.3 to 0.5 μm in size, 90% of which are likely to be inhaled and deposited on the alveolar lung tissue.[58] Therefore the common mask that filters only 5.0-μm particles provides inadequate

---

• BOX 3-2 Example of Charting and Documentation for Laser Periodontal Therapy

10-11-2012: Pt presented for PIT [periodontal infection therapy] UR.

Health history reviewed, no contraindications to treatment.

Administered 20% topical benzocaine followed by 2% lidocaine, with epi 1:100,000, 1.8 mL for local anesthesia of teeth #2-5.

Disclosed #5-8 and instructed on specific daily biofilm removal techniques. Recommended: Bass toothbrush technique twice daily and adding floss to current routine. Review floss technique further at next appointment.

Preprocedural laser decontamination with 980-nm diode, uninitiated 300-μm fiber, power of 0.4 W [watt] in CW administered approx 16 sec/tooth throughout.

Supragingival ultrasonic biofilm removal throughout. Manual and ultrasonic definitive debridement of #2-5.

Laser decontamination of #2-5 with same laser and fiber, 2.0 W in PW on 25 msec/off 50 msec for an average power of 0.7 W administered approx 20 sec/site. Laser coagulation followed with power of 0.8 W in CW administered approx 10 sec/site.

Laser-specific glasses were worn by patient and clinician during laser procedures. No adverse reactions. Postop instructions given in both written and oral forms.

Next visit: PIT for UL area.

CW, Continuous wave [mode]; *epi*, epinephrine; *PW*, pulse width; *UL*, upper left; *UR*, upper right.

filtration. Use of a mask filtering 0.1-μm particles is recommended.[55]

The combination of high-volume evacuation and a high-efficiency filtration mask decreases the exposure risk associated with ultrasonic and laser procedures. These masks are available in tie-on and ear-loop styles through dental supply companies.

> ### CLINICAL TIP
> As an alternative to high-efficiency filtration masks, tuberculosis (TB) masks may be worn.

Technical Aspects of Laser Settings

The treatment objective, fiber size, and existing chromophore concentration should be considered in choosing the settings for a nonsurgical periodontal procedure. For laser-assisted hygiene applications, lower settings are required for thorough decontamination of the tissues. The fiber size can directly affect the amount of energy the target receives with a specific setting. A 320-μm fiber has a smaller spot size, which increases the power density at the target, compared with a 400-μm fiber. With the same setting, a 400-μm fiber delivers only 64% of the power density delivered with a 320-μm fiber.

The concentration of chromophore present in the target tissue also will affect settings. Diseased tissue has an increased amount of hemoglobin and responds well to certain wavelengths, requiring less energy. Fibrotic tissue, with decreased vascularization and hemoglobin, comparatively needs more energy.

Printed parameters from laser manufacturers are only guidelines for treatment. Observed tissue interaction is the key to knowing if the settings are adequate or need adjustment. A rule of thumb is to use the minimum amount of energy to achieve the therapy needed. Reference sources for settings have been added, for convenience, to the suggested parameters in Table 3-1.[59-61] Although each of the listed lasers may be used in nonsurgical periodontal procedures, some are more efficient than others. One laser used for therapy may require more or less treatment time than another, which affects treatment planning. Table 3-2 contrasts the time investment required with three types of lasers. The patient undergoing treatment exhibited 87 "bleeding on probing" sites, 106 sites of 4-mm depth or greater, and 20 involved teeth. Because of treatment protocol, the Nd:YAG and diode lasers reflect treatment of

TABLE 3-1 Suggested Laser Parameters for Nonsurgical Periodontal Therapy*

Laser Type	Fiber/Tip Diameter/Aperture	Preprocedural Decontamination	Debridement	Coagulation
Argon	Fiber diameter: 300 μm	No suggested parameters in literature	0.5 W, 0.05-sec pulse duration, 0.2 sec between pulses[†]	0.7–0.8 W, 0.05-sec pulse duration, 0.2 sec between pulses[†]
Diode (810 nm)	Fiber diameter: 300 μm, initiated	1.0 W, uninitiated fiber, gated 50% duty cycle, 15 sec/tooth[43]	0.4 W, continuous wave, 20 sec/site[†]	0.8 W, continuous wave, 10 sec/site[†]
Nd:YAG (1064 nm)	Fiber diameter: 300 μm	No suggested parameters in literature	30 mJ and 60 Hz, 1.8 W, applied 40 sec/site[†]	100 mJ and 20 Hz, 2.0 W, 20 sec/site[†]
Diode (980 nm)	Fiber diameter: 300 μm	No suggested parameters in literature	2.0 W, pulsed 25 msec on/50 msec off for avg power of 0.7 W, applied 20 sec/site *or* 0.4–0.6 W, continuous applied 20 sec/site[57]	0.8 W, continuous applied 10 sec/site
Micropulsed CO_2	Periotip aperture: 0.25 mm	No suggested parameters in literature	80 mJ, 50 Hz, 1.8–2.0 W; avg of 24 sec/tooth[47] 28 mJ, 30 Hz, 1 W, 350-μsec pulse width, 0.31 msec off; avg of 24 sec/tooth[60]	N/A
Er:YAG	Tip diameter: 0.6 mm	No suggested parameters in literature	80 mJ, 30 Hz, 2.4 W avg power with water spray[21]	N/A
Er,Cr:YSGG	Tip diameter: 0.6 mm	No suggested parameters in literature	1.0 W (50 mJ/pulse)[61]	N/A

avg, Average; *N/A,* not applicable.
*This chart provides only *suggested* parameters. Check the owner's manual for the specific laser being used for more complete information regarding settings.
[†]Data from Raffetto N: Lasers for initial periodontal therapy. In Coluzzi DJ, Convissar RA: *Lasers in clinical dentistry,* Philadelphia, 2004, Saunders.

each site exhibiting disease, whereas the CO_2 laser reflects treatment per tooth.

Fiber

The fibers used with argon, diode, and Nd:YAG lasers are constructed similarly and are manufactured in a variety of diameters, with the 300- to 400-μm fiber most often used for laser-assisted hygiene procedures. The fiber has four parts: the jacket, cladding, fiber, and coupler. The *jacket* is a thick, flexible, clear or translucent, latex-like covering, or in some models, a thin, tougher plastic, that protects the fiber. The *cladding* is a coating on the outside of the fiber that is inwardly reflective, collimating the laser beam completely to the fiber's terminal end. The fiber itself is made of quartz and is crystalline in structure. The *coupler* connects the fiber to the laser.

Proper handling of these parts is critical for optimal power delivery. The extra length of fiber should be loosely coiled and secured away from rolling chairs or sources of entanglement. Manufacturers produce accessories to help manage the extra length of fiber. When preparing the fiber for the handpiece, strip away as little of the jacket as possible. The fiber should be bare through the cannula but not at the point at which the collet nut in the handpiece tightens. Damage to the cladding can occur with use of an improperly sized stripping tool. Overclosing on the fiber during stripping will nick the cladding. Should the cladding become scratched, laser energy will be lost from that site, decreasing the power at the working end. Inspect the fiber for light leaks of the aiming beam before inserting it into the handpiece. If light leaks are present, strip the fiber farther back, and cleave the fiber just behind the point where visible light is detected.

Fiber breakage may occur if the fiber is coiled too tightly or retracted repeatedly in a cassette. Breakage may also occur while working in the pocket. If a metal cannula is used, the side of the fiber may rub against the cannula's edge, inadvertently scoring the fiber and leading to breakage. If such breakage goes undetected, unwanted exposure to laser energy may result. Loss of fiber integrity can waste valuable treatment time, diminish power needed for treatment, and constitute a hazard.

Initiating the Fiber

Initiating the fiber is helpful with some laser-assisted hygiene procedures but is not desired in others. Initiation of the fiber tip is accomplished by activating the laser while touching the fiber to a dark chromophore. Though many practitioners use articulating fiber or cork, neither produces a satisfactory, complete or thorough initiation. The best initiation is performed by using black ink suitable for painting onto glass surfaces (available at any art supply or hobby store) and a good quality, very thin paintbrush. The paintbrush is dipped into the ink and painted onto the tip of the laser fiber and allowed to dry for 30 seconds. The purpose is to concentrate heat energy at the fiber's tip, increasing the thermal interaction with the tissue and accelerating debridement.

Initiation is used with lasers of lower fluence, particularly diode lasers, in the decontamination procedure. Because an initiated fiber concentrates the laser energy at the point of tissue contact, heat can accumulate within the tissues quickly. Application time should be limited to minimize collateral damage in surrounding tissue. Lower settings are used in continuous-wave mode for a shorter duration to accomplish decontamination of the pocket wall. Also, in working with fibrotic tissue exhibiting less chromophoric concentration, initiation is helpful.

If the objective is *penetration of the laser energy* into the tissue beyond the fiber, the fiber is *not* initiated. An uninitiated fiber is used for preprocedural decontamination and coagulation. The Nd:YAG, a free-running pulsed laser, does not require initiating because of its high peak powers and immediate interaction with the tissue. Argon and diode lasers may be used in pulsed or continuous-wave mode, with an uninitiated fiber used for preprocedural decontamination and coagulation. Continuous-wave mode requires less energy and shorter application time, which will minimize heat accumulation

---

CAUTION

If the cladding is damaged but the fiber is not broken, the aiming beam will still be visible at the terminal end, but the power of the working beam will be lessened, sometimes significantly.

TABLE 3-2	Example Case of Time Investment with Three Lasers		
Laser (wavelength)	Duration of Application	Number of Sites Treated	Laser Application (minutes)
Nd:YAG (1064 nm)	40 sec/site*	106	71
	20 sec/site*	106	35 TOTAL: 106
Diode (810 nm)	20 sec/site*	106	35
	10 sec/site*	106	18 TOTAL: 53
CO_2 (10,600 nm)	26 sec/tooth	20 teeth	TOTAL: 8.6

*Data based on suggested parameters from Raffetto N: Laser for initial periodontal therapy. In Coluzzi DJ, Convissar RA: *Lasers in clinical dentistry*, Philadelphia, 2004, Saunders.

within the tissue. The pulsed-wave mode may use higher settings with slightly longer treatment times. The off time between pulses allows heat dissipation within the tissue.

The clinician must have a clear understanding of the laser effects with an initiated or uninitiated fiber and must be proficient in reading tissue–laser interaction.

Cleaving the Fiber

Fiberoptic systems require cleaving for maximum energy delivery. *Cleaving* refers to creating a flat, 90-degree surface at the terminal end of the fiber. This "clean cut" ensures maximum energy delivery from the fiberoptics. Types of cleaving tools include carbide or diamond "pens" held at 90 degrees, 1-inch serrated ceramic tiles held at a 45-degree angle, and scissors, all used to *score* the fiber, not cut through it (Figure 3-11).

To cleave a fiber, lay the fiber down on a firm, flat surface and secure with the nondominant hand. Orient the cleaver appropriately at 2 mm from the end of the fiber. Move the cleaver across the fiber *one* time to score the quartz. When using the scissors design, place the fiber at 90 degrees between the blades, allowing the fiber to scoot along the blades while closing them. With a proper score created by any one of these devices, a "light leak" should be visible and the fiber can be easily snapped away or pulled off.

When checking the fiber for an optimal cleave, hold the fiber perpendicular 1 cm from a flat, light-colored surface (Figure 3-12). The aiming beam should show a well-defined, solid circle. A poor "cleave" creates an uneven or diffuse margin and may have a "comet tail." With an imperfect cleave, the amount of laser energy being delivered to the target tissue is diminished, and trauma is induced when it contacts tissue. The technique for cleaving should

be mastered both to conserve fiber length and to provide efficient laser energy delivery during treatment.

Observe laser safety precautions. Never look directly at the laser light. *Do not activate the laser* when assessing the fiber's cleave, even though it may be in ready mode. The cleaved portion of the fiber, whether contaminated or not, is considered a "sharp," and disposal in an appropriate container is required.

> **CLINICAL TIP**
>
> Cleaving tools are basically nothing more than knives used to cut (score) a glass fiber. One secret of a good chef is to have sharp knives at all times. Chefs are constantly sharpening their knives to obtain the best possible cutting efficiency. Dull knives don't cut well, leading to less-than-ideal results. A cleaving tool must be replaced periodically to ensure creation of cleaves that are always as clean as possible.

Fiber Handpieces

A variety of handpieces may be used with fiberoptic delivery systems; however, it is important that they be compatible with the selected fiber. Just as with hand scalers, handpiece designs include different barrel sizes, textures, and weights (Figure 3-13). The clinician should consider these factors for comfort and working ergonomics.

Properly sized components inside the handpiece will prevent the fiber from slipping during treatment. Most handpieces are designed with a collet nut or chuck that tightens around an inner bushing. The bushing grips the fiber jacket, holding the fiber in place. Some bushings accept only a certain size of jacket, whereas others may be adjusted. If the jacket is stripped away, allowing the bushing to tighten against the bare fiber, the cladding may be damaged, resulting in loss of laser power.

Cannulas

Because the crystalline structure of the fiber will not allow sharp bends in the fiber, the cannula is essential for guiding the fiber to the treatment site. Many different designs of cannula are available: Some are metal and others clear or

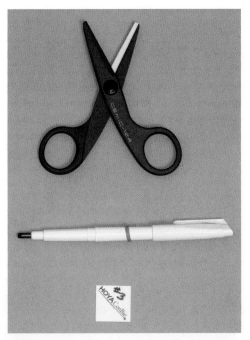

• **Figure 3-11** Three styles of cleaving tools. *From top,* Scissors, glass-cutting pen, and ceramic tile.

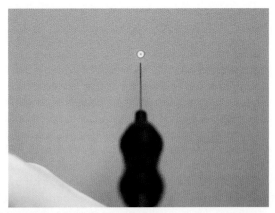

• **Figure 3-12** Example of optimal cleave. Note well-defined, solid circle of light. A less-than-ideal cleave would show an oval or "comet tail" appearance of the light.

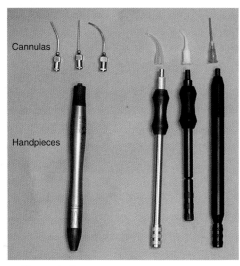

• **Figure 3-13** Various handpieces and cannulas.

translucent plastic (see Figure 3-13). Some screw onto the handpiece, whereas others are tension-retained. Some cannulas are multiuse and sterilizable; others are single-use and disposable. Some can be shaped into a gentle arc, whereas others have a predefined shape. Selecting the best cannula to provide access to the treatment site effectively and efficiently will facilitate periodontal therapy.

Fiber Patency

Before connecting the sterilized fiber to the laser, check the fiber's patency, or openness. Hold the terminal end of the fiber to a light source and look at the connector end. It should show a bright light representing the full diameter of the fiber at the connector. Several conditions may prevent patency. The fiber at the connector may be occluded with oils from sterilization or handling. This can be corrected by cleaning the connector according to the manufacturer's guidelines. Also, the fiber may be broken. Check by installing the fiber and using the aiming beam to locate the "light leak." Strip away the jacket, and cleave the fiber.

> **CAUTION**
>
> Do not install and activate the laser fiber until criteria for patency are met.

Sterilization

Ensuring fiber, handpiece, and cannula integrity throughout the sterilization and installation procedures requires specific care. Manufacturer recommendations should be followed for processing. Avoid sterilizing fibers in autoclaves used for sterilizing oiled handpieces. Oil may accumulate on the connector, causing damage to the laser when activated. Handpieces require minimal maintenance beyond cleaning and sterilizing. Occasionally, plastic bushings break down with heat or chemical processing and must be replaced. Sterilizable cannulas may become occluded with debris

during procedures. The internal aspect should be cleaned with tufted floss or a slightly smaller-diameter cleaning tool and very warm water, then sterilized. Protect metal cannulas from damage when not in use. Proper sterilization and handling of the fiber, handpiece, and cannula will eliminate related cross-contamination and increase longevity of components.

Treating Periimplant Mucositis and Periimplantitis

Treatment of periimplant mucositis and periimplantitis is similar to that discussed earlier for gingivitis and periodontitis. The objective is to preserve attachment or to promote its regeneration by removing pathogens and supporting healing. The attachment of tissue to the implant is a glycoprotein matrix that adheres to the titanium. When the biologic seal is disrupted by inflammation or trauma, the result is an open pathway to the bone supporting the implant.

In periimplant mucositis, the implant often is described as "ailing," with inflammation but no bone loss. The condition warrants therapy to reverse the inflammatory process, with preservation of as much attachment of tissue and bone as possible. As discussed in gingivitis therapy, it is essential to remove biofilm on the implant collar and crown using specialized instruments for implant care. The periimplant tissue is then decontaminated by laser treatment using the previously recommended settings. Therapy should involve at least two sessions 10 days apart. Reappoint at the same interval until conditions resolve.

If the implant is diagnosed as "failing," when half of the implant is still supported with bone and no mobility is detected, other treatment is necessary. Laser therapy can provide immediate decontamination of the surrounding tissue as preparation for a surgical procedure. Nonsurgical therapy is limited because of the inability to fully address the biofilm on the complex implant structure.

Lasers with soft tissue applications can accomplish treatment of periimplant mucositis or periimplantitis. The technique of nonsurgical application with most wavelengths does not aim the laser energy directly toward the implant. Only the soft tissue is treated for decontamination. The laser settings used for nonsurgical therapies are much lower than in surgical procedures. Some wavelengths require more attention than others; for example, a wavelength absorbed in dark chromophores has the potential to cause greater thermal rise and heat transfer. When coated with blood, the implant surface could accumulate heat, which would radiate through the implant body to the bone. An implant coated with hydroxyapatite could absorb another wavelength, resulting in a modified surface.[62] High risk of surface alteration is recognized for the Nd:YAG laser. Much lower risk has been documented with use of the CO_2, Er:YAG, and Er,Cr:YSGG wavelengths. CO_2 laser use in periimplant treatment is well documented in the literature.[63,64] Effectiveness of treatment with the erbium family of lasers is variable, with contradicting results reported. Effectiveness with diodes also is variable as reported for all four diode laser wavelengths (see Chapter 7). CO_2 laser energy is not absorbed at all by implants, so it may be directed toward the implant to remove the biofilm from the implant.

Early detection of disease and good planning with appropriate treatment can result in excellent resolution of inflammation in periimplant tissue. The goal of treatment should be clear to achieve expected outcomes. Even when more advanced care is required, the nonsurgical laser therapy can prepare the site by reducing the inflammatory process and pathogenic load. Laser-assisted periimplant tissue therapy is a valuable treatment.

Diagnosis

Diagnosis and classification of periodontal disease in a given patient depends on accurate assessment. The initial clinical appointment includes the general health history; screening for oral cancer; assessment of hard tissues, occlusion, and the temporomandibular joint (TMJ); complete periodontal and radiographic evaluation; and bacterial testing. Risk assessments from data collected at this appointment help determine the diagnosis of disease and its severity or can serve to confirm periodontal health.

Once periodontal disease is detected, classification and case type are needed for treatment planning. The classification categories as presented at the 1999 World Workshop on Periodontics include the following:

- Gingivitis
- Chronic periodontitis*
- Aggressive periodontitis*
- Periodontitis as a manifestation of systemic disease
- Necrotizing periodontal diseases
- Abscesses of the periodontium
- Periodontitits associated with endodontic lesions

These classification categories are used for diagnosis and third-party billing of insurance, along with the following American Dental Association (ADA) case types[65]:

Healthy—pocket depths of 3 mm or less and no bleeding or inflammation

Type I: *Gingivitis*—pockets 3 mm or less, bleeding on probing, inflammation, and possibly some debris present supragingivally

Type II: *Mild periodontitis*—pockets 4 to 6 mm with slight bone loss, bleeding on probing, inflammation, and debris present subgingivally

Type III: *Moderate periodontitis*—pockets 6 to 7 mm with bone loss, bleeding on probing, inflammation, and debris present subgingivally, with some mobility and possible furcation involvement

Type IV: *Advanced periodontitis*—pockets 7 mm or greater, heavy bleeding on probing, inflammation and suppuration,

and debris present supragingivally and subgingivally, with mobility and furcation involvement

Type V: *Refractory periodontitis*—inflammation and pocket depths of 4 mm or greater in a periodontium previously treated for periodontal disease

Severity also is based on *clinical attachment loss,* graded as follows:
- 1 to 2 mm = slight
- 3 to 4 mm = moderate
- 5 mm or greater = severe

Treatment Planning

Treatment planning may encompass many different strategies based on the patient's needs. Because each case is unique, the following considerations and guidelines are used to develop a customized treatment design rather than fitting each case into a strict, predefined protocol.

Treatment needs are discovered during the process of data collection and the diagnostic workup. Planning should address all issues, ranging from obvious signs of periodontal disease to occlusal problems, and incorporate keys for behavior modification. Factors such as the wavelength being used in therapy and the clinician's level of training and expertise also influence treatment planning. The following treatment plans are suggestions based on our own experiences using Nd:YAG, diode, and CO_2 lasers in periodontal care since 1999.

Considerations in Planning Treatment

1. What are the patient's tolerances concerning physical conditions limiting treatment time, such as temporomandibular disease (TMD) or back problems?
2. Does the patient have moderate or severe anxiety?
3. Will the appointment be conducted with the patient under conscious or intravenous sedation?
4. Will local anesthesia or only topical gel be required?
5. Are there any points of data to be reevaluated (e.g., periodontal charting, radiographs)?
6. Will restorative treatment be accomplished during the same appointment?
7. What is the severity of disease? Is it localized or generalized?
8. Are the biofilm and deposits slight, moderate, or heavy, and what is the tenacity?
9. How large is the surface area to be debrided and decontaminated (both tissue surface and tooth surface)?
10. How motivated and skilled is the patient with daily care?
11. Are there occlusal problems exacerbating the periodontal disease that need to be addressed?

Each treatment session involves much more than instrumentation. The answers to the previous questions will influence the time allowed for treatment, as well as the arrangement of appointments needed for therapy. It must be emphasized that the laser will not overcome poor daily biofilm management.

*Further defined as *localized* (<30% teeth affected) and *generalized* (>30% affected)

Regardless of the degree of periodontal disease, home care is still an essential element of the treatment plan.

Guidelines for Planning Appointments

1. Address only those clinical goals that can be completed in the scheduled appointment time. Issues to be included are patient motivation and skill refinement, complete and thorough debridement, laser treatment, and postoperative instructions.
2. The more severe the disease, the more time required per tooth for treatment.
3. Include time for patient management.
4. The amount of time needed to perform laser treatment of the pocket tissue depends on the laser used, the extent of disease, and the laser–tissue interaction.
5. For each millimeter of optimal attachment gain desired, a session of laser treatment is needed after the original debridement.

   Example: A 6-mm pocket should be decreased to 3 mm.
   - Appointment 1: tooth debridement and laser tissue treatment
   - Appointment 2: ultrasonic biofilm removal on the cervical one third and laser treatment
   - Appointment 3: ultrasonic scaling and laser treatment
   - Appointment 4: ultrasonic scaling and laser treatment

6. Begin therapy in the deepest pockets.[51] This approach allows retreatment of the deepest pockets as the shallow pockets are being treated in successive appointments.
7. In subsequent appointments, areas previously treated will be revisited, with ultrasonic biofilm removal at each tooth's cervical area, and relased. As the patient's daily care improves, less time is spent on biofilm assessment and skill refinement and, typically, more time on laser treatment.

Repetitive therapy is designed to address localized biofilm infection and to promote the regeneration of a strong connective tissue attachment. By decontamination of the periodontal infection site at frequent intervals, the biofilm's community structure is continually weakened, with fewer remnants left to rebuild each time. This strategy optimizes the body's ability to respond. The body will begin to heal when the host is no longer challenged with the inflammatory response initiated by biofilm. (A refractory case will not respond because the host is impaired.) Epithelium covers the surface of a wound in 7 to 10 days.[8] Connective tissue begins regenerating at approximately day 5,[8] maturing for 12 weeks and continuing even up to 1 year.

Assisting the body in balancing the proliferation of these tissue types is the foundation for the following protocols.

Basic Elements of All Appointments

The following basic elements should be included in all appointments:
1. Health history review
2. Concerns of the patient
3. Assessment of oral health
   - Oral cancer screening
   - Evaluation of the TMJ
   - Occlusal evaluation
   - Radiographic survey as needed
   - Periodontal charting (six-point probing, recession, mobility, furcations)
   - Assessment of existing debris, biofilm, and calculus
   - Description of patient's daily dental care routine
   - Evaluation of restorative needs
4. Diagnosis
5. Treatment
6. Supportive care, retreatment, or referral

Gingivitis

General Approach

Gingivitis involves only the gingival tissues, without bone loss. The tissues may exhibit classic signs of erythema, swelling, hemorrhage, blunted papillas, and pseudopocketing. The objective of therapy is to coach the patient in daily cleaning skills and to professionally remove localized factors initiating the inflammatory response. This latter step includes scaling to thoroughly remove biofilm and deposits on the tooth structure and laser decontamination of the sulcus.

At least two appointments are needed in the gingivitis series (Case Study 3-1). The first appointment allows diagnosis, development of patient skills for daily dental care using appropriate tools and techniques to manage biofilm plus nutritional counseling, scaling, and laser decontamination. The second appointment continues refinement of daily cleaning skills, scaling, and laser decontamination.

Full-Mouth Debridement

Full-mouth debridement is indicated when heavy calculus prevents access for probing, or when inflammation with discomfort prevents assessment of the periodontal tissues. This procedure provides gross removal of calculus but is not considered a definitive treatment. The patient should be scheduled for a follow-up appointment in 2 to 4 weeks for thorough periodontal evaluation and determination of further therapy.

Periodontitis

General Approach

Periodontitis is the inflammatory process initiated by the presence of biofilm, with destruction of the tooth's supporting structures, including bone. Clinical attachment loss is apparent with pocketing and with no gingival recession, or recession with no pocketing, or both pocketing and recession. Again, the objective of therapy is to coach the patient in daily techniques to prevent or minimize accumulation of biofilm in the mouth. Professional therapy must address the depth of disease in both the tooth structure and the tissue

CASE STUDY 3-1

Moderate/Severe Gingivitis

Diagnosis of conditions: Negative findings on oral cancer screening; TMJ function is normal; radiographs show no bone loss, and there is no evidence of decay. There is no mobility, and the occlusion is without interferences. Periodontal tissues show moderate to severe gingivitis, moderate generalized hemorrhaging, pseudopocketing, supra- and subgingival plaque, and calculus.

Appointment 1

1. Manage patient discomfort with topical or local anesthesia, if needed.
2. Address daily cleaning needs with use of appropriate tools and technique recommendations.
3. Begin debridement of tooth structures, completing as much as possible at this appointment.
4. Floss to remove additional biofilm and loose calculus.
5. Perform laser decontamination of areas that exhibit signs of inflammation.
6. Give postoperative instructions, and schedule next appointment for 10 days later.

Appointment 2

1. Manage patient discomfort.
2. Review the daily cleaning routine, and refine according to the needs presented.
3. Complete debridement, or provide biofilm removal throughout if debridement has already been completed.
4. Floss.
5. Perform laser decontamination of areas with continued inflammation.
6. Review postoperative instructions.

Continue to schedule subsequent appointments at 10-day intervals until daily skills support health and inflammation is resolved. If systemic health issues are a concern, referral to a physician may be indicated.

Continued Care

This patient is susceptible to recurrence of disease. Once inflammation is resolved, schedule appointments for 3-month intervals to monitor and maintain health. As health is stabilized for an extended time, intervals may be lengthened 2 to 4 weeks more at each visit, as long as health is maintained. If reinfection occurs, the intervals should be shortened.

Necrotizing ulcerative gingivitis (NUG) may be managed with the same therapy as just outlined. It is important to recognize that the patient with NUG may be experiencing intense discomfort; accordingly, it may not be possible to perform periodontal charting or instrumentation at this appointment. Radiographic survey and visual evaluation for diagnosis followed by instruction for daily cleaning at home may be all that is accomplished at this visit. The patient may require systemic antibiotic therapy, as well as analgesics. An appointment to begin gingivitis therapy should be scheduled for within 5 to 10 days.

disinfection or an expanded periodontal infection therapy approach may offer the best treatment for certain patients. With any treatment program, ongoing attention to current severity of and susceptibility to disease is essential in determining intervals of active therapy, evaluation, and continued care.

Full-Mouth Disinfection Therapy

Full-mouth disinfection therapy consists of complete debridement with extensive subgingival irrigation within 24 hours (Case Study 3-2). This treatment program also includes biofilm reduction in the entire oral cavity with a specific twice-daily regimen of flossing, brushing the teeth as well as all accessible oral mucosa, scraping the tongue, rinsing the mouth, and spraying the throat with chlorhexidine.[66] The full-mouth disinfection treatment design requires fewer appointments with longer treatment times.

Advantages

- Quicker reduction of overall microbial load
- Completion of the most difficult part of treatment
- More efficient for sedation appointments
- Restorative concerns may be addressed at the same visit

Disadvantages

- Limited opportunity to work with the patient on daily care skills (with sedation-appointment patients, such opportunity is lacking)
- Patient fatigue
- Psychologically overwhelming for the patient
- Postoperative discomfort increased because all areas are treated
- Clinician fatigue and decreased instrumentation effectiveness
- Follow-up appointments are needed to address recurring biofilm at about 10-day intervals
- Loss of a large amount of production time if the appointment is broken

> **CLINICAL TIP**
>
> Full-mouth treatment would employ the same basic treatment design without adding an antimicrobial, such as chlorhexidine.

Expanded Periodontal Infection Therapy

The expanded-therapy design for management of periodontal infection takes into consideration the *severity* of the disease to be treated. The treatment plan has the flexibility to treat all diseased teeth in a beginning or localized case, or very small sections of teeth in an advanced case. This strategy is structured with more appointments with shorter treatment times (Case Study 3-3).

Advantages

- Repeated reduction of microbial load within the pocket
- Supports the healing process by retarding epithelium and allowing connective tissue growth

wall forming the pocket. This is accomplished through supragingival and subgingival definitive debridement of tooth structure, followed by sulcular debridement.

The series of appointments may be designed in various ways. Some cases can be effectively treated with traditional half-mouth or quadrant therapy; however, full-mouth

CASE STUDY 3-2

Type IV Periodontitis

Diagnosis of conditions: Negative findings on oral cancer screening; TMJ function is normal; radiographs show horizontal bone loss, no decay.

Periodontal condition: Chronic periodontal disease, generalized moderate bone loss (case type III) with moderate to severe gingivitis; moderate generalized hemorrhaging; supra- and subgingival plaque and calculus, horizontal bone loss in posterior with vertical bone loss on #4 and furcation involvement on #2 and 19. Class I mobility of anterior teeth. The occlusion exhibits interferences (Figures 3-14 and 3-15).

Treatment Plan for Full-Mouth Disinfection within 24 Hours (Figure 3-16)
- 5 hours planned for tooth debridement and laser decontamination
- 2 hours for laser decontamination (four 30-minute appointments)
- 30 minutes for reinfection assessment (optional)
- 60 minutes for reevaluation (definitive therapy)

Appointment 1: Upper/Lower Left (UL/LL) (2.5 hours)

1. Administer local anesthesia for left side.
2. Apply disclosing agent in area of left side and recommend tools and techniques for daily care.

3. Remove biofilm with ultrasonic scaling throughout.
4. Debride tooth structure definitively with manual and ultrasonic scaling and extensive irrigation.
5. Floss.

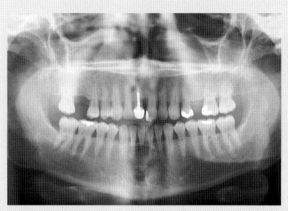

• **Figure 3-15** Panoramic radiograph obtained as part of the initial periodontal evaluation.

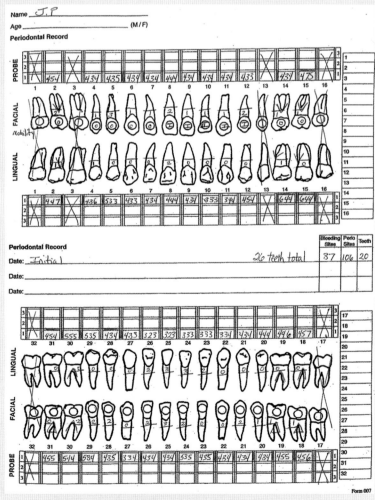

• **Figure 3-14** Initial periodontal probing for baseline evaluation.

CASE STUDY 3-2—cont'd

Type IV Periodontitis

UR UL

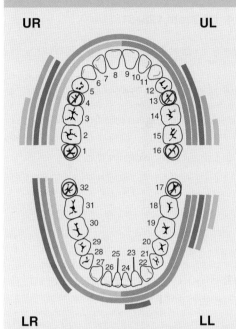

LR LL

	Appt 1	Appt 2	Appt 3	Appt 4	Appt 5	Appt 6 Laser decontamination
Appt 1 UL/LL debride+lase	All UL/LL pockets		Areas 4+mm	Areas 5+mm	Areas 6+mm	Areas 7 mm
Appt 2 UR/LR debride+lase	---------	All UL/LL pockets				
Appt 3 lase	---------	---------	4+mm			
Appt 4 lase	---------	---------	------	5+mm		
Appt 5 lase	---------	---------	------	------	6+mm	
Appt 6 lase	---------	---------	------	------		7+mm

• **Figure 3-16** Graphic representation of treatment plan for full-mouth nonsurgical periodontal laser treatment. Colors in chart at *right* correspond to those in the tooth chart at *left*.

6. Perform laser decontamination.
7. Provide postoperative palliative care (e.g., vitamin E oil).
8. Give postoperative instructions.
9. Confirm appointment for next day.

Appointment 2: Upper/Lower Right (UR/LR) (2.5 hours)

1. Administer local anesthesia for right side.
2. Apply disclosing agent in area of right side and reinforce daily care from the previous day.
3. Remove biofilm with ultrasonic scaling throughout.
4. Debride tooth structure definitively with manual and ultrasonic scaling and extensive irrigation.
5. Floss.
6. Perform laser decontamination (on the right side only, because 7 days have not passed).
7. Provide postoperative palliative care (e.g., vitamin E oil).
8. Give postoperative instructions.
9. Confirm next appointment in 10 days.

Appointments 3 to 6: Laser Decontamination

1. Plan 60 minutes to address all areas; less time may be required for fewer treatment sites.
2. Apply disclosing agent in one area to demonstrate need for improved daily care or in another area to highlight good management.

3. Remove biofilm at the cervical portion of each tooth.
4. Floss.
5. Repeat laser treatment of all areas previously noted with disease.
6. Provide postoperative care and instructions.
7. Confirm next appointment in 10 days.
   The laser decontamination appointments continue until the deepest pockets have been treated enough times to minimize biofilm and inflammatory activity and support connective tissue reattachment.

Appointment 7

Perform reinfection assessment 6 weeks after laser decontamination (optional).

Appointment 8

Provide definitive therapy 8 to 12 weeks after laser decontamination.

Appointment 9

Provide supportive periodontal therapy, retreatment, or referral.

• Continued assessment and refinement of daily care skills (working to form good habits in self-care)
• Decreased postoperative discomfort because smaller areas are treated.
• Increased effectiveness of instrumentation (less clinician fatigue)

• Less patient fatigue
• Restorative concerns may be addressed at same visit
• Repeated biofilm removal at the cervical portion of the tooth
• Less production time lost if the appointment is broken

CASE STUDY 3-3

Treatment Plan for Expanded Periodontal Infection

(Figure 3-17)
- 5 hours planned for tooth debridement and laser decontamination
- 30 minutes for final laser decontamination
- 30 minutes for reinfection assessment (optional)
- 60 minutes for definitive therapy

Appointment 1: UR Teeth #2, 4–8

1. Administer local anesthesia for selected area.
2. Apply disclosing agent in an area and recommend tools and techniques for daily care.
3. Remove biofilm with ultrasonic scaling throughout.
4. Debride tooth structure definitively with manual and ultrasonic scaling.
5. Floss.
6. Perform laser decontamination.
7. Provide postoperative palliative care (e.g., vitamin E oil).
8. Give postoperative instructions.
9. Confirm next appointment at approximately 10 days.

Appointment 2: LL Teeth #18–21

1. Repeat steps 1 to 6 above.
2. At this appointment, repeat laser treatment of #2, 4, 5, 6, 7, and 8.

Appointment 3: UL Teeth #9, 10–12, 14, 15

1. Repeat steps 1 to 6 above.
2. At this appointment, repeat laser treatment of #18–21 and 2, 4, 5 of UR.

Appointment 4: LR Teeth #28–31

1. Repeat steps 1 to 6 above.
2. At this appointment, repeat laser treatment of #9, 10 to 12, 14, 15 and 2, 4, 14, 15, 18, 19.

Appointment 5: LR/LL Teeth #22–27

1. Repeat steps 1 to 6 above.
2. At this appointment, repeat laser treatment of #28–31 and 2, 14, 15, 18, 19.

Appointment 6: Laser Decontamination

1. Plan 30 minutes to address remaining sites needing care.
2. At this appointment, repeat laser treatment of #22–27 and any areas exhibiting inflammation.
· The laser decontamination appointments continue until the deepest pockets have been treated enough times to minimize biofilm and inflammatory activity and to support connective tissue reattachment.

Appointment 7

Perform reinfection assessment 6 weeks after laser decontamination (optional).

Appointment 8

Provide definitive therapy 8 to 12 weeks after laser decontamination.

Appointment 9

Provide supportive periodontal therapy, retreatment, or referral.

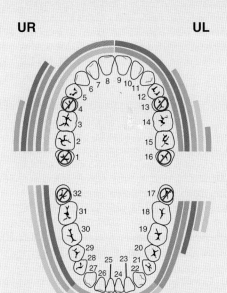

	Appt 1	Appt 2	Appt 3	Appt 4	Appt 5	Appt 6 Laser decontamination	Appt 7 Laser decontamination
Appt 1 UR debride+lase	#2,4–8	Areas 4+mm	Areas 5+mm	Areas 6+mm	Areas 7+mm	----------	----------
Appt 2 LL debride+lase	----------	#18–21	4+mm	5+mm	6+mm	7+mm	----------
Appt 3 UL debride+lase	----------	----------	#9–12, 14,15	4+mm	5+mm	6+mm	7+mm
Appt 4 LR debride+lase	----------	----------	-------	#28–31	4+mm	5+mm	----------
Appt 5 LR/LL debride+lase	--------	----------	-------	-------	#22–27	4+mm	5+mm

• **Figure 3-17** Graphic representation of treatment plan for full-mouth nonsurgical periodontal laser treatment. Colors in chart at *right* correspond to those in the tooth chart at *left*.

Disadvantages

- More visits, requiring coordination of patient and practice schedules
- Not practical for sedation appointments

Apatzidou and Kinane[67] found that both expanded treatment and full-mouth treatment strategies were effective and suggested selecting the treatment modality on the basis of practical considerations related to patient preference and clinical workload.

Sedation Appointment (Intravenous or Conscious)

Sedation appointments require variation in the treatment design, according to the procedures scheduled during the sedation. Patients receiving sedation often will have restorative and periodontal procedures accomplished in the same visit. Because periodontal disease affects the supporting structures of the teeth, it is prudent to give it a high priority in the treatment sequence.

Active periodontal infection therapy with sedation focuses only on definitive debridement of the teeth and decontamination of tissues. Treatment planning must consider the time required for thorough treatment within the practical time available. The clinician should work to completion in sections, so that if an unforeseen complication forces treatment to conclude, each treated section has full benefit of therapy.

Active periodontal infection therapy also involves coaching the patient with customized techniques and recommended tools for removing biofilm effectively on a daily basis. Because this cannot be addressed with the patient in a sedated state, it is helpful to have an appointment concentrating on biofilm management techniques before the sedation appointment, as well as additional "coaching" appointments at intervals after the sedation. Tissue rehabilitation is optimal if the patient can undergo "laser decontamination" procedures, including ultrasonic biofilm removal and continued laser treatents, at 10-day intervals. If the patient cannot tolerate these appointments, the next option is to schedule several appointments at 2-week intervals until effective biofilm control is demonstrated.

The treatment that follows the sedation appointment(s) depends on patient tolerance. If the biofilm is not continually controlled and the healing processes are not supported, rehabilitation of the tissues will not be as effective as with repetitive therapy.

Debridement Appointment

The debridement appointment includes definitive removal of calculus and endotoxins on the tooth surfaces, along with the first application of laser decontamination of the diseased pocket walls. The objective is to greatly reduce the microbial load in the instrumented area. The number of teeth selected and time allowed for each debridement appointment depend on the case severity and treatment design.

Laser Decontamination Appointment

The laser decontamination appointment is provided after thorough debridement of tooth structure, when continued decontamination of the tissue wall, impairment of epithelium, and maturation of connective tissue are required. Laser decontamination appointments continue until each pocket has had sufficient therapy to support healing to ideal resolution.

Again, for each millimeter of attachment gain desired, an additional laser decontamination session should be provided. These sessions are scheduled approximately 10 days apart after the last debridement plus lasing session. Sessions may be 30 to 60 minutes in length, depending on the number of sites and pocket depths to be treated. At completion of the last laser decontamination appointment, the definitive therapy appointment should be scheduled for 6, 8, or 12 weeks (a longer interval allows attachment to mature).

Reinfection Assessment Appointment (Optional)

The purpose of the reinfection assessment appointment is to evaluate tissue rehabilitation, reinforce biofilm removal skills, and maintain patient motivation. It does not include probing or instrumentation, unless an area presents with inflammation. The patient's daily cleansing skills are assessed, and further coaching and motivation are directed at prevention of reinfection. Biofilm removal at the cervical portion of each tooth is provided with ultrasonic scaling. Should an area need further instrumentation, laser decontamination is indicated as the last step of disinfection.

The reinfection assessment appointment should be scheduled as a 30-minute appointment and should follow the last laser decontamination appointment by approximately 6 weeks. The patient should be seen for the definitive therapy appointment after another 6 weeks.

> **CLINICAL TIP**
>
> Reinfection assessment at a separate appointment is indicated when the definitive therapy appointment is scheduled for 12 or more weeks later and the patient is at moderate risk for reinfection.

Reevaluation (Definitive Therapy)

The definitive therapy appointment marks the completion of active phase I periodontal infection therapy and is the occasion for providing evaluative and therapeutic services. This appointment follows the last laser decontamination appointment by 6 to 12 weeks and includes continued evaluation of daily care. Periodontal disease status is reevaluated, with documentation of six-point probing, recession, and mobility. These data are compared with pretreatment charting to determine the extent of rehabilitation. Occlusal stresses and restorative needs also are evaluated, providing important information for indicated treatment recommendations.

Healthy sites are supported with appropriate care as well during this appointment. Treatment includes biofilm removal throughout, instrumentation of areas where calculus is present, and in unresolved areas, further debridement with manual and ultrasonic instruments. Laser decontamination in areas of inflammation and persistent pocketing completes the process for the definitive therapy (reevaluation) appointment.

The clinician must determine whether management of unresolved areas can be addressed during the appointment or if periodontal needs are more extensive. This decision will depend on the number of areas manifesting with inflammation and pocketing, in addition to the contributing factors. With a limited number of unresolved sites, the root surfaces can be debrided again and continued laser decontamination provided. Subsequent appointments for continued supportive periodontal therapy should be scheduled at an appropriate interval.

More extensive needs may include another series of root debridement and laser decontamination appointments, moving ahead with restorative treatment, or pursuing surgery (conventional or laser-assisted). Some patients may require medical referral for systemic evaluation. At any time during the patient's care, it is the clinician's judgment, based on personal knowledge and skill, whether to continue with active phase I periodontal infection therapy or to refer the patient to a specialist.

Supportive Periodontal Therapy

Supportive periodontal therapy appointments maintain the body's stabilization in oral health by eliminating or reducing local microbiologic factors.[8] Clinically, this strategy involves preserving clinical attachment level, maintaining alveolar bone height, eliminating inflammation, and ensuring comfortable function. The patient in whom a satisfactory level of maintenance has been achieved can be treated as previously discussed for the reevaluation (definitive therapy) appointment, and subsequent appointments for continued follow-up can be scheduled at an optimal interval.

The Venn diagram in Figure 3-18 reinforces the concept that periodontal health is maintained when daily (home) care and recommended professional care are implemented. If either daily care or professional care is lessened, periodontal health may decline.

Often, patients believe that their periodontal disease is "fixed," like a healed broken arm. They should be counseled on the chronic nature of the disease, with episodes of activity and remission, and requiring consistent evaluation at shorter intervals and treatment as indicated by activity level. When a patient presents with reinfected sites,

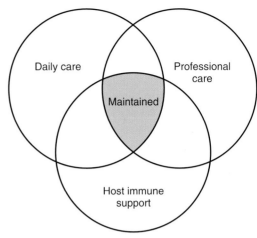

• **Figure 3-18** Venn diagram depicting health maintenance with daily and recommended care.

additional therapy is needed, as discussed for the reevaluation appointment.

Determine whether the patient's needs can be addressed during the supportive therapy appointment. If additional treatment is required, keep in mind that a single session of retreatment usually is insufficient to control biofilm within the pocket or to promote connective tissue reattachment.

Conclusions

Few contraindications to laser treatment exist. There are no concerns regarding development of resistant bacteria or allergic reactions. Lasers may be used in children, pregnant women, immunocompromised patients, and patients with pacemakers or defibrillators or other implanted medical devices. When used within appropriate parameters, lasers provide gentle, yet highly effective decontamination at the target site, thereby promoting healing. Laser wavelengths are bactericidal, with associated improvement in indices related to periodontal health. Laser treatment is an excellent adjunct to thorough root debridement and tissue rehabilitation. Understanding applications and safe techniques of laser-assisted therapy provides a higher standard of care.

In keeping with various trends in dental health, such as an aging population retaining teeth longer, an increase in diabetes and other chronic diseases in all age groups, and diets of poor nutritional value among the general population, the prevalence of periodontal disease is likely to increase. Unless patients are better educated and experience more positive therapies, increasing periodontal disease prevalence will continue. Laser therapy is an improvement on traditional therapeutic modalities. It is less invasive and more efficient, decreasing the time spent in treatment and reducing the need for surgery. As research and clinical study reveal more aspects of periodontal disease, treatment modalities will continue to evolve to provide more successful prevention and healing.

Acknowledgments

We wish to thank Drs. Akira Aoki, Don Coluzzi, Robert Convissar, Jon Julian, and Randall Wolcott for their mentoring and assistance with research and information. Gratitude also is extended to the University of Missouri–Kansas City (UMKC) School of Dentistry Library, Mrs. Corey, and staff for assistance gathering research data.

References

1. American Academy of Periodontology: Epidemiology of periodontal diseases (AAP position paper), *J Periodontol* 76:1406–1419, 2005.
2. Lin D, Moss K, Beck JD, et al.: Persistently high levels of periodontal pathogens associated with preterm pregnancy outcome, *J Periodontol* 78(5):833–841, 2007.
3. Zambon JJ: Periodontal diseases: microbial factors, *Ann Periodontol* 1:879–925, 1996.
4. Paju S, Scannapieco FA: Oral biofilms, periodontitis, and pulmonary infections, *Oral Dis* 13(6):508–512, 2007.
5. Scannapieco FA: Role of oral bacteria in respiratory infection, *J Periodontol* 70(7):793–802, 1999.
6. Hujoel PP, Bergstrom J, del Aguila MA, DeRouen TA: A hidden periodontitis epidemic during the 20th century? *Community Dent Oral Epidemiol* 31:1–6, 2003.
7. Armitage GC: Clinical evaluation of periodontal diseases, *Periodontol* 2000(7):39–53, 1995.
8. Perry D, Beemsterboer P, Taggart E: *Periodontology for the dental hygienist*, ed 2, Philadelphia, 2001, Saunders.
9. Fux CA, Costerton JW, Stewart PS, Stoodley P: Survival strategies of infectious biofilms, *Trends Microbiol* 13:34–40, 2005.
10. Donlan RM, Costerton JW: Biofilms: survival mechanisms of clinically relevant microorganisms, *Clin Microbiol Rev* 15:167–193, 2002.
11. Manor A, Lebendiger M, Shiffer A, Tovel H: Bacterial invasion of periodontal tissues in advanced periodontitis in humans, *J Periodontol* 55(10):567–573, 1984.
12. Rumbaugh K, et al: *Pseudomonas aeruginosa* forms biofilms in acute infection independently of cell-to-cell signaling, 2006, personal communication (in *Wound care practice*, Chapter 29).
13. Wolcott R: Biofilm-based wound care. In Fife CE, Sheffield PJ, editors: *Wound care practice*, ed 2, Flagstaff, Ariz, 2007, Best Publishing.
14. Mertz PM: Cutaneous biofilms: friend or foe? *Wounds Compend Clin Res Pract* 15:1–9, 2003.
15. Aoki A, Sasaki KM, Watanabe H, Ishikawa I: Lasers in nonsurgical periodontal therapy, *Periodontol* 2000(36):59–97, 2004.
16. Schwarz F, Sculean A, Berakdar M, et al.: In vivo and in vitro effects of an Er:YAG laser, a GaAlAs diode laser and scaling and root planing on periodontally diseased root surfaces: a comparative histologic study, *Lasers Surg Med* 32:359–366, 2003.
17. Rechmann P, Henning T: Selective ablation of subgingival calculus. In Loh HS, editor: *4th International Congress on Lasers in Dentistry*, Bologna, 1995, Monduzzi Editore, pp 159–162.
18. Crespi R, Barone A, Covanin U, et al.: Effects of CO_2 laser treatment on fibroblast attachment to root surfaces: an SEM analysis, *J Periodontol* 73:1308–1312, 2002.
19. Moritz A, Schoop U, Goharkhay K, et al.: Treatment of periodontal pockets with a diode laser. Department of Conservative Dentistry, Dental School of the University of Vienna, Austria, *Lasers Surg Med* 22(5):302–311, 1998.
20. Neill ME, Mellonig JT: Clinical efficacy of the Nd:YAG laser for combination periodontitis therapy, *Pract Periodont Aesthet Dent* 9:1–95, 1997.
21. Ando Y, Aoki A, Watanabe H, Ishikawa I: Bactericidal effects of erbium YAG laser on periodontopathic bacteria, *Lasers Surg Med* 19:190–200, 1996.
22. Walsh LJ: Utilization of a carbon dioxide laser for periodontal surgery: a three-year longitudinal study, *Periodontol* 2000(16):3–7, 1995.
23. Finkbeiner RL: The results of 1328 periodontal pockets treated with the argon laser: selective pocket thermolysis, *J Clin Laser Med Surg* 13:273–281, 1995.
24. Crespi R, Barone A, Covani U: Histologic evaluation of three methods of periodontal root surface treatment in humans, *J Periodontol* 76(3):476–481, 2005.
25. Kojima T, Shimada K, Iwasaki H, Ito K: Inhibitory effects of a super pulsed carbon dioxide laser at low energy density on periodontopathic bacteria and lipopolysaccharide in vitro, *J Periodont Res* 40(6):469–473, 2005.
26. Kreisler M, Kohnen W, Marinello C, et al.: Bactericidal effect of the Er:YAG laser radiation on dental implant surfaces: an in vitro study, *J Periodontol* 73(11):1292–1298, 2002.
27. Alling C, Catone G: *Laser applications in oral and maxillofacial surgery*, Philadelphia, 1997, Saunders.
28. Coluzzi DJ, Convissar RA: *Atlas of laser applications in dentistry*, Chicago, 2007, Quintessence.
29. Cobb CM: Non-surgical pocket therapy: mechanical, *Ann Periodontol* 1:443–490, 1996.
30. Manni JG: *Dental applications of advanced lasers*, Burlington Mass, 2004, JGM Associates.
31. Sibbald RG, et al.: Preparing the wound bed: debridement, bacterial balance, and moisture balance, *Ostomy Wound Manage* 46:14–18, 30, 2000.
32. Steed DL, Donohoe D, Webster MW, Lindsley L: Effect of extensive debridement and treatment on the healing of diabetic foot ulcers, Diabetic Ulcer Study Group, *J Am Coll Surg* 183:61–64, 1996.
33. Gans SL, Austin E: The use of lasers in pediatric surgery, *J Pediatr Surg* 23(8):695–704, 1988.
34. Jia YL, Guo ZY: Effect of low-power He-Ne laser irradiation on rabbit articular chondrocytes in vitro, *Lasers Surg Med* 34(4):323–328, 2004.
35. Medrado AP, Soares AP, Santos ET, et al.: Influence of laser photobiomodulation upon connective tissue remodeling during wound healing, *J Photochem Photobiol Biol* 92:144–152, 2008.
36. Schindl A, Schindl M, Schindl L, et al.: Increased dermal angiogenesis after low-intensity laser therapy for a chronic radiation ulcer determined by a video measuring system, *J Am Acad Dermatol* 40(3):481–484, 1999.
37. Garavello I, Baranauskas V, da Cruz-Hofling MA: The effects of low laser irradiation on angiogenesis in injured rat tibiae, *Histol Histopathol* 19(1):43–48, 2004.
38. Reis SR, Medrado AP, Marchionni AM, et al.: Effect of 670-nm laser therapy and dexamethasone on tissue repair: a histological and ultrastructural study, *Photomed Laser Surg* 26(4):305–311, 2008.
39. Karu T: Photobiological fundamentals of low-power laser therapy, *J Quant Elect* 23:1704–1717, 1987.
40. Henry CA, Judy M, Dyer B, et al.: Sensitivity of *Porphyromonas* and *Prevotella* species in liquid media to argon laser, *Photochem Photobiol* 61:410–413, 1995.

41. Gutknecht N, Franzen R, Schippers M, Lampert F: Bactericidal effect of a 980-nm diode laser in the root canal wall dentin of bovine teeth, *J Clin Laser Med Surg* 22(1):9–13, 2004.

42. Sennhenn-Kirchner S, Klaue S, Wolff N, et al.: Decontamination of rough titanium surfaces with diode lasers: microbiological findings on in vivo grown biofilms, *Clin Oral Implants Res* 18(1):126–132, 2007.

43. Watanabe H, Ishikawa I, Suzuki M, Hasegawa K: Clinical assessments of the erbium:YAG for soft tissue surgery and scaling, *J Clin Laser Med Surg* 14:67–75, 1996.

44. Assaf M, Yilmaz S, Kuru B, et al.: Effect of the diode laser on the bacteremia associated with dental ultrasonic scaling: a clinical and microbiological study, *Photomed Laser Surg* 25(4):250–256, 2007.

45. Scannapieco FA: Periodontal inflammation: from gingivitis to systemic disease? *Compend Contin Educ Dent* 25(7 suppl 1):16–25, 2004.

46. UltraSpeed CO_2 Smart US20 D and PerioPulse Dental Hygiene Laser, DEKA, Ft Lauderdale, Fla.

47. Mariotti AJ, Rumpf DA: Chlorhexidine-induced changes to human gingival fibroblast collagen and non-collagen protein production, *J Periodontol* 70:1443–1448, 1999.

48. Guarnelli ME, Fanceschetti G, Manfrini R, Trombelli L: Adjunctive effect of chlorhexidine in ultrasonic instrumentation of aggressive periodontitis patients: a pilot study, *J Clin Periodont* 35(4):333–341, 2008.

49. Lee MK, Ide M, Coward PY, Wilson RF: Effect of ultrasonic debridement using a chlorhexidine irrigant on circulating levels of lipopolysaccharides and interleukin-6, *J Clin Periodont* 35(5): 415–419, 2008.

50. Hoang T, Jorgensen MG, Keim RG, et al.: Povidone-iodine as a periodontal pocket disinfectant, *J Periodont Res* 38(3):311–317, 2003.

51. Raffetto N: Lasers for initial periodontal therapy. In Coluzzi DJ, Convissar RA, editors: *Lasers in clinical dentistry*, Philadelphia, 2004, Saunders, pp 923–936.

52. Wilson TG, Kornman KS: *Fundamentals of periodontics*, ed 2, Chicago, 2003, Quintessence.

53. Newman MG, Takei H, Carranza FA, Klokkevold PR: *Carranza's clinical periodontology*, ed 9, Philadelphia, 2002, Saunders.

54. Harrel SK, Molinari J: Aerosols and splatter in dentistry: a brief review of the literature and infection control implications, *J Am Dent Assoc* 135:429–437, 2004.

55. Douglas OH: Laparoscopic hazards of smoke, *Surg Serv Manage AORN* 3(3), 1997.

56. Ulmer B: Air quality in the operating room, *Surg Serv Manage AORN* 3(3), 1997.

57. Garden J: Viral disease transmitted by laser-generated plume (aerosol), *Arch Dermatol* 138(10):1303–1307, October 2002.

58. Albrecht H, Wasche W: *Evaluation of potential health hazards caused by laser and RF-surgery: analysis of gaseous, vaporized and particulate debris produced during medical treatment*, Eureka Project, EU 642, Stilmed, 1995, German Federal Ministry for Education, Science, Research and Technology (BMBF), European BIOS.

59. KaVoGENTLEray 980 Classic and Premium, KaVo Dental, Lake Zurich, Ill; info.us@kavo.com.

60. Spectra Denta CO_2 laser, Lutronic, Princeton Junction, NJ; office@lutronic.com.

61. Ting CC, Fukuda M, Watanabe T, et al.: Effects of Er,Cr:YSGG laser irradiation on the root surface: morphologic analysis and efficiency of calculus removal, *J Periodontol* 78(11):2156–2164, 2007.

62. Kreisler M, Gotz H, Duschner H: Effect of Nd:YAG, Ho:YAG, Er:YAG, CO_2, and GaAIAs laser irradiation on surface properties of endosseous dental implants, *Int J Oral Maxillofac Implants* 17(2):202–211, 2002.

63. Stubinger S, Henke J, Deppe H: Bone regeneration after peri-implant care with the CO_2 laser: a fluorescence microscopy study, *Int J Oral Maxillofac Implants* 20(2):203–210, 2005.

64. Deppe H, Horch H, Henke J, Donath K: Peri-implant care of ailing implants with the CO_2 laser, *Int J Oral Maxillofac Implants* 16:659–667, 2001.

65. Armitage GC: Development of a classification system for periodontal diseases and conditions, *Ann Periodontol* 4:1–6, 1999.

66. Lyle DM: Full-mouth disinfection: a treatment option, *J Pract Hygiene* 22–24, Sept/Oct 2001.

67. Apatzidou DA, Kinane DF: Quadrant root planing versus same-day full-mouth root planing. I. Clinical findings, *J Clin Periodontol* 31(2):132–140, 2004.

4

Lasers in Surgical Periodontics

SAMUEL B. LOW

Advantages of Laser Surgery

Lasers have multiple uses in surgical periodontics. Advantages of laser therapies over conventional periodontal surgery center on six major areas:

1. Minimal collateral effects result in decreased tissue damage, thereby enhancing healing.

Although an association between use of lasers and altered wound healing has been recognized, with use of optimal settings for a given procedure, laser therapy will result in wound healing comparable to or better than (i.e., accelerated) that observed with conventional surgery (Figure 4-1). Studies on wound healing with lasers (e.g., neodymium-doped yttrium-aluminum-garnet [Nd:YAG], diodes, carbon dioxide [CO_2]) versus the scalpel generally show an initial lag in soft tissue wound healing but equivalence within 2 weeks of postoperative observation.[1,2] Many of these studies were done more than a decade ago with units that emitted much higher fluences than current lasers. Studies performed with more modern equipment by the more knowledgeable researchers of today might show equivalence between scalpel and laser wound healing within 24 h of the incision.

The specific objectives of planned laser procedures must be considered on a wavelength-by-wavelength basis; results of CO_2 laser wound studies cannot be extrapolated to those for Nd:YAG, diodes, or erbium wavelengths. As with all "hi-tech" devices and instruments, the results depend greatly on the expertise of the user, for whom appropriate training is essential to develop the requisite clinical skills (see Chapter 16) and a sound knowledge base that includes optimal settings for watts (W), millijoules (mJ), hertz (Hz), duty cycle, pulse width, hand speed, and other parameters (see Chapter 2).

2. Patient comfort can be enhanced.

Many laser procedures avoid extensive flap reflection and significant trauma to the wound area. Accordingly, with minimal invasive site preparation, the inflammatory response is decreased, resulting in greater patient comfort. Decreased pain and swelling result from laser sealing of the lymphatics and nerve endings.[3,4] Biostimulation of the wound area and enhanced wound healing also may occur[5,6] (see Chapter 15).

3. Hemostasis and coagulation typically are readily achieved, making the laser essential for medically compromised patients.

The Nd:YAG and diode lasers emit wavelengths that are absorbed more readily in pigmented tissues, such as tissues with a high concentration of hemoglobin. Use of these lasers, therefore, creates a hemostatic environment during and immediately after surgery as the hemoglobin absorbs the laser energy.[7] CO_2 lasers accomplish hemostasis through a different mechanism: When collagen in the walls of the blood vessels absorbs the CO_2 wavelength, the helical collagen polymer unravels. With this altered conformation, the collagen fibers shrink, causing the lumens of the blood vessels to shrink, with consequent hemostasis.[3]

Therefore significant hemostasis can be achieved in laser procedures, especially in medically compromised patients (Figure 4-2). Preoperatively, the medical history often reflects extensive pharmaceutical intervention to provide anticoagulation, including prophylactic aspirin and platelet aggregation inhibitors. Patients also may be using many "natural" homeopathic remedies and other preparations that may interfere with clotting. They may not identify the use of these over-the-counter (OTC), nonprescription preparations in the medical or drug history. Such compounds as curry powder, cayenne pepper, cinnamon, and other herbs and spices have a high salicylate content, which can affect clotting. Ginkgo biloba, vitamin E, and other preparations available in health food stores and pharmacies also are associated with impaired clotting.

When scalpel procedures must be avoided in a patient with coagulation considerations, lasers allow surgery to proceed without compromising the patient's overall health. In the past, the anticoagulant therapy regimen would have been modified and extensively monitored. With lasers, anticoagulant therapy is much less of an issue during treatment.

4. Some procedures can be performed with use of topical anesthesia only.

Some superficial soft tissue procedures can be performed with use of commercially available topical anesthetics, such as those containing lidocaine and prilocaine. Orthodontic and pediatric patients requiring frenectomy and gingivoplasty or gingivectomy are especially suitable candidates for laser procedures with topical anesthesia (see Chapters 11 and 12).

5. The concept of minimally invasive dentistry (MID) can be achieved.

With use of loupes with at least 3× magnification, sulcular laser procedures with small-spot-size laser tips can be performed without gingival flap reflection. This may be applied to procedures such as sulcular debridement and some limited crown-lengthening procedures.

6. Lasers are safe to use if the operator adheres to protocols.

Knowledge of laser physics is a prerequisite to successful clinical application and generally is acquired through laser certification courses. Familiarity with the properties of each wavelength, including depth of penetration of different tissue types, is essential for the practitioner in determining the optimal laser treatment, to maximize the quality of results. In addition, implementation of specific safety protocols, including the designation of a laser safety officer, is mandatory in any clinical setting in which a laser is used. Laser safety education is a requirement for all dental surgery team members.

Nonsurgical Applications

Most laser wavelengths have antimicrobial properties. Nd:YAG and diode laser wavelengths are absorbed by bacteria, especially those with pigmentation, thereby reducing

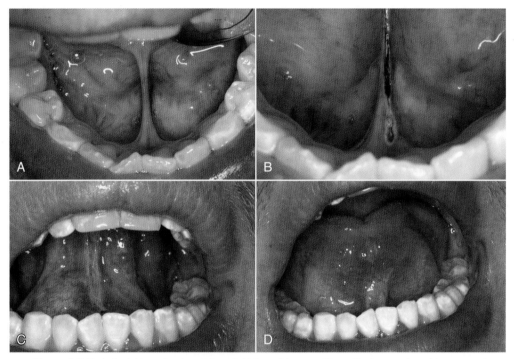

• **Figure 4-1** Periodontal laser treatment for a tight lingual frenum. The patient was referred by a speech pathologist for surgical correction. **A,** Presurgical view of the frenum. **B,** Beginning incision for release of lingual frenum with CO_2 laser. Note excellent hemostasis and conservative incision. **C,** Immediate postoperative view of completed lingual frenectomy. **D,** Lingual frenectomy site 3 days after surgery. Note excellent and rapid healing. © Dr. Robert A. Convissar.

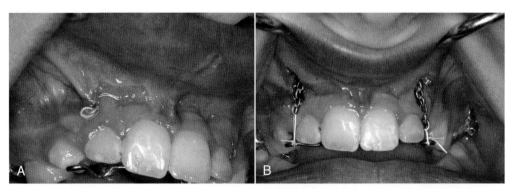

• **Figure 4-2** Use of a laser to gain adequate intraoral surgical access in a medically compromised patient on anticoagulation therapy. **A,** Presurgical view of a buried orthodontic chain. **B,** Immediate postoperative view after exposure of the orthodontic chain accomplished by means of a laser. The laser tip was moved in an apical direction while tension was placed on the exposed chain. With minimal hemorrhage, clear access to the wound area has been obtained. The chain can now be successfully incorporated into the orthodontic appliance.

colonization.[8,9] Decreasing bacterial load in the soft tissue wound site can enhance wound healing, resulting in less postoperative discomfort. CO_2 and erbium laser wavelengths are absorbed by the water content in cells, with consequent vaporization when the temperature of the intracellular water exceeds 100° C.

Although the use of lasers in initial periodontal therapy has significant advantages, it must be emphasized that laser treatment is an *adjunct* to standard therapy rather than a replacement therapy. For example, with standard nonsurgical scaling and root planing, the goals include reduction of the bacterial biofilm, removal of necrotic cementum and subgingival calculus, and deepithelialization of the sulcus. Scaling and root planing should result in decreased inflammation, decreased pocket depth, and attachment gain through a long junctional epithelial attachment.[10] Lasers do not remove necrotic cementum or subgingival calculus but do aid in reduction of the biofilm and deepithelialize tissue more quickly and easily than with conventional techniques. Rossmann et al.[11] emphasized that CO_2 lasers can be used to delay the apical downgrowth of epithelium, and that this technique is less technically demanding and more time-efficient than other techniques.

The Nd:YAG and diode lasers are of limited use in hard tissue root therapy for root detoxification because they are primarily soft tissue lasers. By contrast, erbium lasers demonstrate capability for root debridement by their effect on calculus and necrotic cementum, with reduced endotoxins.[12,13] Also, evidence indicates that these effects can increase the attachment level gain over that achieved with scaling and root planing.[14,15] However, systematic reviews (especially evidence-based) demonstrate minimal differences in nonsurgical periodontal end points between laser and conventional periodontal therapy. Evidence shows that soft tissue laser curettage does not contribute to additional gains in attachment level beyond those obtained with meticulous periodontal root planing in chronic adult periodontitis. Therefore soft tissue lasers such as the Nd:YAG and diode, with their ability to deepithelialize the gingival sulcus and some antibacterial properties, may have limited application for nonsurgical periodontal therapy. The erbium laser, in addition to soft tissue use, may be the device required for calculus removal and hard tissue detoxification, creating a biocompatible surface for attachment of connective or epithelial tissue.[16] Using the CO_2 wavelength, Crespi et al.[17] found that they could increase the quality and quantity of fibroblasts attaching to the root surface.

As an adjunct to periodontal debridement, *photodynamic therapy* may have potential. In one such approach, with use of either a "cold" (low-level) laser or a conventional dental laser with wavelengths absorbed by pigment (e.g., diode, Nd:YAG), methylene blue dye is placed in the sulcus as a subgingival irrigant. These laser wavelengths are attracted to and interact with the dye, disrupting the bacterial cell membranes. The light energy activates the dye, interacts with intracellular oxygen, and destroys the bacteria by lipid peroxidation and membrane damage. Chapters 3 and 15 discuss the use of lasers for initial (nonsurgical) periodontal therapy.

Gingivectomy

Gingivectomy is a time-honored procedure for removal of gingiva. The indications range from access to esthetics. The gingivectomy can be used when suprabony pockets are present and access to osseous structures is not necessarily important. The procedure assists in decreasing gingival tissue in cases of enlargement and in altering fibrotic gingiva (Figure 4-3). However, gingivectomy is contraindicated when (1) access to osseous structure is critical or (2) gingival attachment is inadequate (minimal) or absent.

Clinical observation demonstrates that resecting gingiva with a laser enhances access because of increased visualization resulting from sealing of capillaries and lymphatics during laser irradiation. In the early stage of tissue healing with use of blades, inflammation is noted, along with collagen production and epithelialization, and the wound has a high tensile strength.

The laser wound generally demonstrates delayed epithelialization, collagen production, and inflammation, with a lower tensile strength. In later phases of healing, however, the process accelerates, with collagen production and epithelialization. Myofibroblasts are present in fewer numbers during healing of a laser-resected wound site, which leads to less wound contraction and less scar formation[18] (Figure 4-4).

As discussed earlier, no clear conclusion has emerged regarding healing rates for laser-induced wounds versus conventional scalpel wounds. However, Nd:YAG, CO_2, erbium-doped YAG (Er:YAG), and diode lasers demonstrate wound healing that is either comparable with that achieved after use of conventional scalpel blades or somewhat accelerated.[19] White et al.[20] compared several laser technologies using histologic analysis and determined that wound

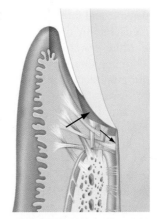

• **Figure 4-3** Excision versus incision. The excisional gingivectomy incision is created on an external bevel *(small arrow)*. If the bevel cannot be created owing to difficulties with access, the incision can be blended into the apical gingiva using the laser tip. The internal incision *(large arrow)* also can be created for purposes of the flap procedure. (Modified from Rose LF, Mealey BL: *Periodontics: medicine, surgery, and implants,* St Louis, 2004, Mosby.)

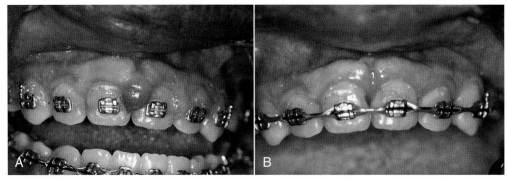

• **Figure 4-4** Laser gingivectomy for treatment of gingival hyperplasia. **A,** Presurgical view. **B,** Ten days after the laser procedure. The cause of the hyperplasia was lack of oral hygiene compliance exacerbated by loading from orthodontic appliances.

healing is influenced by certain instrument settings—W, Hz, pulse duration, and time of exposure. It could be concluded, therefore, that wound healing after a flap or a gingivectomy procedure using laser therapy depends as much on device settings as on the actual laser wavelength used. Also, training often is as important as or sometimes more important than laser wavelength.

An alternative to laser therapy, *electrosurgery* (especially monopolar devices), does not have a defined target tissue as with laser technology. The primary mode of tissue interaction with electrosurgical instruments is by heat ablation. The zone of necrosis after electrosurgery can be 500 to 1500 µm. Diode and Nd:YAG lasers can generate heat in tissue at a depth of up to 500 µm, whereas erbium and CO_2 lasers, because of high water absorption, penetrate from 5 to 40 µm. Bipolar electrosurgery units constitute an improvement over monopolar units in that bipolar units generate less lateral heat and can be used in a wet environment.[21]

Treating noninflamed, fibrotic gingiva with diode and Nd:YAG lasers requires different power settings than for hyperemic or vascular tissue.[22] Lasers are attracted by specific chromophores, so less power is needed to incise tissue if abundant chromophore is present in the tissue. When the gingiva is hyperemic and inflamed, less power is needed because of the high amount of chromophore (hemoglobin) in the tissue. More power is needed to incise fibrotic tissue with less chromophore (hemoglobin) present. The same holds true for gingivectomies in patients with higher melanin content of tissues. *Melanin* is one of the chromophores of Nd:YAG and diode lasers. Tissue that is heavily pigmented with melanin requires much less power than gingiva that is very light, coral pink when theses wavelengths are used.

In performing surgery with CO_2 and erbium lasers, melanin and hemoglobin content is less important. Erbium and CO_2 laser wavelengths are absorbed primarily by water, so both of these lasers will require less power for incising hyperemic tissue than for cutting through fibrotic tissue. An erbium laser can be used for a gingivectomy, but hemostasis can be problematic with this wavelength. Some clinicians may follow an erbium laser procedure with use of a diode, Nd:YAG, or CO_2 laser to achieve coagulation if hemorrhage

is a problem. Others use erbium laser settings that create a so-called *laser bandage* (settings of low wattage, no water, and some air, with fewer pulses per second). In the past, this laser bandage was referred to as a "char layer" or an "eschar." Although older lasers routinely created a char layer because of their high fluences, newer laser units rarely char tissue. Use of a char layer will depend on the clinician's preference, because the findings reported in the literature are equivocal.

The clinician must appreciate both the *emission* spectrum of the laser and the *absorption* spectrum of the tissue. What wavelength is being emitted? What is the primary chromophore of the tissue? How does tissue biotype affect the laser parameters? All of the variables of laser use—power, spot size, pulses per second, and hand speed—must be taken into account, along with wavelength and tissue biotype (see Chapter 2). It is a mistake to consider that increasing power alone may result in quicker cutting through the target tissue. Lasers generate heat that may result in tissue necrosis from lateral thermal damage. Therefore settings are critical in performing laser therapy. Again, it must be emphasized that training should be one of the primary considerations in evaluation of the different laser manufacturers before purchase.

Initial incisions for gingivectomies are similar to that of using a blade with an external bevel approach. The distance of the incision from the coronal gingival margin is based on pocket depth and amount of existing attached gingiva. A gingival chamfer (beveled edge) is achieved, rather than a direct right angle into the gingiva. Thus the initial cut is made slightly apically to the pocket depth measurement. A slow, unidirectional hand motion is used, moving the tip at an external bevel toward the tooth structure. Caution is necessary in approaching the tooth, especially near root structure, because of the possible laser–hard tissue interaction, which could result in tissue damage. Decreasing the power will prevent such injury; if the power is decreased, however, multiple passes over the incision line may be necessary to complete the cut. Delivering laser energy repeatedly over tissue that has already been treated may result in a greater extent of lateral thermal damage.

Some clinicians use a reflective barrier in the sulcus to prevent the wavelength from interacting with the root.

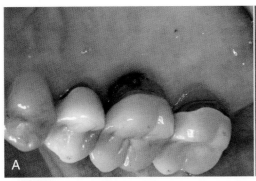
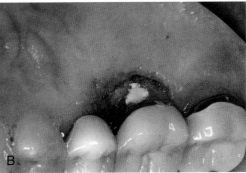

• **Figure 4-5** Laser gingivectomy performed to gain access for restoration prognosis: preoperative **(A)** and immediate postoperative **(B)** views. The patient presented with a possible carious lesion detected subgingivally with an explorer on examination. To determine the extent of the lesion, gingivectomy was performed with a diode laser. Note excellent hemostasis.

Placing a thin, sterile #7 wax spatula or a small periosteal elevator, or even a piece of metal or mylar matrix band, in the sulcus between the tooth and the soft tissue will prevent any laser energy from damaging the hard tissue; the metal or mylar will reflect the laser energy away from the tooth. Once the gingiva has been excised, power-driven ultrasonic scaling is used to debride the root surface.

Because of the sculpting ability of lasers, gingivoplasty can now be performed to smooth the gingival margins for a parabolic appearance. With diode, CO_2, and Nd:YAG lasers, hemostasis is achieved during the procedure. Erbium lasers create hemostasis after the procedure by altering laser parameters to seal blood vessels. Again, some clinicians incorporate the erbium laser bandage as the final procedure. Whether or not to place a dressing is a matter of clinician preference (Figure 4-5).

Frenectomy

Use of the frenectomy procedure in periodontics (unlike in orthodontic or pediatric applications) is limited because of the minimal increase in attached gingiva observed after post-frenectomy wound healing (Figure 4-6). Alveolar mucosa is characterized by a red color and a smooth surface and generally is loose and mobile, whereas attached gingiva is keratinized, pink, stippled, and firm, with no mobility (Figure 4-7).

Gingival surgery in the form of soft tissue augmentation is necessary under the following conditions:

- Marginal gingiva is inflamed.
- Bleeding or exudate is present at the sulcus/pocket.
- Obvious recession is present.
- Pulling of marginal tissue occurs with retraction of the lip.
- As determined by direct measurement, the sulcular depth in millimeters is subtracted from the keratinized zone of gingiva. At least 2 mm of "keratinized attached gingiva" should be present.

Frenectomy procedures with a laser are predictably successful so long as the following steps are incorporated:

1. Creation of a periosteal fenestration at the base of the frenectomy to prevent reattachment of fibers
2. Removal of all impeding muscle fibers

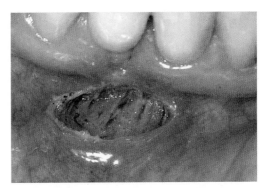

• **Figure 4-6** Immediate postoperative view of laser frenectomy site in a patient in whom the frenectomy was performed without consideration for the extent of gingival attachment, which was minimal to none. A mucogingival graft procedure or vestibuloplasty is indicated to gain an adequate amount of keratinized attached gingiva. Note hemostasis.

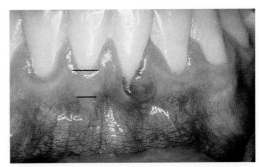

• **Figure 4-7** Comparison of alveolar mucosa and gingiva. Parameters of color, surface, and mobility are used in differentiating mucosa from gingiva. Mandibular left lateral incisor has a cleft that borders on alveolar mucosa. The level of inflammation makes discerning the level of attached gingiva difficult; this determination is best delayed until after health is achieved.

Parameter	Alveolar Mucosa	Gingivae
Color	Red	Coral pink
Surface	Smooth	Stippled
Mobility	Loose	Firm

• **Figure 4-8** **A,** Preoperative view of frenum pull. **B,** Immediate postoperative view of laser frenectomy site. **C,** Postoperative view at 1 week. Note rapid healing.

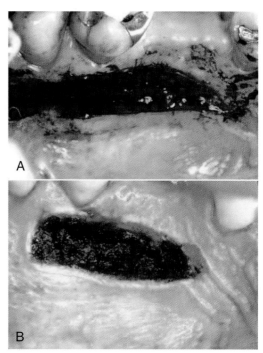

• **Figure 4-9** Use of a laser in a mucogingival procedure to "seal" the surgical wound for control of hemorrhage. **A,** Donor site immediately after harvesting of a graft in conventional fashion with a blade. **B,** Donor site immediately after creation of a "laser bandage" for local hemostasis. (Courtesy Dr. Stuart Coleton.)

All laser wavelengths can be used to perform a frenectomy successfully; however, depth of penetration for diode and Nd:YAG lasers is much higher (500 µm) than for erbium or CO_2 lasers (5 to 40 µm), so settings must be monitored closely to prevent thermal damage to the underlying periosteum and bone.[23] In some patients, topical anesthesia is sufficient to allow performance of a frenectomy, with excellent precision, and with less discomfort and shorter healing time than with conventional techniques. CO_2 laser treatment for frenectomy provides better postoperative patient perceptions of control of pain and improved function than with the scalpel technique.[24] Likewise, use of the Nd:YAG laser may result in less postoperative pain and fewer functional complications.[25]

The technique for a laser frenectomy is similar to that using a blade (Figure 4-8). Local or topical anesthesia is administered. The clinician should first visualize the procedure by forming a mental outline of the incision. This incision begins at the coronal attachment; the laser tip is then moved unidirectionally, with tension achieved by pulling on the lip. With use of the correct parameters (spot size, power, hand speed), one pass of the laser should be sufficient to sever all of the fibers. If multiple passes are necessary, care must be taken to avoid excessive lateral thermal necrosis from reexposure of already-treated tissue. The laser incision is continued to undermine the muscle attachment until the periosteum is reached.

To ensure minimal regrowth and prevent frenum "relapse," the periosteum should be fenestrated with a hand instrument. All lasers are effective for a frenectomy with settings suggested by the manufacturer. Care must be taken not to char the tissue, with consequent thermal tissue damage. The erbium laser creates a wound that may exhibit some hemorrhage, so sealing the wound with the laser bandage (see Fig. 4-9) approach may be required. No suturing or dressing is necessary (see also Chapters 11 and 12).

> **CLINICAL TIP**
>
> The greater the amount of tension placed on the frenum achieved by pulling on the lip, the faster the frenectomy proceeds.

Mucogingival Surgery

Lasers can be used in mucogingival procedures for a variety of therapies. Donor material can be acquired from the palate or other keratinized areas in the oral cavity with laser therapy. Using a laser to "seal" the wound when donor material is taken from these areas using blades can reduce hemorrhage significantly (Figure 4-9).

In some patients, the resulting recipient area may be over-contoured at several weeks postoperatively if an overly thick donor graft was used. Any soft tissue laser can be used to recontour the site, with a positive esthetic result (Figure 4-10).

In other patients, rather than performing a graft procedure, the zone of attached tissue may be increased by a *vestibuloplasty.* Although the preoperative view in Figure 4-11*A* shows an insufficient amount of attached gingiva, the underlying problem is that the fibers are very tightly bound together. A vestibuloplasty releases the tightly bound fibers, resulting in a wider band of attached gingiva, without the need for a graft procedure.

Crown Lengthening

A crown-lengthening procedure is used to gain access to subgingival caries, expose margins, and explore fractures. The procedure allows for developing a proper form for a restoration and increasing surface area for retention. The patient's smile can be enhanced by manipulation of the gingival contour. When considering a crown-lengthening procedure, the clinician must address the following questions (Figures 4-12 and 4-13):

- Can biologic width be maintained?
- Will attached gingiva be preserved?
- Can opening and invading furcations be avoided?
- Is the tooth restorable?
- Will there be loss of support to the adjacent tooth?

Contraindications to crown lengthening include attempting to retain a nonrestorable tooth, compromising adjacent teeth, compromised crown/root ratios, root proximity issues, and unrealistic expense.

The technique of laser crowning lengthening varies with the laser type. If the objective is soft tissue, the diode, Nd:YAG, and CO_2 wavelengths are sufficient. However, to alter underlying osseous structures, erbium lasers and possibly the 9300-nm CO_2 laser are used. Only the erbium wavelengths have received U.S. Food and Drug Administration (FDA) clearance for osseous resection. Few studies have

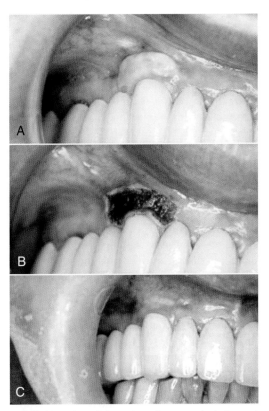

• **Figure 4-10** Use of a soft tissue laser for mucogingival recontouring. **A,** Preoperative view of bulky, unesthetic free gingival graft. **B,** Immediate postoperative view of graft site after laser debulking. **C,** Two-week postoperative view of graft site. Note superior tissue contours and more esthetic result. (Courtesy Dr. Stuart Coleton.)

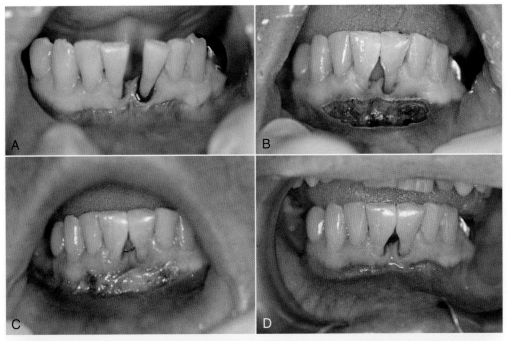

• **Figure 4-11** Laser surgery for enhancing mucogingival attachment. **A,** Preoperative intraoral view showing inflammation around tooth #24, high frenum attachment, and minimal attachment of gingival margin. **B,** Immediately after frenectomy/vestibuloplasty. **C,** Two-day postoperative view of surgical site. Note excellent healing. **D,** Two-week postoperative view showing fully healed site with increase in zone of attached gingiva. (Courtesy Dr. Jon Julian.)

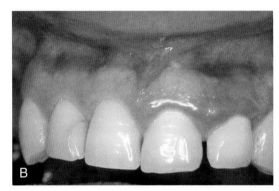

Sulcus

Epithelial
attachment 1.07 mm
} Biological
width
2.04 mm
Connective tissue
0.97 mm

A

B

• **Figure 4-12** Biologic width. **A,** Diagram of relevant anatomy. **B,** Violation of biologic width with resulting inflammation. Standard measurement for biologic width is 2 mm; this includes epithelial and connective tissue attachment. When a restoration is placed into this zone and within 2 mm of the osseous level, a foreign body reaction occurs, resulting in inflammation. (**A,** Modified from Rose LF, Mealey BL: *Periodontics: medicine, surgery, and implants,* St Louis, 2004, Mosby.)

delineated bone response with use of diode and Nd:YAG lasers; however, the chromophores that absorb diode and Nd:YAG (melanin and hemoglobin) are essentially absent in osseous tissue, and it would take great power for these wavelengths to cut hard tissue, producing a large amount of heat during the procedure. This heat would cause at the least delayed healing, with osseous necrosis in some cases.[26,27] Erbium lasers (e.g., Er:YAG, Er,Cr:YSGG) appear to be effective in osseous surgery without inducing significant collateral damage; these lasers emit wavelengths with high absorption coefficients for both water and hydroxyapatite.[28,29]

The primary positive effect of using a laser for bone surgery would be to create a clear removal of the bony defect with minimal charring, melting of mineral, or delayed wound healing. However, the issue becomes whether the clinician can perform a proper ostectomy with a laser and establish a viable biologic width, especially at line angles of teeth, without opening up a flap, as discussed shortly.

The following protocol establishes the necessary biologic width with due consideration of patient esthetics[30]:

1. "Sound" the osseous crest (3.0 mm from osseous crest to proposed gingival margin).
2. Provide zone of keratinized gingival margin (scallop desired lengths if 3 mm or more will be retained).
3. Bevel papillary areas (levels can be apically positioned and adjusted later).
4. Leave papilla intact at base.
5. Thin the osseous crest, but leave at least 1 mm of thickness.
6. Determine whether dentin/root surfaces will be exposed (plan treatment for restorative procedures).

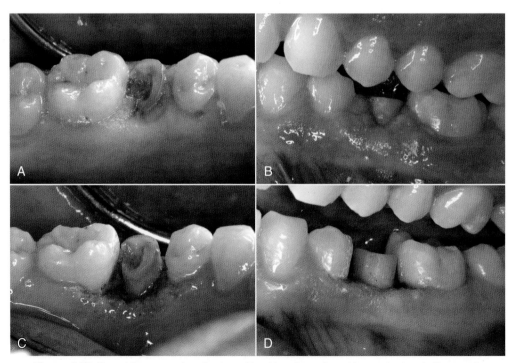

• **Figure 4-13** Closed-flap crown lengthening with erbium laser (to achieve ostectomy). Preoperative views: lingual **(A)** and buccal **(B)**. Immediate postoperative views: lingual **(C)** and buccal **(D)**. The patient presented with a coronal fracture of questionable prognosis. Sounding bone levels determined that osseous levels would require apical alteration to achieve biologic width.

In laser crown-lengthening techniques, first determine the apical extent of the presumed restorative margin. If it is determined that the margin will be within 2 to 3 mm of the osseous crest, osseous surgery inevitably will be required to maintain the biologic width. Therefore a flap reflection will be necessary, or a "closed" flap crown-lengthening procedure must be considered.

Controversy surrounds the closed-flap crown-lengthening procedure when bone is removed. This surgery can be challenging because it involves "blind" sounding of the osseous levels, and removal of bone can be unpredictable. If no osseous surgery is required, and if the end result will maintain adequate attached gingiva, a modified laser

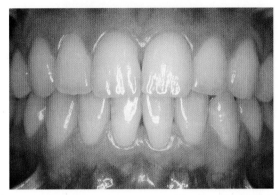

• **Figure 4-14** Rule of "golden proportion" in determining height versus width for anterior teeth. When possible, the clinician strives to achieve an optimal relation between height and width of teeth in the smile line. The necessary alteration can involve changing the gingival parameters and the restorations themselves.

gingivectomy procedure will provide the necessary access for crown length, especially in the anterior esthetic zone.

To begin an esthetic crown-lengthening procedure, the clinician may want to fabricate a surgical guide or stent to assist in determining the apical extent of the gingival margin, using the principles of ideal width and height of respective tooth types (Figure 4-14). After local anesthesia is obtained with infiltration, the following steps can be performed with most dental lasers when osseous surgery is not necessary (Figures 4-15 to 4-18):

1. With the surgical guide in place, an outline of the initial incision can be made with the laser in a slightly defocused mode. As with a conventional blade-initiated gingivectomy, the laser incision is started slightly apical to the stent and at a 45-degree angle to create a gingival chamfer.
2. The stent can be removed after the outline, and with the laser tip moving slowly in a unidirectional manner, the tip is increasingly moved toward the tooth surface. Caution is necessary for preserving the papillae for esthetics.
3. The now-free excised collar can be removed with a curette and the stent replaced to check the accuracy of margin placement.
4. With a relatively lower wattage, the laser tip can now be moved in a sweeping motion to sculpt the margin and enhance the chamfer and to decrease gingival thickness to a more knifelike architecture. Placement of the laser subgingivally is not necessary unless osseous surgery is needed and the erbium laser is required to establish the biologic width.

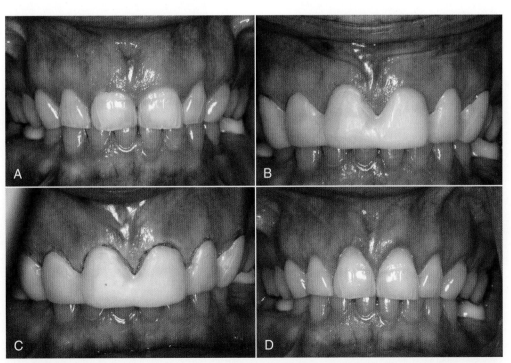

• **Figure 4-15** Laser crown-lengthening procedure for restoration of maxillary and mandibular anterior teeth. **A,** Preoperative view. **B, C,** Closed-flap crown-lengthening approach was used, with creation of a surgical stent. The erbium wavelength was chosen for the required osseous surgery. Note minimal hemorrhage. **D,** Two-week postoperative view.

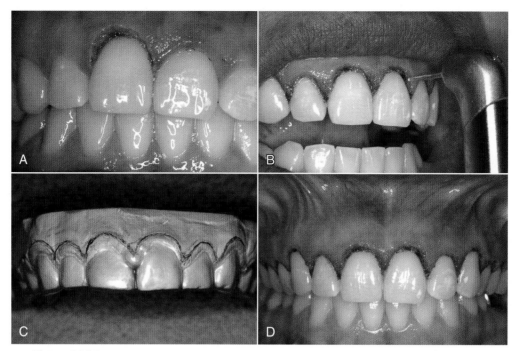

• **Figure 4-16** Performing esthetic osseous crown lengthening with an erbium laser. The patient desired a change in the esthetic appearance of the anterior teeth. Sounding performed with the patient under anesthesia indicated that moving the gingival margins apically would violate the biologic width. **A,** Laser gingivectomy was performed, with contour emphasized at the distal facial line angle. **B,** Continued gingivectomy was done on remaining teeth to ensure balance of gingival contour. **C,** A stent was fabricated to determine the respective heights of the anterior teeth and to be used as a surgical guide. **D,** Completed crown lengthening with closed ostectomy. A parabolic osseous contour is achieved under the gingiva with the erbium tip.

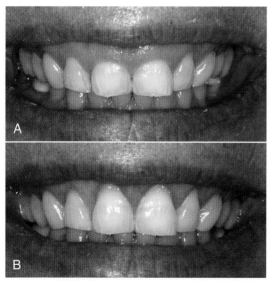

• **Figure 4-17** Closed crown-lengthening procedure with osseous surgery performed using an erbium laser. **A,** Preoperative view of the patient smiling, who elected not to have restorative dentistry. **B,** Postoperative view at 9 months. The reference point for the ideal gingivoincisal length of teeth in this patient was the maxillary canines, and an attempt was made to increase the height of the centrals and laterals to achieve a positive esthetic effect on smiling.

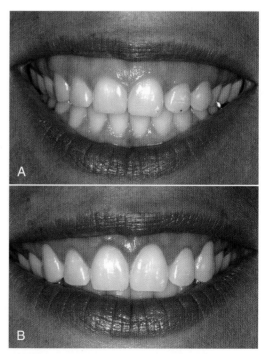

• **Figure 4-18** Osseous crown-lengthening laser procedure. **A,** Preoperative view. The smile/lip line is high, and a "gummy" smile is evident. The patient did not want restorations, and the gingiva was contoured with an erbium laser tip with ostectomy in a closed-flap environment to achieve biologic width. **B,** Postoperative view at 9 months shows stable gingival levels with improved smile profile.

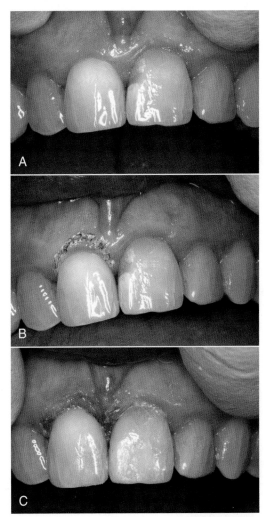

• **Figure 4-19** CO_2 laser gingivectomy to equalize zeniths of adjacent teeth. **A,** Preoperative view of discrepancy between zeniths of teeth #8 and #9. **B,** The laser was used in intermittent mode to outline the planned gingivectomy incision. **C,** Immediate postoperative view after completed gingivectomy. (Courtesy Dr. Robert Convissar.)

5. The resulting wound will exhibit minimal hemorrhage. Again, the laser bandage technique is used at the clinician's discretion.
6. Postoperative care consists of gentle brushing and antimicrobial rinsing for 2 weeks. Whether or not to place a surgical dressing is again the clinician's decision. After 2 weeks, patients return to conventional oral hygiene, with a soft brush for sulcular cleaning and flossing for interproximal hygiene.

Rather than using a stent, some lasers can be used in an *intermittent* exposure mode (not to be confused with pulsed delivery). This intermittent delivery allows the surgeon to outline margins of a gingivectomy before performing an irreversible incision (Figure 4-19). This technique is routinely used in other disciplines of dentistry, especially in outlining margins of a planned biopsy specimen (see Chapter 8).

Periodontitis

The 2000 document "Parameters on chronic periodontitis with advanced loss of periodontal support" from the American Academy of Periodontology[31] provides therapeutic goals that include eliminating microbial contaminants, addressing risk factors, arresting the progression of the disease, and preserving the dentition. In addition, regeneration of the periodontal attachment can be attempted. Periodontal procedures include regenerative therapy with bone grafting, guided tissue regeneration, combined regenerative techniques, and resective therapy, which includes creation of flaps with or without osseous surgery, root resective therapy, and gingivectomy.

Periodontal Surgery

Technique in laser periodontal surgery for pathology depends on whether the goal is strictly alteration of the soft tissue or includes manipulation of the hard tissue. Accurate pocket depth charting, radiographic evaluation, identification of mobility patterns, measurements of the attached gingiva, and occlusal evaluation should preface all procedures. The following issues need to be addressed:
1. **What are the pocket depth measurements? In pocket reduction, how much depth is above and below the cementoenamel junction?**
If suprabony pathology with pseudopocketing is present with significant attached keratinized gingiva, the clinician may consider gingivectomy as the first step. With minimal attached gingiva and no pseudopocketing, the procedures are performed from a sulcular approach with no coronal gingiva removed.
2. **If pockets will be reduced, where is the mucogingival junction, and what are the esthetic considerations?**
If significant attached gingiva and pseudopocketing are present, gingivectomy is considered. The clinician must consider all esthetic end points for gingival reduction.
3. **What is the underlying osseous typography, horizontal or angular?**
If osseous surgery will be performed, the erbium laser will be used for this process. The CO_2, diode, or Nd:YAG laser can be used for the soft tissue phase. However, conventional instrumentation must be included for osteoplasty/ostectomy.

Once the decision points are completed, the clinician can consider the following steps (Figures 4-20 to 4-22):
1. Excise supragingival pseudopocketing with either a conventional blade (e.g., 15/16 Kirkland, 1/2 Orban knife) or a laser, as described earlier for gingivectomy.
2. Sculpt the incised surface to decrease the bulky gingiva; if using a blade for the incision rather than a laser, use the laser to create hemostasis.
3. Beginning at the coronal intrasulcular surface, move the laser tip apically in a back-and-forth motion circumferentially. This movement should be continued until proximity with the apical connective tissue or osseous levels is attained. The laser settings are decreased overall

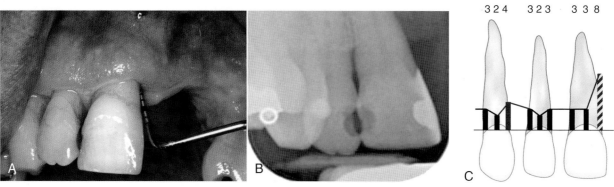

• **Figure 4-20** Preoperative laser data collection in a patient with severe periodontitis and major bone resorption in the maxillary central incisor area. **A,** Clinical probing; **B,** radiographic appearance; **C,** periodontal charting. The patient's history included use of a removable dental appliance for several years without any symptoms, but the pocket depth for the maxillary right central was 8 mm, associated with an angular osseous defect at the base of the lesion.

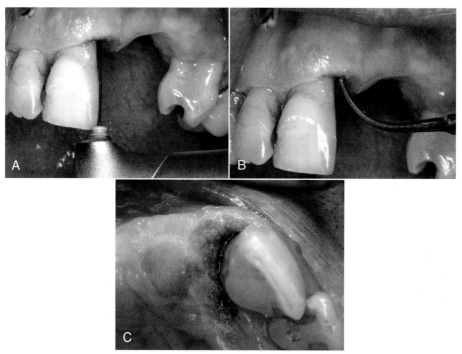

• **Figure 4-21** Laser procedure for periodontitis. **A,** The laser tip is placed in the sulcus after gingivectomy to perform sulcular debridement to achieve deepithelialization and degranulation. **B,** Ultrasound device creates lavage and performs root and osseous debridement. **C,** During the procedure, hemorrhage is minimal, with excellent access obtained. Deepithelialization of coronal gingiva is achieved with the laser to slow down apical migration of advancing epithelium and to enhance soft tissue rather than long-junctional epithelial reattachment.

in energy output compared with gingivectomy settings. The granulation tissue seen moving out of the sulcus should be removed. The clinician must always examine the tip to ensure that it is firing appropriately; it should be cleaned, cleaved, or replaced in accordance with manufacturer recommendations.

4. With use of an erbium laser, the tip can be placed parallel to the root surface, where calculus and possibly root endotoxins can be removed. The root debridement process is completed with a power-driven device (e.g., ultrasound). Again, laser-debrided tissue is flushed out of the sulcus and then removed. Some clinicians prefer to continue

degranulation to the periosteal level of the osseous structures using either a laser or a conventional blade at this point. The erbium laser can degranulate the diseased tissue, decorticate the bone, and detoxify the root if desired. Other wavelengths can simply be used to degranulate the diseased tissue and deepithelialize the area.

5. The final step may consist of placing the laser tip back into the sulcus to decrease hemorrhage from the wound area and to create a clot from heat activation or biomodification of the red blood cells. The rationale for creating the clot is to create a barrier so that epithelium from the coronal wound surface will not migrate apically into the

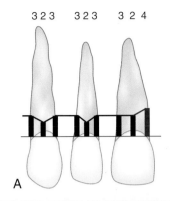

3 2 3   3 2 3   3 2 4

A

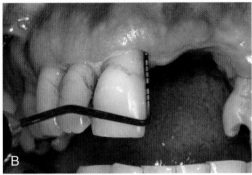

B

• **Figure 4-22** Long-term results with laser surgery for severe periodontitis. **A,** Periodontal charting done postoperatively (compare Figure 4-20*C*). **B,** One-year postoperative clinical view (compare Figure 4-20*A*). After the laser periodontal procedure, a 3-month periodontal maintenance program was instituted, with attention to oral hygiene. Pocket depth is reduced 4 mm, with a slight recession.

surgical area. This allows the wound to be populated with connective cells, enhancing new attachment.

Depending on the wavelength, some clinicians believe in adding a laser deepithelialization step: Practitioners who use the CO$_2$ wavelength rely on the research of Rossmann, Israel, Cettny, Froum, and others, who have provided histologic proof using three different models—beagles, monkeys, and humans—that deepithelialization with this wavelength is more than sufficient to prevent migration of the epithelium, and that it leads to the formation of new soft tissue attachment, rather than a long junctional epithelium.

6. Placing finger pressure on the wound with compression will mold the tissue back to the root-bone interface. Placing a dressing or pack is the clinician's choice.

Postoperative Instructions

The following considerations should be included in postoperative management for the first week:

- Patient must refrain from oral hygiene in the affected area. A very soft brush can be used for superficial coronal plaque removal, but not an electric toothbrush.
- Texture of ingested food should be softer than normal, with chewing restricted mostly to the nonaffected sites.
- Analgesic medication should be taken the day before, day of, and day after the procedure; the medication then is taken on an as-needed basis. A nonsteroidal antiinflammatory

drug (NSAID) may be considered as the analgesic. Because of the minimal discomfort, most laser practitioners no longer advise analgesics before the procedure, instead suggesting OTC medications postoperatively if needed.

- If the patient experiences discomfort, swelling, or bleeding, the clinician should be contacted.
- If a dressing placed during the procedure comes off in the first week or before the next appointment, patients should not be concerned unless it causes discomfort.
- An oral rinse may be considered. Systemic antibiotic coverage is not necessary unless a medical condition requires such.
- After the first week, the patient continues with gentle brushing and proceeds with interdental plaque removal with a soft brush. A rinse is used after the first week only if wound healing is delayed.

From 2 weeks on, the patient resumes normal oral hygiene, with emphasis on interproximal biofilm removal.

Regeneration

Most clinical studies comparing laser with standard therapy in the treatment of periodontitis use scaling and root planing as the control treatment, rather than conventional surgical procedures. The concept of regeneration of the periodontal attachment apparatus as an ultimate goal in the treatment of periodontitis is an end point for which clear data are lacking regarding long-term retention of the dentition. The debate will continue over the regenerated connective tissue attachment versus the long junctional epithelial attachment resulting from many surgical and nonsurgical periodontal procedures.[32,33] For purposes of comparison, however, laser procedures appear to be conducive to regeneration by decreasing bacteria, affecting root surfaces, removing granulation tissue, and deepithelializing the sulcular lining, as previously suggested.

However, when laser therapies are compared with conventional open-flap procedures, with or without the addition of biologic mediators such as enamel matrix protein derivatives, the conclusions are consistent in that no statistical or clinically significant differences have been found between open-flap procedures and laser-mediated periodontal surgeries.[12,34]

In a human histologic study, use of an Nd:YAG laser to remove sulcular epithelium resulted in formation of new cementum and new connective tissue attachment, whereas a control group of patients exhibited development of a long junctional epithelium with no evidence of regeneration.[35] Moreover, no adverse changes were described in the laser group. This report suggests a *laser-assisted new attachment procedure* for the treatment of chronic periodontitis. Of interest, the study did not use stents to aid in clinical measurements. Although manual probing is susceptible to variation, the results achieved nevertheless fall within the range of acceptable measurement error for probing depth and clinical attachment levels of ±1 mm reported in other clinical trials.[36,37] A justifiable conclusion, therefore, is that

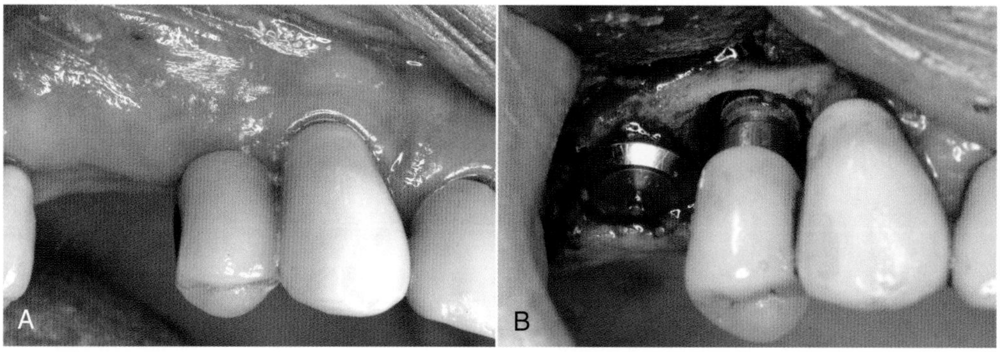

• **Figure 4-23** Laser treatment for impending failure of an endosseous root form implant. **A,** Implant demonstrating periimplantitis. The patient had minimal symptoms; however, suppuration was present, with radiographic bone loss of 20% but no mobility. A flap was reflected to visualize the implant's surface. **B,** An erbium laser was used to prepare the site for osseous grafting. The laser tip was placed in the lesion to remove granulation tissue and to "sterilize" the implant surface.

these two parameters may merely be equal to those observed with scaling and root planing.

Schwarz et al.[38] treated naturally occurring periodontitis in beagle dogs with an erbium laser or with an ultrasonic power-driven device. Both treatment groups exhibited new cementum formation with embedded collagen fibers. The investigators concluded that both therapies supported the formation of new connective tissue attachment. Many other researchers (e.g., Rossmann, Israel, Froum, Cettny) have shown the CO_2 laser's ability to create a new connective tissue attachment, rather than a long junctional epithelium. CO_2 laser manufacturers have received FDA clearance under the 510(K) rule, showing equivalence to the laser-assisted new attachment procedure.

Again, technique in periodontal surgery for periodontitis depends on whether the clinician chooses to alter only soft tissue or both soft and hard tissue. Accurate pocket depth charting, radiographic evaluation, establishment of mobility patterns, and measurements of attached gingiva are required before all procedures.

Lasers in Flap Procedures

Practitioners perform periodontal flap procedures either exclusively or adjunctively with a laser. These procedures will be limited by clinician preference, case consideration, and laser equipment. Therefore an internal bevel incision may incorporate the general principles as discussed earlier for all lasers. Once the flap is reflected, lasers again can be used for sulcular debridement and deepithelialization on the inside of the flap. If root debridement will be done with a laser, it is strongly suggested that only an erbium laser be used, because of possible thermal damage with diode and Nd:YAG lasers. CO_2 lasers may be used according to the protocol of Crespi et al.[5,17] to increase fibroblast attachment to the root surface. When osseous surgery is necessary after flap reflection, again, it can be performed with erbium lasers or conventional instrumentation such as a high/slow-speed handpiece, diamond/carbide burs, and manual devices (e.g., chisel).

It must be noted that although they can cut bone, erbium lasers have not been universally accepted as instruments for this purpose. Oral and maxillofacial surgeons, who work extensively on osseous structures as well as soft tissue, have embraced the CO_2 wavelength for soft tissue treatment but typically do not favor the erbium wavelengths because of their rather slow speed in cutting osseous tissue.

Lasers in Treating the Failing Implant

Although dental endosseous root form implants have an excellent long-term success rate, various complications can result in their loss. A major contributor to failure of dental implants is periimplantitis.[39] Progressive osseous resorption in a failing implant may be due to a microbial inflammatory response or may have a mechanical component (e.g., excessive occlusal loading).[40]

Implant surfaces can become contaminated with microbial patterns similar to those for chronic periodontitis lesions.[41] In such cases, a variety of topographical features (e.g., screw-thread architecture) can present a significant clinical challenge in attempting to decontaminate the surface of a failing implant. Past therapies have consisted of local and systemic antibiotics, mechanical intervention (e.g., debridement), and surface treatments (e.g., with EDTA).[42] Regenerative therapies such as guided bone regeneration also have been used to reverse osseous resorption.[43]

Because good evidence suggests that various laser wavelengths have antimicrobial properties, clinicians have used laser technology to decontaminate failing implant surfaces (Figure 4-23). It is marginally predictable that a laser-treated surface will be free of microbial deposits, an organic smear layer, and a receptive surface for tissue regeneration.[44,45] Recent studies, however, demonstrate promise for use of CO_2, erbium-chromium–doped yttrium-scandium-gallium-garnet (Er,Cr:YSGG), and diode lasers of certain (but not all) wavelengths to repair the failing implant.[46-48] In vitro studies have used other laser wavelengths to determine the potential for charring of the implant surface or increased thermal changes to the implant itself.[49] Although consensus is lacking regarding the most effective wavelength for treating periimplantitis, evidence suggests that using laser technology can be a beneficial adjunct in reversing the failing implant. A complete discussion on the use of lasers for placement of implants and treatment of periimplantitis can be found in Chapter 7.

Conclusions

The laser is a versatile and valuable device to accomplish a myriad of periodontal procedures so long as the principles of fundamental wound healing are applied. Laser applications are associated with a drier operative field through improved hemostasis, with better visibility. Antibacterial properties of laser energy help sterilize the wound. With minimal collateral wound damage, results of surgical laser periodontics include decreased postoperative inflammation and a consequent decrease in patient discomfort. Overall, both the surgical wound and its outcome are more acceptable, with less contraction and scarring.

References

1. Romanos GE, Pelekanos S, Strub JR: A comparative histologic study of wound healing following Nd:YAG laser with different energy parameters and conventional surgical incision in rat skin: general clinical laser surgery, *J Clin Laser Med Surg* 13:11–16, 1995.
2. Strauss RA, Guttenberg SA: Lasers in oral and maxillofacial surgery, *Oral Maxillofac Surg Clin North Am* 16(2):xi–xii, 2004.
3. Catone G, Alling C: *Lasers in oral and maxillosurgery*, Philadelphia, 1997, Saunders.
4. Walinski CJ: Irritation fibroma removal: a comparison of two laser wavelengths, *Gen Dent* 52(3):236–238, 2004.
5. Crespi R, Romanos GE, Cassinelli C, Gherlone E: Effects of Er:YAG laser and ultrasonic treatment on fibroblast attachment to root surfaces: an in vitro study, *J Periodontol* 77:1217–1222, 2006.
6. Strauss RA, Fallon SD: Surgery, *Dent Clin North Am* 48(4):861–888, 2004.
7. Wigdor H, Walsh J, Featherstone JD, et al.: Lasers in dentistry, *Lasers Surg Med* 16:103–133, 1995.
8. Harris DM, Yessik M: Therapeutic ratio quantifies laser antisepsis: ablation of *Porphyromonas gingivalis* with dental lasers, *Surg Med* 35:206–213, 2004.
9. Gutknecht N, Radufi P, Franzen R, Lampert F: Reduction of specific microorganisms in periodontal pockets with the aid of an Nd:YAG laser: an in vivo study, *J Oral Laser Appl* 2:175–180, 2002.
10. Badersten A, Ninvelus R, Eglberg J: Effective nonsurgical periodontal therapy, *J Clin Periodontol* 12:351–359, 1985.
11. Rossmann J, McQuade M, Turunen D, et al.: Retardation of epithelial migration in monkeys using a carbon dioxide laser: an animal study, *J Periodontol* 63:902–907, 1992.
12. Schwarz F, Sculean A, Berakdar M, et al.: In vivo and in vitro effects of an Er:YAG laser, a GaAlAs diode laser and scaling and root planing on periodontally diseased root surfaces: a comparative histologic study, *Lasers Surg Med* 32:359–366, 2003.
13. Schwarz F, Sculean A, Georg T, Becker J: Clinical evaluation of the Er:YAG laser in combination with an enamel matrix protein derivative for the treatment of intrabony periodontal defects: a pilot study, *J Clin Periodontol* 30:975–981, 2003.
14. Ting CC, Fukuda M, Watanabe T, et al.: Effects of Er, Cr: YSGG laser irradiation on the root surface: morphologic analysis and efficiency of calculus removal, *J Periodontol* 78(11):2156–2164, 2007.
15. Folwaczny M, Aggstaller H, Mehl A, Hickel R: Removal of bacterial endotoxin from root surface with Er:YAG laser, *Am J Dent* 16(1):3–5, 2003.
16. Aoki A, Miura M, Akiyama F, et al.: In vitro evaluation of Er:YAG laser scaling of subgingival calculus in comparison with ultrasonic scaling, *J Periodont Res* 35:266–277, 2000.
17. Crespi R, Barone A, Covani U, et al.: Effects of CO_2 laser treatment on fibroblast attachment to root surfaces: a scanning electron microscopy analysis, *J Periodontol* 73:1308–1312, 2002.
18. Fisher S, Frame J, Browe RM: A comparative histological study of wound healing following CO_2 laser and conventional surgical excision of canine buccal mucosa, *Arch Oral Biol* 28:287–291, 1983.
19. Cobb CM: Lasers in periodontics: a review of the literature, *J Periodontol* 77:545–564, 2006.
20. White JM, Gekelman D, Shin KB, et al.: *Lasers and dental soft tissues: reflections of our years of research. Lasers in dentistry*, Amsterdam, 2003, Elsevier Science. 13–19.
21. Livaditis GJ: Comparison of monopolar and bipolar electrosurgical modes for restorative dentistry: a review of the literature, *J Prosthet Dent* 86(4):390–399, 2001.
22. Miserendino L, Pick R: *Lasers in dentistry*, Chicago, 1995, Quintessence. 145–160.
23. Lanigan S: *Lasers in dermatology*, London, 2002, Springer-Verlag.
24. Haytac M, Ozcelik O: Evaluation of patient perceptions after frenectomy operations: a comparison of carbon dioxide laser and scalpel techniques, *J Periodontol* 77(11):1815–1819, 2006.
25. Kara C: Evaluation of patient perceptions of frenectomy: a comparison of Nd:YAG laser and conventional techniques, *Photomed Laser Surg* 26(2):147–152, 2008.
26. McDavid VG, Cobb CM, Rapley JW, et al.: Laser irradiation of bone. III. Long-term healing following treatment by CO_2 and Nd:YAG lasers, *J Periodontol* 72:174–182, 2001.
27. Fontana CR, Kurachi C, Mendonca CR, Bagnato VS: Temperature variation at soft periodontal and rat bone tissues during a medium-powered diode laser exposure, *Photomed Laser Surg* 22:519–522, 2004.
28. Sasaki KM, Aoki A, Ichinose S, et al.: Scanning electron microscopy and Fourier transformed infrared spectroscopy analysis of bone removal using Er:YAG and CO_2 lasers, *J Periodontol* 73:643–652, 2002.
29. Kimura Y, Yu DG, Fujita A, et al.: Effects of erbium, chromium YSGG laser irradiation on canine mandibular bone, *J Periodontol* 72:1178–1182, 2001.
30. Butler B: Personal communication, 2008.
31. American Academy of Periodontology: Parameters on chronic periodontitis with advanced loss of periodontal support, *J Periodontol* 71:856–858, 2000.
32. Beaumont RH, O'Leary TJ, Kafrawy AH: Relative resistance of long junctional epithelium adhesions and connective tissue attachments to plaque-induced inflammation, *J Periodontol* 55:213–223, 1984.
33. Magnusson I, Runstad L, Nyman S, Lindhe J: A long junctional epithelium: a locus minoris resistentiae in plaque infection? *J Clin Periodontol* 10:333–340, 1983.
34. Sculean A, Schwarz F, Berakdar M, et al.: Healing of intrabony defects with or without an Er:YAG laser, *J Clin Periodontol* 31:604–608, 2004.

35. Yukna RA, Carr RL, Evans GH: Histologic evaluation of an Nd:YAG laser–assisted new attachment procedure in humans, *Int J Periodont Restorative Dent* 27:577–587, 2007.

36. Magnusson I, Clark WB, Marks RG, et al.: Attachment level measurements with a constant force electronic probe, *J Clin Periodontol* 15:185–188, 1988.

37. Gibbs CH, Hirschfeld JW, Lee JG, et al.: Description and clinical evaluation of a new computerized periodontal probe: the Florida probe, *J Clin Periodontol* 15:137–144, 1988.

38. Schwarz F, Jeppsen S, Herten M, et al.: An immunohistochemical characterization of periodontal wound healing following non-surgical treatment with fluorescence controlled Er:YAG laser radiation in dogs, *Lasers Surg Med* 39:428–440, 2007.

39. Tonetti MS: Risk factors for osseodisintegration, *Periodontol 2000* 17:55–63, 1998.

40. Esposito M, Hirsch J, Lekholm U, Thomson P: Differential diagnosis and treatment strategies for biologic complications and failing implants: a review of the literature, *Int J Oral Maxillofac Implants* 14:473–490, 1999.

41. Mombelli A, van Oosten MA, Schurch E, Lang NP: The microbiota associated with successful or failing osseointegrated titanium implants, *Oral Microbiol Immunol* 2:145–151, 1987.

42. Klinge B, Gustafsson A, Berglundh T: A systematic review of the effect of anti-infective therapy on the treatment of periimplantitis, *J Clin Periodontol* 29(suppl 3):213–225, 2002.

43. Persson LG, Ericsson I, Berglundh T, Lindhe J: Guided bone regeneration in the treatment of periimplantitis, *Clin Oral Implants Res* 7:366–372, 1996.

44. Schwarz F, Nuesry E, Bieling K, et al.: Influence of an erbium, chromium–doped yttrium, scandium, gallium, and garnet (Er,Cr:YSGG) laser on the reestablishment of the biocompatibility of contaminated titanium implant surfaces, *J Periodontol* 77:1820–1827, 2006.

45. Huang HH, Chuang YC, Chen ZH, et al.: Improving the initial biocompatibility of a titanium surface using an Er,Cr:YSGG laser–powered hydrokinetic system, *Dent Mater* 23:410–414, 2007.

46. Romanos GE: Treatment of the peri-implant lesions using different laser systems, *J Oral Laser Appl* 2:75–81, 2002.

47. Miller RJ: Treatment of the contaminated implant surface using the Er,Cr:YSGG laser, *Implant Dent* 13:165–170, 2004.

48. Romanos GE, Nentwig GH: Regenerative therapy of deep peri-implant infrabony defects after CO_2 laser implant surface decontamination, *Int J Periodont Restorative Dent* 28:245–255, 2008.

49. Oyster DK, Parker WB, Gher ME: CO_2 lasers and temperature changes of titanium implants, *J Periodontol* 66:1017–1024, 1995.

5

Regenerative Laser Periodontal Therapy

ERICA KROHN JANY MIGLIORATI AND DANIEL SIMÕES DE ALMEIDA ROSA

This chapter discusses regenerative periodontal surgery and the use of laser light as an adjunct to regenerative therapy. An important use of lasers in regenerative periodontal surgery is the preparation or modification of the root surface to increase fibroblast attachment. Such preparation promotes regeneration of a fibroblast-mediated new attachment, rather than a long junctional epithelium.

Most forms of periodontal disease are plaque-associated disorders, so it is understood that surgical access procedures can be considered only as adjunctive to specific therapy. In other words, it is imperative to eliminate the causative condition to the extent possible before initiating the surgical phase of treatment. Periodontal diseases are plaque/biofilm-induced chronic inflammatory conditions. The etiology is infection; specific pathogens in supragingival plaque accumulate around the tooth and inside the periodontal pocket subgingivally. The host's susceptibility, manifested by an exaggerated inflammatory response, also is a factor in tissue breakdown. Periodontal pathogenic microorganisms in people with hyperinflammatory genotypes may amplify the local inflammatory response, which may result in the characteristic severe tissue destruction seen in patients with advanced periodontitis.

The increased inflammatory response to plaque accumulation in susceptible hosts increases overgrowth of opportunistic microbiota.[1] Furthermore, environmental and systemic risk factors, such as smoking and diabetes, can worsen the expression of periodontal disease.[2] Smokers and diabetic patients may respond poorly to conventional periodontal treatment. Therefore clinicians have been in search of new techniques to treat advanced periodontal diseases in patients with risk factors associated with an inadequate response to periodontal therapy.

Objectives of Periodontal Treatment

The *immediate* goal of periodontal treatment is to prevent, arrest, control, or eliminate periodontal disease. The ideal goal would be to promote healing through regeneration of lost form, function, esthetics, and comfort. When the ideal cannot be achieved, the *pragmatic* goal of therapy is to repair the damage resulting from disease. The *ultimate* goal of therapy is to sustain the masticatory apparatus, especially teeth, or their analogs, in a state of health.[3]

Achieving any of these goals requires addressing the infectious and inflammatory component of some types of periodontal disease. It is important to eliminate the potentially injurious microbes in plaque/biofilm and to achieve a shift from pathogenic to indigenous flora. Once the early microbial colonizers have been reestablished in the periodontal sulcus, the challenge is to maintain health through home oral hygiene and appropriate dental care at periodic recall appointments and to control the inflammatory response during periodontal treatment.

The clinical objectives of periodontal treatment, therefore, include the following:

- Less than 10% of sites with bleeding on probing
- No sites with probing pocket depths of 5 mm or deeper, preferably at 4 mm or less
- No furcation involvements of degree II or III

According to Haffajee et al.,[4] the elimination of a residual true pocket of 6 mm or greater in probing depth after active periodontal treatment is an important goal of periodontal therapy and aims at arresting further disease progression. Also, it is known that deep periodontal pockets remaining after treatment play a significant role in predicting future periodontal destruction.[5] Claffey et al.[6] suggested that patients with advanced periodontitis associated with multiple residual probing depths (≥6 mm at reevaluation) are at greater risk for developing sites with additional attachment loss than are patients with few such residual pocket depths.

On a biologic/histologic level, the objective of periodontal treatment is to slow down epithelial migration from the gingival margin into the periodontal pocket to promote new *connective tissue attachment* (CTA), instead of generation of a long junctional epithelium.[7]

In an animal study, Caton et al.[8] observed that even with different periodontal treatment modalities, the expected result—formation of new CTA—could not be achieved. The four regenerative treatments were root planing and soft tissue curettage; Widman flap surgery without bone grafting; Widman flap surgery with the placement of frozen autogenous red bone marrow and cancellous bone; and use of beta-tricalcium phosphate in intrabony defects. All of the results showed healing with a long junctional epithelium extending to or close to the same level as before treatment.

In another animal study, Caton and Nyman[9] examined the effect of the modified Widman flap procedure on the CTA level and supporting alveolar bone. Treatment of periodontal pockets using this procedure produced no gain in CTA and no increase in crestal bone height. In angular bony defects, a certain degree of "bone fill" was noted. However, this bone repair was never accompanied by new CTA. Therefore, despite significant previous efforts, researchers are still testing treatment modalities and new materials to achieve the goal of preventing periodontal healing by formation of long junctional epithelium.

Initial Therapy

The following are important steps of the initial periodontal therapy:
1. Oral examination and periodontal health examination
   - Probing pocket depths
   - Attachment level
   - Bleeding on probing
   - Mobility and furcation involvement
2. Radiographic examination that includes periapical and bitewing films
3. Intraoral examination that includes digital photographs
4. Study models for evaluation of the occlusion
5. Determination of a diagnosis (based on data collected) and an initial prognosis
6. Elimination of hopeless teeth and equilibration of occlusal structure

After collection of complete clinical and radiographic data, the next phase of periodontal treatment comprises plaque assessment, oral hygiene instruction, scaling and root planing (SRP), and then reevaluation, assessment of periodontal surgical needs, and maintenance recall appointments.

It is important to keep in mind that the critical determinant of the success of periodontal therapy is not the choice of treatment modality but the detailed thoroughness of the root surface debridement and the patient's standard of oral hygiene. Evidence supports SRP as an essential and effective component of therapy for a majority of inflammatory periodontal diseases.[3] (See Chapter 3 for a complete discussion on use of lasers as an adjunct therapy in this phase of treatment.) If periodontal health cannot be achieved by initial therapy, a surgical approach can be considered.

Periodontal Surgery

Rationale

As mentioned earlier, in assessing risk factors for individual teeth in periodontal patients, the presence of sites with a residual true periodontal pocket depth of 6 mm or deeper after active treatment is considered a strong factor in predicting future periodontal destruction.[4] Therefore an important goal of surgical periodontal therapy is to obtain a reduced pocket depth, to arrest further disease progression.[6] In periodontal health, a pocket is referred to as a *sulcus,* ranging from 1 to 3 mm in depth. Based on this guideline, one of the objectives of periodontal surgery is to provide access for proper instrumentation and cleaning of the root surface when root areas are difficult to reach. Selection of available surgical methods should be based on their potential to facilitate removal of subgingival deposits and self-performed plaque control, enhancing the long-term preservation of the periodontium.

Resective Surgery

Resective periodontal surgery is a technique used for pocket elimination. The objective is to facilitate debridement of root surfaces through access. Resective surgery is indicated for the removal of excessive soft periodontal tissue on the gingival margin (gingivectomy) in pseudopockets, or when there is no loss of attachment (as in gingivitis). It also is used to correct true periodontal pockets (with loss of attachment) in periodontitis when both the pocket epithelial lining and the inflamed connective tissue are removed to promote reattachment of connective tissue fibers to the root surface (see Chapter 4).

An undesirable consequence of periodontal treatment, whether surgical or nonsurgical, is recession of the gingival margin after healing. In severe cases of periodontitis, such recession may lead to poor esthetics in the anterior area of the dentition. It often is associated with surgical procedures of bone recontouring for the eradication of bone defects. Therefore researchers have sought other techniques to avoid or reduce the problems caused by recession. By applying regenerative surgical procedures, the lost periodontal attachment in bone defects can be restored.[10]

Regenerative Periodontal Therapy

In recent years the use of regenerative procedures to restore architecture and function of the lost periodontal apparatus has become more common. These procedures are specifically designed to restore those parts of the tooth-supporting apparatus that have been lost due to periodontitis.

Periodontal regeneration has been reported after a variety of surgical approaches involving root surface biomodification, placement of bone grafts or bone substitutes, and the use of organic or synthetic barrier membranes, or *guided tissue regeneration* (GTR). Evidence suggests that the use of bone grafts and GTR procedures are of equal clinical benefit in treating intraosseous defects. The treatment objective is to obtain shallow, maintainable pockets by reconstruction of the destroyed attachment apparatus, as well as to limit recession of the gingival margin.

Periodontal regeneration surgery is selected to obtain (1) an increase in the periodontal attachment of a severely compromised tooth; (2) a decrease in deep pocket depth to a more maintainable range; and (3) a reduction in the vertical and horizontal components of furcation defects. Current approaches, however, remain technique-sensitive, and clinical success requires application of meticulous diagnostic and treatment strategies.[11]

As stated in the proceedings of the 1996 World Workshop in Periodontics, the attachment of the tooth is considered to have been regenerated when new cementum with inserting collagen fibers has formed on the detached root surface. Regeneration of the periodontal supporting apparatus (periodontium) also includes regrowth of the alveolar bone. Procedures to restore lost periodontal support also have been described as "reattachment" or "new attachment" procedures. With current regenerative techniques, significant regeneration is obtained at localized sites on specific teeth. However, if complete regeneration is to become a reality, additional stimuli to enhance the regenerative process probably are needed and could be provided using combined procedures.[12]

Early Studies and Objectives

In clinically successful regenerative procedures in periodontology, including cases with significant growth of new alveolar bone, histologic examination may show an epithelial lining along the treated root surface, instead of deposition of new cementum.[13]

The search for techniques and materials to promote regeneration in the periodontium began as early as the 1970s, when researchers formulated the following hypothesis: If epithelium and gingival connective tissue were to be excluded from the healing surgical site, progenitor cells migrating from the periodontal ligament would have the potential to form new CTA.[14] Almost all available human histologic evidence to date, however, demonstrates healing by formation of a long junctional epithelium with no or minimal CTA.[3]

The rationale for achieving this goal is to remove the crestal epithelium, to stop migration of the epithelial tissue cells into the pocket. Regeneration could then occur at the expense of the periodontal ligament, with insertion of new fibers to the root surface. Thus removal of sulcular/pocket epithelium has been the foundation of several other treatment modalities, including subgingival curettage, the excisional new attachment procedure (ENAP), and the modified Widman flap procedure. All have the objective of setting up an environment for new CTA.[15-18]

Laser Types

Investigations into a predictable method of epithelial exclusion have applied the unique characteristics of the laser wound in periodontal therapy. Laser techniques can be an excellent adjunct to achieve this goal, and several laser wavelengths have been studied. Evidence of delayed epithelialization found in wounds created by a carbon dioxide (CO_2) laser of 10.6-μm wavelength, for example, emerged from a series of animal and human studies. Earlier animal trials showed the ability of the CO_2 laser to retard epithelial downgrowth after periodontal surgery for up to 14 days,[19]

confirming that use of the CO_2 laser can remove epithelium from the gingiva without causing underlying damage to the connective tissue.[20,21] An early clinical study performed with the CO_2 laser evaluated whether deepithelialization with this type of laser at flap surgery and at 10-day intervals over the first 30 days of healing had the potential to enhance CTA formation. The deepithelialization was repeated on the test side at 10, 20, and 30 days postsurgically. This interval was determined on the basis of knowledge that regeneration of epithelial tissue occurs in 10 to 14 days, when it begins to grow into the pocket, lining the soft tissue wall of the new sulcus. The laser-treated side in one patient showed a fill with CTA and with some repair cementum, which was not seen in control subjects.[22] This preliminary clinical finding led to other laser studies.

The use of a pulsed CO_2 laser to deepithelialize the gingival flaps is an attempt to exclude epithelial cells from the healing wound.[21] This approach has been used with and without the benefit of GTR membranes. Other results from human studies and case reports combined with animal trials indicate a positive benefit in wound healing with the laser deepithelialization technique.[23]

Another clinical study compared conventional periodontal surgery combined with the use of CO_2 laser and conventional periodontal surgery alone with respect to epithelial elimination and degree of necrosis of mucoperiosteal flaps. The results confirmed that (1) a more complete removal of sulcular epithelium was obtained with CO_2 laser than with scalpels and (2) the CO_2 laser technique effectively removes the oral and sulcular epithelium from a gingival flap without damaging the viability of the flap during wound healing.[21]

Some investigators believe that this technique has shown significantly better results than those obtained through conventional osseous grafting alone, and appears to be comparable in efficacy with GTR procedures using barrier membranes. This concept provides a paradigm shift from the conventional use of GTR therapy by acknowledging the difficulty in controlling epithelium during the early wound healing process. It also allows a more comprehensive therapy for periodontal disease that addresses the generalized nature of the condition, with concurrent treatment of multiple lesions in an economical manner. In the patient presenting with generalized advanced periodontal disease, several defects could be treated definitively in one quadrant using the laser deepithelialization technique, without the need for multiple membrane therapies.[23]

Understanding the benefits of the laser light in delaying epithelial growth into the periodontal sulcus during the healing process requires consideration of the wound healing mechanism after laser use. With the pulsed CO_2 laser, for example, researchers have found that this wavelength can create a unique wound in the gingival tissues. The mechanism is not a burn but rather an instantaneous vaporization of the intracellular fluid with resultant disintegration of the cell structure.[24] Laser wounding in skin, mucous membrane,[25] and gingiva causes a delay in reepithelialization because of factors such as reduced inflammatory response and less wound contraction.[26] To explain further the delay in CO_2 laser wound epithelialization, previous studies have proposed the following combination of events:

1. Laser wound margins show thermal necrosis and formation of a firm eschar that impedes epithelial migration.[27]
2. Decrease in wound contraction (caused by fewer myofibroblasts at wound site) compared with scalpel wounds leaves a greater surface area remaining to be epithelialized.[28]
3. The thin layer of denatured collagen found on the surface of the laser wound acts as an impermeable dressing in the immediate postoperative period, which reduces the degree of tissue irritation from oral contents.[29]
4. Reduced inflammation in the laser-induced wound may provide less stimulation for epithelial migration.[30]

The coagulation necrosis produced by pulsed CO_2 laser irradiation with relatively low fluence does not disturb this repair process but rather promotes its steady progress and subsequent tissue remodeling.[31] Regarding its application on skin, the pulsed CO_2 laser is capable of bloodless skin ablation with improved wound healing at relatively low irradiance (2 W). Increasing the repetition rate (100 Hz) of the CO_2 laser helps to achieve a better surgical outcome. This laser may be a valuable instrument for ablation of skin and skin lesions when used in a pulsed mode.[32]

On the basis of the effects of the pulsed CO_2 laser on the periodontal soft tissue wall, the U.S. Food and Drug Administration (FDA) has given clearance for all periodontal applications to some CO_2 laser manufacturers. The clearances are for sulcular debridement and a laser-assisted new attachment procedure, a regenerative technique for periodontal pocket elimination, referred to as "cementum–mediated periodontal ligament new attachment to the root surface in the absence of long junctional epithelium." Of note, these CO_2 lasers are the "conventional" 10,600-nm (10.6-μm) CO_2 devices. The 9300-nm CO_2 laser does not yet have such clearance, nor has peer-reviewed literature justifying its use been accumulated.

Other laser wavelengths have been used on the periodontal soft tissue wall. One manufacturer of a neodymium-doped yttrium-aluminum-garnet (Nd:YAG) laser received FDA clearance for a laser-assisted new attachment procedure.

Because the histologic features of the new healed interface between the soft tissues and the root had not been elucidated, Yukna et al.[33] conducted a study to evaluate wound healing after a laser-assisted new attachment procedure in periodontal pockets. A free-running pulsed Nd:YAG laser was used to treat six single-rooted teeth with moderate to advanced chronic periodontitis associated with subgingival calculus deposits. After 3 months, all treated teeth were removed en bloc for histologic processing. Probing depth reductions and clinical gains in probing attachment level (PAL) were greater for the laser-assisted new attachment procedure–treated teeth than for the control teeth. All laser-assisted new attachment procedure–treated specimens showed new cementum and CTA in, and occasionally coronal to, the bur notch on the root. In the control specimens, five of the six teeth exhibited a long junctional epithelium with no evidence of new attachment or regeneration. There was no evidence of any adverse histologic changes around the laser-assisted new attachment procedure specimens.

These findings support the concept that in clinical practice, a laser-assisted new attachment procedure can be associated with cementum-mediated new CTA and apparent periodontal regeneration of diseased root surfaces.[33] As indicated by current evidence, the pulsed CO_2 and free-running Nd:YAG laser wavelengths are those best supported by the literature for the laser-assisted new attachment procedure. More histologic proof is needed to provide further rationale for use of the free-running Nd:YAG wavelength.

Biomodification of Root Surface

For years, research has been directed at finding novel means of conditioning or altering the periodontitis-involved root surfaces and of preparing them to promote the formation of a new CTA from periodontal ligament cells.

In 1976 Melcher[14] suggested that the type of cell that repopulates the root surface after periodontal surgery determines the nature of the attachment that will form. Ideally, healing of the periodontium should occur from the activity of periodontal ligament cells, which have the potential to form a new CTA, proof of which was recently provided using a novel and unique experimental model in dogs.[34] The purpose of this study was to explore the formation of periodontal tissues around titanium implants. After resection of the crowns of the maxillary canine teeth in nine mongrel dogs, the roots were hollowed to a depth of 5 mm, leaving a thin dentinal wall. Slits were prepared in the cavity wall to create passages from the chamber to the periodontal ligament area. A custom-made titanium implant was placed into the center of each chamber. Machined, titanium plasma–sprayed (TPS) and sandblasted with large grit and acid–attacked (SLA) surfaces were used. A collagen barrier was placed over the submerged chamber. After 4 months of healing, jaw sections were processed for histologic analysis. Newly formed periodontal ligament, alveolar bone, and root cementum filled the space between the implant and the wall of the chamber. Ingrown bone was in contact with neither dentin nor the implant. Thus an interposed soft connective tissue layer was present. Healing by fibrous encapsulation was observed around most implants. As confirmed in this study, strong evidence shows that the progenitor cells for periodontal attachment formation reside in the periodontal ligament and not in the alveolar bone as previously assumed.

Over the years, studies have evaluated several aspects of root surface preparation, starting with simple removal of bacterial deposits, calculus, and endotoxins. It has been well established that these essential steps to support the healing process should be part of initial periodontal therapy. More sophisticated studies, in animal models, showed improved healing response on histologic preparations after citric acid and tetracycline root surface demineralization.[35,36] Additional animal studies demonstrated adverse outcomes with the use of citric acid, such as root resorption and ankylosis.[37,38] In humans, studies have demonstrated histologic new CTA after citric acid demineralization of root surfaces.[39] Other studies showed no statistical difference in clinical conditions after flap surgery when comparing control surfaces with citric acid–treated roots.[40,41] Citric acid and tetracycline for root preparation are rarely used at present because of the contradictory clinical outcomes reported.[11]

Biomodification of the root surface with demineralization achieved through application of ethylenediaminetetraacetic acid (EDTA) followed by a preparation of enamel matrix proteins, Emdogain (EMD), during surgery has been introduced to accomplish regeneration of periodontal tissues. The biologic concept is that the enamel matrix proteins (amelogenins) may promote periodontal regeneration by inducing conditions mimicking events that took place during development of the periodontal tissues.[42,43] It is unclear, however, how this concept stands in accordance with current knowledge about periodontal wound healing, because no evidence shows that the cells derived from the periodontal ligament are those cells encouraged to repopulate the root surface after treatment.[11]

The use of EMD in periodontal regeneration strategies has been extensively studied, with conflicting results. Some trials show ankylosis and root resorption.[44] A recent in vitro study failed to confirm that EMD has any significant effect on periodontal ligament cell proliferation.[45] Better results with the use of EMD appear in case series showing 70% bone fill in intrabony defects and 4 to 4.5 mm of gain in clinical attachment.[46,47] Additional clinical and radiographic evidence showed larger amounts of *probing attachment level* (PAL) gains and statistically significantly more bone gain using EMD versus open-flap debridement only.[48,49]

Compared with GTR, EMD showed similar results for *clinical attachment level* (CAL) gain and PAL gain.[50-53] Further studies evaluated EMD in combination with some bone graft materials, with achievement of clinical improvement.[54-56]

Other investigations failed to demonstrate a beneficial effect of this combined treatment.[57] On the basis of studies with EMD, histologic evidence of new cementum formation can be observed, with collagen fibers inserting into a previously periodontitis-affected root surface and the formation of new alveolar bone in human specimens.[51,58]

Growth regulatory factors for periodontal regeneration may represent a potential aid in attempts to encourage regeneration of the periodontium. Such products include platelet-derived growth factor (PDGF) and insulin-like growth factor (IGF). Some studies show that control sites treated without growth factors healed with a long junctional epithelium and no new cementum or bone formation, whereas regeneration of a periodontal attachment apparatus occurred at the sites treated with growth factors.[59-65]

As stated earlier, creation of surgical access should be considered only as an adjunct to cause-related therapy. A primary rationale for raising a flap is to provide access for proper instrumentation and cleaning of the root surface. If these procedures cannot be done because of tooth anatomy, flap surgery should be considered only after as much of the etiologic agents of the periodontal disease are removed by closed techniques. Case Studies 5-1 and 5-2, with Figures 5-1 and 5-2, respectively, illustrate these points.

CLINICAL TIP

The deepithelialization of the gingival margin of the flap should be performed *after* (not before) suturing. Occasionally, deepithelialization of the flap may cause slight shrinkage of the tissue; if the tissue is deepithelialized before suturing, it may be difficult to gain primary closure.

CASE STUDY 5-1

Pocket Biomodification

The medical history for a 47-year-old female patient requiring pocket modification includes lupus, hypothyroidism, hypertension, and osteopenia, all of which are being controlled with medications. The only medication of clinical relevance to her dental condition is alendronate (Fosamax), 70 mg once weekly.

Figure 5-1A shows a preoperative view of the affected tissue. After conventional SRP, a laser was used to deepithelialize the marginal gingiva, as shown in Figure 5-1B. The reason for this initial step is based on sound biologic principles: In order for a true fibroblast-mediated soft tissue reattachment to the root surface to occur, the epithelium must be prevented from migrating into the pocket. Removal of the marginal epithelium will prevent such migration.

Once the marginal epithelium has been removed, the laser tip is then placed into the pocket parallel to the long axis of the root. The purpose of this step is the reduction or elimination of bacteria (removal of the etiologic agent) from the pocket (see Figure 5-1C). The various protocols for the depth of placement of the laser into the pocket depend on the wavelength used, manufacturer's suggestions, and other criteria. It is important to recognize that some protocols do not address removal of the marginal epithelium before entering the pocket.

Besides the biologic rationale just discussed, the marginal epithelium is removed before laser placement because otherwise,

placing the laser into the pocket is a "blind" procedure; the clinician is not able to see the laser-tissue interaction. For this step, the following considerations are paramount:
- Is there insufficient laser energy to perform its intended therapeutic effect?
- Is there too much laser energy, so that the laser is actually incising the tissue, rather than simply removing the epithelial layer?

There is no way to monitor the laser-tissue interaction unless the clinician can visualize the interaction. Removing the crestal epithelium allows the clinician to see the laser-tissue interaction—the response of the tissue to the laser parameters used—and to possibly modify the laser parameters accordingly. Without this step, as noted, laser tip placement is a blind procedure, with the potential to cause adverse effects on the internal tissue wall.

Figure 5-1D shows the 1-week postoperative view after laser treatment of the upper right quadrant, as well as the immediate postoperative view after laser treatment of the upper left side. Figure 5-1E shows the upper left quadrant immediately after laser treatment. Figure 5-1F shows the 1-month postoperative clinical view. Figure 5-1G shows the preoperative charting, and Figure 5-1H shows the 1-month postoperative charting.

Comparison of Four Lasers: Effects on Root Surfaces and Wound Healing

Lasers have multiple uses in periodontal therapy. This section reviews the current evidence on four different wavelengths and their application in regenerative procedures. Most reported studies used the CO_2 laser, the Nd:YAG laser, the erbium family of lasers, and to a lesser extent the diode lasers.[66] Lasers can be used for root surface biomodification in promoting ligament cell reinsertion or creating a proper surface for reattachment. The modification of cementum and dentin is wavelength-dependent and is discussed for each laser.

CASE STUDY 5-2

Furcation and Biomodification

Surgical access was necessary because of an anatomic problem in a 52-year-old man with no relevant medical history. Figure 5-2A shows an upper left second molar with a diseased furcation. Periodontal probing of the furcation is 10 mm. Because of the fluting and curvature of the mesiobuccal root distally toward the furcation, and the distobuccal root mesially toward the furcation, it was impossible to use conventional instrumentation in this patient to remove the etiological factors.

Figure 5-2B shows the surgical site after elevation of a flap. Exposure of the root surfaces showed a ball of diseased tissue in the furcation, firmly adherent to the roots. After conventional instruments (curettes) were used to remove the bulk of the diseased tissue, a laser was applied to remove the remnants of soft tissue from the root surface and also for biomodification of the root surface to promote attachment of fibroblasts.

Figure 5-2C shows the root surface after laser biomodification. The inner surface of the flap was then deepithelialized. Once again, the purpose of removing the epithelium from the flap is to allow the growth of a fibroblast-mediated soft tissue attachment to the biomodified root surface. Bone analog was placed in the furcation and the flap was sutured into place. The laser was then used to deepithelialize the gingival margin of the flap. The patient was sent home with routine postoperative instructions. At 9 days postoperatively, the patient returned to the office, where the sutures were removed and the flap margin was again deepithelialized. At 19 days the patient returned once more for additional deepithelialization of the gingival margin.

The rationale for three sessions of deepithelialization (on the day of surgery and then at 9 days and 19 days postoperatively) is based on sound biologic principles. The work of Rossmann, Centty, Israel, and their co-workers[19-23] has shown that removal of epithelium at 10-day intervals over the first 30 days enhances a soft tissue attachment.

Figure 5-2D shows the surgical site with a fully healed furcation 90 days postoperatively.

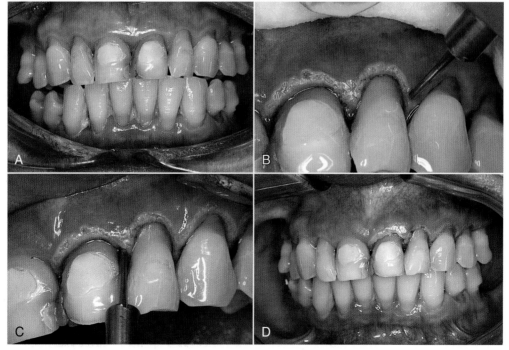

• **Figure 5-1** Laser biomodification of periodontal pocket. **A,** Preoperative view of affected tissue. **B,** *Step 1*: Laser deepithelialization of gingival margin. Note that this is not a cutting procedure; gingival height is not reduced, and no tissue is incised or excised. Surface epithelium is removed so that it does not interfere with formation of a fibroblast-mediated soft tissue attachment. **C,** *Step 2*: Reduction of bacterial contents in periodontal pocket. Laser tip is placed parallel to the long axis of the root. **D,** One-week postoperative view after laser treatment in upper right quadrant and immediate postoperative view after laser treatment of upper left side.

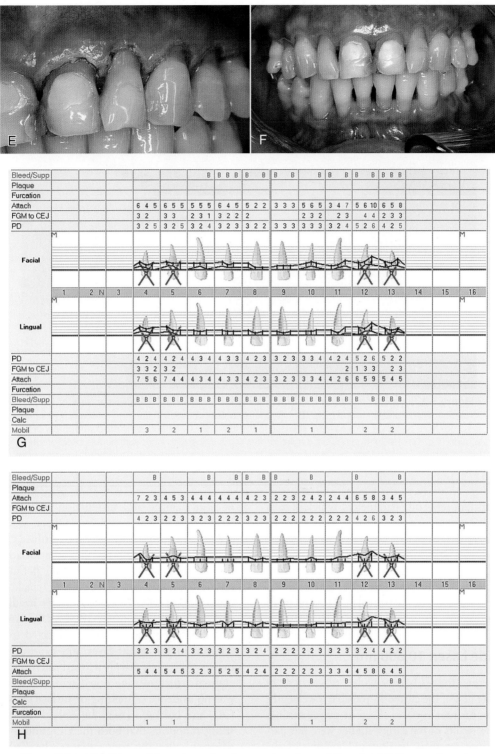

• **Figure 5-1, cont'd** **E,** Immediate postoperative close-up view of upper left quadrant. **F,** One-month postoperative view. **G,** Preoperative periodontal charting. **H,** Periodontal charting 1 month after final treatment session.

The mineral component of both cementum and dentin is a carbonated hydroxyapatite that demonstrates intense absorption bands in the mid-infrared region of the light spectrum. Consequently, of the lasers of various wavelengths studied, the Er:YAG laser appears to be the instrument of choice for effective removal of calculus, for root etching, and for creation of a biocompatible surface for cell or tissue reattachment.[66,67] Research indicates that its safety and effects might be expected to be within the range reported for conventional mechanical debridement.[68]

A meaningful comparison between various clinical studies or between laser and conventional therapy is difficult at best and probably impossible at present. Reasons include different laser wavelengths; wide variations in laser

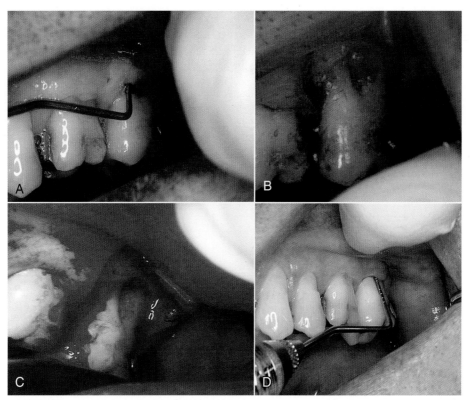

• **Figure 5-2** Surface biomodification in laser treatment of furcation. **A,** Preoperative view of furcation involvement on maxillary second molar. **B,** Intraoperative view of exposed furcation after a flap has been elevated. Note presence of diseased soft tissue in the furcation. **C,** Immediate postoperative view of the surgical site. Diseased tissue has been ablated from the surgical site. Root surface has been prepared for a fibroblast-mediated soft tissue attachment. **D,** Three-month postoperative view of the surgical site shows excellent healing. The furcation can no longer be probed. (**A** and **D** courtesy Dr. Robert Convissar.)

parameters; insufficient reporting parameters, which in turn do not allow calculation of energy density; differences in experimental design; lack of proper controls; variable severity of disease and treatment protocol; and measurement of different clinical end points. Despite these problems and the lack of clinical trials, sufficient data are available to recognize trends in the results of laser-mediated treatment of chronic periodontitis.[67]

Carbon Dioxide Laser: 10,600 nm

In chronologic terms, the CO_2 laser with a wavelength of 10,600 nm was the first of the currently available wavelengths studied for effects on root surfaces. Even at power settings as low as 4 W, the results of the earlier studies were not particularly encouraging, in that charring and melting of the root surface were common side effects. In addition, Fourier-transformed infrared spectroscopy analysis of charred surfaces revealed the presence of cyanamide and cyanate, both cytotoxic chemical residues.[69,70] However, the parameters used in these early studies, as well as the temporal emission mode, were completely different from parameters used today. These early studies used a continuous-wave CO_2 laser, which is known to damage hard tissues more than pulsed CO_2 laser mode.

Another issue is water cooling. It is important to use irrigation during CO_2 laser application, to avoid collateral zones of heat damage and production of toxic substances.[69-71] Israel et al.[71] compared three laser wavelengths—CO_2, Nd:YAG, and Er:YAG—for root surface changes after irradiation with and without air/water surface cooling. Those changes included cavitation defects, globules of melted and resolidified mineral, surface crazing (cracking), and production of a superficial char layer after irradiation with CO_2 and Nd:YAG. By contrast, the Er:YAG laser produced root surface changes that might be expected from acid etching: removal of the smear layer and exposure of the collagen matrix. Although sharply defined microfractures of the mineralized structure were noted with the Er:YAG laser, there was no evidence of melting or surface char, unlike with the CO_2 and Nd:YAG lasers. In view of the parameters of this study, it appears that both the CO_2 and the Nd:YAG lasers adversely alter the root surface. The Er:YAG laser, however, when used at low energy densities, shows sufficient potential for root surface modification to warrant further investigation.

Barone et al.[72] showed that heat-induced cracking of the root surface occurs when the CO_2 laser is used at power settings of 4 W or greater in a continuous-wave mode. However, when used with a pulsed wave in a defocused mode and at low power settings, the CO_2 laser appears to cause minimal damage. Although both laser delivery modes produced changes to the treated root surface specimens, the changes from a defocused beam created a smooth surface, which may present an advantage in periodontal treatment.[72] By contrast, when used in continuous mode, the CO_2 laser (0.5 W, 20 sec continuous circular movements) creates a molten, recrystallized (nonporous, glazed) surface on root dentin, with the tubules almost completely sealed.[73]

It can be concluded, therefore, that using the CO_2 laser is safe in pulsed mode, in the vicinity of root surfaces, for accomplishing bacterial reduction in the periodontal pocket, for example, so long as this laser wavelength is used with low power settings, controlled time of delivery, water coolant spray, and parallel direction of the beam in relation to the root. This conclusion underscores that one of the most important determinants in choosing laser wavelength or manufacturer should be the amount of initial training and education provided for the purchaser, as well as continuing education. With all laser wavelengths, using the correct parameters is critical to the success of the procedure.

After root planing, a surface smear layer containing remnants of dental calculus, contaminated root cementum, bacterial endotoxins, and subgingival plaque invariably covers the instrumented root surface. Studies have investigated alternatives to compensate for the limitations of mechanical root therapy. Crespi et al.[74] found that the resultant root surface had areas devoid of cementum, with completely sealed dentinal tubules. The dentin surface appeared as a melted layer showing a flat, smooth surface with apparent fusion of the smear layer. The dentin layer had the appearance of a glazed surface. No residual bacteria were observed on any roots after CO_2 laser irradiation. Other investigations have shown that the CO_2 laser used in a pulsed defocused mode and at low power settings (1.0 sec at 3 W) completely removed the smear layer, leaving partially exposed dentinal tubules with minimal change in their diameter. Root surface modifiers (e.g., EDTA, citric acid) also were effective in removing the smear layer, but the exposed dentinal tubules showed funnel-shaped widening.[75]

Irradiation with the CO_2 laser, used at low power and in the defocused mode, combined with traditional mechanical instrumentation, could improve root surface debridement of periodontally involved teeth. Open dentinal tubules are a goal in periodontal treatment for optimal reinsertion of new connective tissue fibers to enhance regeneration of lost periodontal attachment.

Recent studies of the biocompatibility of the CO_2 laser with root surfaces show conflicting results, even at low energy densities. Crespi et al.[76] and Pant et al.[77] reported increased in vitro attachment of fibroblasts to laser-treated surfaces compared with control surfaces (with SRP only) or chemically treated surfaces. However, Fayad et al.[78] reported a total lack of fibroblast attachment to surfaces irradiated at only 1.25 mJ/pulse.

Regarding the periodontal soft tissue wall, Gopin et al.[79] evaluated soft tissue attachment to root surfaces after CO_2 laser irradiation in an animal model. After mucoperiosteal flaps were raised, each laser-treated root surface was irradiated until a confluent char layer was visually evident. The settings and parameters were 6 W, 20 Hz, and pulse length of 0.01 second; energy density of approximately 240 J/cm^2; and distance of 2 mm from the target surface, with a focal spot diameter of 0.8 mm. This application promoted a cytotoxic char layer on the root surfaces. Within areas of charring, histologic examination revealed a lack of flap reattachment to the root surface. However, all specimens treated by SRP alone or by laser irradiation followed by SRP exhibited flap reattachment to treated surfaces. These findings led to the clinical use of pulsed CO_2 laser irradiation as an adjunctive modality, along with SRP, in treatment of periodontal pockets.

Regarding the use of the CO_2 laser on bone, in an animal model, osteotomy defects induced by laser (versus rotary bur) exhibited a delayed healing response, apparently related to residual char in the bony tissue.[80] The healing response was severely delayed even with use of a surface cooling spray of air/water.[81] It can be concluded, therefore, that the CO_2 wavelength is not appropriate for use on osseous tissue.[80,81]

Whether the final laser result on dental/periodontal tissues is favorable or damaging, most studies do not mimic the clinical scenario in their material and methods. Therefore the parameters and settings tested in laboratory trials should be evaluated and adapted before clinical application. Important aspects to observe in material and methods in all laser studies are (1) settings and parameters (power density, watts, hertz, exposure time), (2) delivery system, (3) delivery mode, (4) direction of the beam, and (5) use of water cooling.

Besides the physical radiation parameters, the parameters of clinical handling, particularly the angulations of the application tip and hand speed on moving the laser through the pocket, strongly influence the root substance preparation.[82] In a 2007 pilot study, Mullins et al.[83] tested a manufacturer's suggested parameter to treat the periodontal pockets in patients diagnosed with advanced chronic periodontitis. The purpose was to evaluate, by scanning electron microscopy (SEM), the surface effects of a third-generation CO_2 laser (of 10,600-nm wavelength) treatment on the root surfaces and soft tissues and to investigate the effects of this "ultraspeed" laser on periodontal pathogenic bacteria compared with negative control specimens. A one-time irradiation by CO_2 laser at a power of 2.2 W, 50 Hz, 80-msec pulse length, and exposure rate of 1 mm per 5 sec was applied in the periodontal pockets. Data obtained on DNA analysis of eight periodontal bacteria in samples collected from laser-treated and control sites before and immediately after treatment were compared between groups. In addition, block biopsy specimens, including soft tissue, were harvested. SEM examination of test group specimens showed heat damage on the soft tissues in 3 of 17 specimens (17.6%). In addition, 11.7% (2 of 17) of the CO_2 laser–treated teeth exhibited localized slight damage to root surfaces. Microbiologic analysis results for the control sites indicated that 90.6% of the bacterial counts remained the same, 6% increased, and 3% decreased. In the test group, 71.25% of the bacterial counts for the eight different periodontal microbes remained the same, 12.50% increased, and 16.25% decreased.

The study concluded that a one-time use of this particular CO_2 laser in periodontal pockets does not sterilize or substantially reduce subgingival bacterial populations compared with negative control specimens.[83] The damage seen on the root surface of laser-treated teeth can be explained by the excessive time of application. The recommendation is to move the delivery tip in the subgingival area at an exposure rate of 1 mm per 1 sec, for a total time of 16 sec per side of the tooth in a molar area, for example, with reduction in application time for narrow teeth (mandibular anteriors). Regarding the microbiologic results, the lack of pocket "sterilization" may be affected by several variables (e.g., contamination with saliva). However, the investigators agreed that it is unlikely, although unproved, that any significant amount of residual microbial DNA can survive laser irradiation with resulting temperatures in excess of 100° C.

Another conclusion from this investigation is that a one-time use of this CO_2 laser in periodontal pockets did not substantially reduce subgingival bacterial populations.[83] It is therefore the manufacturer's recommendation to repeat the procedure in the periodontal pocket, in cases of moderate to advanced periodontitis, every 7 to 10 days for at least three visits. Again, it must be emphasized that use of the correct laser parameters as well as the correct treatment protocols is critical to the success of the procedure.

An important point in this context is that all of the CO_2 laser studies have been carried out with the 10,600-nm wavelength device. The recently introduced 9300-nm CO_2 has not yet been the subject of any published results on periodontal treatment. Of note, extrapolation of the results from one CO_2 wavelength to another is poor science and never holds up in the face of scrutiny.

Neodymium-Doped Yttrium-Aluminum-Garnet Laser

Since the 1990s, clinical case reports have shown favorable results with the Nd:YAG laser (1064 nm) in periodontology, increasing the interest of clinicians in this wavelength.[84] Early studies looked at removal of periodontal pocket epithelium with a laser. In 1994, Gold and Vilardi[85] showed that the pulsed Nd:YAG laser can remove pocket epithelial lining in moderately deep pockets at 1.25 to 1.75 W of power and 20 Hz. Most samples showed a complete removal of epithelium, with no damage to the underlying connective tissue. In other studies, microbiologic analysis of laser-treated periodontal pocket samples showed a posttreatment reduction in the levels of bacterial types tested—*Aggregatibacter actinomycetemcomitans* (*Aa*) (previously *Actinobacillus actinomycetemcomitans*); *Tannerella forthysia* (*Tf*), formerly *Bacteroides forsythus* (*Bf*); *Porphyromonas gingivalis* (*Pg*); and *Treponema denticola* (*Td*)—compared with pretreatment levels and control specimens.[86-89] In vitro investigations confirmed the finding that the pulsed Nd:YAG laser was able to ablate *Pg* without visible effect on blood agar plates.[90] The 810-nm diode laser destroyed both the pathogen and the gel, indicating that the pulsed Nd:YAG may selectively destroy pigmented pathogens, leaving the surrounding tissue intact.[91]

Reported clinical cases of laser ENAP (i.e., excisional new attachment procedure) demonstrated improved clinical measurements and radiographic evidence of bone regeneration in the areas treated.[92,93] The Nd:YAG laser requires lower doses of infiltration analgesia and promotes better control of operative and postoperative bleeding than that achievable with scalpel surgery.[94] Tissue necrosis was related to laser exposure time, type of laser delivery tip (fiber), and applied laser energy. The most homogeneous and extensive coagulation zone was seen after laser treatment with rather low laser energy applied over a longer period.[95]

Another consideration is the effect of the laser light on root surfaces and bone. In 1996, Radvar et al.[96] showed that the Nd:YAG laser applied in the periodontal pocket caused no damage to the root surface with settings of 50 and 80 mJ, delivery time of 3 min, and orientation of the laser tip parallel to the root surface. However, time of application in the pocket was excessive, with consequent damage to soft tissues. Therefore no improvement was noted on soft tissues treated with the Nd:YAG laser, using these parameters, compared with non–laser-treated control tissues.

Another conclusion in this study is that bacterial reduction can be achieved with SRP and that laser irradiation alone without SRP is not the best treatment option.[96] The combination of lasers with mechanical debridement produces the best results for bacterial reduction, as confirmed by the 1997 investigation of Neill and Mellonig.[87]

Regarding attachment of cultured fibroblasts, several in vitro and in vivo studies showed that applying the Nd:YAG laser to the root surface (per trial settings and delivery time) was damaging to the root surface with less attachment of cultured fibroblasts.[69,97-100] In 1994, Thomas et al.[101] evaluated in vitro the effects of the Nd:YAG laser either alone or combined with root planing or air-powder abrasive treatment on fibroblast attachment to nondiseased root surfaces. The root segments were randomly assigned to four treatment groups: control, laser-only treatment, laser treatment followed by root planing, and laser treatment followed by air-powder abrasive treatment. Laser-treated root specimens were exposed for 1 minute with energy of 75 mJ at 20 pulses/sec using a 320-μm contact fiber. The contact fiber was held parallel to the root segments, which were kept moist with distilled water. The decreased fibroblast attachment observed in the laser-only treatment group suggests a laser-induced biologic incompatibility of the root surface. Observed surface alterations included ablation of cementum with exposure of dentinal tubules and crater formation. In cell counts of fibroblasts attached to specimens, the greatest difference was observed between control (higher attachment) and laser surfaces (lower attachment). However, increased numbers of fibroblasts were seen attached to the laser-treated root segments after root planing or after exposure to an air-powder abrasive, indicating that the laser-induced bioincompatibility is reversible and is most likely to represent a surface phenomenon.

Of interest, in this experiment the laser fiber was held parallel to the target tissue, which is similar to the current suggested clinical application for initial periodontal therapy. Also, removal of the toxic layer on the root surface after Nd:YAG laser application helps create a favorable environment for healing. This study by Thomas et al.[101] confirmed the 1992 findings of Trylovich et al.[100] However, the direction of the beam was perpendicular to the root surface for 1 minute in the latter study (Nd:YAG settings of 80 mJ at 10 Hz), and the organic matrix appeared to have been burned off, leaving a resolidified substance with a lavalike appearance.

In a 2005 in vitro study, Chen et al.[102] examined the long-term effect of Nd:YAG laser irradiation on cultured human fibroblasts. The power delivery was 50 mJ × 10 pps (pulses per second), at 0.5 W, with irradiation duration of 60, 120, 180, or 240 sec. The optical fiber of the laser was kept perpendicular to the root surface at 2 mm from the cell layer. Laser delivery was not static, a major innovation in this study; instead, a timed and controlled movement was used to cover the entire growth surface of the cell culture. The viability and collagen content of laser-irradiated human periodontal fibroblasts (hPFs) were assessed on day 5 after laser treatment using light microscopy and transmission electron microscopy (TEM). Thus, with fixed power output and different exposure time, it was possible to investigate the long-term effect of pulsed Nd:YAG laser on hPFs. The statistically significant decrease in cellular viability and collagen content was noted only in the cells irradiated at higher energy density, but even with power output of 0.5 W, some cell damage and decrease in collagen content occurred. These results suggest that the coexistence of viable cells and progressive degeneration of laser-damaged cells was associated with the in vitro mineralization of hPF cultures. Nd:YAG laser irradiation could induce the formation of mineralized deposits of hPF cells cultured in medium to differentiate further into osteoblast-like cells responsible for in vitro mineralization.[102]

These results were confirmed by another study in which Nd:YAG laser irradiation (20 mJ, 10 Hz, 10 sec) had a stimulatory effect on the cell viability and proliferation of human osteoblast-like cell culture.[103] Increases in the pulse energy, pulse repetition rate, and power output had an inhibitory effect on cell viability and proliferation.

The direction of the laser beam is a major factor in the control of damage to target tissues. Nd:YAG laser irradiation, even at low power settings (0.5 to 1.5 W), but with 1 minute of irradiation in a perpendicular direction of application, altered chemical organization of root structure proteins.[104] As with the diode laser, the Nd:YAG laser beam applied in a parallel direction, for example, produced root surface alterations that included fusion and resolidification of root dentin, with partial smear layer and debris removal at 1.5 W, 15 Hz (100 mJ), and 2 mm/sec.[105]

On the other hand, the Nd:YAG laser caused greater damage on calculus than on cementum or dentin,[106] and at 5 W, it is possible to remove the smear layer on root surface with small changes on the surface but with increased temperature.[107] Several in vitro studies[99,101] have demonstrated heat-induced morphologic changes on the root surface after irradiation with the Nd:YAG laser, ranging from low settings of 156.2 to 166.6 J/cm^2 to a high of 571 J/cm^2. However, even the lowest energy density used in some studies still resulted in melting of the mineral phase, as well as creation of craters and charring of root surfaces. Therefore Nd:YAG laser settings must be adjusted when adapted to an in vivo application.[67]

At least two in vitro studies performed in the early 1990s demonstrated that the Nd:YAG laser, when used at low energy densities or in a combination of low energy density and defocused beam, can remove root surface smear layers without causing collateral damage to underlying cementum or dentin or increasing temperatures to a level that might trigger irreversible pulpal damage.[107,108] Despite their effectiveness for laser smear layer removal, these parameters may not be appropriate for clinical use as an adjunct to conventional periodontal therapy because of the high power delivered (20 W) and distance of the laser beam from the target tissue (5 cm).

Another area of interest in periodontal treatment is the control of inflammatory cytokines with laser light. As mentioned earlier, the exaggerated inflammatory response in periodontitis increases the risk of breakdown. The cytokine interleukin-1 (IL-1), especially in the beta (β) form, has an important catabolic effect on bone tissue[109] and is implicated as the most potent known inducer of bone demineralization.[110] Therefore IL-1 may play a pivotal role in connective tissue remodeling and bone destruction during inflammatory disease, as well as in the pathogenesis of periodontal disease.[111] The purpose of the 1999 study by Liu et al.[112] was to evaluate the in vivo effects of Nd:YAG laser treatment on root surfaces when used alone or in combination with conventional SRP, through measurement of IL-1β levels in crevicular fluid in four different treatment groups, including ultrasonic scaling alone, laser alone, and combinations of treatment modalities. Results show that combined SRP followed by laser (group 4), or vice versa, laser followed by SRP (group 3), appeared to produce prolonged clinical improvement (in gingival index, clinical erythema, and edema) throughout the later periods of the study compared with laser therapy alone. The combination therapy groups (groups 3 and 4) also exhibited a greater reduction in mean crevicular fluid IL-1β in all periodontitis-affected sites than in the laser treatment–only group at 6 to 12 weeks. Of the four modalities tested, inclusion of SRP gave a superior IL-1β response compared with non-SRP therapies, and laser therapy followed by SPR resulted in a more prominent reduction of this cytokine. Differences in results with monotherapies (laser use alone versus ultrasonic scaling) were not statistically significant.[89]

The early studies demonstrating root damage used laser settings detrimental to tissues, with excessive exposure times. Consequently, the current clinical use of lasers applies parameters and settings that differ from those used in the initial clinical trials. It is now known that for bacterial reduction in the periodontal pocket or for root conditioning to occur, the outcome depends not only on the settings but also on duration of application and direction of the beam.[113] Distance from the target tissue also must be considered. For example, when used in contact mode, the laser systems tested produced tissue effects that were highly different from those achieved in noncontact mode. Health care providers performing laser treatments in close boundaries must be aware that changing from noncontact to contact mode in laser application greatly influences the resulting tissue effects.[114]

Relative to regeneration of periodontal supporting tissues, *laser-assisted new attachment procedure* is a novel technique that demonstrates consistently positive histologic responses in periodontal pockets in patients with a diagnosis of periodontitis treated with a free-running pulsed Nd:YAG laser. As discussed earlier, Yukna et al.[33] found apparent periodontal regeneration (in cementum, periodontal ligament, and alveolar bone) on a calculus and plaque–contaminated area of the root on two test teeth and cementum-mediated new attachment on the other four laser-treated teeth.

Diode Lasers

Surgical diode lasers have as their active medium various semiconductor solids, such as aluminum (Al) and gallium arsenide (GaAs). The generated electrical energy becomes the laser beam, emitted in the infrared part of the spectrum, as with the Nd:YAG laser wavelength. The main difference between the two is the light-generating mechanism, which makes the diode unit smaller and more economical.[115] The FDA cleared diodes for use in soft tissue surgery beginning in 1995 and for subgingival curettage in 1998.

Four surgical diode wavelengths are situated between 800 and 1064 nm. The delivery system is through optic fibers of different diameter, typically used in contact with tissues, in continuous-wave or gated-pulse mode. As with the Nd:YAG, the diode laser is highly absorbed by pigmented tissues and hemoglobin. The penetration coefficient is lower, the amount of heat generated higher, and the coagulation deeper (showing surface carbonization) with the diode than with the Nd:YAG laser. Of importance, the experimental results obtained with one diode laser wavelength must not be extrapolated to justify use of the other three wavelengths. The absorption coefficients for the various diode wavelengths in water are quite different, so their effects on soft tissue also will differ. Production of a specific effect or result with a particular diode wavelength does not mean that the other wavelengths will produce similar results.

The strongest indications for use of diode lasers are for management of soft tissues for incision, excision, and coagulation and control of bacterial growth in open wounds.[116] Another indication is for debridement in the periodontal pocket,[117] to address the infectious component of periodontitis.[118] Diode lasers with outputs of 500 mW or less are used in *low-level laser therapy* (LLLT) to provide biomodulation,[119] wound repair,[120,121] and pain relief[115] (see Chapter 15). Because other wavelengths are better suited for periodontal regenerative procedures in regard to root preparation,[122] little peer-reviewed information on use of diode lasers for this application is available.

Research on bacterial reduction with surgical diodes began in the middle to late 1990s. In a 1998 study, Moritz et al.[123] evaluated bacterial reduction after diode laser (805 nm) irradiation compared with SRP alone. Initial and final bacterial counts showed considerable bacterial reduction in the diode laser–irradiated groups, more accentuated for *Aggregatibacter actinomycetemcomitans* (*Aa*), formerly known as *Actinobacillus actinomycetemcomitans*. Also, clinical parameters were improved in the laser group, with more pronounced reduction in bleeding on probing and decrease in pocket depth. In an animal study[124] and in an in vitro–in vivo investigation, Fontana et al.[125] observed some positive laser effects on bacterial levels of *Prevotella* spp. and *Fusobacterium*. When applied at medium power and for controlled irradiation time, the diode laser did not induce temperature variation high enough to cause irreversible thermal damage to the periodontal tissues investigated, establishing thermally safe working parameters.[125] More recent data, however, show no statistically significant difference between the study and control groups, both in clinical aspects (reduced gingival inflammation) and in evaluation of pain during SRP. The conclusion was that using a diode laser as an auxiliary modality in SRP provided no apparent clinical benefit for teeth with shallow to moderate pockets.[126]

As discussed previously, one of the goals of periodontal therapy is to reduce bacterial deposits in the pockets and to enhance clinical attachment. To achieve healing through new CTA, it is necessary to prevent epithelial downgrowth during healing by removing epithelium in the periodontal pocket during SRP. In an animal model, Romanos et al.[127] used a diode laser (980 nm) to accomplish epithelial removal and compared results with those for conventional techniques. No epithelial remnants were found in any irradiated sections. The laser at low power was able to remove the thin pocket epithelium in the same way in all samples. By contrast, irradiation at high-power settings caused significant damage to the underlying connective tissues. The control sites, which were instrumented using conventional curettes, demonstrated significant epithelial remnants in all of the tissues. On histologic examination, instrumentation of the soft periodontal tissues with the 980-nm diode laser was found to lead to complete removal of epithelium, compared with conventional treatment with hand instruments.

A similar investigation in humans showed that applying the diode laser for treatment of inflammatory periodontitis at 1 W, in continuous-wave mode, with 10 sec of irradiation in the pocket, is a safe clinical procedure and can be recommended as an adjunct to conventional SRP.[128] The greater reduction in tooth mobility and probing depth probably is not related in a major way to the bacterial reduction in periodontal pockets achieved in this study, but the clinical improvement is thought to derive from the enhanced CTA secondary to the deepithelialization of the periodontal pockets.

An important caveat, however, is that diode laser irradiation may jeopardize pulp vitality. Limiting power output to 0.5 W (continuous-wave mode) and the time of irradiation to 10 sec is essential in using the laser on the root surfaces of lower incisors and first maxillary premolars. For treatment of other teeth, a power output of 1.0 W (continuous-wave mode) and an exposure time of 10 sec must not be exceeded to ensure a safe clinical application. Temperature elevations are associated in an energy- and time-dependent manner. Dentin thickness has a significant effect on intrapulpal temperature changes.[129]

Only a few studies with the diode laser[122] have addressed root preparation for periodontal regeneration and attachment of periodontal ligament cells.[130] Kreisler et al.[131] evaluated possible morphologic alterations of root surfaces treated with a 809-nm GaAlAs diode laser under standardized in vitro conditions, as well as the effect of a saline solution and a human blood film on the root surface. Irradiation of dry specimens and specimens moistened with saline resulted in no detectable alterations, regardless of exposure time and power output applied. Severe damage to the root surface was noted when segments were covered by a thin blood film with use of higher power settings. At a power output of 1 W or less, however, the result was little to no damage on the root surface, whereas power selections of 1.5, 2.0, and 2.5 W produced various degrees of carbonization (charring) and heat-induced surface cracking at a distance of 0.5 mm to the specimen. The angle of irradiation had a significant effect on the degree of root surface damage.

To avoid damage to the root surface, one alternative is the addition of irrigation. Another possibility is to delay use of the diode laser until 1 to 2 days after SRP, to decrease the possibility of laser-blood interaction. Borrajo et al.[132] applied the diode laser in the periodontal pocket with abundant saline solution irrigation. Settings were as follows: 2 W, pulsed mode, application of the fiberoptic tip parallel to the long axis of the tooth in constant motion, and exposure time of 10 sec per tooth face. Compared with those for SRP alone, results showed lower levels in papilla bleeding index (PBI) and bleeding on probing (BOP) in the laser group, with no significant differences in CAL.

Erbium Family of Lasers

Erbium-doped yttrium-aluminum-garnet (Er:YAG) and erbium plus chromium–doped yttrium-scandium-gallium-garnet (Er,Cr:YSGG) lasers (also referred to as erbium lasers or erbium family lasers) have wavelengths in the near-infrared zone of the spectrum, 2940 nm and 2780 to 2790 nm, respectively. Although similar in wavelength, these two erbium lasers are slightly different in absorption coefficient, extinction length, and other wavelength-dependent parameters. As with diode lasers, it must be emphasized that the results of procedures performed with one of the erbium wavelengths may not be extrapolated to the other wavelength. A critical review of the literature is necessary to delineate the differences in clinical and experimental results for each wavelength.

With both erbium lasers, the energy is delivered through a crystal tip on an articulated arm or hollow guide, or a special fiber and can be applied in contact or noncontact mode to the target tissue. These wavelengths are used preferably on hard tissue but also can be used on soft tissue. Ablation (removal of tissue) occurs when the target tissue absorbs photons and the resulting temperature increase is sufficient to vaporize tissue within the laser beam's path. A basic physical characteristic of tissue ablation by laser energy is that as radiant exposure increases, the depth of tissue removal increases.[133] Erbium laser wavelengths are highly absorbed by water; therefore effective ablation with a very thin surface interaction occurs on the irradiated tissues, with no major thermal damage to the irradiated and surrounding tissues.[134] These laser energies also are highly absorbed by hydroxyapatite,[135] so most recent research on laser-induced root surface modification has involved the erbium lasers.

The use of erbium lasers was cleared by the FDA for several areas of oral care: in 1997 for hard tissue treatment (enamel and dentin),[136] in 1999 for soft tissues surgery and sulcular debridment,[137] and in 2004 for osseous surgery.[138,139]

The erbium lasers are versatile and can be used for many different procedures in dentistry. The excellent ablation effect of these lasers for both soft and hard tissue procedures has generated numerous periodontal investigations. In vitro and clinical studies have already demonstrated an effective application of erbium lasers for calculus removal[140-144] and decontamination of diseased root surface in nonsurgical[145-148] and surgical periodontal procedures.[134] These wavelengths also effectively remove smear layers on root surface cementum after SRP[71,145,149] or inside the root canal.[150-152] Erbium lasers can remove cementum[142,143,145,153,154] and cementum-bound endotoxins.[155,156] Another important property is to promote fibroblast adhesion.[157,158] Several studies show that erbium laser–treated root surface appears to be at least as biocompatible as that produced by SRP[141,143,159-161] or other means (e.g., ultrasonic device).[162-167]

Other studies compared periodontal treatment with erbium laser plus SRP with SRP alone and evaluated clinical parameters only in patients with chronic periodontitis, with no statistical difference between the groups.[168] Long-term, split-mouth studies concluded that the CAL gain obtained after nonsurgical periodontal treatment with erbium laser or SRP can be maintained over a 2-year period.[169] With respect to the bactericidal effect of lasers,[170] even when root surface preparation is comparable to that of conventional SRP, the advantage of using lasers is to promote healing by controlling the infection in the periodontal pocket.

Theoretically, the erbium laser absorption coefficient in water is 10 times higher than that for the CO_2 (10,600-nm) and even higher than for the Nd:YAG (1064-nm) laser. Because the erbium laser energy is highly absorbed in water and other hydrous organic contents, when irradiating tissues with high water content, only a superficial interaction occurs. This limited effect explains less tissue degeneration and thin surface interaction.[139] The mechanism of hard tissue ablation with the erbium lasers is described by the theory of "microexplosions."[171,172] According to this theory, the energy is selectively absorbed in water; some vapor such as steam builds up internal pressure until explosive destruction of inorganic substance occurs before the melting point is reached. These effects probably are not explained completely by thermal phenomena but rather are the result of the microexplosions associated with water evaporation within the hard tissue. In other words, internal pressure increases in the hard tissue, with rupture of the mineral structure. This phenomenon is also referred to as *spallation* or "explosive ablation"[139,171,173] (see Chapters 2 and 10).

When lasers are applied to dental hard tissue, the major problem is heat-related side effects. This thermal effect of the laser beam is based on the absorption of energy by tissue and subsequent transformation of laser energy into heat.[174,175] Heat generation during laser irradiation often causes carbonization, melting, and cracking of the tooth structure, with consequent inflammation and necrosis of the pulp.[174,176] The application of the CO_2 and Nd:YAG lasers for hard tissue treatment tends to result in deleterious effects such as denaturation of proteins,[104] with formation of toxic substances, as well as compositional changes in the irradiated tissue.[174,175]

Compared with the CO_2 and Nd:YAG lasers, erbium lasers show satisfactory results, with faster healing after irradiation of bone than seen with use of a CO_2 laser or mechanical bur. A cell-rich granulation tissue with fibroblasts and osteoblasts was predominant in 7-day specimens of an Er:YAG laser group. Treatment with the erbium lasers may be advantageous for wound healing of bone tissue, with minimal delay observed before healing began and complete replacement by new bone after 56 days.[177] This healing presumably results from a favorable surface for cell attachment consequent to laser irradiation.[178]

The erbium laser family has great potential for cutting hard tissues such as bone by ablation, with minimal thermal damage and a positive effect on the healing process.[179,180] One drawback, however, is their relatively slow cutting speed. Oral-maxillofacial surgeons have embraced the use of CO_2 lasers since the 1960s for soft tissue procedures but have yet to embrace erbium lasers because of the prolonged applications required for hard tissue ablation. A second potential drawback is the size of these units, which are much larger than other dental laser wavelengths. The units themselves, as well as replacement fibers, handpieces, and attachments, also are more expensive than other dental lasers.

The search for ideal parameters and settings has shown that when erbium lasers are used at low energy densities with a water spray surface coolant, the temperature elevation is minimal, with minimal heat-induced tissue damage and with production of smooth surfaces.* The relevant studies indicate that the erbium lasers remove dental hard tissue[183] and bone[184] as well as soft tissue without carbonization. Because of their characteristics of soft tissue ablation, erbium lasers can incise tissue atraumatically, with a bactericidal effect during irradiation.[185] However, erbium lasers cannot promote coagulation to the same degree as that achieved with the other wavelengths (CO_2, Nd:YAG, and diode).[66,67,139,186]

The traditional therapy for periodontal diseases affecting the supporting apparatus of the tooth is SRP. However, complete removal of bacterial deposits and their toxins from the root surface within the periodontal pocket is still difficult and not necessarily achievable with conventional mechanical therapy.[118] Such instrumentation may be associated with extensive cementum removal, leading to increased surface roughness in both supragingival and subgingival areas, which may potentially enhance plaque retention.[187] Achieving a biologically compatible root surface can be a challenge. Factors that increase difficulty of SRP are complex root anatomy, interproximal areas, furcation areas, the cementoenamel junction, multirooted teeth, and distal sites of molars, all of which often are associated with residual calculus and plaque after treatment. Accordingly, erbium laser scaling was recently introduced as an adjunct to conventional SRP procedures because of this laser's property of calculus and smear layer removal as well as a strong bactericidal and detoxification effect.[139,145,188,189]

Other applications for erbium lasers in periodontal treatment include elimination of bacteria in the periodontal pocket and inactivation of bacterial toxins diffused within root cementum.[155,156] Success with these applications suggests a possible advantage of laser periodontal therapy[160] by eliminating contaminated cementum and smear layer, detrimental to periodontal tissue healing after SRP because of the potential to inhibit or impair the reattachment of cells to the root surface.[190,191] Once the treated root surface has been cleaned, it will be biocompatible and properly prepared for the insertion of periodontal ligament fibers in a newly formed connective tissue.[163] In a comparison of an erbium laser–ultrasound system SRP alone, the numbers of attached fibroblast cells per mm^2 were significantly higher for the laser-based modality than for SRP.[157]

In an animal model, periodontal flap surgery was followed by degranulation and root debridement in the furcation areas using an Er:YAG laser or a curette.[192] Histologic and histometric analysis was performed 3 months after surgery. Degranulation and root debridement were effectively accomplished with the Er:YAG laser without major thermal damage and somewhat faster than with a curette. Histologically, the amount of newly formed bone was significantly greater in the laser group than in the curette group, although both groups showed similar amounts of cementum formation and CTA. These findings show that an Er:YAG laser

---

*See references 140, 143, 152, 153, 155, 160, 181, 182.

irradiation technique can be safely and effectively used in periodontal flap surgery, with the potential to promote new bone formation.[193]

Sculean et al.[194] tested a similar design in a 2004 clinical study comparing the healing of intrabony periodontal defects after treatment with access flap surgery, with and without debridement by Er:YAG laser (160 mJ, 10 Hz). In a parallel design, access flap surgery was followed by root surface and defect debridement using Er:YAG laser (test) or hand and ultrasonic instruments (control). The test group displayed a greater tendency for CAL gain, although this did not prove to be statistically significant. Within the limits of this pilot study, it can be concluded that at 6 months after treatment, both therapies led to significant improvements in the investigated clinical parameters, and that the Er:YAG laser may represent a suitable alternative for defect and root surface debridement in conjunction with periodontal surgery.

Erbium lasers also were investigated for their potential to promote root preparation for regeneration, either alone or with materials to enhance healing. When the Er:YAG laser was used with application of enamel matrix proteins (i.e., EMD) and compared with SRP + EMD + EDTA, its combination with EMD did not improve the clinical outcome. Both treatment groups showed similar results.[195]

Recombinant human platelet-derived growth factor BB (rhPDGF-BB) might be a potent stimulator and strong mitogen for human periodontal ligament cells. Er:YAG laser irradiation used alone or in combination with rhPDGF-BB application may offer a promising periodontal therapy for conditioning root surfaces, with the combined application slightly more effective. However, testing laser use at intervals and with parameters less than 60 mJ/pulse and 10 Hz, respectively, is required to verify the minimum threshold values necessary to obtain complete root debridement, and to clarify optimal conditions for fibroblast cell attachment and growth. Further studies are needed to determine ideal parameters for creating the best environment for successful periodontal treatment.[196]

Erbium lasers applied to enhance biocompatibility of root surfaces for fibroblast attachment show promising results.[157] Feist et al.[158] compared adhesion and growth of cultured human gingival fibroblasts on root surfaces either treated by irradiation with Er:YAG laser using two different protocols (groups B and C) or prepared with a curette alone (group A). The two laser treatment groups each received two irradiation sessions—at 60 mJ/pulse and 10 Hz, 10 sec each, with 10-second intervals, 3 J/cm² in group B, and at 100 mJ/pulse and 10 Hz, 10 sec each with 10-sec interval, 5 J/cm², in group C. The tip was applied at a 45-degree angle, in standardized motion and with continuous water spray. Human gingival fibroblasts adhered to and grew on all treated surfaces. Group B demonstrated a significantly higher cell count than the other two groups at days 1 and 2. Three days after seeding, the cultured fibroblasts of groups A and B reached total confluence. The cell count for group B was significantly higher than that for group C.

Treatment of surfaces with Er:YAG laser irradiation of 60 mJ/pulse promoted faster adhesion and growth than treatment with root planing alone or laser irradiation of 100 mJ/pulse. Again, the selection of settings has an impact on treatment outcome.

Low-level laser irradiation has been reported to enhance wound healing by activation of gingival fibroblasts with a potential for early wound healing in periodontal treatment. Low-level Er:YAG laser irradiation stimulates the proliferation of cultured gingival fibroblasts. The optimal stimulative energy density was found to be 3.37 J/cm². This result suggests that this laser technique may be of therapeutic benefit for wound healing.[197]

In analyzing the effect of lasers on cell proliferation to promote healing, at least one other study was conducted by Pourzarandian et al. to investigate if prostaglandin E_2 (PGE_2) and Er:YAG laser irradiation could accelerate wound healing.[198] Cultured fibroblasts were exposed to low-power Er:YAG laser irradiation with an energy density of 3.37 J/cm². Er:YAG laser irradiation appears to exert its stimulative action on gingival fibroblasts proliferation through the production of PGE_2 via the expression of COX-2 (early mediators in the natural healing process). This could be considered as one of the important regulatory pathways to accelerate wound healing after Er:YAG laser irradiation.[198] It can be concluded, therefore, that erbium laser light can be used not only to prepare root surfaces for the attachment of connective tissue fibers but also to promote wound healing of the periodontal soft tissues.

Conditioning of the root surface after SRP has been widely studied. Surface morphology as well as biocompatibility of root cementum was evaluated histologically in regard to adhesion of blood components on these root surfaces[122] and attachment of periodontal ligament fibroblasts.

Connective tissue repair to the root surface seems critically dependent on an attachment between the fibrin clot and the root. The demineralization of root surfaces with acidic agents promotes the establishment of a new connective tissue attachment. Maruyama et al.[199] compared erbium laser irradiation alone with irradiation followed by chemical and/or mechanical conditioning (using tetracycline, EDTA gel, or minocycline paste). Laser irradiation for all test groups was performed at an energy output on the laser control panel of 50 to 60 mJ/pulse, energy density of 10.5 J/cm², and pulse repetition rate of 30 Hz, in the oblique contact mode at a 30-degree angle, in constant motion and for 45 sec for each application. Laser irradiation produced a thin affected layer (5.7 μm in depth) with a superficial microstructure on the cementum. The characteristic microstructures of the irradiated surface were fragile and could be removed by chemical or mechanical conditioning treatments. In the cell attachment assay, the laser-only group exhibited the lowest number of cells, suggesting that laser irradiation alone tends to hinder the early attachment of periodontal ligament cells. However, chemical or mechanical root conditioning treatment may improve and increase the biocompatibility of the Er:YAG laser–treated root cementum by removing the microstructures of the surface and further exposing the collagen fibers.[199] Also with the erbium lasers, studies have shown that roots are better prepared for fibroblast attachment when they are debrided after laser application.

It has been suggested that *pulse duration* is one of the major factors in generating thermal effects on biologic tissues. Single pulse durations above 1 μsec often were associated with considerable thermal effects. The erbium laser system used in several of the studies previously described emitted pulse radiation with single pulse duration of 250 μsec. It can be assumed, therefore, that a certain degree of thermal change is inevitable with use of erbium lasers for treating mineralized tissues, even when the operating field is irrigated with water. Additional mechanical treatment to remove the superficially changed layer, using acid etching or hand instruments, is recommended to enhance periodontal tissue healing.[159,200]

Periimplantitis

An increasing number of studies are investigating the biologic effects of laser irradiation on titanium implant surfaces.[201] The aim of the 2008 study by Lee et al.[202] was to investigate the responses of osteoblast-like cells seeded onto laser-irradiated, anodized titanium discs, using a CO_2 or Er,Cr:YSGG laser, with reference to cellular proliferation and differentiation in vitro. The cells proliferated actively on all substrates; greatest cellular proliferation was observed in the discs treated with Er,Cr:YSGG laser at 300 J/cm. These data show that irradiation with a CO_2 laser or Er,Cr:YSGG laser may induce a measurable positive effect on osteoblast proliferation and differentiation.[203]

The Er:YAG laser with settings of 30 mJ/pulse and 30 Hz with water spray is capable of effectively removing plaque and calculus on the implant abutments without injuring their surfaces, indicating that this laser can be used for debridement of implant abutment surface.[204] Regarding the influence of the Er,Cr:YSGG laser on surface structure and biocompatibility of titanium implants, one study concluded that even though this wavelength exhibited high efficiency in removing plaque biofilm in an energy-dependent manner, it failed to reestablish the biocompatibility of contaminated titanium surfaces.[205]

The use of Er:YAG laser therapy for the treatment of periimplantitis is promising. Implant surface debridement and granulation tissue removal were accomplished effectively and safely with the erbium laser (at 95 to 105 mJ/pulse, with irrigation at a 30- to 45-degree angle) compared with plastic curettes. On histologic examination, a favorable formation of new bone was observed on the laser-treated implant surface, and the laser group showed a tendency to produce greater bone-to-implant contact compared with the curette group.[206] A complete discussion of laser treatment of periimplantitis can be found in Chapter 7.

Also, multiple studies using CO_2 lasers for healing of periimplant defects, without or with bone-grafting material and collagen membrane, show excellent results in vivo.[207]

The effect of diode laser use in periimplantitis is difficult to elucidate because of the different diode wavelengths available and the different experimental protocols and different fluences used. Use of Nd:YAG lasers around implants is contraindicated because they can heat the implant surface and cause sloughing of titanium from the surface.[201]

Chapter 7 further describes treatment of periimplant mucositis and periimplantitis[208] with lasers.

Conclusions

Used in conjunction with or as a replacement for traditional methods, specific laser technologies can be expected to become an essential component of contemporary dental practice over the next decade.[209] Laser light application in regenerative procedures is an excellent tool so long as the operator understands how to use the different wavelengths. Settings, parameters, time of delivery on target tissue, direction of the beam, and water cooling/irrigation all are important aspects of laser use to promote a successful outcome. This unique therapy, used in combination with conventional periodontal techniques, has the potential to revolutionize the field of regeneration of diseased periodontium.

References

1. Nibali L, Tonetti MS, Ready D, et al.: Interleukin-6 polymorphisms are associated with pathogenic bacteria in subjects with periodontitis, *J Periodontol* 79(4):677–683, 2008.
2. Seymour GJ, Taylor JJ: Shouts and whispers: an introduction to immunoregulation in periodontal disease, *Periodontol 2000*(35):9–13, 2004.
3. Cobb CM: Non-surgical pocket therapy: mechanical, *Ann Periodontol* 1(1):443–490, 1996.
4. Haffajee AD, Socransky SS, Lindhe J, et al.: Clinical risk indicators for periodontal attachment loss, *J Clin Periodontol* 18(2):117–125, 1991.
5. Grbic JT, Lamster IB: Risk indicators for future clinical attachment loss in adult periodontitis: tooth and site variables, *J Periodontol* 63(4):262–269, 1992.
6. Claffey N, Egelberg J: Clinical indicators of probing attachment loss following initial periodontal treatment in advanced periodontitis patients, *J Clin Periodontol* 22(9):690–696, 1995.
7. Caton JG, Zander HA: The attachment between tooth and gingival tissues after periodic root planing and soft tissue curettage, *J Periodontol* 50(9):462–466, 1979.
8. Caton J, Nyman S, Zander H: Histometric evaluation of periodontal surgery. II. Connective tissue attachment levels after four regenerative procedures, *J Clin Periodontol* 7(3):224–231, 1980.
9. Caton J, Nyman S: Histometric evaluation of periodontal surgery. I. The modified Widman flap procedure, *J Clin Periodontol* 7(3):212–223, 1980.
10. Isidor F, Karring T, Attstrom R: The effect of root planing as compared to that of surgical treatment, *J Clin Periodontol* 11(10):669–681, 1984.
11. Karring T, Lindhe J: Concepts in periodontal tissue engineering. In Lindhe J, Lang NP, Karring T, editors: *Clinical Periodontology and Implant Dentistry*, ed 5, Blackwell, 2008, Oxford, pp 541–569.

12. Garrett S: Periodontal regeneration around natural teeth, *Ann Periodontol* 1(1):621–666, 1996.

13. Listgarten MA, Rosenberg MM: Histological study of repair following new attachment procedures in human periodontal lesions, *J Periodontol* 50(7):333–344, 1979.

14. Melcher AH: On the repair potential of periodontal tissues, *J Periodontol* 47(5):256–260, 1976.

15. Yukna RA, Bowers GM, Lawrence JJ, Fedi Jr PF: A clinical study of healing in humans following the excisional new attachment procedure, *J Periodontol* 47(12):696–700, 1976.

16. Yukna RA: A clinical and histologic study of healing following the excisional new attachment procedure in rhesus monkeys, *J Periodontol* 47(12):701–709, 1976.

17. Echeverria JJ, Caffesse RG: Effects of gingival curettage when performed 1 month after root instrumentation: a biometric evaluation, *J Clin Periodontol* 10(3):277–286, 1983.

18. Ramfjord SP, Caffesse RG, Morrison EC, et al.: Four modalities of periodontal treatment compared over five years, *J Periodont Res* 22(3):222–223, 1987.

19. Rossmann JA, McQuade MJ, Turunen DE: Retardation of epithelial migration in monkeys using a carbon dioxide laser: an animal study, *J Periodontol* 63(11):902–907, 1992.

20. Rossmann JA, Gottlieb S, Koudelka BM, McQuade MJ: Effects of CO_2 laser irradiation on gingiva, *J Periodontol* 58(6): 423–425, 1987.

21. Centty IG, Blank LW, Levy BA, et al.: Carbon dioxide laser for de-epithelialization of periodontal flaps, *J Periodontol* 68(8): 763–769, 1997.

22. Israel M, Rossmann JA, Froum SJ: Use of the carbon dioxide laser in retarding epithelial migration: a pilot histological human study utilizing case reports, *J Periodontol* 66(3):197–204, 1995.

23. Rossmann JA, Israel M: Laser de-epithelialization for enhanced guided tissue regeneration: a paradigm shift? *Dent Clin North Am* 44(4):793–809, 2000.

24. Hall RR: The healing of tissues incised by a carbon-dioxide laser, *Br J Surg* 58(3):222–225, 1971.

25. Lippert BM, Teymoortash A, Folz BJ, Werner JA: Wound healing after laser treatment of oral and oropharyngeal cancer, *Lasers Med Sci* 18(1):36–42, 2003.

26. Fisher SE, Frame JW, Browne RM, Tranter RM: A comparative histological study of wound healing following CO_2 laser and conventional surgical excision of canine buccal mucosa, *Arch Oral Biol* 28(4):287–291, 1983.

27. Moreno RA, Hebda PA, Zitelli JA, Abell E: Epidermal cell outgrowth from CO_2 laser- and scalpel-cut explants: implications for wound healing, *J Dermatol Surg Oncol* 10(11):863–868, 1984.

28. De Freitas AC, Pinheiro AL, de Oliveira MG, Ramalho LM: Assessment of the behavior of myofibroblasts on scalpel and CO_2 laser wounds: an immunohistochemical study in rats, *J Clin Laser Med Surg* 20(4):221–225, 2002.

29. Pogrel MA, McCracken KJ, Daniels TE: Histologic evaluation of the width of soft tissue necrosis adjacent to carbon dioxide laser incisions, *Oral Surg Oral Med Oral Pathol* 70(5):564–568, 1990.

30. Fisher SE, Frame JW: The effects of the carbon dioxide surgical laser on oral tissues, *Br J Oral Maxillofac Surg* 22(6):414–425, 1984.

31. Yamasaki A, Tamamura K, Sakurai Y, et al.: Remodeling of the rat gingiva induced by CO_2 laser coagulation mode, *Lasers Surg Med* 40(10):695–703, 2008.

32. Wang X, Ishizaki NT, Matsumoto K: Healing process of skin after CO_2 laser ablation at low irradiance: a comparison of continuous-wave and pulsed mode, *Photomed Laser Surg* 23(1): 20–26, 2005.

33. Yukna RA, Carr RL, Evans GH: Histologic evaluation of an Nd:YAG laser-assisted new attachment procedure in humans, *Int J Periodont Restorative Dent* 27(6):577–587, 2007.

34. Parlar A, Bosshardt DD, Unsal B, et al.: New formation of periodontal tissues around titanium implants in a novel dentin chamber model, *Clin Oral Implants Res* 16(3):259–267, 2005.

35. Claffey N, Bogle G, Bjorvatn K, et al.: Topical application of tetracycline in regenerative periodontal surgery in beagles, *Acta Odontol Scand* 45(3):141–146, 1987.

36. Polson AM, Proye MP: Effect of root surface alterations on periodontal healing. II. Citric acid treatment of the denuded root, *J Clin Periodontol* 9(6):441–454, 1982.

37. Magnusson I, Claffey N, Bogle G, et al.: Root resorption following periodontal flap procedures in monkeys, *J Periodont Res* 20(1):79–85, 1985.

38. Bogle G, Adams D, Crigger M, et al.: New attachment after surgical treatment and acid conditioning of roots in naturally occurring periodontal disease in dogs, *J Periodont Res* 16(1):130–133, 1981.

39. Stahl SS, Froum S: Human suprabony healing responses following root demineralization and coronal flap anchorage: histologic responses in 7 sites, *J Clin Periodontol* 18(9):685–689, 1991.

40. Fuentes P, Garrett S, Nilveus R, Egelberg J: Treatment of periodontal furcation defects: coronally positioned flap with or without citric acid root conditioning in class II defects, *J Clin Periodontol* 20(6):425–430, 1993.

41. Moore JA, Ashley FP, Waterman CA: The effect on healing of the application of citric acid during replaced flap surgery, *J Clin Periodontol* 14(3):130–135, 1987.

42. Hammarstrom L, Heijl L, Gestrelius S: Periodontal regeneration in a buccal dehiscence model in monkeys after application of enamel matrix proteins, *J Clin Periodontol* 24(9 pt 2):669–677, 1997.

43. Gestrelius S, Lyngstadaas SP, Hammarstrom L: Emdogain–periodontal regeneration based on biomimicry, *Clin Oral Invest* 4(2):120–125, 2000.

44. Araujo M, Hayacibara R, Sonohara M, et al.: Effect of enamel matrix proteins (Emdogain) on healing after re-implantation of "periodontally compromised" roots: an experimental study in the dog, *J Clin Periodontol* 30(10):855–861, 2003.

45. Chong CH, Carnes DL, Moritz AJ, et al.: Human periodontal fibroblast response to enamel matrix derivative, amelogenin, and platelet-derived growth factor-BB, *J Periodontol* 77(7): 1242–1252, 2006.

46. Heden G, Wennstrom J, Lindhe J: Periodontal tissue alterations following Emdogain treatment of periodontal sites with angular bone defects: a series of case reports, *J Clin Periodontol* 26(12):855–860, 1999.

47. Heden G: A case report study of 72 consecutive Emdogain-treated intrabony periodontal defects: clinical and radiographic findings after 1 year, *Int J Periodont Restorative Dent* 20(2):127–139, 2000.

48. Heijl L, Heden G, Svardstrom G, Ostgren A: Enamel matrix derivative (Emdogain) in the treatment of intrabony periodontal defects, *J Clin Periodontol* 24(9 pt 2):705–714, 1997.

49. Tonetti MS, Lang NP, Cortellini P, et al.: Enamel matrix proteins in the regenerative therapy of deep intrabony defects, *J Clin Periodontol* 29(4):317–325, 2002.

50. Sculean A, Donos N, Chiantella GC, et al.: GTR with bioresorbable membranes in the treatment of intrabony defects: a clinical and histologic study, *Int J Periodont Restorative Dent* 19(5):501–509, 1999.

51. Sculean A, Donos N, Windisch P, et al.: Healing of human intrabony defects following treatment with enamel matrix proteins or guided tissue regeneration, *J Periodont Res* 34(6):310–322, 1999.

52. Silvestri M, Sartori S, Rasperini G, et al.: Comparison of infrabony defects treated with enamel matrix derivative versus guided tissue regeneration with a nonresorbable membrane, *J Clin Periodontol* 30(5):386–393, 2003.

53. Sanz M, Tonetti MS, Zabalegui I, et al.: Treatment of intrabony defects with enamel matrix proteins or barrier membranes: results from a multicenter practice-based clinical trial, *J Periodontol* 75(5):726–733, 2004.

54. Zucchelli G, Amore C, Montebugnoli L, De Sanctis M: Enamel matrix proteins and bovine porous bone mineral in the treatment of intrabony defects: a comparative controlled clinical trial, *J Periodontol* 74(12):1725–1735, 2003.

55. Gurinsky BS, Mills MP, Mellonig JT: Clinical evaluation of demineralized freeze-dried bone allograft and enamel matrix derivative versus enamel matrix derivative alone for the treatment of periodontal osseous defects in humans, *J Periodontol* 75(10):1309–1318, 2004.

56. Trombelli L, Annunziata M, Belardo S, et al.: Autogenous bone graft in conjunction with enamel matrix derivative in the treatment of deep periodontal intra-osseous defects: a report of 13 consecutively treated patients, *J Clin Periodontol* 33(1):69–75, 2006.

57. Sculean A, Pietruska M, Schwarz F, et al.: Healing of human intrabony defects following regenerative periodontal therapy with an enamel matrix protein derivative alone or combined with a bioactive glass: a controlled clinical study, *J Clin Periodontol* 32(1):111–117, 2005.

58. Mellonig JT: Enamel matrix derivative for periodontal reconstructive surgery: technique and clinical and histologic case report, *Int J Periodont Restorative Dent* 19(1):8–19, 1999.

59. Lynch SE, Williams RC, Polson AM, et al.: A combination of platelet-derived and insulin-like growth factors enhances periodontal regeneration, *J Clin Periodontol* 16(8):545–548, 1989.

60. Lynch SE, de Castilla GR, Williams RC, et al.: The effects of short-term application of a combination of platelet-derived and insulin-like growth factors on periodontal wound healing, *J Periodontol* 62(7):458–467, 1991.

61. Rutherford RB, Niekrash CE, Kennedy JE, Charette MF: Platelet-derived and insulin-like growth factors stimulate regeneration of periodontal attachment in monkeys, *J Periodont Res* 27(4 pt 1):285–290, 1992.

62. Giannobile WV, Finkelman RD, Lynch SE: Comparison of canine and non-human primate animal models for periodontal regenerative therapy: results following a single administration of PDGF/IGF-I, *J Periodontol* 65(12):1158–1168, 1994.

63. Giannobile WV, Hernandez RA, Finkelman RD, et al.: Comparative effects of platelet-derived growth factor-BB and insulin-like growth factor-I, individually and in combination, on periodontal regeneration in *Macaca fascicularis, J Periodont Res* 31(5):301–312, 1996.

64. Howell TH, Fiorellini JP, Paquette DW, et al.: A phase I/II clinical trial to evaluate a combination of recombinant human platelet-derived growth factor-BB and recombinant human insulin-like growth factor-I in patients with periodontal disease, *J Periodontol* 68(12):1186–1193, 1997.

65. Lekovic V, Camargo PM, Weinlaender M, et al.: Effectiveness of a combination of platelet-rich plasma, bovine porous bone mineral and guided tissue regeneration in the treatment of mandibular grade II molar furcations in humans, *J Clin Periodontol* 30(8):746–751, 2003.

66. Aoki A, Sasaki KM, Watanabe H, Ishikawa I: Lasers in nonsurgical periodontal therapy, *Periodontol* 2000 36:59–97, 2004.

67. Cobb CM: Lasers in periodontics: a review of the literature, *J Periodontol* 77(4):545–564, 2006.

68. Schwarz F, Aoki A, Becker J, Sculean A: Laser application in non-surgical periodontal therapy: a systematic review, *J Clin Periodontol* 35(8 suppl):29–44, 2008.

69. Spencer P, Cobb CM, McCollum MH, Wieliczka DM: The effects of CO_2 laser and Nd:YAG with and without water/air surface cooling on tooth root structure: correlation between FTIR spectroscopy and histology, *J Periodont Res* 31(7):453–462, 1996.

70. Sasaki KM, Masuno H, Ichinose S, et al.: Compositional analysis of root cementum and dentin after Er:YAG laser irradiation compared with CO_2 lased and intact roots using Fourier transformed infrared spectroscopy, *J Periodont Res* 37(1):50–59, 2002.

71. Israel M, Cobb CM, Rossmann JA, Spencer P: The effects of CO_2, Nd:YAG and Er:YAG lasers with and without surface coolant on tooth root surfaces: an in vitro study, *J Clin Periodontol* 24(9 pt 1):595–602, 1997.

72. Barone A, Covani U, Crespi R, Romanos GE: Root surface morphological changes after focused versus defocused CO_2 laser irradiation: a scanning electron microscopy analysis, *J Periodontol* 73(4):370–373, 2002.

73. Moritz A, Gutknecht N, Goharkhay K, et al.: The carbon dioxide laser as an aid in apicoectomy: an in vitro study, *J Clin Laser Med Surg* 15(4):185–188, 1997.

74. Crespi R, Barone A, Covani U: Histologic evaluation of three methods of periodontal root surface treatment in humans, *J Periodontol* 76(3):476–481, 2005.

75. Misra V, Mehrotra KK, Dixit J, Maitra SC: Effect of a carbon dioxide laser on periodontally involved root surfaces, *J Periodontol* 70(9):1046–1052, 1999.

76. Crespi R, Barone A, Covani U, et al.: Effects of CO_2 laser treatment on fibroblast attachment to root surfaces: a scanning electron microscopy analysis, *J Periodontol* 73(11):1308–1312, 2002.

77. Pant V, Dixit J, Agrawal AK, et al.: Behavior of human periodontal ligament cells on CO_2 laser irradiated dentinal root surfaces: an in vitro study, *J Periodont Res* 39(6):373–379, 2004.

78. Fayad MI, Hawkinson R, Daniel J, Hao J: The effect of CO_2 laser irradiation on PDL cell attachment to resected root surfaces, *Oral Surg Oral Med Oral Pathol Oral Radiol Endod* 97(4):518–523, 2004.

79. Gopin BW, Cobb CM, Rapley JW, Killoy WJ: Histologic evaluation of soft tissue attachment to CO_2 laser-treated root surfaces: an in vivo study, *Int J Periodont Restorative Dent* 17(4):316–325, 1997.

80. Friesen LR, Cobb CM, Rapley JW, et al.: Laser irradiation of bone. II. Healing response following treatment by CO_2 and Nd:YAG lasers, *J Periodontol* 70(1):75–83, 1999.

81. McDavid VG, Cobb CM, Rapley JW, et al.: Laser irradiation of bone. III. Long-term healing following treatment by CO_2 and Nd:YAG lasers, *J Periodontol* 72(2):174–182, 2001.

82. Folwaczny M, Thiele L, Mehl A, Hickel R: The effect of working tip angulation on root substance removal using Er:YAG laser radiation: an in vitro study, *J Clin Periodontol* 28(3):220–226, 2001.

83. Mullins SL, MacNeill SR, Rapley JW, et al.: Subgingival microbiologic effects of one-time irradiation by CO_2 laser: a pilot study, *J Periodont* 78(12):2331–2337, 2007.

84. Myers TD: Lasers in dentistry, *CDS Rev* 84(8):26–29, 1991.

85. Gold SI, Vilardi MA: Pulsed laser beam effects on gingiva, *J Clin Periodontol* 21(6):391–396, 1994.

86. Ben Hatit Y, Blum R, Severin C, et al.: The effects of a pulsed Nd:YAG laser on subgingival bacterial flora and on cementum: an in vivo study, *J Clin Laser Med Surg* 14(3):137–143, 1996.

87. Neill ME, Mellonig JT: Clinical efficacy of the Nd:YAG laser for combination periodontitis therapy, *Pract Periodont Aesthet Dent* 9(6 suppl):1–5, 1997.

88. Cobb CM, McCawley TK, Killoy WJ: A preliminary study on the effects of the Nd:YAG laser on root surfaces and subgingival microflora in vivo, *J Periodontol* 63(8):701–707, 1992.

89. Miyazaki A, Yamaguchi T, Nishikata J, et al.: Effects of Nd:YAG and CO_2 laser treatment and ultrasonic scaling on periodontal pockets of chronic periodontitis patients, *J Periodontol* 74(2):175–180, 2003.

90. Meral G, Tasar F, Kocagoz S, Sener C: Factors affecting the antibacterial effects of Nd:YAG laser in vivo, *Lasers Surg Med* 32(3):197–202, 2003.

91. Harris DM, Yessik M: Therapeutic ratio quantifies laser antisepsis: ablation of *Porphyromonas gingivalis* with dental lasers, *Lasers Surg Med* 35(3):206–213, 2004.

92. Gregg RH, McCarthy DK: Laser ENAP for periodontal ligament regeneration, *Dent Today* 17(11):86–89, 1998.

93. Gregg RH, McCarthy DK: Laser ENAP for periodontal bone regeneration, *Dent Today* 17(5):88–91, 1998.

94. White JM, Goodis HE, Rose CL: Use of the pulsed Nd:YAG laser for intraoral soft tissue surgery, *Lasers Surg Med* 11(5):455–461, 1991.

95. Lippert BM, Teymoortash A, Folz BJ, Werner JA: Coagulation and temperature distribution in Nd:YAG interstitial laser thermotherapy: an in vitro animal study, *Lasers Med Sci* 18(1):19–24, 2003.

96. Radvar M, MacFarlane TW, MacKenzie D, et al.: An evaluation of the Nd:YAG laser in periodontal pocket therapy, *Br Dent J* 180(2):57–62, 1996.

97. Tewfik HM, Garnick JJ, Schuster GS, Sharawy MM: Structural and functional changes of cementum surface following exposure to a modified Nd:YAG laser, *J Periodontol* 65(4):297–302, 1994.

98. Morlock BJ, Pippin DJ, Cobb CM, et al.: The effect of Nd:YAG laser exposure on root surfaces when used as an adjunct to root planing: an in vitro study, *J Periodontol* 63(7):637–641, 1992.

99. Spencer P, Trylovich DJ, Cobb CM: Chemical characterization of lased root surfaces using Fourier transform infrared photoacoustic spectroscopy, *J Periodontol* 63(7):633–636, 1992.

100. Trylovich DJ, Cobb CM, Pippin DJ, et al.: The effects of the Nd:YAG laser on in vitro fibroblast attachment to endotoxin-treated root surfaces, *J Periodontol* 63(7):626–632, 1992.

101. Thomas D, Rapley J, Cobb C, et al.: Effects of the Nd:YAG laser and combined treatments on in vitro fibroblast attachment to root surfaces, *J Clin Periodontol* 21(1):38–44, 1994.

102. Chen YJ, Jeng JH, Jane Yao CC, et al.: Long-term effect of pulsed Nd:YAG laser irradiation on cultured human periodontal fibroblasts, *Lasers Surg Med* 36(3):225–233, 2005.

103. Arisu HD, Turkoz E, Bala O: Effects of Nd:YAG laser irradiation on osteoblast cell cultures, *Lasers Med Sci* 21(3):175–180, 2006.

104. Gaspirc B, Skaleric U: Morphology, chemical structure and diffusion processes of root surface after Er:YAG and Nd:YAG laser irradiation, *J Clin Periodontol* 28(6):508–516, 2001.

105. De Moura-Netto C, de Moura AA, Davidowicz H, et al.: Morphologic changes and removal of debris on apical dentin surfaces after Nd:YAG laser and diode laser irradiation, *Photomed Laser Surg* 26(3):263–266, 2008.

106. Radvar MS, Gilmour WH, Payne AP, et al.: An evaluation of the effects of an Nd:YAG laser on subgingival calculus, dentine and cementum, *J Clin Periodontol* 22(1):71–77, 1995.

107. Wilder-Smith P, Arrastia AM, Schell MJ, et al.: Effect of Nd:YAG laser irradiation and root planing on the root surface: structural and thermal effects, *J Periodontol* 66(12):1032–1039, 1995.

108. Ito K, Nishikata J, Murai S: Effects of Nd:YAG laser radiation on removal of a root surface smear layer after root planing: a scanning electron microscopic study, *J Periodontol* 64(6):547–552, 1993.

109. Gowen M, Wood DD, Ihrie EJ, et al.: An interleukin-1–like factor stimulates bone resorption in vitro, *Nature* 306(5941):378–380, 1983.

110. Stashenko P, Dewhirst FE, Peros WJ, et al.: Synergistic interactions between interleukin 1, tumor necrosis factor, and lymphotoxin in bone resorption, *J Immunol* 138(5):1464–1468, 1987.

111. Page RC: The role of inflammatory mediators in the pathogenesis of periodontal disease, *J Periodont Res* 26(3 pt 2):230–242, 1991.

112. Liu CM, Hou LT, Wong MY, Lan WH: Comparison of Nd:YAG laser versus scaling and root planing in periodontal therapy, *J Periodontol* 70(11):1276–1282, 1999.

113. Harris DM, Gregg 2nd RH, McCarthy DK, et al.: Laser-assisted new attachment procedure in private practice, *Gen Dent* 52(5):396–403, 2004.

114. Janda P, Sroka R, Mundweil B, et al.: Comparison of thermal tissue effects induced by contact application of fiber guided laser systems, *Lasers Surg Med* 33(2):93–101, 2003.

115. Coluzzi DJ: Fundamentals of dental lasers: science and instruments, *Dent Clin North Am* 48(4):751–770, 2004.

116. Nussbaum EL, Lilge L, Mazzulli T: Effects of low-level laser therapy (LLLT) of 810 nm upon in vitro growth of bacteria: relevance of irradiance and radiant exposure, *J Clin Laser Med Surg* 21(5):283–290, 2003.

117. Renvert S, Wikstrom M, Dahlen G, et al.: Effect of root debridement on the elimination of *Actinobacillus actinomycetemcomitans* and *Bacteroides gingivalis* from periodontal pockets, *J Clin Periodontol* 17(6):345–350, 1990.

118. Takamatsu N, Yano K, He T, et al.: Effect of initial periodontal therapy on the frequency of detecting *Bacteroides forsythus*, *Porphyromonas gingivalis*, and *Actinobacillus actinomycetemcomitans*, *J Periodontol* 70(6):574–580, 1999.

119. Carnevalli CM, Soares CP, Zangaro RA, et al.: Laser light prevents apoptosis in Cho K-1 cell line, *J Clin Laser Med Surg* 21(4):193–196, 2003.

120. Do Nascimento PM, Pinheiro AL, Salgado MA: Ramalho LM: A preliminary report on the effect of laser therapy on the healing of cutaneous surgical wounds as a consequence of an inversely proportional relationship between wavelength and intensity: histological study in rats, *Photomed Laser Surg* 22(6):513–518, 2004.

121. Whelan HT, Buchmann EV, Dhokalia A, et al.: Effect of NASA light-emitting diode irradiation on molecular changes for wound healing in diabetic mice, *J Clin Laser Med Surg* 21(2):67–74, 2003.

122. Theodoro LH, Sampaio JE, Haypek P, et al.: Effect of Er:YAG and diode lasers on the adhesion of blood components and on the morphology of irradiated root surfaces, *J Periodont Res* 41(5):381–390, 2006.

123. Moritz A, Schoop U, Goharkhay K, et al.: Treatment of periodontal pockets with a diode laser, *Lasers Surg Med* 22(5):302–311, 1998.

124. Fontana CR, Kurachi C, Mendonca CR, Bagnato VS: Microbial reduction in periodontal pockets under exposition of a medium power diode laser: an experimental study in rats, *Lasers Surg Med* 35(4):263–268, 2004.

125. Fontana CR, Kurachi C, Mendonca CR, Bagnato VS: Temperature variation at soft periodontal and rat bone tissues during a medium-power diode laser exposure, *Photomed Laser Surg* 22(6):519–522, 2004.

126. Ribeiro IW, Sbrana MC, Esper LA, Almeida AL: Evaluation of the effect of the GaAlAs laser on subgingival scaling and root planing, *Photomed Laser Surg* 26(4):387–391, 2008.

127. Romanos GE, Henze M, Banihashemi S, et al.: Removal of epithelium in periodontal pockets following diode (980 nm) laser application in the animal model: an in vitro study, *Photomed Laser Surg* 22(3):177–183, 2004.

128. Kreisler M, Al Haj H, d'Hoedt B: Clinical efficacy of semiconductor laser application as an adjunct to conventional scaling and root planing, *Lasers Surg Med* 37(5):350–355, 2005.

129. Kreisler M, Al-Haj H, d'Hoedt B: Intrapulpal temperature changes during root surface irradiation with an 809-nm GaAlAs laser, *Oral Surg Oral Med Oral Pathol Oral Radiol Endod* 93(6):730–735, 2002.

130. Kreisler M, Meyer C, Stender E, et al.: Effect of diode laser irradiation on the attachment rate of periodontal ligament cells: an in vitro study, *J Periodontol* 72(10):1312–1317, 2001.

131. Kreisler M, Al Haj H, Daublander M, et al.: Effect of diode laser irradiation on root surfaces in vitro, *J Clin Laser Med Surg* 20(2):63–69, 2002.

132. Borrajo JL, Varela LG, Castro GL, et al.: Diode laser (980 nm) as adjunct to scaling and root planing, *Photomed Laser Surg* 22(6):509–512, 2004.

133. Walsh Jr JT, Deutsch TF: Er:YAG laser ablation of tissue: measurement of ablation rates, *Lasers Surg Med* 9(4):327–337, 1989.

134. Ishikawa I, Aoki A, Takasaki AA: Clinical application of erbium:YAG laser in periodontology, *J Int Acad Periodontol* 10(1):22–30, 2008.

135. Featherstone JD: Caries detection and prevention with laser energy, *Dent Clin North Am* 44(4):955–969, 2000.

136. Sulewski JG: Historical survey of laser dentistry, *Dent Clin North Am* 44(4):717–752, 2000.

137. Watanabe H, Ishikawa I, Suzuki M, Hasegawa K: Clinical assessments of the erbium:YAG laser for soft tissue surgery and scaling, *J Clin Laser Med Surg* 14(2):67–75, 1996.

138. Sasaki KM, Aoki A, Ichinose S, et al.: Scanning electron microscopy and Fourier transformed infrared spectroscopy analysis of bone removal using Er:YAG and CO_2 lasers, *J Periodontol* 73(6):643–652, 2002.

139. Ishikawa I, Aoki A, Takasaki AA: Potential applications of erbium:YAG laser in periodontics, *J Periodontal Res* 39(4):275–285, 2004.

140. Aoki A, Ando Y, Watanabe H, Ishikawa I: In vitro studies on laser scaling of subgingival calculus with an erbium:YAG laser, *J Periodontol* 65(12):1097–1106, 1994.

141. Schwarz F, Sculean A, Berakdar M, et al.: In vivo and in vitro effects of an Er:YAG laser, a GaAlAs diode laser, and scaling and root planing on periodontally diseased root surfaces: a comparative histologic study, *Lasers Surg Med* 32(5):359–366, 2003.

142. Schwarz F, Putz N, Georg T, Reich E: Effect of an Er:YAG laser on periodontally involved root surfaces: an in vivo and in vitro SEM comparison, *Lasers Surg Med* 29(4):328–335, 2001.

143. Folwaczny M, Mehl A, Haffner C, et al.: Root substance removal with Er:YAG laser radiation at different parameters using a new delivery system, *J Periodontol* 71(2):147–155, 2000.

144. Crespi R, Romanos GE, Barone A, et al.: Er:YAG laser in defocused mode for scaling of periodontally involved root surfaces: an in vitro pilot study, *J Periodontol* 76(5):686–690, 2005.

145. Crespi R, Barone A, Covani U: Er:YAG laser scaling of diseased root surfaces: a histologic study, *J Periodontol* 77(2):218–222, 2006.

146. Folwaczny M, Mehl A, Aggstaller H, Hickel R: Antimicrobial effects of 2.94 micron Er:YAG laser radiation on root surfaces: an in vitro study, *J Clin Periodontol* 29(1):73–78, 2002.

147. Folwaczny M, George G, Thiele L, et al.: Root surface roughness following Er:YAG laser irradiation at different radiation energies and working tip angulations, *J Clin Periodontol* 29(7):598–603, 2002.

148. Derdilopoulou FV, Nonhoff J, Neumann K, Kielbassa AM: Microbiological findings after periodontal therapy using curettes, Er:YAG laser, sonic, and ultrasonic scalers, *J Clin Periodontol* 34(7):588–598, 2007.

149. Crespi R, Barone A, Covani U: Effect of Er:YAG laser on diseased root surfaces: an in vivo study, *J Periodontol* 76(8):1386–1390, 2005.

150. Schoop U, Moritz A, Kluger W, et al.: The Er:YAG laser in endodontics: results of an in vitro study, *Lasers Surg Med* 30(5):360–364, 2002.

151. Schoop U, Goharkhay K, Klimscha J, et al.: The use of the erbium, chromium:yttrium-scandium-gallium-garnet laser in endodontic treatment: the results of an in vitro study, *J Am Dent Assoc* 138(7):949–955, 2007.

152. Schoop U, Barylyak A, Goharkhay K, et al.: The impact of an erbium, chromium:yttrium-scandium-gallium-garnet laser with radial-firing tips on endodontic treatment, *Lasers Med Sci* 24(1):59–65, 2009.

153. Frentzen M, Braun A, Aniol D: Er:YAG laser scaling of diseased root surfaces, *J Periodontol* 73(5):524–530, 2002.

154. Krause F, Braun A, Brede O, et al.: Evaluation of selective calculus removal by a fluorescence feedback-controlled Er:YAG laser in vitro, *J Clin Periodontol* 34(1):66–71, 2007.

155. Yamaguchi H, Kobayashi K, Osada R, et al.: Effects of irradiation of an erbium:YAG laser on root surfaces, *J Periodontol* 68(12):1151–1155, 1997.

156. Folwaczny M, Aggstaller H, Mehl A, Hickel R: Removal of bacterial endotoxin from root surface with Er:YAG laser, *Am J Dent* 16(1):3–5, 2003.

157. Schwarz F, Aoki A, Sculean A, et al.: In vivo effects of an Er:YAG laser, an ultrasonic system and scaling and root planing on the biocompatibility of periodontally diseased root surfaces in cultures of human PDL fibroblasts, *Lasers Surg Med* 33(2):140–147, 2003.

158. Feist IS, De Micheli G, Carneiro SR, et al.: Adhesion and growth of cultured human gingival fibroblasts on periodontally involved root surfaces treated by Er:YAG laser, *J Periodontol* 74(9):1368–1375, 2003.

159. Aoki A, Miura M, Akiyama F, et al.: In vitro evaluation of Er:YAG laser scaling of subgingival calculus in comparison with ultrasonic scaling, *J Periodont Res* 35(5):266–277, 2000.

160. Sasaki KM, Aoki A, Ichinose S, Ishikawa I: Morphological analysis of cementum and root dentin after Er:YAG laser irradiation, *Lasers Surg Med* 31(2):79–85, 2002.

161. Moghare Abed A, Tawakkoli M, Dehchenari MA, et al.: A comparative SEM study between hand instrument and Er:YAG laser scaling and root planing, *Lasers Med Sci* 22(1):25–29, 2007.

162. Sculean A, Schwarz F, Berakdar M, et al.: Periodontal treatment with an Er:YAG laser compared to ultrasonic instrumentation: a pilot study, *J Periodontol* 75(7):966–973, 2004.

163. Schwarz F, Jepsen S, Herten M, et al.: Immunohistochemical characterization of periodontal wound healing following non-surgical treatment with fluorescence controlled Er:YAG laser radiation in dogs, *Lasers Surg Med* 39(5):428–440, 2007.

164. Noori ZT, Fekrazad R, Eslami B, et al.: Comparing the effects of root surface scaling with ultrasound instruments and Er,Cr:YSGG laser, *Lasers Med Sci* 23(3):283–287, 2008.

165. De Mendonca AC, Maximo MB, Rodrigues JA, et al.: Er:YAG laser, ultrasonic system, and curette produce different profiles on dentine root surfaces: an in vitro study, *Photomed Laser Surg* 26(2):91–97, 2008.

166. Tomasi C, Schander K, Dahlen G, Wennstrom JL: Short-term clinical and microbiologic effects of pocket debridement with an Er:YAG laser during periodontal maintenance, *J Periodontol* 77(1):111–118, 2006.

167. Crespi R, Cappare P, Toscanelli I, et al.: Effects of Er:YAG laser compared to ultrasonic scaler in periodontal treatment: a 2-year follow-up split-mouth clinical study, *J Periodontol* 78(7):1195–1200, 2007.

168. Lopes BM, Marcantonio RA, Thompson GM, et al.: Short-term clinical and immunologic effects of scaling and root planing with Er:YAG laser in chronic periodontitis, *J Periodontol* 79(7):1158–1167, 2008.

169. Schwarz F, Sculean A, Berakdar M, et al.: Periodontal treatment with an Er:YAG laser or scaling and root planing: a 2-year follow-up split-mouth study, *J Periodontol* 74(5):590–596, 2003.

170. Schwarz F, Sculean A, Berakdar M, et al.: Clinical evaluation of an Er:YAG laser combined with scaling and root planing for non-surgical periodontal treatment: a controlled, prospective clinical study, *J Clin Periodontol* 30(1):26–34, 2003.

171. Hibst R, Keller U: Experimental studies of the application of the Er:YAG laser on dental hard substances. I. Measurement of the ablation rate, *Lasers Surg Med* 9(4):338–344, 1989.

172. Sasaki KM, Aoki A, Ichinose S, Ishikawa I: Ultrastructural analysis of bone tissue irradiated by Er:YAG laser, *Lasers Surg Med* 31(5):322–332, 2002.

173. Keller U, Hibst R: Experimental studies of the application of the Er:YAG laser on dental hard substances. II. Light microscopic and SEM investigations, *Lasers Surg Med* 9(4):345–351, 1989.

174. Wigdor HA, Walsh Jr JT, Featherstone JD, et al.: Lasers in dentistry, *Lasers Surg Med* 16(2):103–133, 1995.

175. Jeffrey A, Rossmann C: Lasers in periodontal therapy, *Periodontol 2000* 9(1):150–164, 1995.

176. Frentzen M, Koort HJ: Lasers in dentistry: new possibilities with advancing laser technology? *Int Dent J* 40(6):323–332, 1990.

177. Wang X, Zhang C, Matsumoto K: In vivo study of the healing processes that occur in the jaws of rabbits following perforation by an Er,Cr:YSGG laser, *Lasers Med Sci* 20(1):21–27, 2005.

178. Pourzarandian A, Watanabe H, Aoki A, et al.: Histological and TEM examination of early stages of bone healing after Er:YAG laser irradiation, *Photomed Laser Surg* 22(4):342–350, 2004.

179. Kimura Y, Yu DG, Fujita A, et al.: Effects of erbium, chromium:YSGG laser irradiation on canine mandibular bone, *J Periodontol* 72(9):1178–1182, 2001.

180. Yoshino T, Aoki A, Oda S, et al.: Long-term histologic analysis of bone tissue alteration and healing following Er:YAG laser irradiation compared to electrosurgery, *J Periodontol* 80(1):82–92, 2009.

181. Ishikawa I, Sasaki KM, Aoki A, Watanabe H: Effects of Er:YAG laser on periodontal therapy, *J Int Acad Periodontol* 5(1):23–28, 2003.

182. Theodoro LH, Haypek P, Bachmann L, et al.: Effect of Er:YAG and diode laser irradiation on the root surface: morphological and thermal analysis, *J Periodontol* 74(6):838–843, 2003.

183. Kimura Y, Yu DG, Kinoshita J, et al.: Effects of erbium, chromium:YSGG laser irradiation on root surface: morphological and atomic analytical studies, *J Clin Laser Med Surg* 19(2):69–72, 2001.

184. Stubinger S, von Rechenberg B, Zeilhofer HF, et al.: Er:YAG laser osteotomy for removal of impacted teeth: clinical comparison of two techniques, *Lasers Surg Med* 39(7):583–588, 2007.

185. Ando Y, Aoki A, Watanabe H, Ishikawa I: Bactericidal effect of erbium YAG laser on periodontopathic bacteria, *Lasers Surg Med* 19(2):190–200, 1996.

186. Kreisler M, Kohnen W, Marinello C, et al.: Bactericidal effect of the Er:YAG laser on dental implant surfaces: an in vitro study, *J Periodontol* 73(11):1292–1298, 2002.

187. Schwarz F, Bieling K, Venghaus S, et al.: Influence of fluorescence-controlled Er:YAG laser radiation, the Vector system and hand instruments on periodontally diseased root surfaces in vivo, *J Clin Periodontol* 33(3):200–208, 2006.

188. Schwarz F, Sculean A, Georg T, Reich E: Periodontal treatment with an Er:YAG laser compared to scaling and root planing: a controlled clinical study, *J Periodontol* 72(3):361–367, 2001.

189. Eberhard J, Ehlers H, Falk W, et al.: Efficacy of subgingival calculus removal with Er:YAG laser compared to mechanical debridement: an in situ study, *J Clin Periodontol* 30(6):511–518, 2003.

190. Hatfield CG, Baumhammers A: Cytotoxic effects of periodontally involved surfaces of human teeth, *Arch Oral Biol* 16(4):465–468, 1971.

191. Aleo JJ, de Renzis FA, Farber PA, Varboncoeur AP: The presence and biologic activity of cementum-bound endotoxin, *J Periodontol* 45(9):672–675, 1974.

192. Gaspirc B, Skaleric U: Clinical evaluation of periodontal surgical treatment with an Er:YAG laser: 5-year results, *J Periodontol* 78(10):1864–1871, 2007.

193. Mizutani K, Aoki A, Takasaki AA, et al.: Periodontal tissue healing following flap surgery using an Er:YAG laser in dogs, *Lasers Surg Med* 38(4):314–324, 2006.

194. Sculean A, Schwarz F, Berakdar M, et al.: Healing of intrabony defects following surgical treatment with or without an Er:YAG laser, *J Clin Periodontol* 31(8):604–608, 2004.

195. Schwarz F, Sculean A, Georg T, Becker J: Clinical evaluation of the Er:YAG laser in combination with an enamel matrix protein derivative for the treatment of intrabony periodontal defects: a pilot study, *J Clin Periodontol* 30(11):975–981, 2003.

196. Belal MH, Watanabe H, Ichinose S, Ishikawa I: Effect of Er:YAG laser combined with rhPDGF-BB on attachment of cultured fibroblasts to periodontally involved root surfaces, *J Periodontol* 78(7):1329–1341, 2007.

197. Pourzarandian A, Watanabe H, Ruwanpura SM, et al.: Effect of low-level Er:YAG laser irradiation on cultured human gingival fibroblasts, *J Periodontol* 76(2):187–193, 2005.

198. Pourzarandian AH, Ruwanpura SM, Aoki A, et al.: Er:YAG laser irradiation increases prostaglandin E_2 production via the induction of cyclooxygenase-2 mRNA in human gingival fibroblasts, *J Periodont Res* 40(2):182–186, 2005.

199. Maruyama H, Aoki A, Sasaki KM, et al.: The effect of chemical and/or mechanical conditioning on the Er:YAG laser-treated root cementum: analysis of surface morphology and periodontal ligament fibroblast attachment, *Lasers Surg Med* 40(3):211–222, 2008.

200. Folwaczny M, Benner KU, Flasskamp B, et al.: Effects of 2.94 micron Er:YAG laser radiation on root surfaces treated in situ: a histological study, *J Periodontol* 74(3):360–365, 2003.

201. Kreisler M, Gotz H, Duschner H: Effect of Nd:YAG, Ho:YAG, Er:YAG, CO₂, and GaAIAs laser irradiation on surface properties of endosseous dental implants, *Int J Oral Maxillofac Implants* 17(2):202–211, 2002.

202. Lee JH, Heo SJ, Koak JY, et al.: Cellular responses on anodized titanium discs after laser irradiation, *Lasers Surg Med* 40(10):738–742, 2008.

203. Romanos G, Crespi R, Barone A, Covani U: Osteoblast attachment on titanium disks after laser irradiation, *Int J Oral Maxillofac Implants* 21(2):232–236, 2006.

204. Matsuyama T, Aoki A, Oda S, et al.: Effects of the Er:YAG laser irradiation on titanium implant materials and contaminated implant abutment surfaces, *J Clin Laser Med Surg* 21(1):7–17, 2003.

205. Schwarz F, Nuesry E, Bieling K, et al.: Influence of an erbium, chromium–doped yttrium, scandium, gallium, and garnet (Er,Cr:YSGG) laser on the reestablishment of the biocompatibility of contaminated titanium implant surfaces, *J Periodontol* 77(11):1820–1827, 2006.

206. Takasaki AA, Aoki A, Mizutani K, et al.: Er:YAG laser therapy for peri-implant infection: a histological study, *Lasers Med Sci* 22(3):143–157, 2007.

207. Romanos GE, Nentwig GH: Regenerative therapy of deep peri-implant infrabony defects after CO₂ laser implant surface decontamination, *Int J Periodont Restorative Dent* 28(3):245–255, 2008.

208. Renvert S, Roos-Jansaker AM, Claffey N: Non-surgical treatment of peri-implant mucositis and peri-implantitis: a literature review, *J Clin Periodontol* 35(8 suppl):305–315, 2008.

209. Walsh LJ: The current status of laser applications in dentistry, *Aust Dent J* 48(3):146–155, quiz 198, 2003.

6

Lasers in Fixed Prosthetic and Cosmetic Reconstruction

JAMES C. DOWNS, ROBERT A. CONVISSAR, EUGENIA ANAGNOSTAKI,
GRACE SUN, AND CHARLES R. HOOPINGARNER

This chapter describes the clinical applications of laser dentistry with respect to soft tissue and hard tissue alterations for fixed prosthetic and cosmetic reconstruction. The clinical advantages of laser use, for both the patient and the dentist, are well recognized: Major benefits associated with laser surgery include reduced bleeding, less postoperative discomfort, and remarkably less edema compared with conventional techniques or electrosurgery. In addition, a clear field of vision resulting from excellent hemostasis and moisture control allows much greater precision in performance of the reconstructive procedure.

Many procedural techniques are routinely incorporated into fixed prosthetic and cosmetic reconstruction, such as

- Exposure of clear margins for impression taking
- Hard and soft tissue crown lengthening
- Creation of a physiologic emergence profile
- Cleansable ovate pontic site creation
- Melanin depigmentation
- Laser bleaching

Before any of these procedures is considered for use, the role of various laser wavelengths and biologic width considerations should be fully understood.

Laser Wavelengths for Cosmetic/Prosthetic Procedures

Carbon Dioxide Lasers

The carbon dioxide (CO_2) laser wavelengths of 10,600 nm and 9300 nm are delivered using an articulated arm or waveguide that terminates at a handpiece. Most CO_2 laser manufacturers offer multiple handpieces with different angles (straight and contra-angle) and different focal points to perform procedures such as vaporization, coagulation, or tissue modification (see Chapter 2).

Oral soft tissue is 90% to 97% water. The CO_2 laser wavelength is highly absorbed by water, as are the erbium laser wavelengths. CO_2 lasers are therefore highly efficient when they are used on soft tissue. Soft tissue excision or incision is accomplished at 100° C, at which vaporization of intracellular and extracellular water causes ablation of biologic tissue.[1]

The mode of operation for 10,600 nm CO_2 lasers historically has been as a continuous wave: Energy is emitted constantly for as long as the laser is activated. Mechanical and electrical controls can produce chopped, gated, "superfast," or ultrafast bursts of energy with relatively long relaxation intervals. This controlled delivery minimizes the heat transferred to the collateral tissue, which in turn reduces unwanted thermal damage to the surrounding tissue.

Erbium Lasers

Two erbium wavelengths are currently available: the erbium-doped yttrium-aluminum-garnet (Er:YAG) wavelength at 2940 nm and the erbium-chromium–doped yttrium-scandium-gallium-garnet (Er,Cr:YSGG) wavelength at 2780 nm. Erbium laser wavelengths are transmitted through semiflexible hollow waveguides, low-OH⁻ fiberoptic cables, or articulated arms. All of the delivery methods terminate in a handpiece that may use sapphire, quartz, or hollow metal tip to transmit the energy to the target tissue. These wavelengths are highly absorbed by the water molecules in both soft and hard tissues.[2] Erbium lasers cut soft tissue, but with much less hemostatic ability than for other soft tissue lasers.[2] With newer technology providing for longer pulse durations and wave configurations, however, the hemostatic ability has improved.

Erbium and 9300 nm CO_2 lasers are safe for ablating diseased tooth structure. Patients may not need traditional injectable anesthetic; however, this requirement is driven as much by the patient's perception of dental treatment as by the procedure itself. Laser cavity preparation is less traumatic to the tooth's pulpal tissues than techniques that involve traditional rotary instrumentation. The vibration and heat produced by rotary instruments, which are the main reasons for discomfort during procedures, do not occur as much with the erbium wavelengths as with traditional rotary instruments.[3]

To obtain increased bond strengths over conventional techniques, the finished preparation should be etched in the traditional manner. Techniques that involve adhesion to the smear layer should be avoided, because these lasers remove smear layers.[4]

One disadvantage is that these wavelengths similar to all lasers cannot remove gold or metal crowns, vitreous porcelain, or amalgam restorations (see Chapter 10).

Diode Lasers

Diode lasers deliver wavelengths ranging from 810 to 1064 nm. Diode lasers are compact and portable solid-state units. They are used strictly for soft tissue procedures and penetrate 2 to 3 mm or more into soft tissue, depending on the wavelength and tissue biotype. Diode laser wavelengths are absorbed by pigmented structures, making them ideal for cutting melanotic or highly vascularized soft tissues and providing hemostasis.[5]

The usefulness of the diode laser can be greatly expanded by proper carbonization of the fiber tip. This preparation allows for vaporization with limited peripheral damage to nonpigmented tissue.[6]

Neodymium:Yttrium-Aluminum-Garnet Laser

The neodymium-doped yttrium-aluminum-garnet (Nd:YAG) wavelength of 1064 nm delivered in a free-running mode can be used for numerous soft tissue procedures. As with diode and CO_2 lasers, the advantages of the Nd:YAG laser include a relatively bloodless surgical field, minimal swelling, reduced surgical time, excellent coagulation, and in most cases, reduced or no postoperative pain.[7]

The main disadvantage of the Nd:YAG laser is the greater depth of penetration into the target tissue. The Nd:YAG wavelength penetrates deeply into tissue because it is poorly absorbed by water, the main component of gingival tissue. The clinician must be alert to the risk of unnecessary collateral tissue damage, particularly to underlying bone or pulpal tissues. Tissue vaporization is slower than with other, better-absorbed laser wavelengths (e.g., CO_2). Application of a topical photoabsorbing dye can shorten the lag time for absorption of the laser energy.[8] Nd:YAG laser light directed at the clinical crown or root surface of the tooth for any length of time is a concern. Consequent heating of the pulp may be of sufficient magnitude to cause inflammation and possibly irreversible tissue damage.[9] Such damage would occur only if incorrect laser parameters were used. This risk highlights the critical role of proper training for performing laser-enhanced dentistry (see Chapter 16).

Biologic Width

Gargiulo first described the biologic protection of the dentogingival junction as being a combined function of the connective tissue, fibrous attachment, and epithelial attachment of the gingival tissues to the dentition.[10] It was determined that the length of the epithelial attachment was 0.97 mm

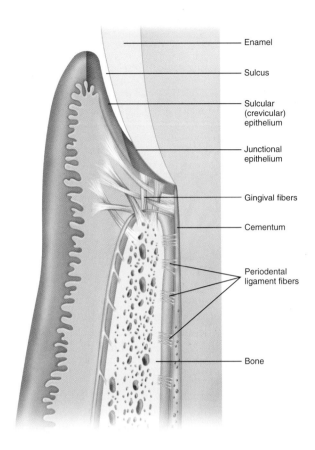

• **Figure 6-1** The tooth is attached to the surrounding gingival tissue and alveolar bone by fibrous attachments. The gingival fibers run from the cementum into the gingiva immediately apical to the junctional epithelium attachment, and the periodontal ligament fibers run from the cementum into the adjacent cortex of the alveolar bone. (Modified from Rose LF, Mealey BL: *Periodontics: medicine, surgery, and implants*, St Louis, 2004, Mosby.)

and the connective tissue attachment was 1.07 mm. This 2-mm functional unit has been described as the biologic width of the attachment. *Biologic width* is defined, in a restorative context, as the combined height of connective tissue and epithelial attachment plus 1 mm. This should be the most apical extension of dental restoration toward the osseous crest necessary to maintain periodontal health. The 1-mm added depth of sulcus establishes a good margin of safety to avoid unnatural inflammatory response to the restoration (Figure 6-1). This distance is important to consider when fabricating dental restorations because the dentist must respect the natural architecture of the gingival attachment to avoid an inflammatory response to the restoration. The problem is not the restoration but rather the bacteria that will always find shelter in the interface between the restorative margin and the tooth structure. When restorative procedures fail to take these considerations into account, with consequent violation of biologic width parameters, three possible issues may arise: (1) pocketing develops, with progression of periodontal soft tissue loss; (2) gingival recession and localized bone loss occur; most dramatically in cases with thin

Enamel
Sulcus
Sulcular (crevicular) epithelium
Junctional epithelium
Gingival fibers
Cementum
Periodontal ligament fibers
Bone

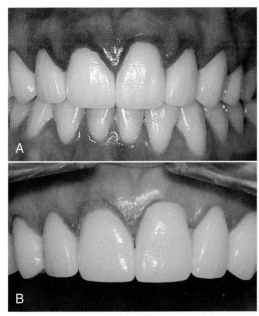

• **Figure 6-2** Laser correction of biologic width. **A,** Biologic width impingement in the anterior segment. Note localized gingival hyperplasia, redness, and inflammation surrounding the porcelain veneers. **B,** Photograph of site 2 weeks after correction of biologic width using an erbium laser in a closed-flap procedure to establish new bone level.

labial bone; or (3) localized gingival hyperplasia develops, with possible bone loss as well (Figure 6-2). This standard remained for many years until Vasek suggested that the connective tissue attachment had a more variable width with a more narrow distribution and range than the epithelial attachment. Although the mean attachment measurements for both epithelial attachment and connective tissue attachment remained remarkably similar to those as described by Gargiulo, a range was given of 0.32 to 3.27 mm for epithelial attachment and 0.29 to 1.84 mm for connective tissue attachment. These findings suggest the need for more thorough analysis of each patient's individual biologic width before a determination of restoration placement is made. As described further on, these attachment levels may be altered with crown-lengthening procedures, using dental lasers.

Soft Tissue Troughing with and without Gingivoplasty

The *gingival trough* is defined as the narrow space between the free margin of the gingival epithelium and the adjacent enamel of a tooth.[11] At times, permanent alteration of the gingival contours around a tooth or teeth is necessary to ensure a superior, long-lasting cosmetic restoration. The successful outcome of a direct or indirect restoration is related to the dentist's ability to control the surgical site. In controlling the site for delivery of a superior restoration, lasers provide the following functions:

1. Enable the dentist to access and visualize the operative site and all of the margins clearly, especially when the margins are subgingival

2. Create a blood-free environment and achieve hemostasis if necessary
3. Control moisture content of the field
4. Ensure bacterial decontamination of the field, leading to superior gingival health around the margins
5. Control the soft tissue contours for a harmonious esthetic and functional relationship between the soft tissues of the periodontium and the restored hard tissues of the teeth and underlying bone

These steps are essential for the fabrication of precise impressions, for digital scanning, or for direct placement of restorative materials. Whenever the restorative interface is subgingival, the displacement of gingival tissue is critical for finalizing tooth preparation and impression taking or restorative material placement.[12] With older restorative materials, a common challenge to the dentist was placement of the preparation "finish line" at or below the crest of the gingiva so that the margin did not show. Retraction of the gingival tissues usually was performed mechanically, with retraction cord impregnated with medicaments for hemostasis. Packing of retraction cord around the circumference of the tooth to reflect the gingiva away from the tooth and to absorb crevicular fluids was the conventional technique used for recording the finished preparation margin or to complete placement of the direct restorative material.

Conventional Techniques

A technique widely used for gingival retraction is a *double-cord technique* for subgingival reflection of tissue. Removing the second (top) retraction cord before injecting the impression material or creating an optical impression allows for complete capture of the finish line. This time-consuming technique has its disadvantages, including potential injury to the periodontal ligament if excessive force is used; difficulty in removing the retraction cord without creating shredding of the cord or bleeding, and postoperative discomfort.[13]

Another conventional gingival troughing technique, use of *electrosurgery* or radiosurgery, allows for contouring of gingival tissues and hemorrhage control. The electrosurgery procedure may be associated with delayed wound healing, with asymmetric gingival heights, crestal bony recession, and moderate postoperative discomfort.[14] In a study of electrosurgical gingival troughing with a fully rectified current on rhesus monkeys, Wilhelmsen et al.[15] showed statistically significant recession of the gingival margin along with apical migration of the junctional epithelium. Deep soft tissue resections close to bone typically produced gingival recession, bone sequestration and necrosis, loss of bone height, furcation involvement, and tooth mobility. Electrosurgery (or radiosurgery) is contraindicated around dental implants[16] and must not be used in patients with any of the following:

• Pacemakers
• A history of radiation to the jaws
• Poorly controlled (or uncontrolled) diabetes
• Blood dyscrasias
• Immunodeficiencies
• Other diseases that cause delayed or poor healing[17]

Scalpel techniques are used primarily to resect tissue to provide access and visualization of the target site. Scalpel incision surgery may result in gingival attachment loss with apical repositioning, exposure of sensitive root surface to the oral environment, asymmetric gingival margins, and the postoperative pain and discomfort typically associated with periodontal surgery.[18]

Laser Troughing

In contrast with conventional techniques, laser troughing allows for clear, clean visualization of gingival margins. Most lasers are excellent coagulation devices, with minimal to no bleeding. Unlike blade or electrosurgical techniques, laser gingival troughing with a laser gingivectomy can be performed at the same appointment as impression taking. The patient saves a trip to the office, greatly reducing valuable chair time. The ease with which necrotic tissue debris is removed from around the preparation finish line simplifies impression taking. Retraction cord is not necessary for reflection around the tooth or teeth; no placement or removal of cord from multiple pockets is required for taking impressions of multiple teeth or a full arch. Laser treatment causes no recession or repositioning of the gingival margin.[19] Laser troughing promotes an ideal environment for use of current impression scanning devices.

Dentists who practice laser surgery and laser gingival troughing have reported high patient acceptance and comfort. Neill's survey[20] on self-reported patient comfort after laser gingival troughing revealed that 3 h after treatment, patients were comfortable, with half "extremely" comfortable. The overall pain rating was 1.9 (on a scale of 0.0 to 10.0), indicating that patients experienced minimal to no pain.

Laser vaporization of fibrotic tissue around crown margins is extremely fast, with no bleeding, swelling, or postoperative pain. Predictable stability of the gingival tissue on healing is the rule, with the additional benefit of elimination of pathogens from the periodontal pocket.[21,22]

Slightly different techniques are used for each wavelength. The laser dentist must learn the specific procedure and follow the specific protocols for the particular device employed. Once again, it must be emphasized that training is critical in using this technology.

CLINICAL TIP

The novice laser dentist should never start with procedures in the esthetic zone. Gingival troughing should start with molars, where the tissue is slightly thicker. Once proficiency with molars has been attained, development of laser surgery skills can be furthered with procedures in more anterior areas, until the confidence and technical expertise necessary for successful surgery in the esthetic zone have been acquired.

Beginner-level laser users should always start with power settings at the lower end of suggested parameters until they become experienced with the modality of treatment. Thermal tissue damage in the anterior region associated with inappropriate use of higher-power settings could potentially result in undesirable gingival contours.

Erbium lasers use thin tips made of sapphire, quartz, or hollow metal for troughing. For use of erbium lasers on soft tissue, the water spray usually is turned off. This precaution aids in hemostasis. CO_2 lasers have thin hollow metal or ceramic tips for troughing. The Nd:YAG and diode lasers use optical fibers of various diameters to perform gingival troughing.

Procedure

The laser troughing procedure is simple to perform. With CO_2, erbium, and Nd:YAG lasers, the laser tip is placed parallel to the long axis of the tooth, barely into the periodontal sulcus. The tip should glide circumferentially around the margin of the tooth, with slight to no resistance. Watch for any yellowing of the gingival tissue, which will indicate thermal collateral damage. With diode lasers, the fiber may be directed from the gingival crest toward the tooth just apical to the margin, removing a thin layer of tissue and opening more of a wedge-shaped trough for easier flow of the impression material.

To maximize its efficiency, the tip must be kept free of debris. With CO_2 lasers, a stream of air blown through the hollow tip keeps it patent. Debris may accumulate on the outside of the tip, however, in which case the tip should be wiped down with gauze or replaced. Nd:YAG and diode lasers use glass or quartz fibers, which become dulled and scratched after multiple uses. A dull tip may cut tissue poorly, much like a broken piece of glass, leaving tissue tags.[7] The tip must therefore be cleaved periodically to ensure optimal results. Some diode lasers are supplied with disposable tips, but the cost of tips is much greater than that incurred with simple recleaving of a standard 3-m optical fiber. The tip also must be "initiated" so that the depth of penetration of the wavelength is minimized, with no deep thermal damage.

During troughing to establish gingival proportions with the diode and Nd:YAG lasers, the clinician may note carbonization on the tissues.[8,23] This layer can be quickly removed using a 3% hydrogen peroxide solution in a mini-brush tip syringe (Figures 6-3 and 6-4).

CLINICAL TIP

An important point of technique is that the laser tip should "glide" through the tissue, with minimal to no resistance. If the Nd:YAG or diode fiber meets resistance or moves irregularly through the sulcus, the tip needs to be cleaved or replaced. When using the laser for hemostasis of previously inflamed tissue, remember to treat the area that is bleeding, which may be coronal to the depth of the trough itself.

Crown-Lengthening Procedures

The performance of crown-lengthening procedures has become progressively more driven both by esthetics, reflecting the increasing popularity of "smile enhancement" procedures, and by practitioners' better understanding of the principles of biologic width preservation in the restoration

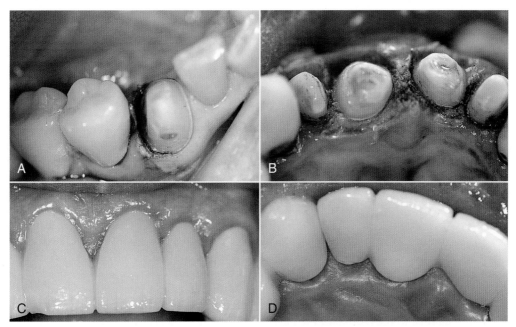

• **Figure 6-3** Gingival troughing of soft tissue with a CO_2 laser. **A,** Treatment of deep distal decay in tooth #28 involves use of CO_2 laser to create gingival trough around entire tooth and minor gingivoplasty of tissue on distal surface of tooth. Note dry field and excellent visualization of gingival margin. **B,** Soft tissue troughing and soft tissue crown lengthening to expose tooth structure without violating biologic width dimensions in an 83-year-old man with traumatic mouth injury. **C,** Anterior facial view of final splinted prosthesis 1 month after delivery. **D,** Lingual-incisal view of final restoration 1 month after delivery. Gingival tissues responded well to treatment.

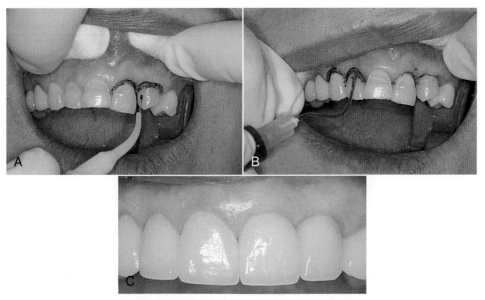

• **Figure 6-4** Gingival troughing of soft tissue with a diode laser. **A,** In this procedure, the diode laser fiber tip glides along the axial surface of the tooth for precision. Technique uses slow, continuous strokes, with care taken not to blunt interproximal papillae. **B,** During gingival troughing to establish gingival proportions with diode laser, carbonization may be seen on the tissues. This layer can be quickly removed using 3% hydrogen peroxide solution in a diffusing-brush syringe. Keep the laser tip parallel to the tooth surface or slightly angled away from the surface, to avoid absorption of the wavelength by hard tissue. **C,** Final postoperative facial view of healthy tissue after gingival troughing and placement of restorations.

of the broken-down dentition. Crown lengthening is a surgical procedure performed to expose a greater gingivoincisal length of tooth structure, before restoring the tooth prosthetically. Such exposure involves predictably excising a small amount of *only* gingival tissue around the tooth (*soft tissue* crown lengthening), or of *both* gingival tissue and alveolar bone (*osseous* crown lengthening). Although many general dentists perform this procedure, many others refer patients requiring crown lengthening to a periodontist or oral surgeon. Conventional techniques of osseous crown lengthening generally involve a full-thickness flap procedure to establish the new gingival level.[17]

Soft Tissue

The crown-lengthening procedure is basically an excision of gingival soft tissue. Conventional methods of executing this technique involve the use of surgical scalpels or periodontal knives or electrosurgery. Recommended placement of the excision is at least 2 mm coronal to the bottom of the gingival attachment, to reduce the risk of root exposure and violation of biologic width principles.[24]

Hard Tissue

Surgical crown-lengthening procedures may involve the hard tissue as well. To provide adequate biologic width from the margin of the restoration, a minimum of 3 mm of attached gingiva must remain over the underlying bone to create a healthy periodontal environment.

Use of flap surgery with osseous resection is the traditional method of choice when crown margins will impinge on the biologic width. Rotary instruments have long been used to recontour the alveolar structure. Bone recontouring can be achieved conventionally with fissure or diamond burs, using copious amounts of water, or with bone chisels. Thinning of the bone around the tooth or teeth reduces craters or ridges that create sharp, uneven soft tissue topography. Sufficient bone is removed to create a 3-mm space between the crest of the bone and the new restoration's finishing-line margin. However, poor esthetics may result from enlarged gingival embrasures, root sensitivity, transient mobility, or root resorption.[24]

In some cases, the need for osseous recontouring may be localized to one specific area because of the presence of a subgingival restoration, carious lesion, or fractured cusp. Erbium lasers may be useful in localized osseous tissue removal for establishing a new biologic width without raising a gingival flap. In allowing for careful removal of osseous tissue in a closed-flap technique, along with soft tissue removal, the clinician can create the biologic width for the final restoration and complete the impressions for the indirect restoration in the same appointment.[25] The closed-flap, hard tissue crown-lengthening procedure is very technique-sensitive and is not recommended for the novice laser dentist; advanced training in open-flap periodontal surgery is highly recommended.

Erbium lasers have end-cutting tips with a water spray that prevents the surgical site from overheating, in contrast with the rotary friction heat released by conventional burs. Collateral thermal tissue damage when using erbium lasers is less than with conventional techniques.[4] The use of rotary diamond or carbide burs for osseous tissue removal risks possible damage to adjacent tooth structure. Healing after conventional osseous surgery is associated with swelling and postoperative pain.[26] Bleeding from a conventional (blade) incision typically will compromise visualization of the surgical site, in contrast with a laser incision, and visualization is critical in working on osseous structure. The risk of bony damage caused by dissipated heat from rotary burs outweighs the risk of trauma from a water-cooled erbium laser when correct parameters are used.

The procedure starts by measuring the amount of needed reduction of the bony crest. End-cutting then commences. While maintained in parallel orientation with the root surface, the laser tip is advanced to penetrate the crestal bone to the desired depth. Miniature osteotomies are produced with the laser tip. Once at the desired depth, the laser tip is withdrawn and moved 1 to 2 mm laterally, and the next osteotomy is performed to the desired depth. This sequence continues across the facial or buccal, mesial, distal, and lingual walls until the entire circumference is treated, if necessary.[25]

Once the cut is completed, the laser tip is inserted into the osteotomy site. A swiping motion in the mesial or distal direction is performed to remove any osseous tags between osteotomy sites. Soft smoothing of the underlying bone removes troughs or craters and creates a scalloped topography from the facial surface to interproximal surface.[25] The gingival tissue is essentially a marker of underlying bone, and preservation of the interproximal bone height will prevent loss of the interproximal papillae. A literature review revealed that the contact area between teeth should be positioned 5 mm incisal to the height of the interproximal bone to maintain the papillae.[27] Provisionalize the area, and allow 3 to 4 weeks for healing before taking the final impression. Once again, it must be pointed out that a closed-flap osseous procedure is a "blind" procedure and is not recommended for laser dentists to perform until they have extensive experience and training with their units.

If conventional (rotary or bone chisel) open-flap osseous recontouring is performed, any laser wavelength (or a scalpel) may be used to open and reflect the flap. With a laser incision for full-thickness flap reflection rather than conventional techniques, visualization of the bony crest is enhanced because bleeding is minimal. The surgical site is cleaner, free of blood, and more "sterile," because the laser destroys bacteria as it incises the soft tissue.

The bone should be contoured so that the bone structure has no craters or ledges. If any of these defects are present, the overlying soft tissue will become thick, hindering good impression taking, in addition to resulting in deep probing depth after the restoration is cemented. Before suturing, it is essential to ensure that the flaps are without tension and

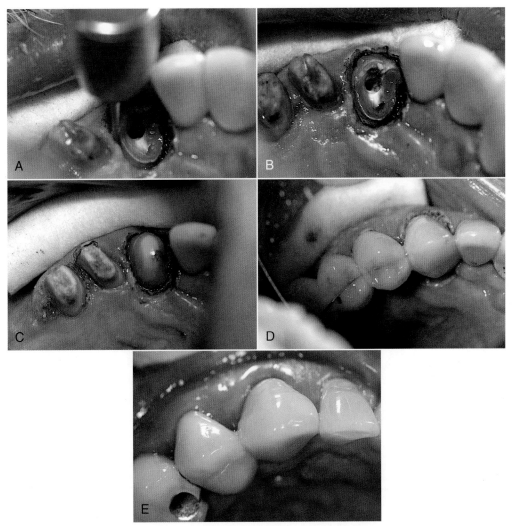

• **Figure 6-5** Hard tissue crown-lengthening procedure. **A,** Miniature osteotomies are produced with the laser tip. Once at desired depth, laser tip is withdrawn and moved 1 to 2 mm laterally, and the next osteotomy is performed. Osseous tissue is dropped to desired depth to create a biologic width zone. Osseous troughing is done circumferentially with Er,Cr:YSGG laser, followed by soft tissue contouring with diode laser to expose tooth structure. **B,** Incisal view after hard tissue and soft tissue crown lengthening on tooth #11. **C,** Dry field has been established for post-and-core buildup, and the site is ready for taking impressions. **D,** Provisional restoration with opened interproximal papilla development. **E,** Final restoration 5 years postoperatively.

preferably covering where the eventual crown margin will be placed. Flaps will not lie correctly if the bone is not contoured properly.[11]

Sutures should be removed within 7 to 10 days. If crown lengthening is performed correctly, the impression can be made 3 to 6 weeks after the open-flap surgery for posterior teeth and a few weeks later for anterior teeth, for which soft tissue esthetics is critical (Figure 6-5) (see also Chapter 4).

Emergence Profile

Emergence profile is defined as the axial contour of a tooth or crown as it relates to the adjacent soft tissue.[28] In developing an optimal emergence profile during procedures that close spaces between teeth (e.g., diastema closure,

ovate pontic site formation, implant placement), presence of interproximal tissue that has no papilla point is typical. This characteristically fibrotic tissue can present an esthetic challenge in treatment plans incorporating crowns and veneers. The clinician needs to measure the periodontal pocket to establish a biologic width requirement. The general rule for creating the ideal emergence profile of the restoration is that for every millimeter of additional width added to each tooth to close a diastema, the margin of the restoration must be prepared an additional 1 mm subgingivally.[29]

Emergence profile is critical for gingival health and esthetic contours. Axial contours of the prepared tooth structure will be reflected in the final restoration contours as well. The contact point of the restoration(s) will influence the overall appearance of the gingival tissue and restoration. Proximal contacts between the posterior teeth are located in the occlusal to middle third of the crowns. The contact must be more than just a point occlusogingivally; it also must not extend too far gingivally to encroach on the gingival embrasure. The axial surface of the restoration cervical to the proximal contact point should be flat or slightly concave to prevent encroachment on the interdental papilla.[27]

Overcontouring of the proximal surfaces apical to the contact area creates convex surfaces, which in turn violates the space of the interproximal papilla, creating biologic width encroachment issues. The most common error with regard to axial inclination is the creation of a bulge or excessive convexity, especially at the gingival third of the restoration. Dental technicians frequently overemphasize this feature. Overcontouring promotes the accumulation of food debris and plaque, and gingival inflammation is encouraged rather than prevented.[30]

Provisional restorations should be used to create and preview the acceptable gingival contours of the final restorations. The provisional restorations may be used to guide the healing contours of the gingival tissue and to fabricate a similar emergence profile in the definitive prosthesis[24] (Figure 6-6).

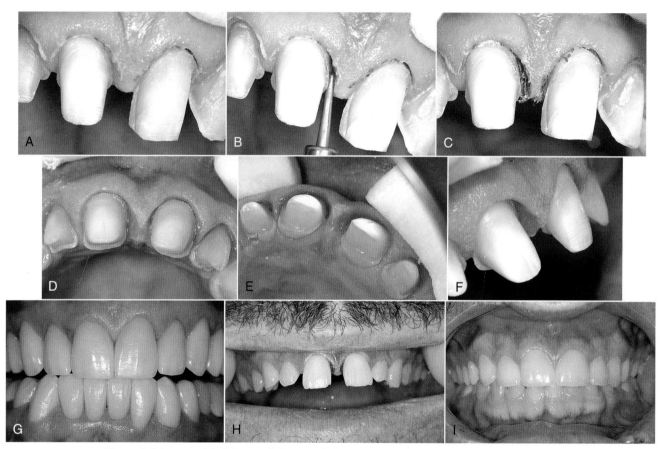

• **Figure 6-6** Laser-assisted closure of diastema. **A,** Preoperative view showing the patient with old porcelain veneers removed. Diastema between teeth #8 and #9 is 2.5 mm wide. Periodontal probing reveals gingival pocket depth of 3 mm. Each tooth will be widened by 1.25 mm to close the diastema. **B,** Gingival trough 1.25 mm deep is created on tooth #8 for lowering preparation margin to establish new emergence profile of restoration. Laser tip is guided along the axial tooth surface for precise control, using slow, continuous strokes from facial-mesial-lingual. Soft tissue wall is tapered toward new papilla point. **C,** Continue creating gingival trough on #9 with same 1.25-mm depth as on #8. Slope tissue trough toward new interdental papilla, and always leave 1 mm of tissue island. Apically position preparation margin on mesial side of #8 and #9 for new emergence profile. Impressions can be taken at this appointment and provisional restorations placed. Allow space for papilla to develop while the patient is wearing provisional restorations. **D,** Facial-incisal view after removal of provisional restorations. Note well-developed, healthy stippled interproximal papilla. **E,** Incisolingual view of developed interproximal tissue before final placement of restorations. **F,** Anteromesial view of interproximal papillae with stippled tissue. **G,** Try-in of final restorations. Note slight blanching of interproximal tissue between #8 and #9. On final cementation, firm pressure is applied to seat the restorations fully before tack curing. **H,** Diastema 3 mm in width in a similar case. Emergence profile will begin 1.5 mm subgingivally on mesial aspect of both #8 and #9. **I,** Postoperative facial view of diastema closure in patient in **H.** Gingival tissue framing is proportionate to the teeth, and restorations have been fabricated with long contact points incisogingivally.

Advanced Emergence Profile Dilemma

The goal of reconstructing an alveolar ridge is to restore the health of the periodontal apparatus so that the patient can continue to function normally. Success is based on not only the final state of health of the gingival tissues but also the stability and esthetics of the case. Some restorative cases may feature irregular bone loss. As bone loss progresses, the anterior ridges become knife-edged, with loss of papillae and the normally scalloped gingival contour.[31]

The absence of the interproximal papilla has adverse effects on esthetic and phonetic results. Restoring the papilla requires surgical precision and soft tissue manipulation to create the desired outcome. Any mistake may be catastrophic because of the small size and meager blood supply of the papilla. Even the use of vasoconstrictors in anesthetics and in conventional retraction cords may lead to necrosis. A laser procedure reduces the risk of gingival migration while not affecting the blood supply necessary to support the interdental papilla.[22]

Ovate Pontic Design

Ovate pontic design enhances esthetics to make the pontic appear to be emerging from the gingival crest, as would a natural tooth, unlike a ridge lap design. The cosmetic advantage of the ovate pontic is its ability to replicate natural contours, maximizing esthetics. The clinical advantages of the ovate pontic include excellent emergence profile for natural contours, ease of cleaning, its function as an effective seal to prevent food entrapment under the prosthesis, and elimination or minimization of the "black triangle" gingival embrasures.[32]

The conventional ovate soft tissue design was classically created by means of gingivoplasty using either a round carbide bur or a football-shaped diamond bur. Major disadvantages with this technique are the potential for tissue mutilation, bleeding, inability to take the final impression immediately after the procedure, and delayed tissue development and healing.[32]

To prevent development of a poor pontic site, immediately after removal of a tooth, a socket preservation procedure (the socket is filled with bone material) is performed to maintain the tissue height.[33]

An ovate pontic site requires a significant facial-lingual width (depending on location in the dental arch) and apical-coronal thickness to surround the ovate pontic within the edentulous space. A thin, knife-edge ridge often is a contraindication to an ovate-type pontic; however, if the dimensions mentioned are inadequate, a surgical augmentation procedure can be considered. Various soft tissue augmentation

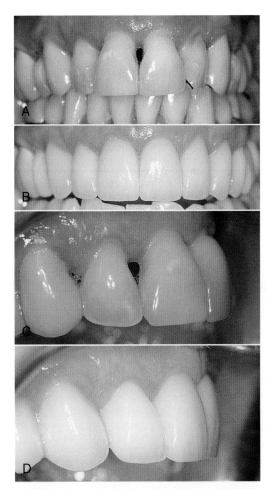

• **Figure 6-7 A,** After periodontal surgery, wide gingival embrasures are evident. Absence of interproximal papilla has adverse esthetic and phonetic results. **B,** Final restorations in place with long incisogingival contacts. Serrated interproximal papilla creates esthetic soft tissue framing of restorations. **C,** Lateral incisor–central incisor embrasure. Treatment technique is the same as for diastema closure between teeth #8 and #9 (see Figure 6-6). **D,** Lateral view of interproximal papillae with healthy stippled tissue.

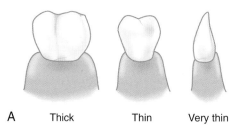

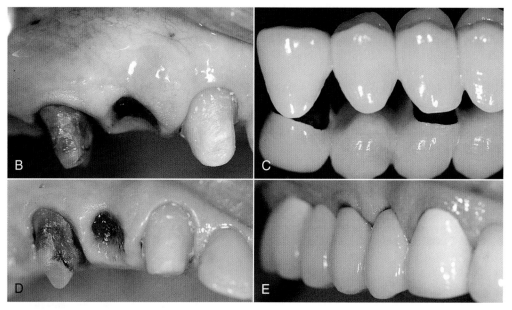

• **Figure 6-8** **A,** *From left*: posterior ovate site placement in center of ridge; bicuspid ovate site placement toward midbuccal area of ridge; anterior ovate site placement to facial area of ridge. **B,** Provisional restoration removed to expose ovate site for try-in of fixed bridge. Note development of interdental papilla mesial and distal to pontic site. **C,** Note ovate pontic fabricated by dental laboratory technician to sit into ovate site. **D,** Occlusobuccal view of interdental papilla development. The ovate site is red and inflamed as a consequence of no plaque control while the patient was wearing the provisional restoration. **E,** Prosthesis try-in. Note slight blanching of ovate site at teeth #5 and #3. These sites may need to be modified at this visit by deepening the ovate site with a laser before cementing the prosthesis.

techniques can be used for this purpose, depending on the complexity of the ridge defect (Figure 6-8).

A molar pontic requires the ovate site to be designed in the middle of the ridge. With more anterior sites, the ovate site design should be closer to the buccal-facial aspect. Aligning the adjacent gingival heights can be accomplished so that the pontic tooth does not appear to be a short clinical crown. Alteration of the gingival edentulous site is started in the middle of the ridge. Sounding the bony ridge to determine gingival thickness allows for evaluation of the biologic width. The center of the convex ovate will be the deepest segment.

The formation of an ovate pontic site using a laser starts with the removal of tissue from the center of the site. In a circular manner, the diameter of the ovate site is then slowly increased, ending it 2 mm from the adjacent abutment tooth in its mesial and distal aspects. The gingival tissue of the ovate site should now begin to slope so that the deepest portion is the center; for this component of the procedure, it is helpful to visualize an egg and how it will be able to sit into that divot. By leaving 2 mm of gingival

tissue mesially and distally, the interproximal papillae can be developed[33] (Figures 6-9 and 6-10). The procedural steps are as follows:

The sculpting of gingival tissue is exceptionally precise with the laser. Use of controlled laser energy for these procedures minimizes postoperative swelling, decreases postoperative pain, and reduces healing time.[18,21] These procedures all are performed at initial treatment, whereas using conventional methods would mean completing these soft tissue alterations several weeks before preparation/impression day.

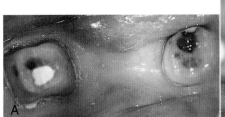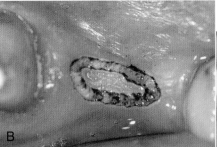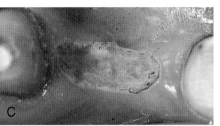

• **Figure 6-9** **A,** Posterior ovate site between teeth #18 and #20. The ovate pontic should be placed in center of the ridge for a molar site. **B,** First, mark the site by outlining planned ovate area. **C,** Start by applying laser energy in center of ovate site and then swirl outward to peripheral boundary of ovate pontic site. Slope the deepest part of ovate *(center)* up to interproximal area of adjacent teeth. Leave the slope 2 mm from adjacent teeth to create interproximal papillae.

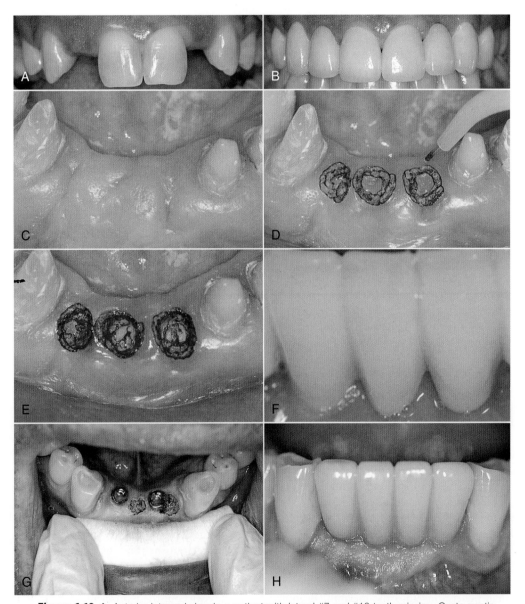

• **Figure 6-10** **A,** Anterior intraoral view in a patient with lateral #7 and #10 teeth missing. Ovate pontic designed to facial aspect of gingival ridge and to match adjacent apical gingival heights. Leave 1 to 2 mm of interproximal tissue to create papillae mesial and distal to the pontic. **B,** Seated three-unit bridges #6 to #8 and #9 to #11. Note gingival heights and interproximal papillae on ovate pontics #7 and #10. **C,** Anterior lower ridge site for ovate pontic development with diode laser. **D,** Mark ridge with diode laser for ovate pontic site. Stay to facial side of ridge. Deepen center portion of pontic and slope up to interproximal papillae. **E,** Deepen ovate sites for pontics to sit within gingival ridge, as opposed to overlapping it. Check for overheating of gingival tissue. If tissues acquire a yellowish tint during the procedure, correct by reducing the wattage. **F,** Ovate pontic site on lower anterior ridge at 5 years. **G,** Ovate pontic site developed around implants in anterior lower segment. Site is deepened for the ovate pontic. **H,** Final restoration in place at 6 months shows excellent interproximal papillae.

A two-stage soft tissue treatment would be likely with conventional techniques because of the swelling associated with electrosurgery, rotary instrumentation, or soft tissue scalpel surgery. Soft tissue results would be unpredictable if these methods were used at the preparation/impression appointment.[14,21]

Hard Tissue Ovate Pontic Site Formation

If less than 2 mm of gingival tissue is present between the bony crest and the pontic site, other treatment modalities must be considered. Using an erbium laser to remove bone from the pontic site would be the solution. Sufficient bone must be removed so that there is no violation of the biologic width. A provisional restoration is placed in the area, and at least 2 mm of space is left between the tissue side of the pontic and the crestal bone, to allow the gingival tissue to granulate inward before proceeding with the final impression.[25]

Laser Depigmentation

Deeply melanotic gingiva can be a social stigma in many cultures; accordingly, laser melanin depigmentation of a patient's gingiva is becoming more common. All of the current dental lasers can accomplish gingival depigmentation, and as with most procedures, dentists have their preferences regarding which wavelength is "best." Some clinicians prefer Nd:YAG and diode laser wavelengths because of their affinity for pigment such as melanin. Others prefer the erbium and CO_2 laser wavelengths because these are easily attracted to the water in the gingival tissue. Most dentists who perform gingival depigmentation believe that laser treatment is the most reliable and satisfactory method.[34–38]

Diode and Nd:YAG lasers use the same basic technique: Because the aim is not to cut the tissue but rather to deliver the laser energy deep to the epithelium, to be absorbed by the pigment, a low power is used. Nd:YAG and diode lasers may be used out of contact with a noninitiated tip; the energy will then not be absorbed by the superficial layers of tissue but will penetrate the tissue until it is absorbed by the melanin. As the laser energy is absorbed by the melanin, the tissue lightens in color. Alternatively, the diode and Nd:YAG lasers can be used in light contact with very light, brushstroke-like movements of the beam through the tissue. If this technique is used, care must be taken that the tip does not accumulate tissue debris. Once debris accumulates on the tip, the laser becomes "activated" and will work superficially, rather than penetrating into the melanin. Erbium and CO_2 lasers interact with surface tissue, so it is necessary to "peel" the tissue down to the level containing the pigmentation.[37] Care should be taken to preserve the marginal gingiva. Because most pigmentation is in the basal and suprabasal areas relatively close to the surface, both techniques can be effective.[36] Regardless of the wavelength used,

laser gingival depigmentation usually is performed with use of only topical anesthetic.

> ### CLINICAL TIP
>
> Diode and Nd:YAG lasers usually come with just one size of fiber, usually a 300- or 400-μm diameter fiber; however, manufacturers make many different sizes of fibers, ranging from 100 μm to 1000 μm in diameter. For dental use, the 100-μm and 200-μm fibers are too thin and fragile to be useful for many procedures. Attempts to use these fibers in periodontal pockets led to breakage of fibers within the pocket. A 300- to 400-μm fiber is an "all-purpose" fiber, capable of performing most routine dental tasks. For melanin depigmentation when the goal is to cover a large surface area quickly, availability of a 600-, 800-, or even 1000-μm fiber will make this procedure much more efficient.

Carbon dioxide lasers may be used to perform a deepithelialization procedure. Again, the goal is not to cut the tissue but to remove the epithelial layer that contains the melanocytes. Low power is used with a large spot size; this combination minimizes the power density and enables the dentist to cover a large area more quickly. In like manner, erbium lasers can be used in contact with the tissue, gently removing the tissue layer by layer until the epithelial layer containing the melanocytes is removed (Figure 6-11).

Laser Bleaching

The pursuit of whiter teeth and use of bleaching techniques have been documented since the nineteenth century. Chemicals used for bleaching vital teeth have included oxalic acid, ether peroxide, hydrogen dioxide, and hydrogen peroxide (H_2O_2). In the early twentieth century, 35% H_2O_2 was recognized as the most effective bleaching agent. In 1918, Abbot used high-intensity light, raising the temperature of H_2O_2 rapidly to accelerate the bleaching process. In the late 1960s, Klusmier noted that a 10% carbamide peroxide solution placed in a nightguard to improve the gingival health of his patients also resulted in bleaching. In 1989, Haywood and Heymann[39] introduced and published this technique. By the 1990s, this procedure had become commonplace in dentistry.

Some patients cannot complete the home bleaching process because of the lengthy time investment, discomfort or irritation from the trays, or discomfort from the bleaching agents associated with gingival recession. For these patients, a single-visit in-office procedure produces good results quickly without these problems.

"Power bleaching," which originated with Abbot in 1918 and progressed to use of heat lamps and heated spatulas in the 1980s, has been effective, but with many side effects, including pulpal necrosis related to the inability to control the highly reactive and caustic 35% H_2O_2 solution. The goal of a single-visit power-bleaching procedure

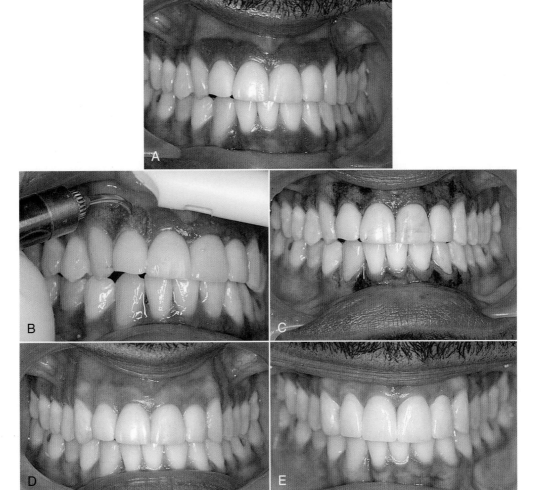

• **Figure 6-11** Laser depigmentation of deep melanotic gingiva. **A,** Preoperative view. **B,** Erbium laser performing melanin depigmentation. **C,** Immediate postoperative view. **D,** Two-week postoperative view. **E,** Six-week postoperative view with new anterior crowns in place.

is to whiten efficiently using controlled temperature elevation of the H_2O_2 on the tooth to prevent pulpal necrosis. The development of bleaching agents that combine H_2O_2 or its analogs with thickening agents, buffers, catalysts, or coloring agents has made power bleaching safer and more reliable.

The objective of laser power bleaching is to excite the bleaching agents using a very efficient source of light energy—a laser. Many studies have shown a relationship between exposure time and adverse pulpal responses: the greater the exposure time of the bleaching agent to the tooth, the greater the risk of pulpal necrosis. With use of photons of one specific wavelength that approximates the absorption spectrum of the bleaching agent, rather than using a light source that emits multiple wavelengths, the chemical reaction proceeds at a faster rate, thereby decreasing exposure time of the bleaching agent to the tooth.

Wetter et al.[40] evaluated bleaching performed using no light source, a light-emitting diode (LED), and a diode laser.

The best overall results were obtained with laser activation of the bleaching agent. Zhang et al.[41] reported similar results in comparing a potassium titanyl phosphate (KTP) laser, a diode laser, and an LED. The selection of laser wavelength is not important; any laser wavelength will successfully bleach tooth structure so long as the emission spectrum of the laser matches the absorption spectrum of the bleaching material.

Torres et al.[42] evaluated the amount of coloring agent placed in bleaching agents. Their results showed that bleaching was more intense when double and triple the amount of coloring agent was placed in the gels. The light energy from the laser excites the highly reactive H_2O_2 molecules, and as the molecules absorb the laser energy, the peroxide decomposes, with ionization into the following compounds:

Hydroxyl ions (OH^-)
Perhydroxyl ions (HOO^-)
Water (H_2O)

Oxygen ions (O^{2-})
Hydrogen ions (H^+)
Oxygen (O_2)

The perhydroxyl ions are considered to be the strongest free radicals formed during the breakage of the H_2O_2 bonds. Using a laser maximizes the perhydroxyl concentration without increasing exposure time (i.e., increased concentration of bleaching free radical without increased contact time). Free radicals are unstable and immediately seek an available target with which to react. These free radicals react with the chromophilic structures of the larger, longer-chained, darker organic compounds in the tooth. As a result, the compounds dissociate into smaller, shorter-chained molecules with different optical properties. The cosmetic result is a visually whitened tooth structure.

General Protocol

After a general review of the medical history, the patient's oral habits, diet, and lifestyle must be ascertained, along with expectations regarding the outcome of treatment. A patient who drinks four cups of black coffee daily and one or two glasses of red wine with dinner every night will have different results from those for a patient who drinks neither coffee nor red wine.

Patients with severe tetracycline staining must be informed that their treatment may take multiple applications and appointments; treatment alternatives should be discussed. Evaluate the teeth for presence of fluorosis and white-spot lesions, and review the kinds of results that can be expected with these lesions.

Confirm the starting shade of the patient's dentition by arranging the Vitapan Classical Shade Guide values in the following order (Figure 6-12):

B1 – A1 – B2 – D2 – A2 – C1 – C2 – D4 – A3 –
D3 – B3 – A3.5 – B4 – C3 – A4 – C4

Document this aspect of the evaluation with photographs.

A detailed discussion with the patient is recommended. Identify the existing restorations and clarify the necessity to replace composite restorations after the bleaching process, because these restorations will not change color during bleaching. Point out any posterior stains, such as amalgam "shining through" on the buccal surfaces of posterior teeth, that will not change without replacing the restoration. Discuss possible treatment problems, such as sensitivity during and after the procedure, associated with gingival recession and exposed root surfaces. The use of take-home trays to complement the in-office treatment may be offered if appropriate.

For the bleaching procedure, assemble the following:
- First-aid kit, including vitamin E ointment or aloe vera gel for accidental exposure of soft tissue to the bleaching agent
- Laser safety glasses
- Bibs
- Cotton rolls
- Cheek retractors
- Preparation kit
  - Pumice and a prophylaxis angle
  - Floss
  - Interproximal strips
  - Fluoride gel and/or potassium nitrate gel
  - Rubber dam (conventional or paint-on)
- Bleaching kit
  - Bleaching agent
  - Brushes, mixing pad, spatula

PROCEDURE

1. Make certain that all personnel are wearing wavelength-appropriate safety glasses.
2. Pumice all surfaces to be bleached. Do not use conventional prophy paste; such pastes usually contain fluoride and oils, which will interfere with the bleaching process.
3. Isolate teeth with rubber dam or light-cured dam.
4. Prepare the bleaching agent and carefully place on the enamel.
5. Activate the laser and follow manufacturer's instructions for exposure time. Be sure to use the recommended wavelength for the bleaching material. Many power-bleaching materials change color when the oxidation process is complete. *Do not continue to expose the bleaching agent to any more laser energy once the color change of the bleaching agent has been completed.*
6. Wipe off the used bleaching agent with wet gauze/cotton and reapply fresh material. *Do not rinse with water between applications.* Use just enough water on the gauze/cotton to remove the used agent.
7. Reapply fresh agent and reactivate the laser.
8. Wipe off the used agent, and reapply fresh agent for the third time, or apply according to manufacturer's instructions.
9. When the third application is complete, wipe off all of the used agent, irrigate with water, remove the isolation material, and rinse thoroughly for 1 min with a fluoride rinse. Apply a nonstaining fluoride solution.
10. Confirm new shade with the shade guide, and photograph the result.
11. Provide a home bleaching kit, or schedule a follow-up appointment if necessary.

CLINICAL TIP

As an objective method for validating the color changes achieved with bleaching processes, a fully calibrated spectrophotometer can used to determine all tooth shade values preoperatively and postoperatively, as in the cases shown in Figures 6-12 to 6-15.

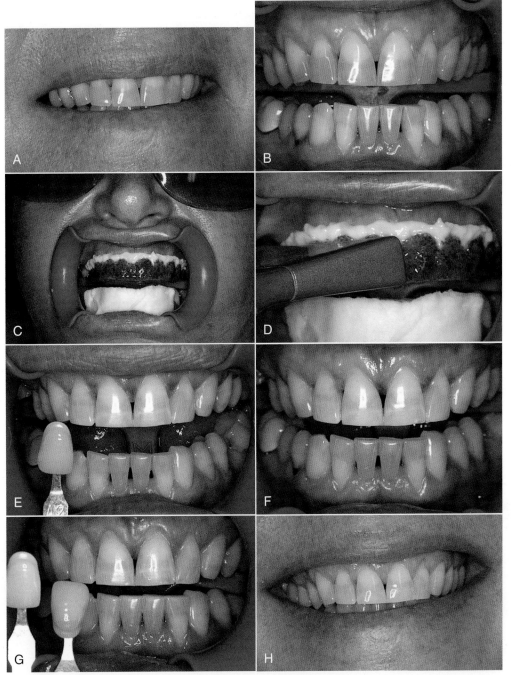

• **Figure 6-12** Laser-assisted bleaching versus home bleaching. **A, B,** Appearance of teeth before and after home bleaching procedure. **A,** The initial shade of upper teeth was A3 on the Vitapan Classical Shade Guide on gingival and middle thirds and A4 on the incisal third. Lower teeth were graded as C4. **B,** Lower arch after 10 days of home tooth whitening (upper arch before bleaching) with cheek retractors in place. Lower teeth improved from C4 to D3, a six-step change on the value-oriented Vitapan shade guide. **C to H,** Laser-assisted bleaching procedure and result. **C,** Laser-assisted bleaching of upper arch. Paint-on dental dam is in place, and bleaching material has been applied to teeth. Note cotton protecting lower arch and safety glasses protecting the patient's eyes. **D,** Diode laser handpiece applying laser energy to bleaching material. **E,** Completed laser bleaching of upper arch. **F,** Postoperative view of laser bleaching results at 48 h. Upper teeth were graded as A1 on the gingival and middle thirds (seven-step change) and as B2 on the incisal third (10-step change). **G,** Immediate postoperative view of second laser bleaching on upper arch and first laser bleaching on lower arch. Upper arch teeth improved from A1 for the gingival and middle thirds and B2 for the incisal third to A2 for the gingival third and A1 for the middle and incisal thirds. Ten days after laser bleaching, lower teeth shade improved from D3 to D2, a six-step change. These results show that one laser-assisted bleaching session of the lower arch produced the same degree of change (six steps) as 10 days of home bleaching. **H,** Six-month postoperative view of laser bleaching result.

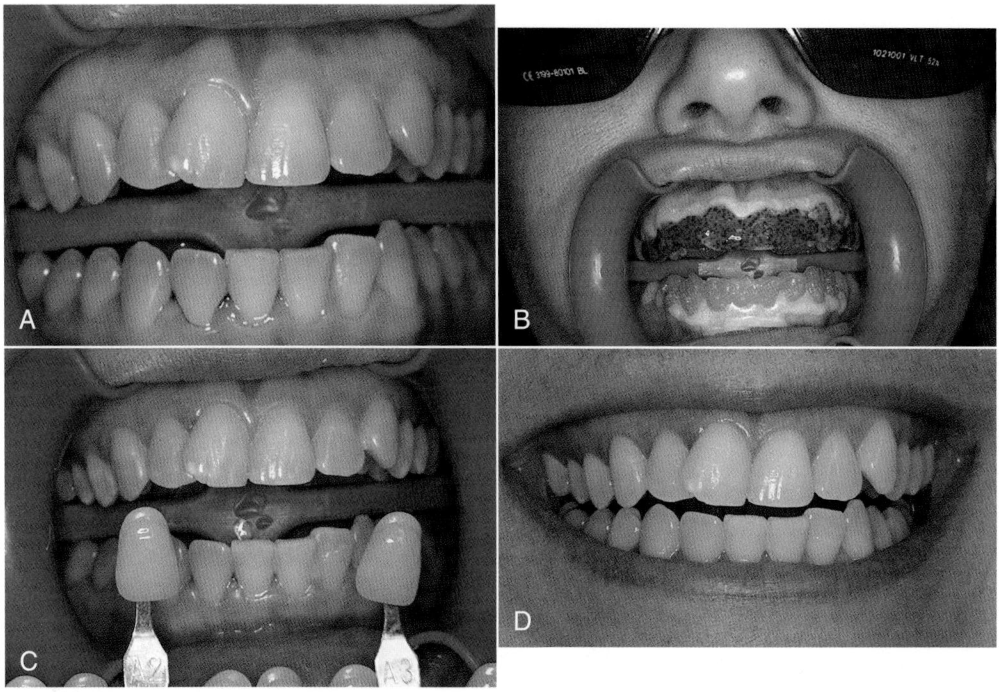

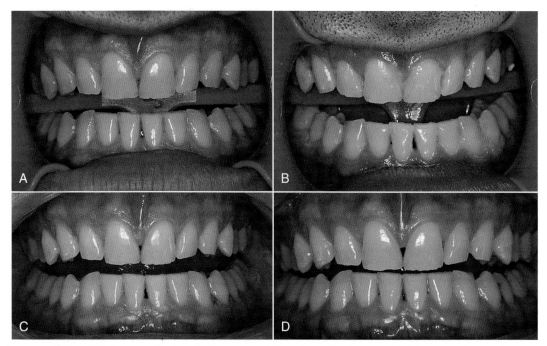

• **Figure 6-13** **A,** Preoperative view of laser-assisted bleaching of upper arch (shade A4) and LED bleaching of lower arch. **B,** Paint-on dental dam in place and bleaching material on teeth. Note mouth prop in place and laser safety glasses protecting the patient's eyes. Bleaching material for upper arch is wavelength specific for the diode laser to be used, and bleaching material for lower arch is wavelength specific for the LED unit. **C,** Immediate postoperative view of laser bleaching of upper arch and LED bleaching of lower arch. Upper arch shade was B2, representing a change of 12 steps on the Vitapan value-oriented scale. **D,** Six-month postoperative view shows two-step rebound to A2.

• **Figure 6-14** A male patient elected to undergo 810-nm laser bleaching on the right side of the mouth and 940-nm laser bleaching on the left side. **A,** Preoperative view. Preoperative shade of upper arch was A4. **B,** Immediate postoperative view. **C,** Postoperative view at 48 h. Final shade was A2, a 10-step difference. **D,** Postoperative view at 3 weeks. The upper arch was completed in two sessions. The lower arch was completed in one session. The maximum results were visible at 48 h, although a slight relapse was noted after 3 weeks.

Soft tissue lasers are especially increasing in popularity because of their potential value in prosthetic and cosmetic gingival procedures. The ability to control moisture and facilitate hemostasis for both soft tissue and hard tissue lasers appears particularly promising for dentists excising or recontouring gingival tissues. The ability to address biologic width issues and maintain same-day impression capabilities enhances the effectiveness and efficiency with which esthetic procedures can be performed.

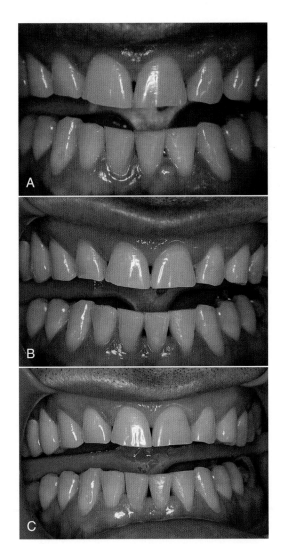

• **Figure 6-15** The patient's treatment plan included 532-nm laser bleaching of upper arch and 810-nm diode laser bleaching of lower arch. **A,** Preoperative view. Preoperative shade of upper left canine was A3.5 and of lower left canine, B4. **B,** Immediate postoperative view. **C,** Postoperative view at 2 months. Final shade of upper left canine was A2, a seven-step difference, and of lower left canine, also A2, an eight-step difference.

Conclusions

Laser-based techniques have been in use for many years with extremely predictable results. The advantage of laser prosthetic/cosmetic reconstruction surgery over traditional techniques is documented strongly in the literature. Ongoing refinements will continue to improve the overall healing time and the patient's postoperative comfort as well as expand the areas where lasers can be used. The addition of laser treatment modalities will enhance the dentist's ability to perform more clinical procedures, increase confidence and experience, and keep the procedures in office instead of referral to specialists. In general, increased awareness of laser treatments as reported in today's media has intensified the contribution of the patient, within the patient–dentist relationship, in determining comprehensive treatment.

References

1. Luomanen M, Meurman JH, Lehto VP: Extracellular matrix in healing CO_2 laser incision wound, *J Oral Pathol* 16:321–331, 1987.
2. Bornstein E: Proper use of Er:YAG lasers and contact sapphire tips when cutting teeth and bone: scientific principles and clinical application, *Dent Today* 23:84, 86–89, 2004.
3. Takamori K, Furukawa H, Morikawa Y, et al.: Basic study on the vibrations during tooth preparations caused by high-speed drilling and Er:YAG laser irradiation, *Lasers Surg Med* 32(1):25–31, 2003.
4. Wan-Yu Tseng, Min-Huey Chen, Hui-Hsin Lu: Tensile bond strength of Er,Cr:YSGG laser irradiated human dentin to composite inlays with resin cements, *Dent Mater J* 26(5):746–755, 2007.
5. Romanos G, Nentwig G: Diode laser (980 nm) in oral and maxillofacial surgical procedures: clinical observations based on clinical applications, *J Clin Laser Surg Med* 17:193–197, 1999.
6. Janda P, Sroka R, Mundweil B, et al.: Comparison of thermal tissue effects induced by contact application of fiber guided laser systems, *Lasers Surg Med* 33:93–101, 2003.
7. Pick RM, Colvard MD: Current status of lasers in soft tissue dental surgery, *J Periodontol* 64:589–602, 1993.
8. Dederich DN, Bushick RD: Lasers in dentistry: separating science from hype, *J Am Dent Assoc* 135(2):204–212, 2004.
9. Von Fraunhofer JA, Allen DJ: Thermal effects associated with the Nd:YAG dental laser, *Angle Orthod* 63(4):299–304, 1993.
10. Gargiulo A, Wentz F, Orban G: Dimensions and relations of the dentogingival junction in humans, *J Periodontol* 32(3):261–267, 1961.
11. *Merriam-Webster's medical dictionary*, Dictionary.com; http://dictionary.reference.com/browse/gingivaltroughs. Accessed October 2008.
12. Shillingburg H, Hobo S, Whitsett LD: *Fundamentals of fixed prosthodontics*, ed 2, Chicago, 1981, Quintessence, pp 195–218.
13. Anneroth G, Nordenram A: Reaction of the gingiva to the application of treads in the gingival pockets for taking impressions with elastic material, *Odont Rev* 20(3):301–310, 1969.
14. Glickman I, Imber LR: Comparison of gingival resection with electrosurgery and periodontal knives: biometric and histologic study, *J Periodontol* 41:142, 1970.
15. Wilhelmsen NR, Ramfjord SP, Blankenship JR: Effects of electrosurgery on the gingival attachment in rhesus monkeys, *J Periodontol* 47(3):160–170, 1976.
16. Wilcox CW, Wilwerding TM, Watson P, Morris JT: Use of electrosurgery and lasers in the presence of dental implants, *Int J Oral Maxillofac Implants* 16(4):578–582, 2001.
17. Takei HH, Azzi RR, Han TJ: Preparation of the periodontium for restorative dentistry. In Newman MG, Takei HH, Carranza FA, editors: *Carranza's clinical periodontology*, ed 9, Philadelphia, 2002, WB Saunders, p 945.

18. Curtis JW Jr, McLain JB, Hutchinson RA: The incidence and severity of complications and pain following periodontal surgery, *J Periodontol* 56:597–601, 1985.

19. Gold SI, Vilardi MA: Pulsed laser beam effects on gingiva, *J Clin Periodontol* 21:391–396, 1994.

20. Neill ME: Sulcular debridement and bacterial reduction with the PulseMaster dental laser: clinical evaluation of the effects of pulsed Nd:YAG laser on periodontitis and periodontal pathogens [master's degree thesis], San Antonio, 1997, University of Texas Graduate School of Biomedical Sciences, pp 123–125.

21. Luomanen M: A comparative study of healing of laser and scalpel incision wounds in rat oral mucosa, *Scand J Dent Res* 95:65–73, 1987.

22. Fisher SE, Frame JW, Browne RM, Tranter RM: A comparative study of wound healing following CO_2 laser and conventional excision of canine buccal mucosa, *Arch Oral Biol* 28:287–291, 1982.

23. Sarver DM, Yanosky M: Principles of cosmetic dentistry in orthodontics. Part 2. Soft tissue laser technology and cosmetic gingival contouring, *Am J Orthod Dentofac Orthop* 127:85–90, 2005.

24. Maynard LG Jr, Wilson RD: Physiological dimensions of the periodontium significant to restorative dentist, *J Periodontol* 50:170–177, 1979.

25. Lowe RA: Clinical use of the Er,Cr:YSGG laser for osseous crown lengthening: redefining the standard of care, *Pract Proc Aesthet Dent* 18(4):S2–S9, 2006.

26. De Mello ED, Pagnoncelli RM, Munin E, et al.: Comparative histological analysis of bone healing of standardized bone defects performed with the Er:YAG lasers and steel burs, *Lasers Med Sci* 23(3):253–260, 2008.

27. Tarnow D, Elian N, Fletcher P, et al.: Vertical distance from the crest of the bone to the height of the interproximal papilla between adjacent implants, *J Periodontol* 74(12):1785–1788, 2003.

28. *Mosby's dental dictionary*, ed 2, St Louis, 2008, Mosby-Elsevier; http://medical-dictionary.thefreedictionary.com/emergence+profile. Accessed April 2009.

29. Downs J: Prep design determines smile design, *Aesth Dent* 4:8–10, 2005.

30. Morris ML: Artificial crown contours and gingival health, *J Prosthet Dent* 12:1146–1156, 1962.

31. Stahl SS: *Periodontal surgery: biologic basis and techniques*, Springfield, Ill, 1976, Charles C Thomas, Publisher.

32. Garber DA, Rosenberg DS: The edentulous ridge in fixed prosthodontics, *Compend Contin Educ Dent* 2:212–224, 1981.

33. Spears F: Maintenance interdental papilla following anterior tooth removal, *Pract Periodontics Aesthet Dent* 11:21–28, 1999.

34. Adams T, Pang P: Lasers in esthetic dentistry, *Dent Clin North Am* 48:838–860, 2004.

35. Atsawasuwan P, Greethong K, Nimmanov V: Treatment of gingival hyperpigmentation for esthetic purposes by Nd:YAG laser: report of 4 cases, *J Periodontol* 72:315–321, 2007.

36. Eses E, Haytac MC, et al.: Gingival melanin pigmentation and its treatment with the CO_2 laser, *Oral Surg Oral Med Oral Pathol Oral Radiol Endod* 98:522–527, 2004.

37. Rosa D, Aranha A, DePaola E: Esthetic treatment of gingival melanin hyperpigmentation with Er:YAG laser: short term clinical observations and patient follow-up, *J Periodontol* 78(10): 2018–2025, 2007.

38. Tal H, Oegiesser D, Tal M: Gingival depigmentation by erbium YAG laser: clinical observation and patient responses, *J Periodontol* 74(11):1660–1667, 2003.

39. Haywood VB, Heymann HO: Nightguard vital bleaching, *Quintessence Int* 20:173–176, 1989.

40. Wetter NU, Barrosco MC, Pelino JE: Dental bleaching efficacy with diode laser and LED irradiation: an in vitro study, *Lasers Surg Med* 35(4):254–258, 2004.

41. Zhang C, Wang X, Kinoshita J, et al.: Effects of KTP laser irradiation, diode laser, and LED on tooth bleaching: a comparative study, *Photomed Laser Surg* 25(2):91–95, 2007.

42. Torres CR, Batista GR, Cesar PD, et al.: Influence of the quantity of coloring agent in bleaching gels activated with LED/laser appliances on bleaching efficiency, *Eur J Esthet Dent* 4(2):178–186, 2009.

7

Lasers in Implant Dentistry

JON JULIAN

Progress in the design and engineering of dental implants has continued over the past several decades. These improvements have led to a success rate of 95% or greater at 10 years and beyond.[1–3] Thus placement of implants has become an extremely successful treatment for the replacement of missing teeth.[4,5]

In the field of dental education, a survey of the curricula of graduate programs shows that dental implantology is taught in oral and maxillofacial surgery (OMS), periodontics, endodontics, and prosthodontics. Most general dentistry residency programs and advanced education in general dentistry (AEGD) programs also include dental implants as part of their curricula. Even orthodontic programs are using dental implants as anchors to aid in moving teeth.[6]

As dental implants become more common in practices worldwide, the question becomes how to improve the means of delivering and supporting dental implant treatment.

This chapter discusses the therapeutic role of dental lasers in improving the presurgical, surgical, postsurgical, and prosthetic phases of implant dentistry. Lasers can be particularly useful in dealing with complications of implant therapy. From surgical placement to prosthetic delivery to treating infected periimplant tissues, lasers have proved to be beneficial in many ways. The different wavelengths of lasers each exhibit unique characteristics that enhance the clinician's approach to implants, as well as the patient's experience. However, the clinician must understand the benefits that each laser wavelength can provide, to match the desired goals of a given procedure to the correct wavelength(s). Both soft tissue lasers, such as diode and 10.6-μm carbon dioxide (CO_2) lasers, and hard tissue lasers, including erbium-doped yttrium-aluminum-garnet (Er:YAG), erbium-chromium–doped yttrium-scandium-gallium-garnet (Er,Cr:YSGG), and 9.3-μm CO_2 lasers, may play a role in implant dentistry.

Generally, lasers aid in obtaining better visualization of the surgical site by decreasing bleeding,[7–9] thus often reducing the duration of a given procedure.[10] Lasers also create more sterile conditions both during and after surgery, so that complications and infections are reduced significantly.[11]

Figure 7-1 shows an incision for a sinus lift made using a 10.6-μm CO_2 laser, with the expected excellent postoperative result. Had this same incision been created with more conventional methods, such as with a scalpel, postoperative redness and swelling would have been major elements of the clinical picture. For the patient, the benefits of reduced pain and swelling and more rapid healing[10,12,13] are invaluable.

Laser Wavelengths

Diode Lasers

Diodes are manufactured in different wavelengths, with 810, 940, 980, and 1064 nm the most common. The energy from these lasers targets pigments such as hemoglobin and melanin in the soft tissue. The energy generally is delivered by a fiber in contact mode. By conditioning, or *carbonizing*, the fiber, the tip heats up to between 500° and 800° C.[14] This heat is transferred to the tissue and effectively cuts by vaporizing the tissue. The tissue is vaporized because of the physical contact of the heated tip of the laser with the tissue, rather than from the optical properties of the laser light itself.[14,15] The 980-nm wavelength is absorbed into water at a slightly higher rate than the 810-nm wavelength. This higher absorption makes a 980-nm diode laser potentially safer and therefore more useful around implants.

Absorption of the wavelength is the primary desired laser–tissue interaction; the better the absorption, the less the collateral thermal heat directed toward the implant.[7] According to Romanos,[16] the 980-nm diodes are safe to use near titanium surfaces even at higher power settings. Studies show that the 810-nm diode laser creates a high temperature rise at the implant surface.[17] Romanos[18] also reported that 810-nm diode lasers may damage the surface of the implant. Use of the 940-nm diode wavelength in the setting of implant therapy has not been documented in the literature. For the purposes of this chapter, the 980-nm diode is the only diode considered useful in implant therapy.

Diode lasers are considered to be similar to neodymium-doped yttrium-aluminum-garnet (Nd:YAG) lasers in dental applications. The advantage of a diode is less depth of penetration than with the Nd:YAG.[7] This more limited effect allows the operator greater control of the laser and reduces

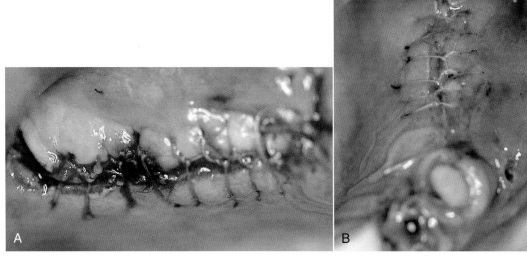

• **Figure 7-1 A,** Large surgical incision made with an ultraspeed CO_2 laser for a sinus lift, closed with continuous, sling-locking sutures. **B,** Photograph of site 48 h postoperatively. Note normal tissue color and relaxed sutures, with minimal evidence of swelling.

the risk of lateral thermal damage. Disadvantages include slowness in speed of cutting and a gated-pulse delivery mode that translates into potential heat buildup in tissue, leading to lateral thermal damage. The clinician should therefore be aware of the power density of the diode, especially when working close to the surface of implants.[17]

The fiber delivery system of diode and Nd:YAG lasers allows debris to build up on the fiber tip. Consequently, frequent cleaning and cleaving of the tip are necessary.[19] Uncovering implants, if the tissue is relatively thin, is an appropriate use for a diode. A full-thickness flap or incision down to the periosteum to place implants is much more difficult with a diode than with a CO_2 laser.

In summary, a 980-nm diode laser can be used safely for some implant procedures, but with limitations in the depth of cut, speed of cut, and efficiency of cutting. The major advantages of a diode laser are its small size and relatively low cost.

Neodymium:Yttrium-Aluminum-Garnet Lasers

The Nd:YAG lasers operate at a wavelength of 1064 nm. These lasers are fiberoptic-delivered contact lasers that generate a free-running pulsed beam of energy. This pulsing mechanism is more sophisticated and the potential for heat penetration even greater than with a diode laser. The 1064-nm wavelength is poorly absorbed in water but readily absorbed into tissue pigments such as hemoglobin and melanin. The Nd:YAG laser is effective at producing coagulation and hemostasis but, because of its penetrating depth of up to 4 mm, has the greatest potential for damaging soft and hard tissues as well as implant surfaces.[16] The energy is delivered through the carbonized tip of a fiber, as with a diode laser. However, the maximum peak power emitted by the Nd:YAG is much greater than for a diode and therefore could penetrate the carbonized debris at the laser tip.[20]

The Nd:YAG laser is useful in periodontal therapy and has had positive effects in pocket therapy.[21] However, Block et al.[22] report that the Nd:YAG laser energy can melt the surface of implants or remove the surface layer from plasma-coated titanium implants. This laser also produces craters and cracks on different surfaces of titanium. Furthermore, Walsh[23] and Chu et al.[24] found contraindications to the use of Nd:YAG lasers near implants. Although anecdotal reports have described use of this wavelength in periimplant therapy, and one manufacturer is promoting a specific laser-assisted periimplantitis protocol, to date, no studies showing the safety of this wavelength when used on implants have been performed. Use of this wavelength, therefore, is considered inherently unsafe for implant-related procedures or periimplant surgery. Nd:YAG lasers will continue to be used successfully in periodontal therapy.[16]

Carbon Dioxide Lasers

The conventional CO_2 laser has a wavelength of 10,600 nm. Its energy can be delivered in continuous-wave mode or gated-pulse mode and more recently, in extremely short pulses of high peak power, labeled "superpulsed" and "ultrapulsed" (i.e., ultraspeed) modes. This wavelength is highly absorbed in water, collagen, and hydroxyapatite[19] and is therefore extremely efficient for soft tissue vaporization. The delivery system usually is a mirrored handpiece (making this a noncontact application) at the end of an articulated arm or a waveguide. The following discussion focuses on this wavelength of CO_2 lasers and its various pulse parameters.

CO_2 lasers have been used for decades in surgical procedures because of their speed and efficiency in cutting soft tissue.[25] They also offer strong hemostatic and bactericidal effects and create minimal wound contraction, thereby minimizing scarring. CO_2 lasers also have minimal depth of penetration, reducing lateral thermal damage.[12,16] The early devices produced significant carbonization because of the high energy densities created. With the newer pulsed models, however, the energy density is reduced to between 180 and 300 mJ/cm^2, delivered at an average speed of 400 to 800 μsec. These settings create less carbonization and charring of tissue and improve the working speed and efficiency of the CO_2 laser. This technology has been further refined with the advent of even shorter pulsing with higher peak powers. By increasing the speed of transmission and decreasing the pulse width, the laser can cut deeper and carbonize less tissue. Thus energy density is now reduced to between 50 and 300 mJ/cm^2, delivered in speeds of 30 to 80 μsec. These improvements have created an extremely versatile CO_2 laser that can safely treat tissue in periodontal pockets and also make surgical incisions up to 4 to 5 mm deep rapidly and efficiently.

The CO_2 laser is safe to use around implants because the energy is absorbed into water and not pigments.[26,27] With its effect restricted to the intracellular water of bacteria, the CO_2 wavelength can safely and effectively treat periimplantitis and mucositis,[28] because the energy is not absorbed into the implant's surface. At the same time, this laser's hemostatic properties are excellent, allowing better visualization of the surgical field, often decreasing procedure time and limiting or preventing postoperative complications (pain, swelling).[29]

With the newer devices, the energy is safe when it comes into contact with bone. When exposed to CO_2 laser energy, the water molecules on the surface of the bone are dehydrated, forming a thin carbon layer of approximately 0.1 mm. The resulting surface will no longer absorb energy, and the damage to bone is clinically insignificant.[30] However, if the CO_2 energy causes hemostasis of bony structures during surgery, curetting the bone to reestablish bleeding for healing is indicated. In my experience, the CO_2 laser is the most versatile of all of the soft tissue lasers available for implant therapy.

A new wavelength of CO_2 laser was recently introduced to the dental market. This wavelength of 9300 nm is delivered by means of an articulating arm. To date, no studies describing the use of this laser in periimplantitis treatment have been published; therefore great caution is advised regarding this clinical application. It is dangerous to extrapolate results with the 10.6-μm CO_2 laser to justify the use of the 9.3-μm CO_2 laser. For the purposes of this chapter, the only CO_2 laser considered appropriate for treatment of implant/periimplant problems is the conventional 10.6-μm CO_2 laser.

Erbium Lasers

The erbium family of lasers includes two similar wavelengths: the Er:YAG laser emitting at 2940 nm and the Er,Cr:YSGG laser at 2780 nm. Both lasers are operated in a free-running pulsed mode. The method of delivery is by mirrored handpiece and articulated arm, waveguide, or trunk fiber and handpiece with a quartz or sapphire fiber tip. The delivery systems include a water spray to prevent heat buildup and to rehydrate the target tissues so that the energy will be absorbed more efficiently.

The erbium wavelengths are highly absorbed in water and hydroxyapatite. They are good for ablating hard tissues such as tooth structure and bone. When first introduced to the market, the U.S. Food and Drug Administration (FDA) cleared the erbium lasers only for hard tissue procedures. By vaporizing water molecules within the hard tissues, erbium lasers create microexplosions in the hydroxyapatite that break down the hard tissue during the ablation process. This effect is achieved without charring or carbonization, and the heat generated is minimal (see Chapter 10). The erbium lasers also will ablate soft tissue, but with limitations. It is most effective in lightly vascularized tissue where bleeding will not be an issue. The erbium wavelength is the least effective of all of the dental laser wavelengths in achieving hemostasis.

Because its energy is absorbed into water, the erbium laser is safe to use around implants and can treat periimplantitis and mucositis safely.[31,32] This laser will leave the bony surface bleeding (for healing), so curettage is not necessary, but it will not harm the implant's surface.[33] Erbium lasers have excellent bactericidal properties because the energy ruptures the cell membranes of bacteria when absorbed into intracellular water.

In summary, erbium lasers are versatile, with good hard tissue applications, although their soft tissue applications are limited compared with true soft tissue lasers because of poor hemostasis.[13,34]

Laser Applications in Clinical Practice
Preoperative Frenectomy and Tissue Ablation

In certain instances, the clinician may need to alter the soft tissue architecture adjacent to the surgical site before the implant is placed. For example, a patient with a high muscle attachment too close to the surgical site would benefit from a frenectomy, to alleviate any tension on the tissue around the implant site. The more complex the surgery, such as bone grafting with creation of a flap, the more important it is to release the muscle tension. The release of muscle tension provides a greater opportunity for success, without sutures pulling, with less postoperative pain and swelling. A frenectomy can be accomplished using any of the soft tissue lasers discussed earlier (Figure 7-2).

Before tooth extraction, the clinician also may need to alter the soft tissue if it is too thick or uneven in thickness. In Figure 7-3, by ablating 2 to 3 mm of tissue in a broad area distal and palatal to the upper right second molar, the resulting tissue thickness can then conveniently accommodate the abutment and crown with hygienically manageable architecture. The ability to remove tissue easily without bleeding, swelling, or postoperative pain is a tremendous advantage to both the clinician and the patient.

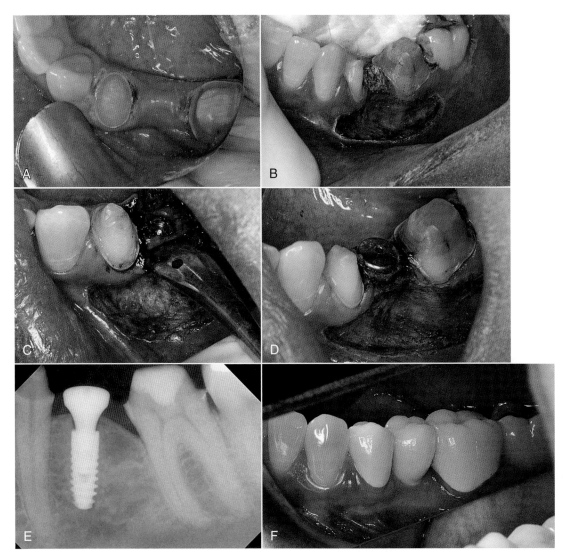

• **Figure 7-2** **A,** Pretreatment occlusal view of planned implant surgery site. **B,** Immediately after muscle release and frenectomy. Note that periosteum is intact. **C,** Midcrestal incision performed with an ultraspeed CO_2 laser and placement of the implant. **D,** Tissue former is placed and tissue sutured into place with two single sutures. No dressing was placed on the tissue. **E,** Radiograph of the implant with tissue former in place. **F,** Final crown seated on implant 4 months after placement.

Preparation of Surgical Site

Site preparation is the first step of implant surgery. To prevent contamination of the surgical site, clinicians have used a variety of antimicrobial rinses, including chlorhexidine, before the procedure.[35,36] Such decontamination efforts have been only partially effective, however, because of the immense bacterial load in the oral cavity. Furthermore, if the site were to become contaminated with saliva during surgery, it would not be practical or effective to stop and rinse again.

Lasers present an excellent solution to the problem of surgical site contamination. All lasers are bactericidal. The clinician simply needs to expose the surgical site to the laser energy for a few seconds. The bactericidal effects are profound and almost instantaneous, and an implant site can be sterilized.[37] Before osteotomy development, the soft tissue can be sterilized much more effectively with a laser than with rinsing or swabbing. Furthermore, with accidental

contamination of the surgical site by saliva during the procedure, simply reapplying the laser in the area will reestablish sterility, so that the procedure can continue with the greatest chance for success. The erbium and diode wavelengths can accomplish decontamination if the contact laser physically "touches" every square millimeter of the surface to be sterilized.[7,38] For this purpose, a slow, deliberate application technique is required; the larger the osteotomy site, the longer the sterilization procedure.

CLINICAL TIP

With a contact laser, the best way to speed up the sterilization procedure is to use a large-diameter fiberoptic cable. Most clinicians who own Nd:YAG or diode lasers have just one- or two-fiber diameters, usually 300 to 400 μm. A decontamination procedure is most effective with use of a fiber diameter of 800 or 1000 μm.

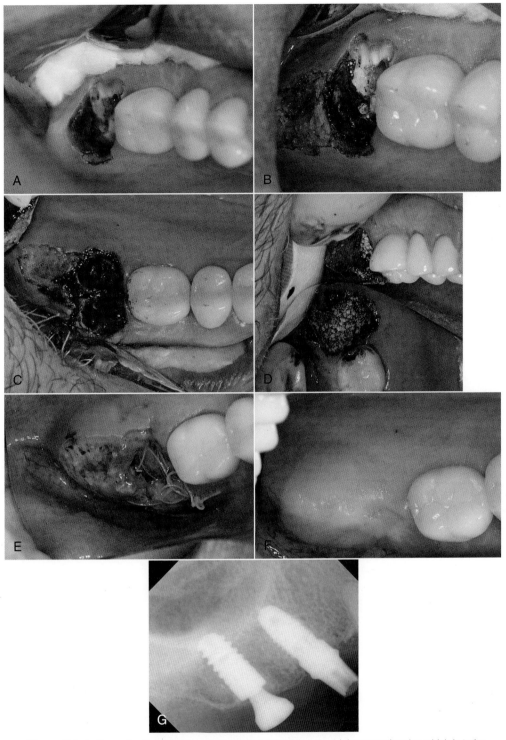

• **Figure 7-3 A,** Excessive tissue thickness distal and palatal to upper right second molar, which is to be extracted and replaced with an implant. **B,** Ultraspeed CO_2 laser was used to reduce the tissue contours where indicated. **C,** Extraction socket immediately after extraction of root. **D,** Socket with osseous grafting material in place. **E,** Postoperative view of extraction/graft site and tissue reduction at 24 h. Note good pink color of tissue and lack of tension on sutures. **F,** Surgical site at 5 months postoperatively. **G,** Radiograph of implant with tissue former.

Decontamination and Implant Placement

A CO_2 laser has a distinct advantage over contact lasers: Because CO_2 lasers are noncontact, it is a simple procedure to place a wide-aperture handpiece on the CO_2 laser to apply the laser beam out of focus, which would increase the spot size on the tissue even more. Sterilization of a large osteotomy site with a CO_2 laser takes mere seconds. As the surgery progresses, the clinician and the assistant should be diligent in keeping the surgical site free of saliva. In most single-implant scenarios, this aim can easily be accomplished. In large-scale surgical procedures with multiple implants or large incisions, however, it may be difficult to maintain a sterile environment. When necessary, laser energy can be redirected to the tissues to decontaminate the surgical site as often as the surgeon deems necessary, using an appropriate power setting for sterilization (Figure 7-4).

Another clinical situation requiring decontamination involves extraction of teeth followed by immediate placement of implants into the extraction site. In some cases, the presence of infected tissues is obvious, and the clinician notices soft tissue around the apices of roots or in the furcation area of molars. Even if infection is not readily apparent, however, a prudent approach is to assume that it might compromise the results of the procedure. The surgical goal is to eliminate all diseased soft tissues in the extraction site and to decontaminate all bony surfaces within the site. A spoon curette can be used to remove gross amounts of soft tissue easily and quickly, with subsequent laser excision to remove any tissue tags. The entire inner surface of the extraction socket can then be decontaminated with a laser.

As with decontaminating the soft tissue of the surgical site immediately before raising the flap, it is difficult to "touch" all of the surfaces of the socket with a diode or Nd:YAG fiber. Of course, neither diode nor Nd:YAG lasers are indicated for use on bone. The erbium wavelengths are effective in removing the remaining soft tissue and decontaminating the bony surfaces at lower power settings with a water-coolant spray.[13] Because they are not as effective as other wavelengths in creating hemostasis, erbium wavelengths would leave the bone surfaces bleeding, which enhances healing of the socket, whether an implant or a graft is placed, or the socket may simply be left to fill in. The CO_2 lasers also are a good choice because they also will remove soft tissue tags and decontaminate bony surfaces, again at low power densities.[39] However, CO_2 laser energy is an excellent hemostatic wavelength, so the effect of hemostasis[39] on the tissues must be overcome for healing.[35]

The clinician should gently curette the bone to reestablish bleeding and maximize the healing potential of the implant or graft site. The laser energy must be delivered to *all* of the bony surfaces within the extraction site. If a severely dilacerated root poses a barrier to the operative line of sight for access of the laser beam, the clinician should make the decision to allow the body's natural defense mechanisms to heal the site over weeks and make it safe for reentry to perform the implant or grafting procedures. Figure 7-5 illustrates the procedure for decontaminating a surgical site and socket, involving an upper left central incisor planned for extraction. An important consideration in this scenario is the proximity of the frenum to the surgical site. A laser frenectomy is performed to ensure no tension on the tissues immediately surrounding the site. After sterilization of the bony crypt and surrounding marginal tissue, the implant is placed with confidence that the soft and hard tissues of the surgical area are free of disease and bacteria.

Figure 7-6 illustrates a similar situation with an upper left first premolar planned for extraction and implant placement. Both the internal and the external aspects of the surgical site are decontaminated with the laser. An abutment is placed so that the patient can wear a temporary fixed prosthesis in that quadrant. A soft tissue troughing procedure is performed on the molar. At 4 months, the soft tissue surrounding the implant is recontoured for a better esthetic result.

Osteotomy
Soft Tissue

The next objective in laser implant surgery is the preparation of the osteotomy, with different considerations for cutting through soft tissues versus hard tissues. The clinician must first decide on the desired pattern of entry through the soft tissue. In some cases a minimal entry, often referred to as a "punch procedure," is the goal. The soft tissue is removed as a 3- to 4-mm-diameter "plug" down to the crest of bone. This soft tissue may be 1 to 2 mm or 3 to 4 mm thick, depending on location and biotype. If the tissue is relatively thin (1 to 2 mm), any wavelength is acceptable. If the tissue is thicker, using a diode or Nd:YAG laser may take minutes versus seconds for erbium and CO_2 lasers. Depending on the tissue quality, bleeding may be an issue with erbium lasers. By quickly and efficiently cutting through the tissue and creating optimal visibility for the surgeon, the duration of the procedure often may be reduced compared with that for conventional techniques.

Other designs for tissue entry include small envelope flaps, often used to gain tissue height (as in anterior implants and other areas) and to provide better-quality tissue around the abutment-crown complex (Figure 7-7).

As the entry site increases in size and the flap design becomes more complex, going through multiple layers of both attached (keratinized) and nonattached (mucosal) tissues becomes a significant consideration in choosing the proper wavelength. Speed of cutting reduces procedure time, as does hemostasis, which also enhances vision. Thus, as more soft tissue is involved, diode and Nd:YAG lasers become less effective—these are *contact* lasers, so to cut through larger amounts and more layers of soft tissue, more time is required to make the incision. Erbium lasers do not provide hemostasis as well as other wavelengths for larger incisions. The unobstructed vision, excellent hemostasis, and efficiency of cutting through all tissue biotypes and thicknesses make the CO_2 laser most suitable for these procedures.[39]

Laser Advantages
Using laser energy to make any incision has several benefits. First, a sterile cut is less likely to become infected. Lasers incise tissue without creating the cascade of events that leads to swelling and inflammation. Because lasers seal off lymphatics and blood vessels, a clinically measurable reduction in pain, swelling, and other postoperative complications has been documented for these incisions.[40,41] With

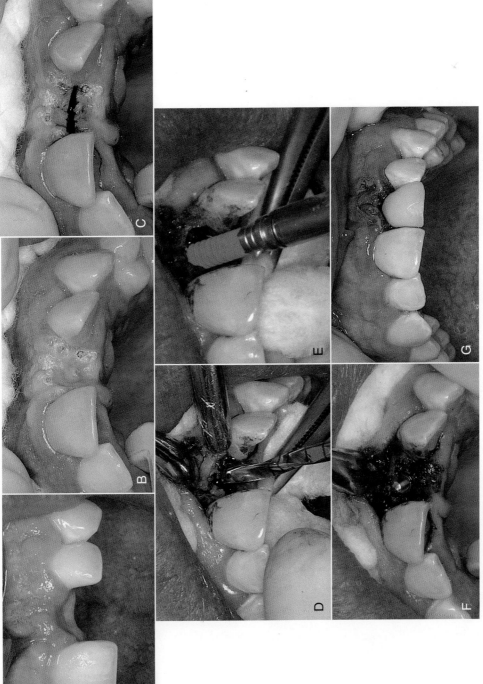

• **Figure 7-4** **A,** Preoperative photograph of implant site for replacing upper left central incisor. **B,** Surgical site decontaminated with an ultraspeed CO_2 laser. **C,** Midcrestal incision made with the laser. **D,** The flap is elevated and the osteotomy site is being prepared. Note excellent visualization of the surgical site with no bleeding to obscure the surgeon's vision. **E,** Implant being placed into osteotomy site. **F,** Completed implant placement. **G,** Immediate temporization of implant with abutment and temporary crown, and tissue reapproximated with two single sutures.

reduced swelling, sutures will not pull through the tissue or are less likely to come undone. Analgesics and antibiotics are needed less frequently, and often in less potent formulations (with fewer drug interactions), because patients experience a significantly less traumatic postoperative course. These benefits apply for both minor and major surgical procedures.

Hemostasis

Another advantage of laser use is the relative safety of such approaches in patients who are anticoagulated with common medications such as aspirin, clopidogrel (Plavix), and warfarin (Coumadin). Some patients also take herbal remedies that can significantly alter their clotting time. The main question with anticoagulated patients is whether their

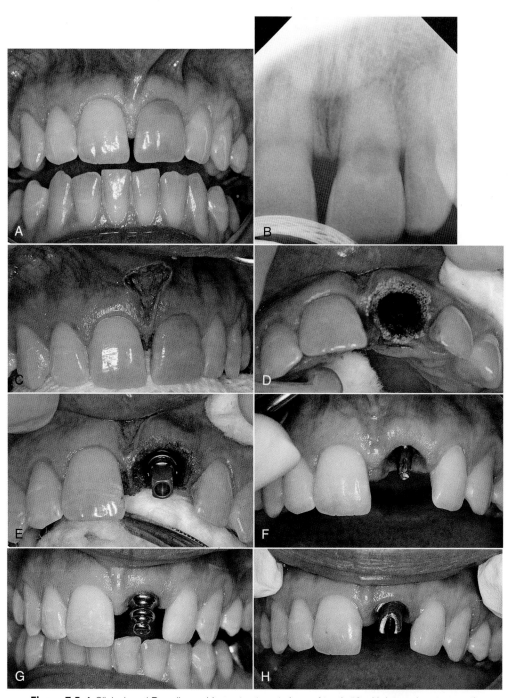

• **Figure 7-5** **A** Clinical, and **B,** radiographic, pretreatment views of tooth #9 with internal root resorption and inevitable extraction. **C,** Tissue recontouring and frenectomy performed with an ultraspeed CO_2 laser. **D,** Postextraction view. Bony crypt is sterilized with surrounding marginal tissue using an ultraspeed CO_2 laser. **E,** Implant is placed immediately after the extraction. **F,** Before impression taking 3 months later, site is evaluated for tissue height and thickness. **G,** Impression coping is in place. **H,** Abutment is seated 4 months after extraction.

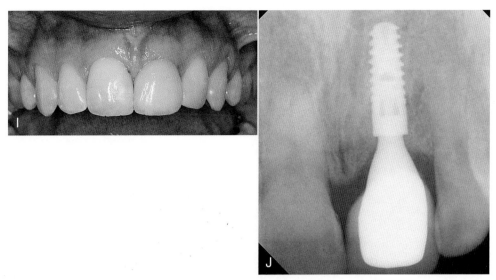

• **Figure 7-5, cont'd** I, Final crown is seated; clinical view shows excellent soft tissue contours. **J,** Radiograph shows excellent bone height.

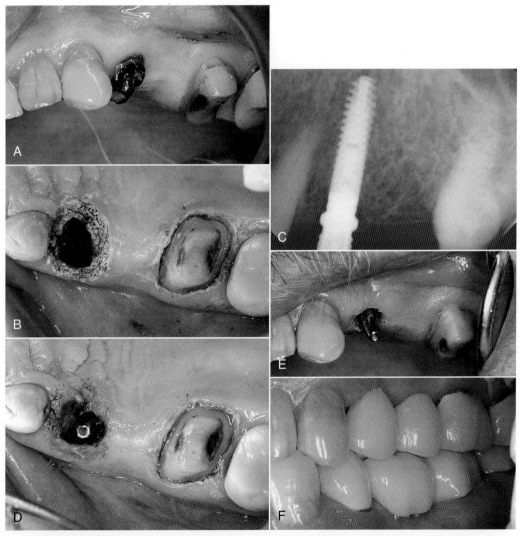

• **Figure 7-6** **A,** Pretreatment site where tooth #12 is to be extracted and an implant placed. **B,** Tooth has been extracted, and laser decontamination of the site is performed both externally and internally. **C,** Radiograph of the immediately placed implant. **D,** Abutment is placed and temporary bridge seated from #14 to the implant. **E,** At 4 months after initial treatment, the necessary tissue modifications were achieved using the same settings as for previous troughing. **F,** Final three-unit bridge cemented in place.

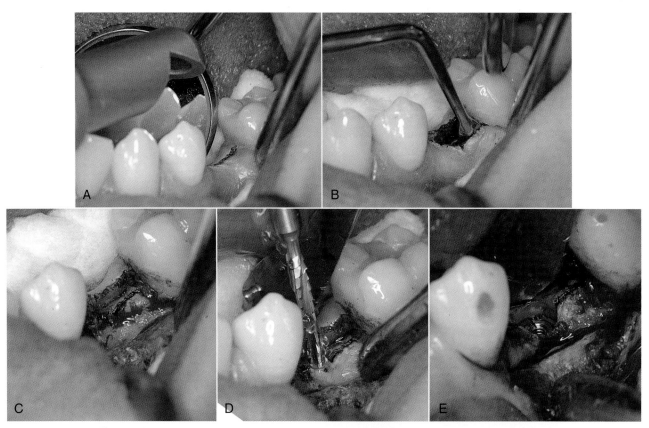

• **Figure 7-7 A,** An ultraspeed CO_2 laser creating incision for implant placement for tooth #20. **B,** Reflecting small envelope flap with minimal bleeding. **C,** Flap reflected. Note excellent visualization of surgical site. **D,** Beginning osteotomy site with bone drills. **E,** The 3.5-mm implant is placed 2 mm below the crest of bone, with excellent visualization maintained throughout the procedure.

medication should be stopped before surgery. The clinician needs to be aware of the individual patient's circumstances and consult with the primary care physician. Before any dental surgery, the patient's health history must be reviewed and updated. With any concern regarding the patient's medications, the appropriate laboratory work, including an international normalized ratio (INR), must be ordered. Recent studies on altering a patient's medications before dental surgery reveal few if any reasons to change the anticoagulant regimen if the INR is less than 4.0,[42,43] although the final decision rests with the primary care physician. Patients receiving anticoagulant therapy will benefit more from the use of lasers in dental surgical procedures than healthier patients. Most lasers have excellent hemostatic properties that lead to decreased bleeding, so intraoperative hemorrhage control is less of an issue.

Also, the use of lasers leads to decreased postoperative swelling and superior tissue healing. This benefit can be attributed to decreased tissue damage, a less traumatic wound, more precise control of the depth of tissue damage, and fewer myofibroblasts in laser wounds compared with scalpel wounds.[25] The traditional scalpel does not induce hemostasis, so the control of bleeding must be addressed by more conventional means. For example, application of pressure by biting on gauze or tea bags, suturing, placing oxidized cellulose, applying topical thrombin, and using

tranexamic acid mouthwashes all can be used to help control hemorrhage.[42] These treatments become unnecessary during laser surgery. The lack of hemorrhage control with the scalpel leads to obstruction of vision at the surgical site and the need for more assistant time suctioning the area and maintaining a dry field.[39]

Figure 7-8 shows an elevated flap with excellent visualization and an essentially bloodless incision in a patient in whom the upper right lateral incisor is congenitally missing. The implant is placed after bone grafting for a facial osseous defect. A laser also is used to make a bloodless releasing incision at the distal aspect of the upper right canine.

Hard Tissue

Once access is gained through the soft tissue, the clinician must decide how to deal with the hard tissue. To ablate bone, the erbium family of lasers is used. An erbium laser can remove bone to begin the osteotomy. Laser ablation of bone is less damaging to osseous tissues than conventional techniques, because this is a noncontact procedure with no friction between laser tip and bone. Friction from the bone-cutting drills may overheat the bone and potentially cause necrosis at the bone-implant interface. The temperature increase in osseous tissue associated with use of an erbium laser is minimal as long as the clinician is familiar with the proper laser parameters and uses an adequate water

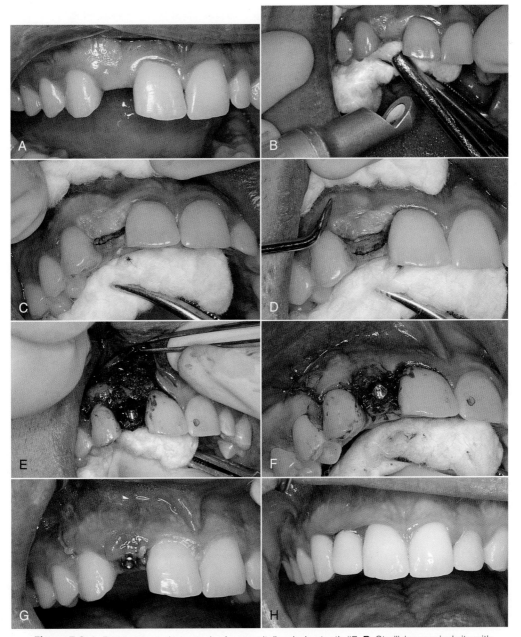

• **Figure 7-8** **A,** Pretreatment photograph of congenitally missing tooth #7. **B,** Sterilizing surgical site with an ultraspeed CO_2 laser, 2.0 W at 80 Hz for 10 sec. **C,** By increasing power to 4.5 W at 80 Hz, a midcrestal incision is accomplished. **D,** Bloodless incision allows good vision as flap is elevated. **E,** Implant placement with bone grafting for a facial defect. Note releasing incision distal to #6, also done with the laser. **F,** Flap is closed and sutured. **G,** At 72 h, tissue color is normal and swelling nonexistent. **H,** At 2 weeks, temporary crown is in place and tissue is healing uneventfully.

spray. Thus controlled ablation without thermal damage is achieved. Studies show better healing and faster new bone formation when erbium lasers are used versus conventional bone drills[13,44–46] (Figure 7-9). In time, it may be possible to use the 9.3-μm CO_2 laser for these procedures as well; to date, however, research on the safety and efficacy of this wavelength in implant osteotomies has yet to be done.

Laser technology has not yet advanced to the point that the entire osteotomy can be completed with lasers. However, manufacturer-based research is under way, with the goal of replacing bone drills with erbium "drills" for osteotomies.

Block Graft Procedure

In the performance of any surgical procedure, focused concentration on each step is essential. For example, while measuring points on a bony surface to cut or prepare, the clinician who looks away even for a moment may lose orientation, necessitating remeasuring and refocusing with the potential for loss of precision. If, however, the measurements could be "drawn" on the bone with an indelible marker, the procedural map thus created could guide all subsequent steps and also allow the clinician to regain focus in the event of distraction.

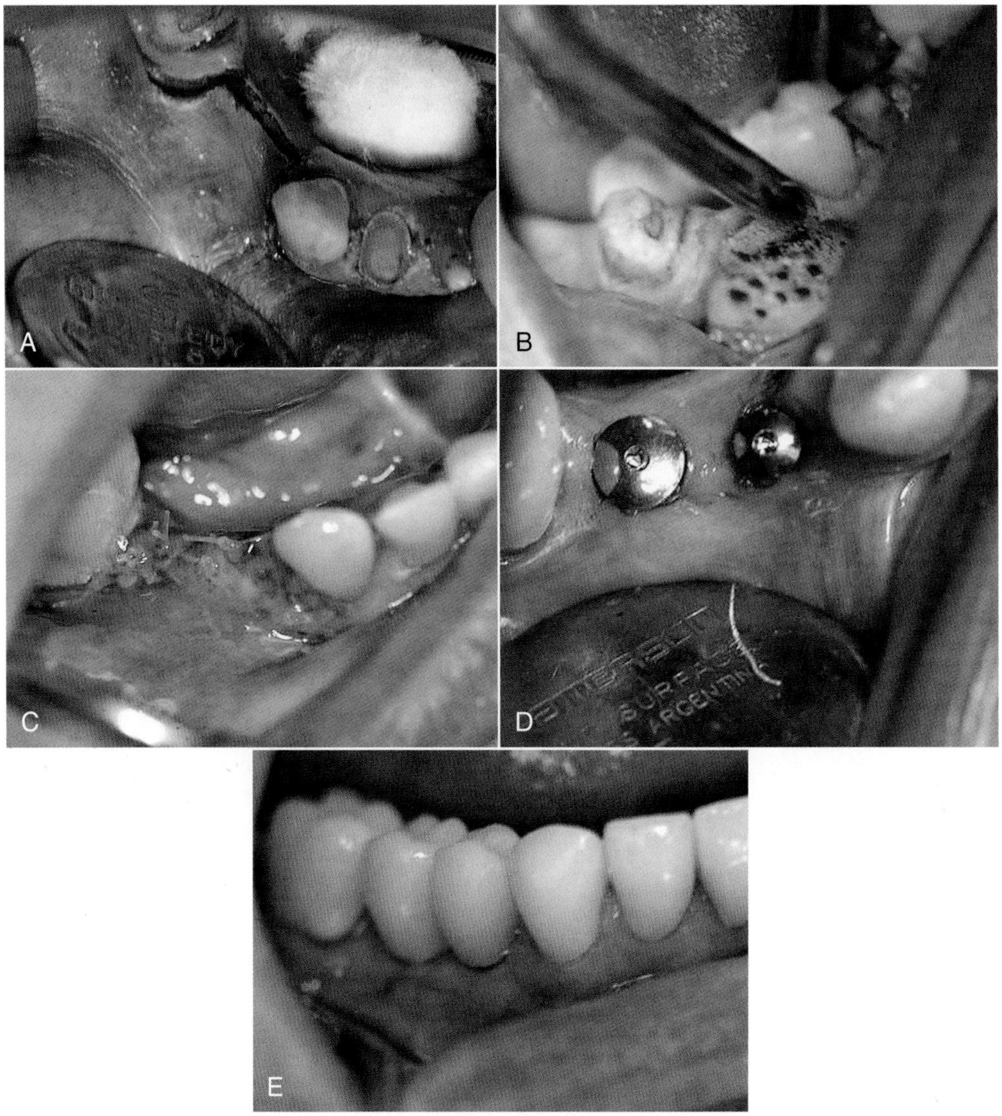

• **Figure 7-9 A,** Laser incision for osseous graft procedure. **B,** Decortication of bone using erbium laser. **C,** At 24 h, postoperative photograph shows good color and relaxed sutures with no swelling. **D,** Implants placed 4 months after graft procedure. **E,** Final restorations in place.

Either CO_2 or erbium wavelengths can be used at a low energy setting to mark measurements on the bone surface, creating an indelible marking. An "x marks the spot" placement of implants can then be accomplished. The receptor site for a block graft can be visualized with this technique, and the donor block can be outlined and measured before cutting.

After the block of bone is cut and sized, the screw holes can be created with an erbium laser, thus eliminating the mechanical and frictional stresses of using a drill. The block can be sanded and modified with the erbium laser as well, also eliminating the mechanical and frictional trauma from a bur.

Lateral Window Sinus Lift

Lasers can enhance the sinus surgery that builds a foundation of bone for the eventual placement of dental implants. A typical *lateral window* approach in a posterior edentulous ridge involves a long incision starting from the distal aspect of the second molar and extending along the crest of the ridge mesially to the cuspid area.[47] Here, a vertical releasing incision is made. The CO_2 laser is most efficient for making such an incision.

After the flap is elevated and the bony aspect of the surgical site visualized, the clinician prepares to cut a window in the bone. By drawing this window outline, as previously discussed for the bony surface, the surgeon is then prepared to cut the bone with a bur in a handpiece, or with a piezotome, to enter the sinus cavity. Using the CO_2 or erbium laser to "draw" on the bone creates a visible marking on the surface without damaging the bone's integrity.[48] The erbium lasers are then used to cut through the bone, especially if the bone covering the sinus is thin, approximately 1 mm in thickness; however, the erbium laser also will cut soft tissue, a potential problem.[49]

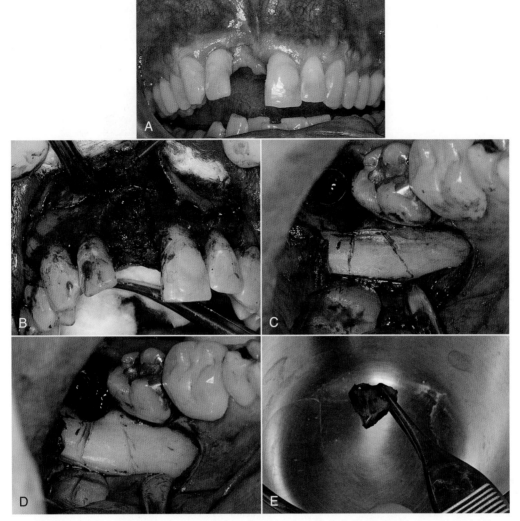

• **Figure 7-10 A,** Pretreatment view of recipient site for block graft. **B,** Releasing incisions performed with laser. Large flap exposes the bony defect. **C,** Flap is created at donor site, which is measured and marked with the laser. Slight char layer on bone could be described as an indelible marker. **D,** Bone saw cutting on laser-drawn lines to obtain block of bone. **E,** Donor block removed from donor site.

The first goal of a well-performed sinus lift is to gain access through the bone without damaging the schneiderian membrane (nasal mucous membrane). The second goal is to deposit graft material in sufficient quantities to support the future implant placement.[50] Once exposed, the schneiderian membrane is carefully and gently elevated away from the inferior and medial surface of the sinus floor. If kept intact, this membrane helps to contain the graft material and prevent migration of the graft particles freely in the sinus cavity. If this membrane is cut or damaged, however, the graft material can migrate elsewhere to cause a foreign body response, leading to complications or infection and possibly a failed graft procedure. Although a damaged membrane can be repaired, this issue simply complicates the procedure and introduces more risk.[51,52]

The erbium lasers cut hard tissue and soft tissue, so it is not possible to penetrate bone without penetrating the soft tissue that is intimately attached to the bone. Cutting the bone with a bur and a handpiece requires skill and practice to create the window without damaging the membrane. Perhaps the most promising tools for this purpose are the piezo surgical devices, which cut by vibration through the bone and will not cut soft tissue.[53]

The true benefit of lasers in the block graft procedure lies in the postoperative effects. The minimal inflammatory response by the soft tissues increases patient comfort and minimizes swelling. Sutures stay relaxed and intact. Prophylactic antibiotics may be used against postoperative sinus infections as the clinician sees fit, but localized infections at the surgical site are rare (Figures 7-10 and 7-11).

Uncovering Implants

When the clinician needs to uncover an integrated implant after healing is complete, occasionally the implant body is covered not only by soft tissue but also by newly formed

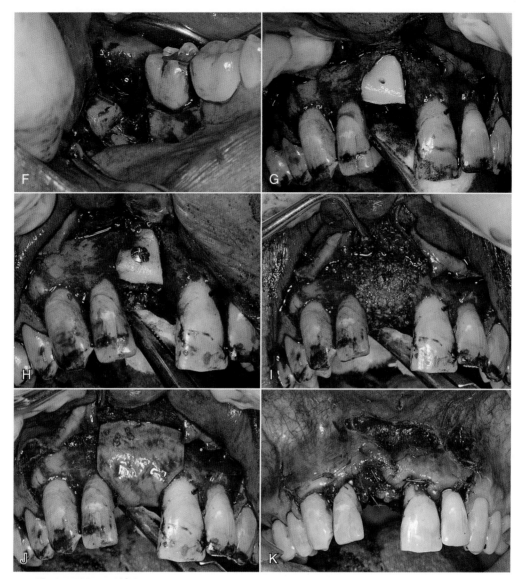

• **Figure 7-10, cont'd** **F,** Donor site after harvesting of the graft. **G,** Screw hole created safely in the block with erbium laser. **H,** Screw in place to secure block. **I,** Particulate graft placed over block. **J,** Resorbable barrier membrane fitted over graft site. **K,** Flap is sutured in place, and frenectomy is performed to prevent tension on surgical site.

bone up to 2 to 3 mm thick. After location of the implant has been ascertained radiographically, the soft tissue must be removed. This removal can be accomplished with any laser wavelength except the Nd:YAG, because of its adverse effects on implants. If the tissue is not too thick (1 to 2 mm), all wavelengths except Nd:YAG work well. With significantly deeper tissue, the diode laser would become too slow and inefficient. With extremely vascular tissue, the erbium laser may be a poor choice because bleeding might impair visibility. For thick tissue, the CO_2 wavelength is most efficient to remove significant tissue quickly and to maintain excellent visualization of the surgical site (Figures 7-12 and 7-13).

If bone has formed over the top of the implant, the clinician must decide on the best approach. The CO_2 laser could affect a thin layer of bone to facilitate its removal with a hand instrument.[39] For any thickness of bone, however, the erbium lasers can efficiently and safely accomplish the

uncovering process. The bone and the implant surface will remain unharmed (Figure 7-14).

In implant dentistry, having too much soft tissue architecture has not been a common problem. In fact, the most common issue is trying to preserve more soft tissue. With some implant designs, however, the characteristic result includes large volumes of soft tissue. This tissue must be sculpted and shaped to allow for impression taking, abutment seating, and crown cementation. Maintaining a dry, clear visual field is imperative. Lasers are excellent tools for these cases (Figure 7-15).

Mucositis and Periimplantitis

The most serious complication in implant dentistry may be a late-stage infection after the implant has integrated with the bone. *Mucositis* is simply a soft tissue infection around the

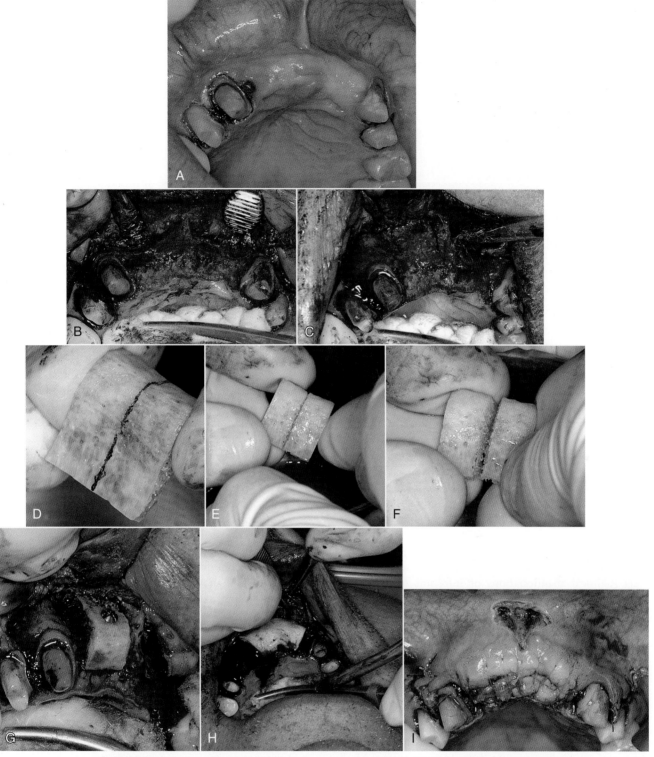

• **Figure 7-11** **A,** Pretreatment view of recipient site for block grafts. **B,** Recipient site marked with laser. Note the light, indelible markings on the bone. **C,** Recipient site for a J-graft showing light indelible char marking on the bone. **D,** J block marked with laser. **E,** J-graft block being cut with erbium laser. **F,** J-graft block cut complete. Note that complete cut is smooth and atraumatic to the bone. **G,** J-graft block segment secured into recipient site with one screw; screw hole created with erbium laser. **H,** Membrane over J-graft block. **I,** Dual-block graft site with flap sutured. Note laser frenectomy to prevent tension on flap.

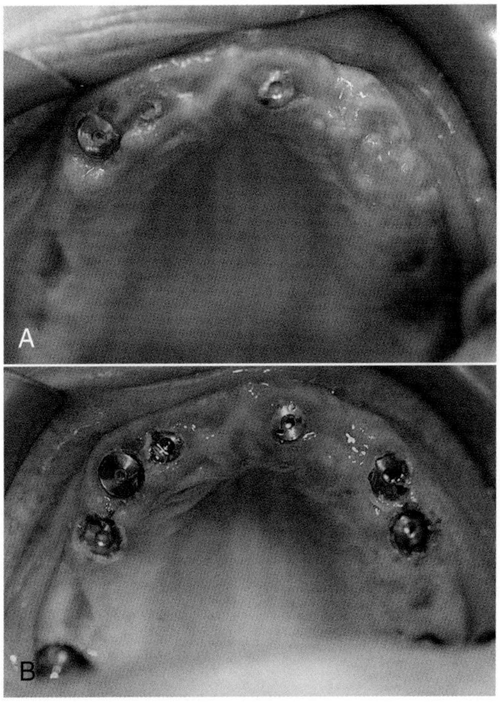

• **Figure 7-12 A,** Multiple implants partially covered by soft tissue. **B,** Implants exposed with laser.

abutment-crown-implant complex, typically at the cervical third of the implant. *Periimplantitis* is an infection around the body or apex of the implant that leads to loss of bone.[54] Both of these conditions are characterized by an inflammatory reaction to anaerobic plaque bacteria associated with a biofilm. Typically, this results in swelling and inflammation of the soft tissues and loss of bone surrounding the implant.

Many causative factors include tissue quality surrounding the implant, design of the implant, surface texture of the implant, alignment of the implant, mechanical loading of the implant in occlusion, and the presence of bacteria. Clinical manifestations of infection may include inflammatory or color changes in the surrounding tissue, bleeding, suppuration, possibly fistula formation, and radiographic bone loss. In severe cases, the implant may need to be removed.

Conventional Therapy

If the implant is still stable and the bone loss is not too severe, the infection can be treated. Surgery with debridement is the treatment of choice, accompanied by administration of antibiotics, attempted mechanical removal of all diseased tissues from around the implant, and eradication of as much bacteria as possible. Therapeutic tools include plastic instruments, citric acid, chlorhexidine, and topical tetracycline.[55–57] After debridement, bone grafting material is placed in the void in the bone in an attempt to regenerate the periimplant hard tissues. The dentition is evaluated for possible mechanical overload, which is corrected if present. Finally, the patient's oral hygiene is reevaluated and possibly improved.

Unfortunately, the success rates with conventional technologies are not good. Leonhardt[58] reported a 42% implant failure rate with conventional therapy for periimplantitis.

Laser-Assisted Therapy

Lasers provide a new treatment modality for patients with mucositis and periimplantitis. If an erbium laser is used, the steps may proceed as follows:
• Access to the implant is obtained through an appropriate laser incision.[59]
• Once the implant and the surrounding bone are exposed, the diseased tissue is vaporized by laser energy.
• The implant surface and bony crypt are decontaminated by the laser.[60]
• By ablating a thin layer of bone, necrotic bone is removed and the area decontaminated.

Thus debridement and decontamination are accomplished with a single instrument. Bone grafting, if necessary, can then be performed. Healing is enhanced because of reduced inflammation and postoperative pain.[12]

If a CO_2 laser is used, the procedure begins with an appropriate laser incision to expose the implant body, the bone, and the diseased soft tissue. This tissue is easily ablated and the implant surface safely decontaminated. The bony surfaces also are decontaminated, but CO_2 laser energy causes carbonization of the bone, with resulting hemostasis. Before grafting, the bony surface is mechanically scraped free of the carbonization layer with a curette, and bleeding is reestablished. Bone grafting may then be performed. The success rate is greatly improved because a more sterile environment has been created. Figure 7-16 shows CO_2 laser debridement of a periimplantitis site, with healthy tissue response.

A diode laser also can be used to remove the granulation tissue and decontaminate the implant surface. Figure 7-17 shows diode laser debridement and decontamination at the site of a fistula above an upper left cuspid implant, with excellent healing at 1 year.

Nonsurgical Therapy

Nonsurgical treatment of crestal mucositis with bone loss also has been studied. Deppe and Horch[39] explored sterilizing exposed implant surfaces with lasers to rehabilitate "ailing implants." In a clinical study of 16 patients with 41 ailing implants, a CO_2 laser was used in a closed (nonflap) procedure. After 4 months, statistically better results were demonstrated for the implant sites decontaminated with a CO_2 laser and soft tissue resection than for the sites decontaminated by conventional means.

Erbium Laser

Schwarz et al.[61] used an Er:YAG laser to treat lesions in 20 patients who had at least 1 implant with moderate to advanced periimplantitis, for a total of 40 implants. An Er:YAG laser was used on half the implants and mechanical debridement with plastic curettes and antiseptic therapy with chlorhexidine

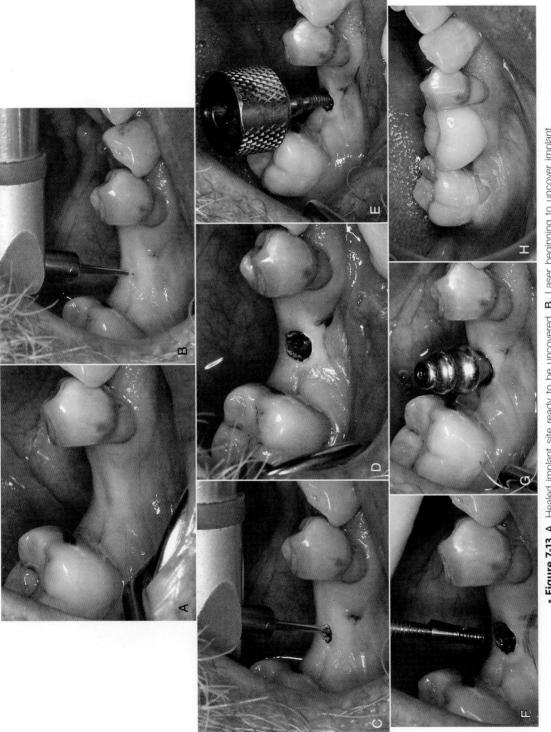

• **Figure 7-13 A,** Healed implant site ready to be uncovered. **B,** Laser beginning to uncover implant. **C,** Tissue being ablated by laser. **D,** Implant uncovered after 30 sec of exposure to laser energy. **E,** Device to remove sealing screw in position. **F,** Sealing screw easily removed. **G,** Impression coping placed easily with no hemorrhaging. **H,** Final crown seated 4 weeks later.

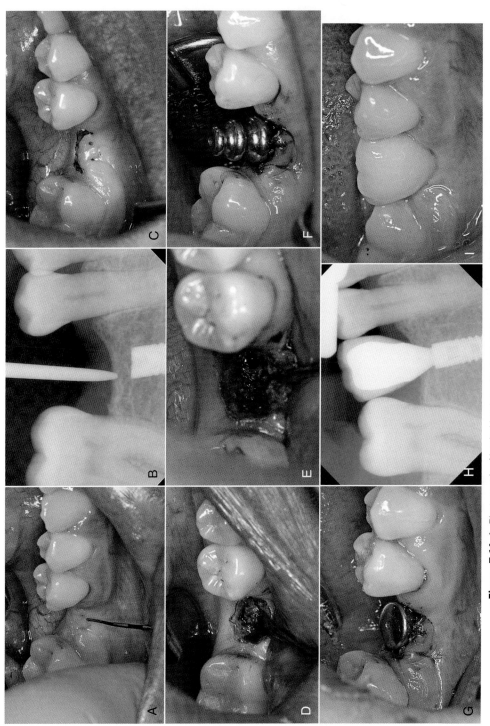

• **Figure 7-14 A,** Photograph of healed implant site ready to be uncovered. **B,** Radiograph of site is used to help locate the integrated implant and reveals bone growth over implant. **C,** Incision in soft tissue down to bone with single pass of laser. **D,** Bone over implant exposed. **E,** Removal of bone with erbium laser. Total laser exposure time was 2 min. **F,** Transfer coping in place. **G,** Tissue former in place. No suturing was done. **H,** Final radiograph of abutment and crown placed into integrated implant 1 month after uncovering. **I,** Clinical photograph of final crown on day of cementation.

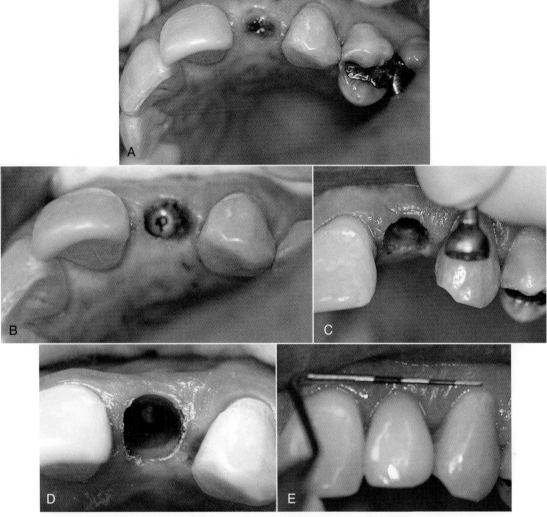

• **Figure 7-15 A,** Laser uncovering an implant. **B,** Incisal view of modified tissue. Sufficient tissue was removed to allow placement of larger-diameter tissue former without blanching tissue. **C,** Tissue former removed and tissue recontoured. **D,** Contour resulting from the new tissue former. **E,** Restoration cemented in place.

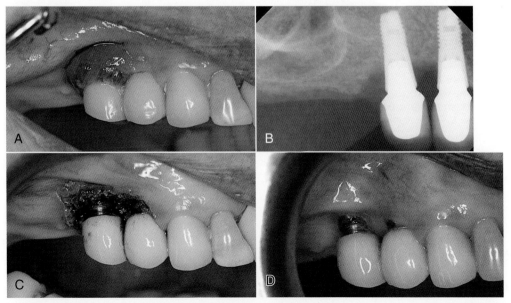

• **Figure 7-16 A,** Periimplantitis affecting implant in upper right second premolar space. **B,** Radiograph of bone loss. **C,** Area after closed ultraspeed CO_2 laser debridement of periimplant tissue. **D,** Excellent tissue response to laser and healthy periimplant tissue.

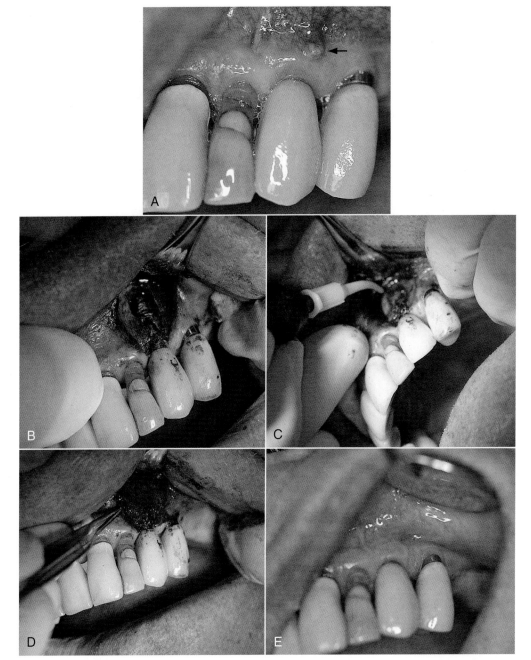

• **Figure 7-17 A,** Fistula *(arrow)* above the upper left cuspid implant. **B,** After conventional access was obtained using a scalpel, the site was exposed. **C,** Diode laser (980 nm) is used to debride soft tissue and decontaminate site. **D,** Osseous graft placed over decontaminated site with a resorbable membrane in place. **E,** Postoperative photograph at 1 year shows excellent healing.

digluconate (0.2%) on the other half. The criteria evaluated were plaque index, bleeding on probing, probing depth, gingival recession, and clinical attachment level. After 3 and 6 months, the sites decontaminated with the laser exhibited more improvement than conventionally treated sites.

Carbon Dioxide Laser

Romanos[16] showed that a power setting of approximately 3 W with a CO_2 laser will decontaminate a periimplantitis-affected restoration. He theorized that the CO_2 laser may be reflected off the implant surface and vaporize the bacteria in

deep bony lesions, leading to a more thorough decontamination of the implant site. This creates better conditions for healing and reosseointegration.

Deppe et al.[26] showed in beagle dogs that decontamination of ailing implants is optimized with the CO_2 laser and can lead to periimplant bone growth. The procedure is performed by placing a CO_2 tip into the sulcus. The laser energy is delivered circumferentially around the implant body. The diseased soft tissue is vaporized and the bacterial count significantly reduced. No bone grafting procedure is done and no flap raised. As suggested by my own clinical

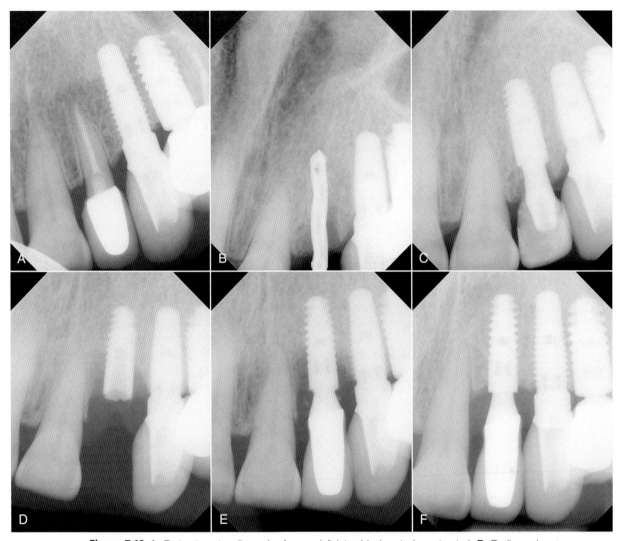

• **Figure 7-18** **A,** Pretreatment radiograph of upper left lateral incisor to be extracted. **B,** Radiograph showing implant site being prepared immediately after extraction. **C,** Radiograph of immediately placed implant loaded with temporary crown. **D,** Bone loss to fourth thread. **E,** Radiograph at 1 month after treatments. **F,** Radiograph at 10 months after cementation. Bone has regenerated to within 1 mm of top of implant. No flap was raised and no grafting was performed.

experience, this procedure, which takes only minutes to perform, should be repeated three or four times every 7 to 10 days. This interval coincides with the time it takes for a complex subgingival biofilm to form.[62] With repeated interruption of formation of this biofilm over 3 to 4 weeks, the body's natural defenses and immune response are able to heal the lesion. With resolution of any other causative factors, such as mechanical overload and suboptimal oral hygiene, the pathologic process will be stopped, and in some cases, regeneration of bone will occur. Although the extent is not yet predictable, with decontamination of "ailing implants" with bone loss of up to 6 mm, regeneration of 1 to 4 mm of new bone has been demonstrated, with restoration of healthy periimplant soft tissue as well.[26,63]

To conclude, the most conservative early- to middle-stage treatment of a mucositis involving bone loss at the cervical aspect of the implant is a nonsurgical approach using laser energy, without an incision or flap and not requiring

a bone grafting procedure. If the problem is more complex or involves the apical portion of the implant, a laser-assisted surgical approach is appropriate, typically involving incisions, flaps, and bone grafting. With either approach, the results to date are promising and appear to have a higher success rate than for traditional methods.[39,64]

Figure 7-18 shows an implant with temporary crown for a left lateral incisor. When the patient returned for dental care after having left the area for 6 months, mucositis was evident, and nonsurgical treatment with a CO_2 laser was instituted. The laser tip was positioned circumferentially and laser energy was applied for 30 sec on the facial, lingual, mesial, and distal aspects of the involved soft tissue. Three additional treatments were given at 1-week intervals. At 1 month, the final abutment and crown were seated and the tissue was treated once more. After another extended absence, the patient again returned for clinical evaluation; bone regeneration was seen at 10 months after cementation (see Figure 7-18*F*).

Diode Versus Carbon Dioxide Laser Treatment Scenarios

If an implant was placed below the crest of the bone and the bone remained intact at the crest, the result would be a large volume of tissue surrounding the implant body. This tissue might need to be sculpted in one of several approaches: simply seating a tissue former or healing abutment; changing to a larger-size tissue former after initial healing; seating the final abutment, depending on its size and shape; or seating the final crown. In each case, hemorrhage control indicates that use of a diode or CO_2 wavelength would be most appropriate. The CO_2 laser would have the benefit of speed and efficiency over the diode instrument.

Also, if an impression was needed of an abutment in place whose margins were below the tissue crest, a *troughing* procedure with a CO_2 or diode laser would create a good environment for obtaining an impression, while being less traumatic to the tissue than the traditional retraction cord technique (see Chapter 6). Furthermore, cementation of crowns below the tissue crest can irritate the tissue if some cement was not removed beforehand. In such cases, a troughing procedure around the crown to visualize all of the margins would be beneficial. The CO_2 wavelength would be the logical choice because of its hemostatic effects, because it is less traumatic to tissue than other soft tissue lasers, and because it is less likely to alter the marginal tissue, so that esthetics would be preserved.

Future of Lasers in Implant Dentistry

As clinicians become more experienced with laser technology in their practice, the adjunctive uses expand. The use of lasers in implant dentistry is even more promising. The ability to control depth of cutting would allow the use of erbium lasers in osteotomy site preparations, instead of bone drills. The mechanical action of a drill creates friction with the potential for overheating the bone.[47] A nonsterile drill can contaminate the surgical site. An erbium laser could make the same cut in the bone without mechanical trauma. Also, because lasers sterilize as they cut, using a laser in the osteotomy site would reduce the risk of postoperative infection and promote a successful outcome.[13]

El-Montaser et al.[65] showed that healing in an implant site prepared with an erbium laser was better than a bur-prepared site. Their results demonstrated that bone ablation with the Er:YAG laser promotes ingrowth of new bone around titanium metal implants and that osseointegration can occur. For erbium lasers to replace current implant drills, precision in the depth and diameter of cut is necessary.

In another area of application, low-level laser techniques are thought to improve wound healing, with evidence of accumulated collagen fibrils, accelerated cell reproduction, and increased prostaglandin levels.[66] More studies are needed, but the science is sufficiently encouraging to support the likelihood that such laser technology will accelerate wound healing and enhance patient comfort (see Chapter 15).

Conclusions

Lasers bring significant benefits to modern clinical dentistry, especially implant dentistry. Diode, CO_2, and erbium lasers have the potential to improve the clinician's ability to deliver the highest quality of care while providing a more comfortable experience for the patient, with fewer postoperative problems. Each laser emits a different wavelength in the electromagnetic spectrum, and each has unique effects on hard and soft tissues. Therefore each wavelength has advantages and disadvantages, depending on the clinical goals, skill, and experience of the dental practitioner and on the target tissue type.

As emphasized in this chapter, most if not all of the steps in implant procedures can be accomplished or enhanced with lasers. It is incumbent on the clinician to learn about the available choices. An embrace of laser technology by the dental profession will lead to impressive clinical benefit with improved patient outcomes, and experienced clinicians undoubtedly will find further uses for lasers as technology continues to improve. Any dentist placing or restoring dental implants will find lasers invaluable in making procedures easier and more successful.

References

1. Marder MZ: Treatment planning for dental implants: a rationale for decision making. Part 1. Total edentulism, *Dent Today* 24(5):74–76, 78, 80–83, 2005.
2. Karoussis I, Brägger U, Salvi G, et al.: Effect of implant design on survival and success rates of titanium oral implants: a 10-year prospective cohort study of the ITI Dental Implant System, *Clin Oral Implants Res* 15(1):8–17, 2004.
3. Lindh T, Gunne J, Tillberg A, Molin M: A meta-analysis of implants in partial edentulism, *Clin Oral Implants Res* 9(2):80–90, 1998.
4. Jivraj S, Chee W: Rationale for dental implants [abstract], *Br Dent J* 200:661–665, 2006.
5. American Academy of Implant Dentistry: *Dental implants preferred option for aging bridges* [news release], May 2008; http://www.aaid-implant.org.
6. Ismail S, Johal A: The role of implants in orthodontics, *J Orthod* 29(3):239–245, 2002.
7. Swick M: Laser-tissue interaction. I, *J Laser Dent* 17(1):28–32, 2009.
8. Adibi S: Er,Cr:YSGG laser use for soft tissue management during the restoration of an implant: a case report, *J Laser Dent* 17(1):34–36, 2009.
9. Coluzzi DJ: Soft tissue surgery with lasers: learn the fundamentals, *Contemp Esthet Restorative Pract*, 1–2, May 2007.
10. Convissar R: The top ten myths about CO_2 lasers in dentistry, *Dent Today* 28(4):70, 2009.
11. Raffetto N, Gutierrez T: Lasers in periodontal therapy, a five-year retrospective, *Calif Dent Hyg Assoc J* 16:17–20, 2001.
12. Aoki A, Mizutani K, Takasakim AA, et al.: Current status of clinical laser applications in periodontal therapy, *Gen Dent* 56(7): 674–684, 2008.
13. Bornstein ES: The safety and effectiveness of dental Er:YAG lasers: a literature review with specific reference to bone, *Dent Today* 22(10):129–133, 2003.

14. Gregg R: Laser resource and reference guide, *Dent Today*, March 2006. http://www.dentistrytoday.com/technology/lasers/1366. Accessed October 2014.
15. Fasbinder D: Dental laser technology, *Compend Contin Educ Dent* 29(8):459, 2008.
16. Romanos G: Laser surgical tools in implant dentistry for the long-term prognosis of oral implants, *Int Congress Series* 1248:111, 2003.
17. Yousif A, Zwinger S, Beer F, et al.: Investigation on laser dental implant decontamination, *J Laser Micro/Nanoeng* 3(2):119–123, 2008.
18. Romanos G: Question 1: is there a role for lasers in the treatment of peri-implantitis? *J Can Dent Assoc* 71:117–118, 2005.
19. Coluzzi D: Fundamentals of dental lasers: science and instruments, *Dent Clin North Am* 48:751–770, 2004.
20. Coleton S: Lasers in surgical periodontics and oral medicine, *Dent Clin North Am* 48:937–962, 2004.
21. Cobb CM: Lasers in periodontics: a review of the literature, *J Periodontol* 77:545–564, 2006.
22. Block CM, Mayo JA, Evans GH: Effects of the Nd:YAG dental laser on plasma-sprayed and hydroxyapatite-coated titanium dental implants: surface alteration and attempted sterilization, *Int J Oral Maxillofac Implants* 7:441–449, 1992.
23. Walsh LJ: The use of lasers in implantology: an overview, *J Oral Implantol* 18:335–340, 1992.
24. Chu RT, Watanabe L, White JM, et al.: Temperature rises and surface modification of lased titanium cylinders (special issue), *J Dent Res* 71:144, 1992.
25. Strauss R, Fallon S: Lasers in contemporary oral and maxillofacial surgery, *Dent Clin North Am* 48:861–868, 2004.
26. Deppe H, Horch H, Helmut G, et al.: Peri-implant care with the CO_2 laser: in vitro and in vivo results, *Med Laser Appl* 20:61–70, 2005.
27. Pang P: Lasers in cosmetic dentistry, *Gen Dent* 56(7):663–664, 2008.
28. Swift J, Jenny J, Hargreaves K: Heat generation in hydroxyapatite-coated implants as a result of CO_2 laser application, *Oral Surg Oral Med Oral Pathol* 79(4):410–415, 1995.
29. Israel M: Use of the CO_2 laser in soft tissue and periodontal surgery, *Pract Periodont Aesthet Dent* 6:57–64, 1994.
30. Forrer M, Frenz M, Romano V, et al.: Bone-ablation mechanism using CO_2 lasers of different pulse duration and wavelength, *Appl Phys B Lasers Opt* 56(2):104–112, 1993.
31. Schwarz F, Bieling K, Sculean A, et al.: Treatment of periimplantitis with laser or ultrasound: a review of the literature, *Schweiz Monatsschr Zahnmed* 114(12):1228–1235, 2004.
32. Kresiler M, Al Haj H: d'Hoedt B: Temperature changes at the implant-bone interface during simulated surface decontamination with an Er:YAG laser, *Int J Prosthodont* 15(6):582–587, 2002.
33. Lee D: Application of laser in periodontics: a new approach in periodontal treatment, *Hong Kong Med Diary* 12(10):23–25, 2007.
34. Walsh L: The current status of laser applications in dentistry, *Aust Dent J* 48(3):146–155, 2003.
35. Fonseca R: *Oral and maxillofacial surgery*, vol 6, Philadelphia, 2000, WB Saunders.
36. Scortecci G, Misch C, Benner K: *Implants and restorative dentistry*, New York, 2001, Martin Dunitz.
37. Kojima T, Shimada K, Iwasaki H, Ito K: Inhibitory effects of a super pulsed carbon dioxide laser at low energy density on periodontopathic bacteria and lipopolysaccharide in vitro, *J Periodont Res* 40(6):469–473, 2005.
38. Stuart C: The use of lasers in periodontal therapy, *Gen Dent* 56(7):612–616, 2008.
39. Deppe H, Horch H: Laser applications in oral surgery and implant dentistry, *Lasers Med Sci* 22:217–221, 2007.
40. Dederich D, Bushick R: Lasers in dentistry: separating science from hype, *J Am Dent Assoc* 135(2):204–212, 2004.
41. Locke M: Clinical applications of dental lasers, *Gen Dent* 57(1):47–59, 2009.
42. Wahl M: Myths of dental surgery in patients receiving anticoagulant therapy, *J Am Dent Assoc* 131(1):77–81, 2000.
43. Pototski M, Amenabar J: Dental management of patients receiving anticoagulant or antiplatelet treatment, *J Oral Sci* 49(4):253–258, 2007.
44. Matjaz L, Marincek M, Grad L: Dental laser drilling: achieving optimum ablation with the latest generation Fidelis laser systems, *J Laser Health Acad* 7(1):1–3, 2007.
45. Kesler G, Romanos G, Koren R: Use of Er:YAG laser to improve osseointegration of titanium alloy implants: a comparison of bone healing, *Int J Oral Maxillofac Implants* 21:375–379, 2006.
46. Walsh Jr JT, Flotte TJ, Deutsch TF: Er:YAG laser ablation of tissue: effect of pulse duration and tissue type on thermal damage, *Lasers Surg Med* 9:314–326, 1989.
47. Miloro M, Ghali GE, Larsen P, Waite P: *Peterson's principles of oral and maxillofacial surgery*, vol 2, Hamilton, Ohio, 2004, BC Decker.
48. Rayan G, Pitha J, Edwards J, Everett R: Effects of CO_2 laser beam on cortical bone, *Lasers Surg Med* 11(1):58–61, 1990.
49. Van As G: Erbium lasers in dentistry, *Dent Clin North Am* 48:1017–1059, 2004.
50. Kaufman E: Maxillary sinus elevation surgery, *Dent Today*, September 2002.
51. Pikos MA: Maxillary sinus membrane repair: report of a technique for large perforations (abstract), *Implant Dent* 8(1):29–34, 1999.
52. Shlomi B, Horowitz I, Kahn A, et al.: The effect of sinus membrane perforation and repair with Lambone on the outcome of maxillary sinus floor augmentation: a radiographic assessment (abstract), *Int J Oral Maxillofac Implants* 19(4):559–562, 2004.
53. Vercellotti T, De Paoli S, Nevins M: The piezoelectric bony window osteotomy and sinus membrane elevation: introduction of a new technique for simplification of the sinus augmentation procedure, *Int J Periodont Restorative Dent* 21(6):561–567, 2001.
54. Chen S, Darby I: Dental implants: maintenance, care and treatment of peri-implant infection, *Aust Dent J* 48(4):212–220, 2003.
55. Mombelli A, Lang NP: The diagnosis and treatment of peri-implantitis, *Periodontol* 2000(17):63–76, 1998.
56. Mombelli A: Microbiology and antimicrobial therapy of peri-implantitis, *Periodontol* 2000(28):177–189, 2002.
57. Santos V: Surgical anti-infective mechanical therapy for peri-implantitis: a clinical report with a 12-month follow-up, *Gen Dent* 57(3):230–235, 2009.
58. Leonhardt A: Five-year clinical, microbiological, and radiological outcome following treatment of peri-implantitis in man, *J Periodontol* 74(10):1415–1422, 2003.
59. Yung F: The use of an Er:YAG laser in periodontal surgery: clinical cases with long-term follow up, *J Laser Dent* 17(1):13–20, 2009.
60. Miller R: Treatment of the contaminated implant surface using the Er,Cr:YSGG laser, *Implant Dent* 13(2):165–170, 2004.
61. Schwarz F, Bieling K, Bonsmann M, et al.: Nonsurgical treatment of moderate and advanced periimplantitis lesions: a controlled clinical study, *Clin Oral Invest* 10:279–288, 2006.

62. Quirynent M, Vogels R, Pauwels M, et al.: Initial subgingival colonization of "pristine" pockets, *J Dent Res* 84(4):340–344, 2005.

63. Stubinger S, Henke J, Donath K, Deppe H: Bone regeneration after peri-implant care with the CO_2 laser: a fluorescence microscopy study, *Int J Oral Maxillofac Implants* 20(2):203–210, 2005.

64. Deppe H, Horch HH, Neff A: Conventional versus CO_2 laser–assisted treatment of periimplant defects with the concomitant use of pure-phase beta-tricalcium phosphate: a 5-year clinical report, *Int J Oral Maxillofac Implants* 22(1):79–86, 2007.

65. El-Montaser M, Devlin H, Dickinson M, et al.: Osseointegration of titanium metal implants in erbium-YAG laser prepared bone, *Implant Dent* 8(1):79–85, 1999.

66. Sun G, Tunér J: Low-level laser therapy in dentistry, *Dent Clin North Am* 48:1061–1076, 2004.

8

Use of Lasers for Minor Oral Surgery in General Practice

TODD J. SAWISCH, GEORGE R. DEEB, AND ROBERT A. STRAUSS

New advances in the field of dentistry are continually changing the patient experience. These changes ideally decrease treatment time, lead to better outcomes, and improve patient comfort. One area of dental practice that is constantly undergoing technological innovation is the use of lasers in dentistry, and in minor oral surgery in particular. Many general practitioners, as well as specialists from a variety of disciplines, are taking advantage of this continually evolving field and using lasers for many of their in-office procedures.

The specialty of oral and maxillofacial surgery has benefited from the use of lasers since the mid-1960s,[1] with the first documented use of a laser for such surgery in 1977.[2] Laser techniques often are considered the standard of care for many surgical procedures, reflecting the proven advantages of improved visualization, hemostasis, and reduced discomfort. The introduction of lasers that incorporate computer interface technology has made these devices much more "user-friendly," contributing to their popularity in the dental profession. Manufacturers also are addressing the need for mobility both within the office and between clinical facilities and are designing lighter, more portable equipment. Laser handpieces have interchangeable components that are more ergonomic and versatile, allowing better control in performing exacting procedures within the confines of the oral cavity.

Intraoral Lasers for Minor Oral Surgery

Understanding laser physics and laser light's biologic interaction with tissues is essential in determining the appropriate laser for any given procedure. A wide array of active laser media with unique radiant-energy wavelengths have been successfully used for various indications and types of tissue, including the carbon dioxide (CO_2), erbium-doped yttrium-aluminum-garnet (Er:YAG), erbium-chromium–doped yttrium-scandium-gallium-garnet (Er,Cr:YSGG), holmium-doped YAG (Ho:YAG), neodymium-doped YAG (Nd:YAG), potassium titanyl phosphate (KTP), pulsed dye, and diode

lasers.[3] The diode, Nd:YAG, erbium, and CO_2 lasers are the most commonly used intraoral lasers because of their wavelength-specific properties (see Chapter 2).

Diode Laser—805 to 1064 nm

Many manufacturers produce diode lasers, delivering wavelengths in the range of 805 to 1064 nm. These devices are compact and portable in design and are relatively inexpensive surgical units, with efficient and reliable benefits for use in minor soft tissue oral surgical procedures. In fact, several diode laser units now available are entirely self-contained within a small handpiece-sized, wireless, delivery system. Although these lasers are not as efficient as the CO_2 laser for soft tissue procedures, their relative safety, comparatively low cost (many are commercially available for less than $4000, compared with $12,000 to $60,000 for CO_2 lasers), ease of use, and versatility have made them a common choice for minor surgery in the general dentistry office. Diode lasers can be used in continuous-wave or gated-pulse mode, either in contact or out of contact with tissue. Because most diode laser wavelengths are absorbed primarily by tissue pigment, in normal mucosa, the laser tip must be "initiated" by touching the fiber to a pigmented item (articulating paper) to pick up some pigment, which then absorbs the beam to produce a thermal effect. The 980-nm diode laser demonstrates significantly higher absorption in water, allowing it to cut more optically than thermally (as is typical with other diode wavelengths, which are mostly absorbed by pigments), with an optical penetration of less than 300 μm. Romanos and Nentwig[4] found that the 980-nm diode laser produced more precise incision margins when compared with other laser wavelengths. In addition to their use in various soft tissue oral surgical procedures, 980-nm diode lasers have become as popular as CO_2 lasers for the treatment of periimplantitis because they offer a bactericidal effect without causing implant surface alterations[5] (see Chapter 7).

Neodymium:Yttrium-Aluminum-Garnet Laser—1064 nm

The Nd:YAG laser's active medium is a crystal of yttrium, aluminum, and garnet doped with neodymium ions.[6] By functioning in the near-infrared part of the spectrum at 1064 nm, the Nd:YAG laser exhibits minimal surface tissue absorption and maximal penetration; this property allows for coagulation of tissue in depth.[7] The optical delivery is free-running but must be in the "pulsed" mode because of Nd:YAG's ability to penetrate deeply into soft tissues. Romanos[8] believed that most procedures could be performed without local anesthesia because the pulse duration is shorter than the time required to initiate a nerve action potential.

Comparing Nd:YAG laser surgery with conventional scalpel surgery, White et al.[9] concluded that the laser could be used successfully for intraoral soft tissue applications without anesthesia and with minimal bleeding. When the procedure involves significant ablation or resection of tissue, local anesthesia is necessary for patient comfort.[7]

As with the diode lasers, the Nd:YAG laser can be used in a contact (excision) and a noncontact (coagulation) mode. These properties have led to its use in a variety of maxillofacial procedures, including coagulation of angiomatous lesions, hemostasis in bleeding disorders, arthroscopic surgery of the temporomandibular joint (TMJ), resections in vascular tissues (in combination with CO_2 wavelength), and palliation of advanced neoplasms.[10] The Nd:YAG laser has demonstrated some benefit for use with minimally invasive periodontal therapies, including sulcular debridement and bacterial decontamination, resulting in potential new attachment of gingival tissues, regeneration of supporting bone, and regrowth of periodontal ligament[11] (see Chapters 3 to 5). In general, however, the deeper penetration depth makes this laser less useful in minor oral surgical procedures, where surface effects for cutting and ablating are desired.

Erbium Lasers—2780 to 2940 nm

Owing to their optical properties, the erbium family of lasers, including those with two similar wavelengths, has gained popularity in dental implant surgery as well as other minor surgical procedures. The erbium lasers are free-running pulsed lasers with thermal effects that interact solely with the surface layers of soft and hard tissue, much like the CO_2 laser.[12] They are popular with general practitioners because they can be used both on hard tissue for caries removal and on soft tissue for minor oral procedures. The beams are reflected by polished metal surfaces such as titanium, so they have no adverse effects on dental implants.[13] Application of the erbium lasers in dental implant surgery has been advocated for the preparation of hard tissue, second-stage surgery, revision of soft tissue, and treatment of periimplantitis.[14–16]

Although the erbium lasers are capable of osseous surgery, such as for crown lengthening, harvesting autogenous bone grafts, and sectioning teeth, these procedures require more time than traditional methods. For this reason, oral surgeons, for whom treatments involving osseous tissue remain a primary concern, have not embraced erbium laser technology.

Carbon Dioxide Laser—10,600 nm

The CO_2 laser has become the workhorse for intraoral soft tissue surgery. The emitted wavelength of 10,600 nm has ideal absorption by soft tissue because soft tissue is composed of 90% water, and CO_2 has excellent absorption in water. Cellular rupture occurs from the photothermal effect when intracellular water absorbs the energy from the CO_2 laser. The cellular vaporization is the basis for the CO_2 laser to function as a surgical tool.[3] The wavelength allows for absorption into soft tissue, rapidly generating heat that is then conducted into the surrounding tissue, creating a very narrow zone of thermal necrosis of approximately 500 μm or less.[17] Limiting lateral thermal damage to such a small area is an excellent advantage of CO_2 laser use, because this effect results in coagulation of vessels up to 500 μm in diameter and is clinically manifested by hemostasis and sealing of the lymphatics, which has been found to reduce postsurgical bacteremia compared with other methods of incision.[18]

The learning curve tends to be slightly steeper with the CO_2 laser because it is the only soft tissue laser used without direct tissue contact. The delivery system is either an articulated arm or a flexible hollow waveguide. The hollow waveguide requires the use of higher power because significant laser energy is absorbed internally by the laser delivery system. These delivery systems are acceptable for use in procedures affording direct vision within the confines of the oral cavity. However, for endoscopic and microscopic surgical procedures in which visibility is limited, a flexible core system can provide a needed advantage. The recently developed BeamPath (Wave Form Systems, Inc., Tualatin, Oregon) fiber allows laser energy to be transmitted by an innovative photonic band-gap omnidirectional dielectric mirror lining, which guides the light through a flexible hollow core.[19]

The CO_2 laser energy can be transmitted in several different modes, including continuous-wave, chopped/gated-pulse wave, and various "superspeed" and "ultraspeed" modes. Lasers generally are perceived as a continuous beam of light. Dispersion of CO_2 laser energy in this manner is associated with a continuous wave. Continuous-wave CO_2 lasers were the forefront of technology in the 1970s and proved to be successful for applications in medicine. However, the constant emission of laser energy was associated with very high-energy densities, causing unnecessary injury to the soft tissues. As this technology progressed, a shutter was integrated into continuous-wave lasers, causing interruption (gating, or chopping) of the continuous wave. These units delivered fluences of approximately 1200 to 1500 mJ/cm^2 of energy density. This development limited the use of these lasers in microsurgical applications. Newer laser technology also can operate in a pulsed-wave mode, meaning the energy bursts on and off very quickly. Pulsed-wave laser energy creates an instant burst of light energy, achieving a greater peak power than the continuous-wave mode.

"Superpulsed" CO_2 lasers are designed to regulate the energy density transmitted to soft tissue. By changing the radiofrequency of the pumping mechanism in the laser, the pulse width and speed of transmission could now be predetermined. The "superpulsed" mode of transmitting CO_2 energy improved the working speed of pulses to 400 to 800 μsec and decreased the energy density to 180 to 300 mJ/cm^2 on soft tissue. A direct result of the decreased pulse width is less time for lateral spread of heat, leading to less carbonization and charring, resulting in more consistent healing in soft tissue procedures.

The latest generation of lasers currently on the market can create pulses of 20 to 80 msec while generating a peak power greater than 300 W, with an extremely small beam diameter. This technology can produce an extremely thin incision at depths of up to 4 to 5 mm in a single pass without carbonization or tissue damage. With many superficial soft tissue procedures using this technology, the amount of injectable anesthetics required is greatly reduced because of an absorption depth of only 0.10 mm, associated with decreased lateral thermal damage and frequently minimal or no bleeding, discomfort, or swelling during surgery and in the postoperative period.

Carbon Dioxide Laser—9300 nm

Although the carbon dioxide laser traditionally has been used at the 10,600-nm wavelength and only for soft tissue surgery, another variant of this laser at 9300 nm (9.3 μm) also is now being used in dentistry owing to its purported ability to work on both hard and soft tissue. Enamel ablation with a microsecond-pulsed 9.3-μm CO_2 laser was reported by Staninec et al.[20] in 2009 as an alternative to use of the high-speed handpiece. These investigators prepared immediately extracted third molars with conventional high-speed handpieces as well as the 9300-nm CO_2 laser and compared the pulpal effects with findings in control teeth. They concluded that the CO_2 laser could ablate enamel safely without harming the pulp under the energy deposition conditions of their study.[20] Recently, the first FDA-cleared 9300-nm CO_2 laser for the cutting of both hard and soft tissues in intraoral locations was introduced for use in dentistry. Further research and clinical experience with the 9300-nm CO_2 laser can be expected to lead to new uses in dentistry and oral surgery involving the cutting of both hard and soft tissues.

Advantages and Disadvantages of Laser Surgery

Benefits

The benefits of using lasers in oral surgical procedures are significant, both for the dental surgeon and for the patient.

Laser light is monochromatic, coherent, and collimated; it therefore delivers a precise burst of energy to the targeted area. Laser energy incises tissue more efficiently than the scalpel, generates complete vaporization, and coagulates blood vessels. For contouring procedures, the laser is perhaps the surgical instrument of choice because of its ability to sculpt soft tissues by selective ablation.

The hemostatic effect created when the laser's energy interacts with the soft tissue eliminates excessive bleeding, a risk factor that traditionally has discouraged dentists from performing surgery, and creates a clean surgical field, allowing increased precision and accuracy and greatly improving visualization of the surgical site, making laser surgery as straightforward as other dental procedures.

Examined histologically, laser wounds have been found to contain a significantly lower number of myofibroblasts.[21] This results in less wound contracture or scarring and, ultimately, improved healing.[22,23] Mobility of the dynamic tissues (lips, tongue, floor of mouth, soft palate) is attained more readily postsurgically. As a result of improved healing and hemostasis, intraoral laser wounds often can be left without sutures, for healing by secondary intention, except when cosmesis is a concern.

With laser technology, the patient typically experiences less postoperative swelling and pain.[24,25] A compromised airway during oral surgery is less of a concern, partly because of the decreased swelling. Although not always predictable, the decreased postoperative pain often can be managed with over-the-counter (OTC) nonnarcotic oral analgesics (e.g., ibuprofen) for most laser procedures. The physiologic mechanism of this effect is still unknown but probably involves decreased tissue trauma and alteration of neural transmission.[7]

Because of the characteristically much less painful surgical experience and minimal postoperative complications with use of lasers, more procedures can be performed on an outpatient basis. Patients often can return to work within 1 day or even immediately after many surgeries.

Drawbacks

Despite the laser's many advantages, when determining the appropriate treatment for a patient, the clinician also must consider its drawbacks. Although the healing process after laser surgery generally is marked by decreased scarring and increased function, some investigators have found that the speed of healing is slightly prolonged compared with other types of wounds.[26] This delay in healing is undoubtedly caused by the sealing of blood vessels and lymphatics and subsequent need for neovascularization. Typical intraoral healing after laser surgery may take as long as 2 weeks for wounds that would otherwise take 7 to 10 days. If sutures are indicated, delayed healing times must be taken into account in considering suture removal, to prevent premature dehiscence of the wound.[25]

Nonsutured CO_2 laser wounds heal by forming a fibrinous coagulum that functions as a biologic dressing. Because of the slow epithelialization of CO_2 laser wounds, the fibrinous coagulum may be present beyond 2 weeks.[24] A clinician new to lasers should not confuse this healing process for infection and unnecessarily perform a wound debridement or prescribe antibiotics when there is no indication. Unlike postsurgical healing after conventional techniques, an increase in pain 4 to 7 days postoperatively may occur, which normally can be controlled with minimal oral analgesics (e.g., ibuprofen). The clinical appearance and anticipated discomfort after laser surgery should be discussed with patients to avoid confusion or perceived complications.[25]

Virtually all laser wavelengths used for surgery to vaporize, coagulate, or cut tissue may produce particulate debris called the *laser plume*. Clinicians, assistants, and patients may be at risk for ill effects from exposure to laser plume. Laser plume may contain carcinogens, irritants, dusts, viruses, and bacterial spores, depending on the procedure. It also may contain carbon monoxide, polyaromatic hydrocarbons, various toxic gases, and chemicals such as formaldehyde, hydrogen cyanide, and benzene. Currently, no potential chronic health effects from long-term exposure to laser plume have been recognized; however, the literature on infectious transmission of laser plumes in medicine is equivocal. Several studies of patients seropositive for human papillomavirus type 2 (HPV-2) deoxyribonucleic acid (DNA) revealed no viable viral particles in the laser plume.[27–32] Other studies have shown HPV DNA in the plume of laser-vaporized tissue.[33–36] None of these studies involved treatment within the oral cavity. A review of the literature reveals no cases of illness in any dental personnel resulting from inhalation of laser plume. In any case, contaminants generated by lasers can and should be controlled by ventilation, safe work practices, and personal protective equipment.

Laser Techniques and Procedures

Although the diode, Nd:YAG, and, to a lesser extent the erbium wavelengths may be used in minor office oral surgical procedures, the focus of this chapter is primarily on surgeries performed with the CO_2 laser. The CO_2 laser, the workhorse of oral-maxillofacial surgery, is the most frequently used wavelength for these procedures, with more than 30 years of peer-reviewed literature justifying its use in the oral cavity. No other laser wavelength has been as extensively researched and studied in this field of practice as the CO_2 laser. That said, for the typical general dental practioner who wishes to perform these procedures, the use of an inexpensive diode laser will work reasonably well in most cases. Typically, procedures that involve incisions are easily done with the diode laser, whereas ablative procedures are better managed with the CO_2 laser.

The basis of good laser technique starts with a thorough familiarity with the ins and outs of the laser system to maximize its use and prevent complications. Laser systems are equipped with an operator's manual, detailing the safety features. The operator and all assistants should thoroughly review the manual before using the laser and should strictly adhere to

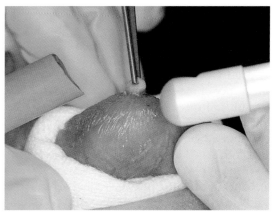

• **Figure 8-1** Moistened gauze surrounding surgical site to absorb stray laser energy and protect surrounding structures before removal of a tongue lesion.

the indications. No health care personnel should attempt to use a laser in a patient without proper training (see Chapter 16).

The most frequent adverse sequelae resulting from the use of lasers are caused by laser energy emitted beyond the working area and striking the surrounding soft tissues. Such misdirection typically occurs when a specimen is transected, because the laser energy passing beyond the margin may redirect off a reflective metal surface of an instrument in or near the oral cavity (e.g., a mirror or other flat retractor). These events usually result in minimal or no injury, but the patient's initial response to the stimulus may be interpreted as pain. This problem can easily be avoided by obstructing the distant tissues with moist gauze or a wet tongue blade and by using matte-finished, nonreflective instrumentation.[3]

Wavelength-specific eyewear is mandatory, protecting the user from misdirected or reflected laser energy. During laser operation, high-speed suction or evacuator devices should be used and high-filtration masks should be worn to prevent illness from inhalation of the plume released at the site of energy–tissue interaction. To prevent ignition with flammable gases, nitrous oxide and oxygen should ideally be temporarily discontinued during laser use, to prevent serious harm to the patient. Because CO_2 laser energy is well absorbed by hydroxyapatite, a major component of tooth enamel, significant amounts of laser energy absorbed by the teeth can cause etching and pitting, weakening enamel[37] and increasing pulpal temperature.[38] When in proximity to the tip during a CO_2 laser procedure, the teeth can be protected with moistened gauze or a fabricated tooth guard to absorb errant energy from the laser beam (Figure 8-1).

In general dentistry practice, the following three fundamental photothermal techniques for CO_2 laser applications can be used to perform various intraoral procedures:
- Incision/excision surgery (Figure 8-2)
- Ablation/vaporization procedures (Figure 8-3)
- Hemostasis/coagulation techniques (Figure 8-4)

All minor office-based oral surgical procedures are based on these three techniques. The first procedure discussed here is biopsy; however, the incisional techniques used to perform biopsies are applicable to virtually every intraoral procedure.

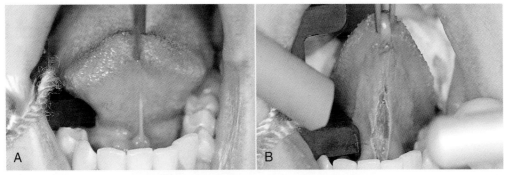

• **Figure 8-2** Example of incision/excision procedure: lingual frenectomy. **A,** Preoperative view; **B,** immediate postoperative view.

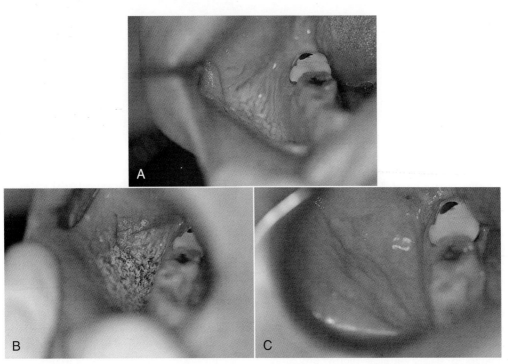

• **Figure 8-3** Example of ablation/vaporization of a previously biopsied leukoplakic lesion. **A,** Immediate preoperative view; **B,** intraoperative view; **C,** 12-day postoperative view.

It is important to recognize that one or more techniques may be necessary for any given clinical scenario, depending on three surgeon-controlled laser parameters: energy, time, and spot size.[3] These parameters equate at the focal point of the laser energy emitted from any given laser handpiece. Altering the distance of the handpiece from the tissue serves to focus and defocus the laser beam's focal point, thereby altering the effect of the laser on the target tissue. A laser in focus will excise and incise with the most efficiency. When the laser is out of focus, depth of effect will be less, but with a wider field of effect for ablation and coagulation.

Incision/Excision Techniques and Procedures

With *focused mode,* the focal point of the laser beam is at such a distance as to exactly focus on the tissue to be affected

(but not in contact with the handpiece), maximizing the power per unit to a pinpointed area. Using the CO_2 laser in focused mode allows for increased depth, yet the laser can produce an incision similar to that made by a scalpel, essentially functioning as a "light" scalpel. The characteristics of the CO_2 laser make it ideal for most intraoral procedures traditionally performed with a scalpel, such as incision and excision, lesion removal, and flap elevation.[3,7,39]

Biopsy Procedure

Every patient requires a screening for cancer, which is accomplished by performing a thorough oral, head, and neck examination. Oral examinations can be made more efficient by inspecting high-risk sites, where 90% of oral squamous cell cancers arise: floor of the mouth, ventrolateral aspect of the tongue, and the soft palate complex.[40] Many screening and detection aids can be used as adjunctive tools to identify

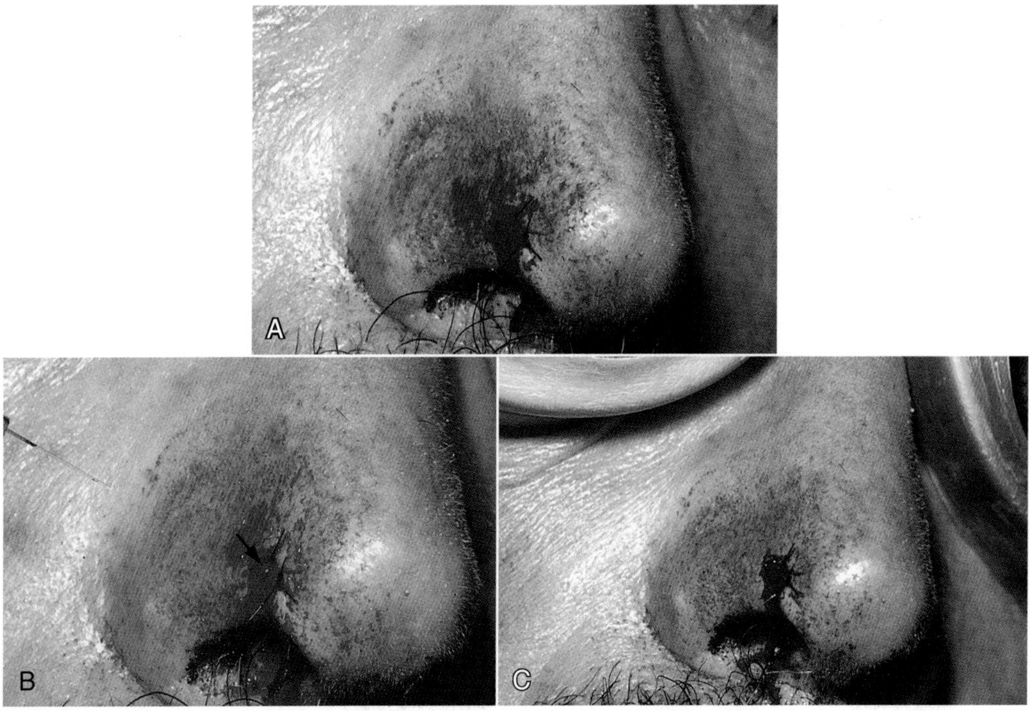

• **Figure 8-4** Example of hemostasis/coagulation procedure in a patient on "blood thinner" medication. **A,** Preoperative view showing bleeding from a sutured excision biopsy of lesion on the nose. **B,** Intraoperative view. Note Nd:YAG laser fiber on the left side and the aiming beam shining on bleeding site *(arrow)*. **C,** Immediate postoperative view after use of laser to coagulate the bleeding site. (Courtesy Dr. Robert Convissar.)

precancerous and cancerous tissues early and before they become visible to the naked eye, expediting diagnosis and improving the patient's prognosis. Oh and Laskin[41] noted visual accentuation of some lesions when patients used acetic acid rinse, but with no significant improvement in detection. Also, examination with chemiluminescent systems can produce reflections that make visualization more difficult.

When cellular changes are detected, the limitation of all adjunctive techniques is that a surgical biopsy procedure remains necessary to obtain a diagnosis.[42–44] Biopsy is the process of removing a sample of tissue from the patient for diagnostic examination. This procedure is required to determine the underlying process within the tissues that is causing changes in their clinical appearance. The pathologic diagnosis obtained ranges from "normal" to an inflammatory process to a benign or malignant neoplasm. Ultimately, an accurate diagnosis guides the clinician in determining the necessary treatment. The five intraoral biopsy techniques are aspiration biopsy, cytologic biopsy, brush biopsy, excision biopsy, and incision biopsy.

The brush biopsy technique has improved the sensitivity (92.3%) and specificity (94.3%) for detection of oral squamous cell carcinoma or dysplasia when tested on visually identified lesions.[45–47] Of note, brush biopsies in particular should be used only as a *screening* tool, and atypical cell identification or a positive result from such biopsies will necessitate an additional step: implementing a surgical procedure to confirm a diagnosis.[48] The main problem with brush biopsy is inadequate depth of the specimen resulting from operator error.

Formulating a definitive diagnosis generally requires the acquisition of a tissue specimen histologically representative of the lesion, using one of the two surgical biopsy techniques. Until recently, most surgical biopsies have been performed with "cold steel"—the scalpel. The disadvantage of this approach is that patients frequently experience significant intraoperative and postoperative sequelae.

The preferred modality for the intraoral surgical biopsy is the laser, for several reasons. The laser's hemostatic nature creates a blood-free surgical field compared with the scalpel. This is critical with vascular lesions or in treating patients who tend to bleed excessively; the laser minimizes blood loss. Other advantages of using a laser are reduced surgery time (superior precision of incision) and unparalleled visualization of the surgical site (lack of blood in surgical field). Decreasing the duration of surgery reduces tissue manipulation and potential wound contamination. The laser's thermal effect produces minimal lateral thermal necrosis but provokes enough response to attain a bactericidal effect. Patients are comfortable during the procedure with minimal local anesthesia. After laser surgery, patients quickly return to their daily routine, experiencing no bleeding or swelling. Discomfort usually is minimal and generally can be treated with OTC nonnarcotic analgesics such as ibuprofen. Surgical biopsies with a laser often can be performed on the patient's initial visit, accelerating the diagnostic process and expediting treatment.

Incision Technique

The location and size of the lesion dictate whether incision or excision surgical biopsy technique should be used. The incision technique removes only a representative portion or portions of a lesion as well as adjacent normal tissue.

Superficial lesions described as being leukoplakic and erythroplakic, with histologic features consistent with hyperkeratosis, lichen planus, leukoedema, epithelial dysplasia, carcinoma in situ, or squamous cell carcinoma, usually are treated with this technique. Frequently, multiple incision biopsies at several locations are required to obtain tissue for microscopic examination when oral cancer is suspected.

The incision biopsy specimen obtained using a scalpel typically is elliptical in shape and should be of sufficient depth and width for obtaining a deep tissue margin, taking into account the infiltrating properties of a carcinoma. When incising the lesion with the laser, it is imperative to generate an adequate specimen. Consideration must be given to the local extent of both healthy and diseased tissue, with careful attention to the possibility of lateral thermal necrosis. The biopsy specimen should extend down into the submucosa to permit determination of depth of invasion, to maximize the possibility of removing the lesion, and to decrease the likelihood of seeding cancerous cells into the surrounding cells.

Excision Technique

Excision technique requires the removal of the entire lesion with at least 2 to 3 mm of peripheral margin (Figure 8-5 A–C). This technique is preferred for oral lesions 1 cm or less and for minor, solid, and exophytic lesions. Localized discrete lesions such as fibroma, papilloma, mucocele, and pyogenic granuloma are most often excised with a laser.

When surgeons perform their first laser biopsy, they should take slightly wider margins than they would take with a blade, to decrease the possibility of thermal necrosis (a beginner's mistake in biopsy technique) at the incision margins.[39]

When an excision biopsy is confirmed to contain a positive margin of disease, this procedure is classified as an "incision" biopsy. Additional treatment is then required to eradicate the disease.

Documentation

Digital photography is invaluable in dental practice today. A clinical photograph should be captured before administering anesthetic to preclude capturing any distortion in the involved tissues. It is vital to document all aspects of a patient's treatment, including presurgical and postsurgical photographs, surgical margins, any surgical defects, and the biopsy specimen (see Figure 8-5 E). A specimen submitted for review should contain any pertinent medical and clinical history, with photographs attached to assist the pathologist in formulating a diagnosis. If a diagnosis is questionable or a malignancy is suspected, it is best to discuss concerns with the pathologist and always perform another biopsy as appropriate.

Anesthesia

Local anesthesia should be used to ensure optimal comfort for the patient. If local anesthetic is placed directly on the lesion or planned incision margin, the fluid content in the tissue from the injection may lead to both altered tissue removal and inconsistent cutting secondary to absorptive properties of the laser energy. Performing neural blocks, deep infiltration, or infiltration at least 1 cm away from the lesion is ideal and will minimize distortion to the surgical area.

PROCEDURE

1. **Outline the planned surgical margins** with incremental spacing using an intermittent laser setting before making the actual incision.

   Such mapping is good practice when performing a biopsy, because it ensures accuracy and allows the clinician to make any necessary changes before the point at which a mistake will become irreversible. This step also allows the clinician to evaluate the laser–tissue interaction so that the speed of incision and energy settings can be changed if deemed necessary.

2. **Connect the outlined margins** with one to two passes using a controlled and rapid motion.

   Maintaining a constant spot size will achieve an incision with a uniform depth. A slower motion increases the depth of the incision, energy absorbed by the tissue, and lateral thermal damage. When further depth to the incision is indicated, this is best achieved by increasing the level of energy or performing additional passes, moving the laser tip further into the incision. To make a shallow incision, increase the controlled motion of the handpiece instead of decreasing the level of energy. Once the maximal speed of motion is reached, reducing the setting may be appropriate.[3,25] Incision depth is lesion-dependent; with superficial lesions, a 2- to 4-mm-thick specimen of soft tissue from the surface is required to permit an accurate microscopic examination by the pathologist. Impingement on the lesion usually occurs at the deepest margin from improper

   angulation of the laser, frequently from attempting to use direct vision. A successful approach is achieved by maintaining a perpendicular position to the surface of the tissue until the desired depth of incision is obtained.

3. **Undermine the lesion.**

   The biopsy procedure culminates with gentle retraction away from the attached surface of the margin of the specimen using a surgical instrument or a retraction suture. As tension is applied to the retracted tissue, the focused, absorbed laser energy facilitates the separation of the specimen from the native tissue. Particular attention should be paid during undermining of the specimen; the laser tip must be carefully directed into the margin, parallel to the base of the lesion, maintaining the desired depth. In this circumstance it is easy for the operator to become misdirected during the excision, leading to accidental transection of the lesion and potentially leaving pathologic cells in the native tissues, resulting in a deficient biopsy specimen. Blocking the surrounding tissues with a moistened gauze or tongue blade during the horizontal laser dissection will help prevent injury from errant laser energy.

4. **Tag and label the specimen** at the margin to ensure that correct orientation of the specimen is maintained.

   Accurate orientation facilitates treatment of suspicious margins and establishes a baseline for discussion of patient care between the pathologist and the clinician.

Continued

PROCEDURE—cont' d

5. **Obtain hemostasis,** if necessary.
The surgical wound is inspected and any bleeding is controlled. Lasers normally provide excellent hemostasis; occasionally, however, bleeding may occur due to one of two reasons: it may arise from a blood vessel larger in diameter than 0.5 mm (the approximate upper limit of hemostatic effectiveness for lasers), or it may occur as a result of moving the handpiece too rapidly over the surgical site, resulting in insufficient time for lateral thermal diffusion and coagulation to take effect.[39] In either case, applying pressure with sterile gauze will gain immediate control. Definitive control with the hemostatic technique is reviewed later.

6. **Sutures** are rarely indicated with use of laser biopsy techniques.
If sutures are necessary, it is best to undermine the peripheral margins to facilitate a tension-free closure and optimize healing. Initially, laser wounds demonstrate a delayed epithelialization compared with scalpel wounds, although studies show that the tensile strength will ultimately be the same.[37] Therefore sutures placed in laser wounds should be removed 7 to 10 days after surgery, versus 5 to 7 days for scalpel wounds (see Figure 8-5).

7. **Place a physiologic bandage on the wound.**
Correct laser technique allows formation of a carbonized layer over the surgical wound. This is accomplished by defocusing the laser and exposing the entire surgical area to laser energy. Deciding whether to place a thin, protective layer over the surgical site or to leave the site directly exposed is a subjective decision facilitated by sufficient clinical experience. The literature on the use of this technique is equivocal, being advocated in the past with continuous-wave CO_2 laser techniques, but probably unnecessary with superpulsed and ultrapulsed CO_2 laser delivery systems. Some clinicians coat the lesion with petroleum jelly, others with vitamin E oil, and still others leave the wound as is. With minor variations in technique, these procedures generally can be performed with a diode or erbium laser as well as the CO_2. This is not generally true, however, of ablation/vaporization procedures.

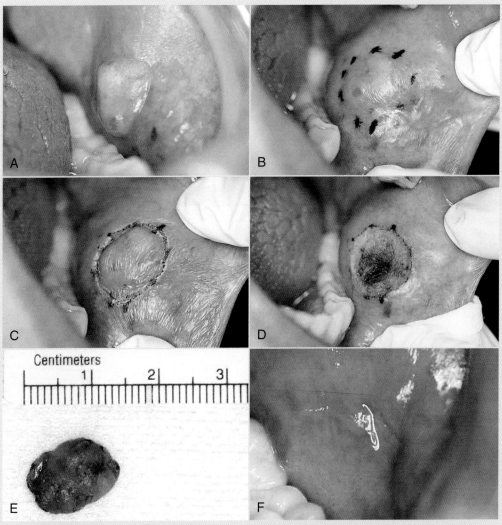

• **Figure 8-5** Excision biopsy technique. **A,** View of the presenting lesion shows surrounding anatomy. **B** and **C,** Outlining the planned incision with a marking pen or with the laser at a lower power setting allows for greater control with incision placement. **D,** Ideal hemostasis within surgical defect. **E,** Photographic documentation of specimen. **F,** One-week postoperative view.

Other Incision/Excision Procedures

Laser incision and excision techniques also are applicable to other intraoral procedures. These techniques are lesion-independent; any lesion or tissue requiring incision or excision is treated using the same basic method previously outlined.[7] Lasers have proved to be successful in correcting many oral soft tissue anomalies.[49,50]

The parameters for incision and excision procedures vary by laser, as well as by type of tissue being treated and the experience of the clinician. Adherence to "cookbook" parameters occasionally recommended in the literature should be avoided; these may not be consistent with the expected tissue effect in a particular case (Case Studies 8-1, 8-2, and 8-3).[3]

Ablation/Vaporization Techniques and Procedures

The CO_2 laser is unique in its ability to function as a "light scalpel" and a photothermal vaporizer. Tissue ablation/vaporization is a technique performed with lasers in defocused mode and achieved by moving the laser away from the tissue beyond the focal point, causing an increase in spot size that directly decreases power density and depth of the cut. The absorbed energy vaporizes the tissue in a controlled, predictable manner. Cryosurgery and chemical peeling are similar but unpredictable because of the inability to achieve a constant depth and the difficulty of applying these modalities intraorally. The noncontact nature of the CO_2 laser makes this wavelength the best of those available for ablation, although the use of wide optical fibers (e.g., 800 μm) may allow other lasers to be used as well.

Laser vaporization is the safest, fastest, and most predictable surgical modality available today. The ablation technique often is used to treat discrete intraoral lesions, benign and premalignant surface lesions, and inflammatory disease, as well as for contouring gingival tissues for functional and esthetic purposes. Other common applications include the management of epithelial hyperkeratosis, hyperplasia, dysplasia, lichen planus, and nicotine stomatitis.

Vaporization Technique

Vaporization of a lesion precludes a histologic diagnosis. Accordingly, vaporization should be performed only in areas for which biopsy specimens have already been obtained or when a reasonable presumed diagnosis has been made.[3]

Vaporization is ideal for removal of large surface lesions confined to the epithelium, located in areas such as the floor of the mouth, where incisions are likely to compromise the underlying anatomy. In such cases, traditional biopsy techniques using a scalpel would be considered aggressive because they eradicate too much tissue and may cause bleeding, scarring, and injury to adjacent structures. With most CO_2 lasers, each pass during tissue ablation penetrates from a few hundred micrometers down to 1 to 2 mm. By selectively removing each cellular layer, laser ablation can be completed in a conservative fashion, with minimal insult to the underlying tissue and structures. After laser ablation, tissue elasticity remains resilient, scarring is reduced, and fundamental function is preserved.[22,23]

Lesion Treatment

Superficial lesions that demonstrate leukoplakia, erythroplakia, or a combination are more likely to undergo malignant transformation. Affected patients have a 50- to 60-fold greater risk of developing oral cancer.[7] Laser ablation of these lesions is considered controversial. Interventional laser excision or ablation of precancerous oral epithelial lesions offers unique advantages, including elimination of diseased tissue, control of blood loss, favorable patient acceptance, low morbidity with reduced complications, and successful healing.[51]

Studies have demonstrated that laser ablation with regular follow-up evaluations is effective in controlling dysplastic lesions of all grades. The recurrence rates for premalignant lesions are not significantly different for scalpel excision and for laser vaporization. Vedtofte et al.[52] reported a 20% recurrence rate over 4 years in patients who underwent scalpel excision. Horch et al.[53] reported a 22% recurrence rate over 37 months in patients who underwent laser vaporization. Thompson and Wylie[54] reviewed data for 57 consecutive laser-treated patients presenting over a 4-year period with histologically confirmed dysplastic lesions. Over 44 months, findings showed 76% of patients remained disease-free, comparable to the 80% success rate in patients treated with surgical excision.

Laser vaporization is an effective, nonmorbid, inexpensive, quick, and relatively painless method of managing premalignant lesions. Many clinicians believe that the hemostatic effect of the laser results in decreased tendency for hematogenous or lymphatic seeding of the malignant cells.[55,56] The low morbidity and minimal pain generally associated with laser ablation make it a valuable tool in the management of premalignant mucosal lesions.

Ablation Technique

Regardless of the type of ablative laser used to perform this procedure, the ablation technique is accomplished using a defocused mode, which increases the spot size and decreases the power density and depth of cut. The depth of ablation is increased by using a higher power setting and decreased by moving the handpiece faster or by increasing the spot size. The size and depth of the lesion help determine the power setting and spot size for treatment.

As with excision biopsy, the clinician should begin by outlining the circumferential margins. The outlined margins serve as surgical boundaries, extending 0.5 cm beyond the identifiable lesion. Ablation of the lesion is accomplished through a continuous series of connecting parallel

CASE STUDY 8-1

Excision of Pyogenic Granuloma

A 46-year-old white female patient presented with a bothersome soft, fleshy, raised mass on the lower lip, which developed after a fall 2 weeks earlier in which she struck her lip on cement (Figure 8-6 *A* and *B*). A ¾ carpule of 2% lidocaine with 1:100,000 epinephrine was given by local infiltration. An excision biopsy was indicated. An elliptical incision followed the outside of the lesion with the laser beam positioned perpendicular to the tissue, to prevent undercutting at the deeper margin (see Figure 8-6 *C* and *D*). Once the orbicularis oris muscle was identified, the specimen was gently lifted from one side of the outlined incision and the excision is performed following the supramuscular plane (see Figure 8-6 *E*). Incising into the muscle will cause increased soreness and create potential for increased bleeding or unnecessary wound contracture. After excision, the specimen should be measured,

photographed, and sent to a pathologist for microscopic examination. Suturing the wound generally is not necessary unless achieving a cosmetic result is a primary concern. A softer diet is recommended to avoid lip movement after the procedure. The 10-day postoperative photographs show an excellent cosmetic result (see Figure 8-6 *F* and *G*).

The mass was diagnosed as a pyogenic granuloma. These granulomas frequently manifest as soft red masses, possibly ulcerated, with fibrinopurulent casings, located intraorally on the gingiva between teeth, or occasionally on the face. Growth of pyogenic granulomas is initiated by irritants such as calculus, rough restorations, or foreign bodies. They tend to bleed easily when traumatized. Surgical excision with 2-mm margins at the periphery is curative if the causative factors are removed. Recurrence is unlikely unless a local irritant remains present.

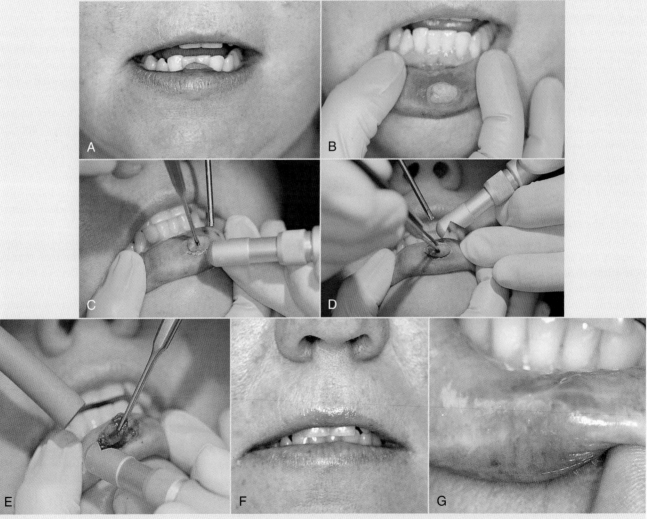

• **Figure 8-6** *A* and **B,** Pyogenic granuloma is a clinically recognizable lesion and usually manifests as an inflammatory soft, red, raised mass that often bleeds when traumatized. **C** and **D,** Incision is performed after delineation of the surgical margins at lesion's periphery. **E,** Complete excision at base of lesion. **F** and **G,** At 10 days, suture removal is completed. An early esthetic result is evident.

CASE STUDY 8-2

Excision of Tongue Lipoma

A 51-year-old white male patient presented with an asymptomatic, slow-growing mass on the left dorsum of the tongue that he first noticed 3 months earlier. Clinical examination demonstrated a nontender, soft, doughy mass 1 cm in diameter, with healthy overlying tissues (Figure 8-7 A). One carpule of 2% lidocaine with 1:100,000 epinephrine was administered by infiltration at the periphery and deep margins of the tongue mass.

The tip of tongue was retracted using gauze. A curvilinear "trapdoor" incision was made using a CO_2 laser. Once the initial incision was made, tissue forceps were gently applied to support the tongue flap, with the laser used to dissect along the capsular plane of the yellow, doughy mass (see Figure 8-7 B). A second retractor was used to grasp the round mass and retract away from the connected tissues. Dissection around the perimeter of the mass in all directions completed the excision biopsy (see Figure 8-7 C). The exposed cavity was irrigated with a sterile

saline solution. Hemostasis was achieved by defocusing the laser. The tongue flap was approximated and primarily closed with 3-0 chromic gut interrupted sutures (see Figure 8-7 D). The specimen should maintain a pericapsular lining, visible on the photograph (see Figure 8-7 E). The specimen was placed in formalin, prepared, and sent for microscopic examination.

Histopathologic analysis identified the mass as a solitary lipoma. Lipomas are proliferations of mature fat cells that arise in the submucosa. These frequently occur in adults 40 to 60 years of age. Intraorally, they typically arise in the buccal vestibules and mucosa, floor of the mouth, and tongue. Solitary lipomas require exploration and local excision. The fatty nature of the tumor will cause bulging from the wound during treatment. The pericapsular lining is best left intact to ensure a complete excision. Because the density of fat is less than that of formalin or water, a lipoma should float when placed in either solution[48] (see Figure 8-7 F).

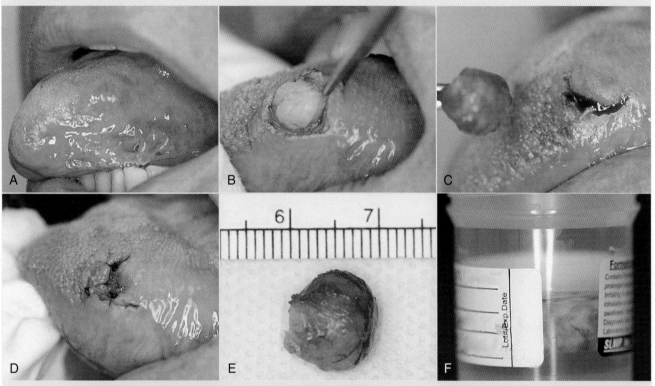

• **Figure 8-7 A,** Soft mass (1 cm) without mucosal ulceration bulging from left dorsal surface of tongue. **B,** Using retraction with tissue forceps while dissecting the mass with the laser will facilitate the separation. **C,** Complete excision of lipoma. **D,** Closure of "trapdoor" flap with interrupted sutures. **E,** Specimen photograph demonstrating pericapsular lining. **F,** Mass is floating in container filled with formalin, suggesting a diagnosis of lipoma.

Us within the delineated margins, taking care not to leave any lesion present. This method ensures an evenly ablated surface. Overlapping ablative passes can result in greater lateral thermal damage and increased depth. Ablated tissues easily become dehydrated; therefore, with retreatment of a previously irradiated area, increased lateral thermal damage may occur. To minimize the likelihood of a poor outcome, the tissues should be rehydrated with water spray, and any surface carbonization should be gently wiped away with moist gauze between passes.[3] To achieve deeper penetration, additional passes may be performed perpendicular to the initial ablative pattern, to ensure complete coverage of the lesion (Figure 8-9 and Case Studies 8-4 to 8-6 with Figure 8-7).

CASE STUDY 8-3

Excision of Tongue Papilloma

A 72-year-old white male patient who had smoked heavily for 25 years presented with a suspicious stalk-like lesion at the right posterior ventrolateral border of the tongue. The patient could not recall how long the lesion had been present. The lesion was 1.0×0.5 cm in size, with peripheral leukoplakic changes but no ulceration or bleeding (Figure 8-8 *A*). One carpule of 2% lidocaine with 1:100,000 epinephrine was given by local infiltration. A marking pen was used to delineate the margins, and an excision biopsy was performed with a CO_2 laser. An elliptical incision was made on the perimeter of the lesion, with the laser energy aimed perpendicular to the tissue to prevent undercutting at the deep margin. After the skeletal muscle of the tongue was identified and isolated, the specimen was gently lifted at the anterior margin and excision performed following the supramuscular plane (see Figure 8-8 *B*). Once slight elevation of the specimen was achieved, the anterior margin was tagged with an interrupted 3-0 silk suture.

With a high likelihood of malignancy, the margins should be tagged and identified by their location: anterior, posterior, medial, lateral, superficial, and deep. Tagging the specimen margins during the procedure will accurately identify the location of any residual tumor and ensure accuracy in the event that additional treatment is indicated. Biopsy specimens are tagged using sutures with "tails" of various lengths to indicate the specimen's anatomic orientation. After excision, the tagged specimen should be positioned on paper, labeled, and photographed (see Figure 8-8 *C*). Closure of intraoral wounds is not necessary with CO_2 laser treatment unless local irritation or bleeding is a concern. In this patient, primary closure was necessary to prevent rubbing of the wound edges on the adjacent dentition. Complete healing should occur in approximately 2 to 4 weeks.

Microscopic examination diagnosed the lesion as a squamous papilloma. Papillomas are common oral lesions with a predilection for the mucosa of the hard and soft palate, including the uvula and vermilion border of the lips. The lesion is not transmissible or threatening based on current studies and is not directly associated with HPV. Its clinical appearance frequently raises concern because it sometimes mimics an exophytic carcinoma, verrucous carcinoma, or condyloma acuminatum, a transmissible viral disease. Excision with 1-mm margins at the base into the submucosa should be curative. Recurrence should raise suspicions for retransmission of condyloma acuminatum or carcinoma.[48] The tongue heals completely, while maintaining function, within 2 to 4 weeks, with minimal to no discomfort (see Figure 8-8 *D*).

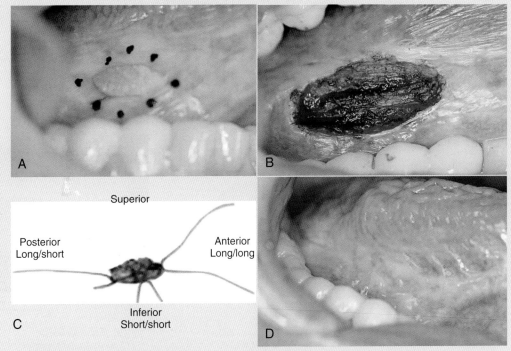

• **Figure 8-8** **A,** Stalklike lesion located on posterior right lateral border of tongue and floor of mouth is a suspected carcinoma. A marking pen delineates margins for the excision biopsy procedure. **B,** Complete excision of specimen at the supramuscular plane. Proximity of adjacent teeth will lead to direct irritation during the healing phase if the incision is not primarily closed. **C,** Specimen tagged with interrupted sutures of various lengths ("suture tails") to indicate correct positioning of the excised lesion. **D,** One-month postoperative view demonstrates complete healing.

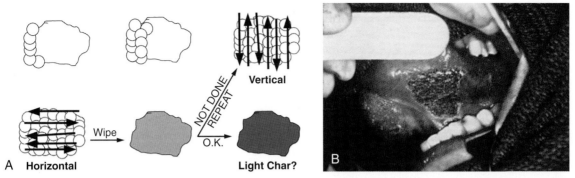

• **Figure 8-9** Ablation technique showing proper use of inverted Us. (From Strauss RA: Laser management of discrete lesions. In Catone G, Alling C, editors: *Laser applications in oral and maxillofacial surgery,* Philadelphia, 1997, WB Saunders.)

CASE STUDY 8-4

Ablation of Asymtomatic leukoplakia

A 71-year-old white male patient presented for evaluation of a whitish plaque, 1.5 × 1.0 cm, located on the left lateral soft palate and present for an unknown duration (see Figure 8-10 *A*). The patient was a 50-year half-pack/day smoker with a history of moderate consumption of alcohol. Clinical examination confirmed a nonremovable plaquelike leukoplakia with irregular borders. A complete medical history was obtained and a thorough head and neck examination performed. No cervical lymphadenopathy was palpable. Incision biopsy performed using local anesthesia resulted in a diagnosis of mild dysplasia. Laser ablation was used to eradicate the mild dysplastic tissues. One carpule of 2% lidocaine with 1:100,000 epinephrine was administered by local infiltration. The laser was used in a defocused mode.

For laser ablation of such lesions, it is recommended to start at the peripheral margin and systematically work back and forth, covering the entire lesion without overlapping. Once the initial pass is completed, the wound is debrided with moist gauze, removing necrotic tissues. Additional passes may be necessary, depending on the severity of the pathologic process. Inspection of the tissues must confirm absence of residual lesion. A thin eschar layer is left over the wound, and healing is complete in 2 to 4 weeks (see Figure 8-10 *B*). Chlorhexidine oral rinse is recommended to reduce infection, and OTC nonsteroidal medication should provide adequate relief of any pain. Follow-up examinations are critical to monitor for recurrence and to ensure early detection of new lesions (see Figure 8-10 *C*).

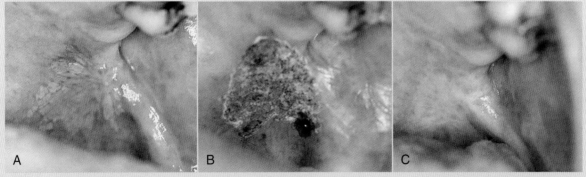

• **Figure 8-10 A,** Asymptomatic leukoplakic plaquelike lesion located on soft palate. **B,** Treatment using CO_2 laser involves two ablative passes with debridement, leaving a thin layer of eschar to help protect the area during initial healing. **C,** Two-month postoperative view demonstrates complete healing with no evidence of active disease.

Inflammatory Conditions

The inflammatory response typically is associated with swelling, pain, and possible systemic disease and infection. Inflammatory conditions such as periodontitis, implantitis, alveolitis, papillary hyperplasia, herpetic lesions, and aphthous ulcerations may be managed with laser vaporization therapy. Vaporization of herpetic and aphthous ulcers is an alternative to use of regularly prescribed medications, which provide temporary palliation at best (see Chapter 11). Laser therapy provides relief of symptoms and establishes an optimal wound for healing, selectively eliminating pathogens and disease through the photothermal tissue interaction in these potentially recurrent lesions.[56] Palliation of the painful symptoms associated with aphthous and herpetic stomatitis.[57–60] and treatment of the oral manifestations of acquired immunodeficiency syndrome (AIDS) can be effectively accomplished with laser therapy.[61]

CASE STUDY 8-5

Ablation of Mucocele

A 19-year-old white male patient presented with a painless, soft, fluid-filled vesicle in the mucosa of the lower lip (Figure 8-11 *A*). He first noted the lesion approximately 4 months earlier, after a blow to the face. He complained of intermittent swelling. The history and clinical presentation are consistent with mucus extravasation phenomenon, with the resulting lesion commonly known as a mucocele.

Mucoceles most often are observed in the younger population, frequently arising after a traumatic injury that severs the minor salivary ducts, forcing extravasated mucus into the mucosa and eliciting an inflammatory reaction that causes localized fibrosis. Mucoceles are easily identified given their bluish color and may occur anywhere a minor salivary gland exists. They most often are found in the lower lip, palpated in the tissues near the midline, and usually measure 1 cm or less across (see Figure 8-11 *B*). Although these lesions frequently are treated by local excision, the ablation technique can be implemented if findings on repeated excisions with histologic confirmation are consistent with the clinical presentation of a mucocele.

The laser ablation technique is a predictable, minimally invasive treatment. Local anesthesia is achieved with administration of one carpule of 2% lidocaine with 1:100,000 epinephrine, by local infiltration. The CO_2 laser is used in a defocused mode. It is recommended to begin ablation of the lesion at the peripheral margin of the mucosa, working in a circular spiral motion toward the epicenter (see Figure 8-11 *C*). This technique helps ensure complete removal of damaged glands, whereas starting from the center may cause shrinkage of damaged glands and partial vaporization, leaving damaged salivary glands with the potential for recurrence. Once the mucosa is ablated and the epicenter has been reached, applying finger pressure on the lesion frequently causes the enlarged fibrotic minor salivary gland to protrude, allowing complete vaporization of the damaged glandular tissues (see Figure 8-11 *D*).

Inspection and palpation of the underlying tissues should confirm the absence of residual lesion. Further ablation is performed by defocusing the energy and working from the epicenter slowly toward the periphery, shrinking the size of the surgical wound by thermal contraction, with no bleeding noted (see Figure 8-11 *E*). The wound is left to granulate. Figure 8-11 *F* shows the surgical site 1 week postoperatively. A nonsteroidal OTC medication should provide adequate relief of any pain.

Alternatively, many surgeons prefer to excise the mucocele with its associated gland. This assures complete treatment and minimizes recurrence. The technique is identical to the biopsy techniques previously discussed.

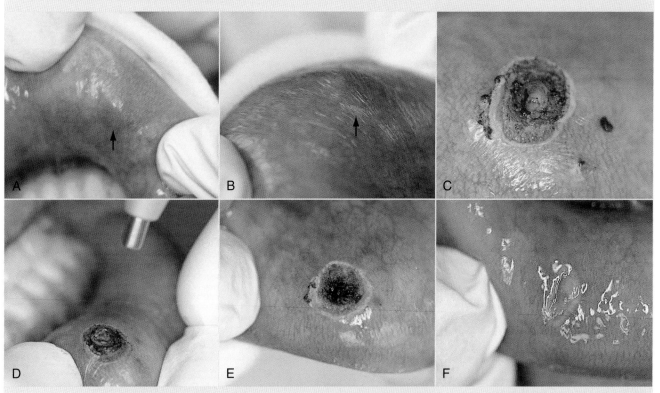

• **Figure 8-11 A** and **B,** Mucoceles frequently are noted in the lower lip and have a distinctive raised, rounded, and bluish appearance. **C,** Superficial ablation is performed starting from peripheral margin and working toward center. **D,** Applied finger pressure causes fibrotic glandular tissue to emerge, allowing complete ablation therapy. **E,** Ablation causes thermal contracture, decreasing the size of the open wound left to granulate, which expedites the healing process. **F,** One-week postoperative view demonstrates rapid healing.

CASE STUDY 8-6

Excision/Ablation of Peripheral Odontogenic Fibroma

A 9-year-old white female patient presented with a painless, firm, soft tissue mass on the gingiva. The growth was noted 8 months earlier, after the eruption of the lower incisors. The gingival mass prevented tooth #23 from appropriate alignment, interfering with normal function (Figure 8-12 A). Radiographic examination demonstrated no intraosseous component. Local anesthesia was obtained using 1/4 carpule of articane hydrochloride with 1:100,000 epinephrine (Septocaine), administered by local infiltration. An excision biopsy procedure was performed using the laser. An incision was made with the laser in focused mode, with the tip parallel to the facial surface placed into the sulcus, while reflecting the mass away from the tooth. With tension applied to the mass in a superior direction, excision of the mass was completed at the level of the gingival crevice, to maintain the scalloped appearance. Proximity of the mass to the tooth increases the potential for injury to the tooth. A matrix band can be placed around the tooth as an extra precaution. Sculpting of irregular tissue, intrasulcular ablation, and hemostasis are accomplished by defocusing energy.

If persistent oozing is encountered, pressure with moist gauze is applied for several minutes, and additional hemostasis is provided as necessary (see Figure 8-12 B). In this case, the 1-week and 2-month postoperative visits demonstrate rapid healing and significant improvement in the tooth position (see Figure 8-12 C and D).

A diagnosis of peripheral odontogenic fibroma was made based on location of the mass and the histologic features. The fibroma manifests as a painless, firm, soft tissue mass with an intact mucosa, emerging directly from the gingival sulcus. These lesions frequently are found in the premolar or canine region and most often in females. The fibroma is less than 2 cm in diameter, and it demonstrates no invasion or destruction to surrounding tissues. Radiographs will not show bony resorption as a reaction to its presence. On histologic examination, odontogenic epithelia are present, making this lesion appear to originate from the periodontal membrane.[48]

Diagnosis and treatment of a peripheral fibroma require excision with 1- to 2-mm mucosal margins, including the attached periodontal ligament from which it arises. The recurrence rate is very low, and regrowth of the lesion typically is associated with residual odontogenic epithelia. Excision performed with a scalpel often results in a periodontal defect because of the inability to excise at the depth of the gingival sulcus. Performing laser excision at the gingival margin and then completing the procedure with intrasulcular ablation of the remnants of the periodontal membrane will minimize potential recurrence and improve the cosmetic outcome.

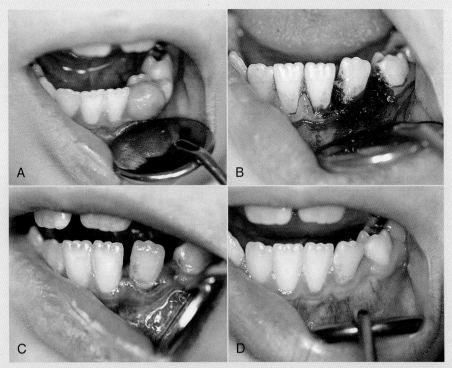

• **Figure 8-12** **A,** Painless, firm, soft tissue mass emerging from gingival sulcus of tooth #23. **B,** Localized laser excision and ablation of gingival mass with hemostasis. **C,** At the 1-week postoperative visit, the characteristic rapid healing after laser surgery is evident. **D,** Two-month postoperative view demonstrates the natural drifting of tooth #23 into appropriate alignment can be seen.

The ablation technique is useful in managing other functional and esthetic concerns in the oral cavity. Laser ablation in the hands of a skilled clinician has revolutionized soft tissue manipulation. Patients who present with fibrous tuberosities and gingival hyperplasia resulting from inflammation or drug therapy are now treated predictably with minimally invasive surgery.

Dental Implants

Many surgeons believe that using the CO_2 laser for dental implant surgery is as important as cone-beam computed tomography (CBCT) and three-dimensional volumetric rendering, implant planning software. The ability to evaluate the underlying bony foundation before implant placement is invaluable. In many cases, implants can be placed with a flapless laser-assisted approach, reducing contamination to the implant from adjacent mucosal tissue. The gingival tissues are decontaminated by the photothermal effect, and the emergence profile is sculpted for the indicated healing abutment without bleeding or swelling, improving the patient's dental implant experience.

Recently, high-energy lasers have been proposed as an alternative to the conventional surgical drill for the preparation of implant osteotomies. Panduric et al.[62] studied the changes in bone volume and bone surface as well as procedure time with use of an erbium-doped yttrium-aluminum-garnet (Er:YAG) laser versus a conventional slow-speed handpiece for the preparation of implant osteotomies. Their conclusions were that the Er:YAG laser produced preparations with regular and sharp-edged contours, without bone fragments and debris, in a shorter time, and with less generated heat. Thermal alterations in the treated surface were minimal.[62] This promising study carried out on porcine ribs may very well lead to research that gives the clinician an alternative to the conventional implant slow-speed hand piece.

Ailing implants also benefit from the photothermal properties of the laser. Local decontamination eliminates infection, optimizing the periimplant tissues, and prolonging the implant's ability to function (see Chapter 7).

Hemostasis/Coagulation Techniques and Procedures

One of the greatest advantages of laser surgery is the ability to achieve hemostasis. Laser surgery is essentially performed in a bloodless field, improving visualization. Hemostasis is not caused by coagulation of blood but by contraction of the vascular wall collagen, which results in constriction of the vessel opening.

Although the argon, copper vapor, KTP, tunable dye, and Nd:YAG lasers have proved to be successful in the treatment of vascular lesions because their wavelengths are highly absorbed by hemoglobin,[63] they generally are not part of the dental armamentarium. Rather, these lasers more often are used to treat extraoral vascular lesions or intraoral lesions for which excision with a CO_2 laser would be precluded. On the other hand, CO_2 lasers can be used to excise many types of intraoral vascular lesions. As previously mentioned, the normal lateral thermal damage created by the laser results in contraction of collagen; therefore sealing of vessels up to 500 μm in diameter occurs. In particular, capillary hemangiomas, cavernous hemangiomas, venous lakes, small telangiectasias, and varicosities are ideally treated using the hemostatic technique, because vessels that supply capillary and small venous vascular lesions are coagulated, allowing for en bloc excision of such lesions.[3]

For the hemostatic technique, the laser is used in defocused mode, which increases the spot size, dispersing the energy over a wider area. The laser tip is passed over the tissue until bleeding ceases. This simple exercise decreases the temperature of the energy absorbed by the lased tissues, causing coagulation. For direct hemostasis, the laser beam can be aimed at a specific bleeding area. These techniques are effective only if the surgical field remains absolutely dry of saliva and blood. Any surrounding body fluids will absorb the energy, thus reducing the laser's effect on the tissues. Continued bleeding indicates a vessel greater in diameter than the spot size of the laser; other, more conventional hemostatic techniques (Gelfoam, Surgicel, sutures) may be required. Other treatment modalities, such as topical thrombin and a tranexamic acid rinse, should always be available in the event that postoperative bleeding persists and additional hemostatic measures need to be taken.

Blood loss with use of a CO_2 laser is significantly less than with the traditional scalpel in treating patients with coagulation disorders[64] and those who take relevant herbal preparations or anticoagulant medication. Patients taking oral anticoagulants can be treated with the CO_2 laser, without the need to discontinue medication, for routine oral soft tissue procedures. In fact, because the risk of postoperative bleeding is outweighed by the higher risk of thromboembolism after cessation of anticoagulant therapy, continuation of the anticoagulant regimen is encouraged. Laser-assisted oral surgery in daily practice has enabled surgeons to achieve controlled hemostasis and minimize intraoperative and postoperative hemorrhage without discontinuing anticoagulants.[65] Of course, a conversation with the primary care physician and knowledge of the patient's international normalized ratio (INR) value are strongly suggested.

Hemangioma

Hemangiomas, most commonly seen in infants, are benign proliferations of blood vessels that resemble normal vessels. One half of all hemangiomas occur in the head and neck area, especially the tongue, buccal mucosa, and lips, and they have a predilection for females. The lesion can manifest as flat or exophytic, smooth-surfaced or lobular, or localized or diffuse and may be single or multiple. Types of hemangiomas include atriovenous, juvenile capillary, cavernous, cherry, and varix.

The type of treatment modality for a hemangioma depends on its size, rate of blood flow, and proximity to other structures. When a hemangioma does not spontaneously involute, nonsurgical therapy consists of corticosteroid injection, with a 75% success rate, and interferon alfa-2a. Surgical procedures include excision scalpel surgery for small lesions and laser removal for large lesions. Many other lesions can be treated in a fashion similar to that for the lip hemangioma described in Case Study 8-7, with Figure 8-13, including aphthous ulcers and herpetic gingivostomatitis[57–61] (see Chapters 11 and 15).

Tooth Extractions

The removal of teeth varies in degree of difficulty. Teeth exposed in the oral cavity may be easily removed when structurally sound, but caries compromises the integrity of the tooth, which usually results in its crumbling into many fragments on attempted extraction. Incompletely erupted or impacted teeth require access to the tooth roots for removal.

Regardless of the circumstance, any tooth removal defined as a "surgical extraction," requiring an incision through mucosal tissue with flap reflection to achieve access for tooth removal, can benefit from the use of the diode, erbium, or CO_2 laser. Advantages include the absence of blood from the tissue incision, improved visibility, reduced swelling and discomfort to the patient, and decontamination of the surgical site secondary to the photothermal effects of the laser. Patients who tend to bleed or have coagulopathies benefit from the laser's hemostatic effect in the extraction site at surgery[66] (Figure 8-14).

Exposing teeth that require extraction frequently necessitates a releasing incision for extended reflection of the soft tissue flap. The laser causes less bleeding than that seen with traditional scalpel techniques, thereby improving visibility in the surgical field. With reflection of the periosteum off the underlying bone, however, the perforating capillaries are torn, and osseous bleeding generally is noted. The bleeding encountered during this procedure usually is slight oozing, requiring no intervention other than intraoperative suctioning for visibility.

Adjunctive procedures such as sectioning the tooth or bone removal may be necessary to facilitate removal. Although an erbium laser can be used for tooth sectioning, traditional sectioning with a bur is faster and makes this one of the few procedures in which traditional methods are preferred over laser use.

Once a tooth has been removed, the laser can serve an important ancillary function: Localized infection within the extraction socket or surrounding gingival tissues can be treated using the photothermal effects of the laser. Laser irradiation at a reduced power setting can be used to decontaminate areas of concern. This technique ultimately reduces bacterial infiltrate within the mucosal tissue or periodontal ligaments within the socket. Caution must be taken to maintain steady movement of the laser tip, to prevent injury to the bone from the thermal insult. Socket curettage with complete removal of granulation tissues should be performed, followed by irrigation with copious amounts of sterile saline into the socket.

Postsurgical bleeding from the socket walls is not unusual. Ancillary grafting procedures can be used at the clinician's discretion, as appropriate. Approximation of the soft tissue flap to cover the underlying bone using sutures is indicated.

Apicoectomy

Teeth that are compromised secondary to endodontic failure may be salvaged with endodontic retreatment. Extirpation of the compromised pulpal tissue and treatment of the localized infection routinely lead to resolution of disease without the need for tooth extraction. If periapical disease persists, however, an adjunctive surgical procedure known as *apicoectomy* is necessary to eradicate the affected tissues and improve the therapeutic outcome.

Apicoectomy procedures involve a soft tissue incision followed by removal of localized diseased tissue and frequently require apical sealing of the endodontically treated tooth. The diode, erbium, or CO_2 laser can be used for sterilization and removal of the infected root apex, as well as for enhanced hemostasis.[67] After surgical access is obtained with exposure of the apex of the involved tooth, whether through a laser or conventional incision, the surrounding cavity can be curetted with a small instrument, to remove the infected tissues or radicular cystic lesion (Figure 8-15).

Evaluation of the offending tooth and the apical seal from the endodontic procedure must be confirmed. If the seal appears inadequate, a retrograde filling is imperative for the best prognosis. Root amputation with a high-speed drill and small, crosscut bur can be used with cooled irrigation to prevent thermal damage to the nonvital tooth. Removal of gutta-percha or filling material is achieved using a slow-speed drill and a small, round bur. Adequate retrograde access into the root canal is necessary for retention of the filling material. CO_2 laser treatment optimally prepares the tooth for final intraoperative filling because of sealing of the dentinal tubules, the resultant elimination of niches for bacteria, and the sterilizing effect of the laser beam.[68]

Alternatively, the erbium laser can be used to amputate the tooth and prepare the root end for a retrograde filling.

Conclusions

The spectrum of oral disease involves systemic, infectious, mucosal, and neoplastic processes. These processes can be treated with multiple surgical modalities currently available. The results of surgery using CO_2 lasers have been consistent, particularly in treating soft tissue. Patients have minimal "down time" and generally experience no bleeding, swelling, or pain after routine procedures. Laser technology continues to advance the dental profession; therefore it is imperative to incorporate lasers into surgical practice.

CASE STUDY 8-7

Ablation of Lip Hemangioma

A laser ablation technique was used to treat a white female patient with a hemangioma of the lip (see Figure 8-13 *A*). Local anesthesia was obtained with one carpule of 2% lidocaine with 1:100,000 epinephrine, administered by local infiltration deep within the tissues, after aspiration to prevent intravascular injection. Of note, local anesthetic injected into the vasculature will cause a blanching appearance to the tissues, posterior to the injection site (see Figure 8-13 *B* and *C*). The laser was used in a defocused mode. Again, for ablation of the lesion, it is recommended to begin at the surface of the mucosa at the peripheral margin, working in a circular spiral motion toward the epicenter (see Figure 8-13 *D–F*). This technique ensures complete removal at its widest dimension. Debridement between passes with moist gauze allows for improved penetration of laser energy. Additional ablative passes are then made by defocusing the energy and working from the epicenter slowly toward the periphery, shrinking the size of the surgical wound by thermal contraction; no bleeding should be evident. Charring of the tissues in a vascular lesion is more prevalent because of the absorptive properties of hemoglobin but does not seem to affect the healing process. The wound is then left to granulate, with the patient instructed in performing daily care. Wound care consists of cleaning the area with diluted hydrogen peroxide and applying a thin layer of petroleum jelly four times daily. Prophylactic antibiotics are used with ablation of vascular lesions, to reduce the risk of bacteremia. A nonsteroidal OTC medication will provide adequate relief of pain. Complete healing is achieved in 2 to 6 weeks, resulting in an esthetic outcome (see Figure 8-13 *G–L*).

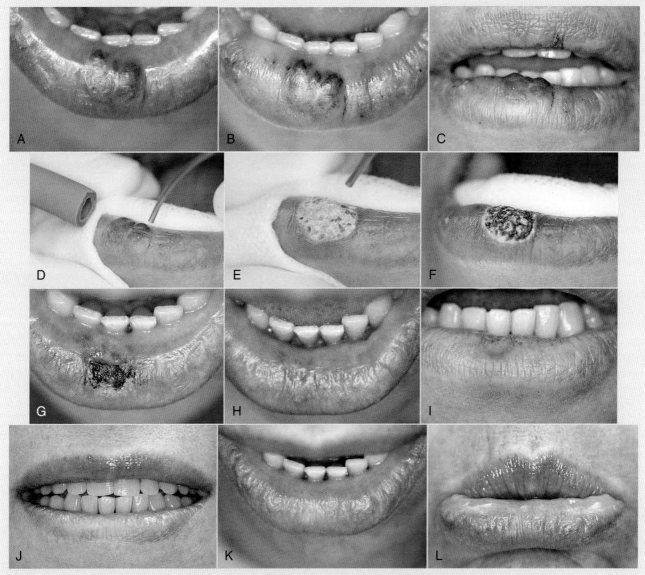

• **Figure 8-13** **A,** Hemangioma of lower lip. **B** and **C,** Localized blanching secondary to injection of local anesthetic with epinephrine into the vascular tissue. **D** to **F,** Multiple sequences of ablation and debridement achieve extension into normal healthy tissue, without demonstrating persistent oozing. **G,** One-week postoperative view demonstrates rapid healing. **H** and **I,** Two-week postoperative view demonstrates minimal irregularity with complete epithelialization. **J** to **L,** Complete healing, maintaining elasticity, with excellent esthetic result.

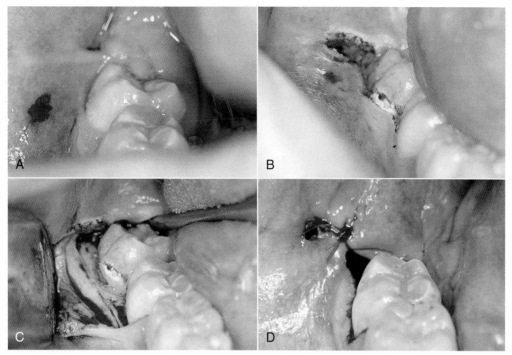

• **Figure 8-14 A,** Soft tissue–impacted third molar, #32, with operculum. **B,** CO_2 laser incision extending from mesial #31 with buccal release at the distal line angle of #32. **C,** Reflection of full-thickness mucoperiosteal flap, allowing access for small elevator distal to #31 to permit luxation and extraction of the tooth without causing trauma to adjacent soft tissue. **D,** Approximating and securing flap with 3-0 chromic gut suture.

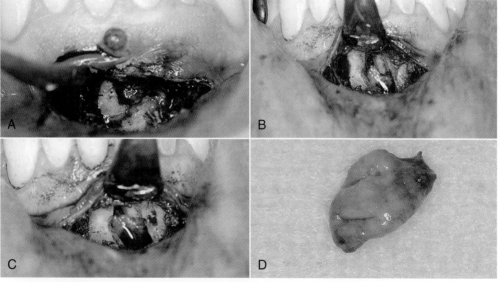

• **Figure 8-15 A,** Fistula below sulcus of tooth #25. The CO_2 laser was used to incise through freely movable mucosa below the mucogingival junction; apical resorption was noted. **B,** Complete curettage of periapical pathology. **C,** Amputation of exposed root tip with retrofilling completed. CO_2 laser at low energy was used to decontaminate the intraosseous cavity. **D,** Specimen removed was confirmed to be a radicular cyst.

References

1. Gaspar L: The use of high-power lasers in oral surgery, *J Clin Laser Med Surg* 12:281–285, 1994.
2. Shafir R, Slutzki S, Bornstein LA: Excision of buccal hemangioma by CO_2 laser beam, *Oral Surg Oral Med Oral Pathol* 44(3):347–350, 1977.
3. Wlodawsky R, Strauss R: Intraoral laser surgery, *Oral Maxillofac Surg Clin North Am* 16:149–163, 2004.
4. Romanos G, Nentwig G: Diode laser (980 nm) in oral and maxillofacial surgical procedures: clinical observations based on clinical applications, *J Clin Laser Med Surg* 17:193–197, 1999.
5. Kreisler M, Gotz H, Duschner H, d'Hoedt B: Effect of Nd:YAG, Ho:YAG, Er:YAG, CO_2, and GaAIAs laser irradiation on surface properties of endosseous dental implants, *Int J Oral Maxillofac Implants* 17:202–211, 2002.
6. Bradley P: A review of the use of the neodymium YAG laser in oral and maxillofacial surgery, *Br J Oral Maxillofac Surg* 35:26–35, 1997.

7. Strauss R, Fallon S: Lasers in contemporary oral and maxillofacial surgery, *Dent Clin North Am* 48:861–888, 2004.

8. Romanos G: Clinical applications of the Nd:YAG laser in oral soft tissue surgery and periodontology, *J Clin Laser Med Surg* 12:103–108, 1994.

9. White J, Goodis H, Rose C: Use of the pulsed Nd:YAG laser for intraoral soft tissue surgery, *Lasers Surg Med* 11:455–461, 1991.

10. White JM, Chaudhry SI, Kudler JJ, et al.: Nd:YAG and CO_2 laser therapy of oral mucosal lesions, *J Clin Laser Med Surg* 16:299–304, 1998.

11. Gregg RH, McCarthy DK: Laser periodontal therapy for bone regeneration, *Dent Today* 21(5):54–59, 2002.

12. Li Z, Reinisch L, van de Merwe W: Bone ablation with Er:YAG and CO_2 laser: study of thermal and acoustic effects, *Lasers Surg Med* 12:79–85, 1992.

13. Arnabat-Dominguez J, Espana-Tost AJ, Berini-Aytes L, Gay-Escoda C: Erbium:YAG laser application in the second phase of implant surgery: a pilot study in 20 patients, *Int J Oral Maxillofac Implants* 18:104–112, 2003.

14. El-Montaser M, Devlin H, Dickinson MR, et al.: Osseointegration of titanium metal implants in erbium-YAG laser-prepared bone, *Implant Dent* 8:79–85, 1999.

15. Walsh L: The use of lasers in implantology: an overview, *J Oral Implantol* 18:335–340, 1992.

16. Kreisler M, Kohnen W, Marinello C, et al.: Bactericidal effect of the Er:YAG laser on dental implant surfaces: an in vitro study, *J Periodontol* 73:1292–1297, 2002.

17. Pogrel MA, McCracken KJ, Daniles TE: Histologic evaluation of width of soft tissue necrosis adjacent to carbon dioxide incisions, *Oral Surg* 70:564–568, 1990.

18. Kaminer R, Liebow C, Margarone JE, Zambon JJ: Bacteremia following laser and conventional surgery in hamsters, *J Oral Maxillofac Surg* 48:45–48, 1990.

19. Temelkuran B, Hart S, Benoit G, et al.: Wavelength-scalable hollow optical fibres with large photonic bandgaps for CO_2 laser transmission, *Lett Nature* 420:650–653, 2002.

20. Staninec M, Darling C, Goodis H, et al.: Pulpal effects of enamel ablation with a microsecond pulsed 9300nm CO_2 laser, *Lasers Surg Med* 41:256–263, 2009.

21. Zeinoun T, Nammour S, Dourov N, et al.: Myofibroblasts in healing laser excision wounds, *Lasers Surg Med* 28(1):74–79, 2001.

22. Fisher SE, Frame JW, Browne RM, Tranter RM: A comparative histological study of wound healing following CO_2 laser and conventional surgical excision of canine buccal mucosa, *Arch Oral Biol* 28:287–291, 1983.

23. Roodenburg JL, ten Bosch JJ, Borsboom PC: Measurement of the uniaxial elasticity of oral mucosa in vivo after CO_2 laser evaporation and surgical excision, *Int J Oral Maxillofac Surg* 19:181–183, 1990.

24. Fisher S, Frame J: The effects of the carbon dioxide surgical laser on oral tissues, *Br J Oral Maxillofac Surg* 22:414–425, 1984.

25. Strauss RA: Lasers in oral and maxillofacial surgery, *Dent Clin North Am* 44(4):851–873, 2000.

26. Frame JW: Treatment of sublingual keratosis with the CO_2 laser, *Br Dent J* 156:243–246, 1984.

27. Bellina JH, Stjernholm RL, Kurpel JE: Analysis of plume emissions after papovavirus irradiation with the carbon dioxide laser, *J Reprod Med* 27:268–270, 1982.

28. Mullarky MB, Norris CW, Goldberg ID: The efficacy of the CO_2 laser in the sterilization of skin seeded with bacteria: survival at the skin surface and in the plume emission, *Laryngoscope* 95:186–187, 1985.

29. Walker NPJ, Matthews J, Newson SWB: Possible hazards from irradiation with the carbon dioxide laser, *Lasers Surg Med* 6:84–86, 1986.

30. Byrne PO, Sisson PR, Oliver PD, Inghan HR: Carbon dioxide laser irradiation of bacterial targets in vitro, *J Hosp Infect* 9:265–273, 1987.

31. Hughes PS, Hughes AP: Absence of human papillomavirus DNA in the plume of erbium:YAG laser–treated warts, *J Am Acad Dermatol* 38(3):426–428, 1998.

32. Kunachak S, Sithisam P, Kulapaditharom B: Are laryngeal papillomavirus-infected cells viable in the plume derived from a continuous mode carbon dioxide laser, and are they infectious? A preliminary report on one laser mode, *J Laryngol Otol* 110(11):1031–1033, 1996.

33. Garden JM, O'Banion MK, Shelnitz LS, et al.: Papillomavirus in the vapor of carbon dioxide laser–treated verrucae, *JAMA* 259:1199–1202, 1988.

34. Sawchuk WS, Weber PJ, Lowy DR, Dzubow LM: Infectious papillomavirus in the vapor of warts treated with carbon dioxide laser or electrocoagulation: detection and protection, *J Am Acad Dermatol* 21:41–49, 1989.

35. Andre P, Orth G, Evenou P, et al.: Risk of papillomavirus infection in carbon dioxide laser treatment of genital lesions, *J Am Acad Dermatol* 22:131–132, 1990.

36. Ferenczy A, Bergeron C, Richart RM: Human papillomavirus DNA in CO_2 laser–generated plume of smoke and its consequences to the surgeon, *Obstet Gynecol* 75:114–118, 1990.

37. Teeple E: Laser safety in anesthesia and oral and maxillofacial surgery. In Catone G, Alling C, editors: *Laser applications in oral and maxillofacial surgery*, Philadelphia, 1997, WB Saunders, pp 46–63.

38. Powell GL, Wisenat BK, Morton TH: Carbon dioxide laser oral safety parameters for teeth, *Lasers Surg Med* 10:389–392, 1990.

39. Strauss R: Laser management of discrete lesions. In Catone G, Alling C, editors: *Laser applications in oral and maxillofacial surgery*, Philadelphia, 1997, WB Saunders, pp 115–156.

40. Mashberg A, Barsa P: Screening for oral and oropharyngeal squamous carcinomas, *CA Cancer J Clin* 34(5):262–268, 1984.

41. Oh E, Laskin D: Efficacy of the ViziLite system in the identification of oral lesions, *J Oral Maxillofac Surg* 65(3):424–426, 2007.

42. Missmann M, Jank S, Laimer K, Gassner R: A reason for the use of toluidine blue staining in the presurgical management of patients with oral squamous cell carcinomas, *Oral Surg Oral Med Oral Pathol Oral Radiol Endod* 102(6):741–743, 2006.

43. Kerr AR, et al.: Clinical evaluation of chemiluminescent lighting: adjunct for oral examination, *J Clin Dent* 17(3):59–63, 2006.

44. Epstein JB, Silverman S Jr, Epstein JD, et al.: Analysis of oral lesion biopsies identified and evaluated by visual examination, chemiluminescence and toluidine blue, *Oral Oncol* 44(6):538–544, 2008.

45. Sciubba JJ: Improving detection of precancerous and cancerous oral lesions: computer-assisted analysis of the oral brush biopsy. US Collaborative OralCDx Study Group, *J Am Dent Assoc* 130(10):1445–1457, 1999.

46. Scheifele C, Schmidt-Westhausen AM, Dietrich T, et al.: The sensitivity and specificity of the OralCDx technique: evaluation of 103 cases, *Oral Oncol* 40(8):824–828, 2004.

47. Hall RR: The healing of tissue incised by a CO_2 laser, *Br J Surg* 58:222–225, 1971.

48. Marx R, Stern D: *Oral and maxillofacial pathology: a rationale for diagnosis and treatment*, Chicago, 2003, Quintessence.

49. Kravitz ND, Kusnoto B: Soft-tissue lasers in orthodontics: an overview, *Am J Orthod Dentofacial Orthop* 133(4):S110–S114, 2008.

50. Tamarit-Borrás M, Delgado-Molina E, Berini-Aytés L, Gay-Escoda C: Removal of hyperplastic lesions of the oral cavity: a retrospective study of 128 cases, *Med Oral Patol Oral Cir Bucal* 10(2):151–162, 2005.

51. Schoelch M, Sekandari N, Regezi J, Silverman S: Laser management of oral leukoplakias: a follow-up study of 70 patients, *Laryngoscope* 109:949–953, 1999.

52. Vedtofte P, Holmstrup R, Hjorting-Hansen E, Pindborg JJ: Surgical treatment of premalignant lesions of the oral mucosa, *Int J Oral Maxillofac Surg* 16(6):656–664, 1987.

53. Horch HH, Gerlach KL, Johaefer HE: CO_2 laser surgery of oral premalignant lesions, *Int J Oral Maxillofac Surg* 15(1):19–24, 1986.

54. Thompson P, Wylie J: Interventional laser surgery: an effective surgical and diagnostic tool in oral precancer management, *Int J Oral Maxillofac Surg* 31:145–153, 2002.

55. Lanzaframe RJ, Rogers DW, Naim JO, et al.: The effect of CO_2 laser excision on local tumor recurrence, *Lasers Surg Med* 6:103–105, 1986.

56. Lanzaframe RJ, Rogers DW, Naim JO, et al.: Reduction of local tumor recurrence by excision with the CO_2 laser, *Lasers Surg Med* 6:439–441, 1984.

57. Colvard M, Kuo P: Managing aphthous ulcers: laser treatment applied, *J Am Dent Assoc* 122(7):51–53, 1991.

58. Convissar R, Massoumi-Sourey M: Recurrent aphthous ulcers: etiology and laser ablation, *Gen Dent* 40(6):512–515, 1992.

59. Colvard M, Kuo P: Managing aphthous ulcers: laser treatment applied, *J Am Dent Assoc* 122(6):51–53, 1991.

60. Parkins F: Lasers in pediatric and adolescent dentistry, *Dent Clin North Am* 44(4):821–830, 2000.

61. Convissar R: Laser palliation of oral manifestations of human immunodeficiency virus infection, *J Am Dent Assoc* 133(5):591–598, 2002.

62. Panduric D, Bago I, Katanec D, et al.: Comparison of Er:YAG laser and surgical drill for osteotomy in oral surgery: an experimental study, *J Oral Maxillofac Surg* 70:2515–2521, 2012.

63. Sexton J: Laser management of vascular and pigmented lesions. In Catone G, Alling C, editors: *Laser applications in oral and maxillofacial surgery*, Philadelphia, 1997, WB Saunders, pp 167–169.

64. Santos-Dias A: CO_2 laser surgery in hemophilia treatment, *J Clin Laser Med Surg* 10(4):297–301, 1992.

65. Chrysikopoulos S, Papaspyridakos P, Eleftheriades E: Laser-assisted oral and maxillofacial surgery–anticoagulant therapy in daily practice, *J Oral Laser Appl* 2:79–88, 2006.

66. Kaddour Brahim A, Stieltjes N, Roussel-Robert V, et al.: Dental extractions in children with congenital coagulation disorders: therapeutic protocol and results, *Rev Stomatol Chir Maxillofac* 107(5):331–337, 2006.

67. Miserendino LJ: The laser apicoectomy: endodontic application of the CO_2 laser for periapical surgery, *Oral Surg Oral Med Oral Pathol* 66(5):615–619, 1988.

68. Moritz A, Gutknecht N, Goharkhay K, et al.: The carbon dioxide laser as an aid in apicoectomy: an in vitro study, *J Clin Laser Med Surg* 15(4):185–188, 1997.

9

Laser-Enhanced Removable Prosthetic Reconstruction

ROBERT A. CONVISSAR, TODD J. SAWISCH, AND ROBERT A. STRAUSS

Before fabrication of a fixed prosthesis, the clinician routinely ensures that (1) both the hard tissue and the soft tissue foundation for the prosthesis are solid; (2) the teeth are firm with minimal pockets or bone loss, and (3) the periodontal apparatus surrounding the abutments is capable of supporting a prosthesis. When the treatment plan for a patient involves a *removable* device, however, the health of the supporting apparatus is not always considered. This dichotomy between fixed and removable prosthetic care results from many factors, including the recognition that a fixed prosthesis will fail if the supporting structure is not in optimal shape, but a removable prosthesis will function (although poorly) even with insufficient or inadequate support. Dental school curricula focus more on the health of the oral cavity when teeth are present than when the oral cavity is edentulous. With the success of implant dentistry as a superior alternative to removable prostheses, treatment planning for a partially or fully edentulous patient before removable prosthetic reconstruction has become less important in dentistry.

Use of a removable prosthesis, however, may be the only treatment plan available for many patients, because of finances or underlying medical conditions. Blanchaert[1] lists diabetes, disorders of bone metabolism, radiotherapy, and chemotherapy as important factors in the decision to place implants. Smoking is also a significant contraindication to implant treatment. Holahan et al.[2] found that implants placed in smokers were 2.6 times more likely to fail than implants placed in nonsmokers. Mundt et al.[3] found similar results in their study of 663 implants placed in 159 patients. Michaeli et al.[4] reported an increased risk for failure in diabetic patients. A diagnosis of Paget's disease or other disease of bone also may contraindicate placement of implants, depending on the quality of the bone.[5] Of course, with the use of bisphosphonates increasing drastically, the number of patients eligible for implant reconstruction unquestionably will likewise decrease drastically due to the risk in these patients of developing bisphosphonate-related osteonecrosis of the jaws (BRONJ) during surgical placement of implants.

Bisphosphonates historically were prescribed mostly for postmenopausal females to prevent osteoporosis.[6,7] Today, these drugs are prescribed for patients with prostate cancer,[8] rheumatic diseases,[9] breast cancer,[10] and kidney cancer,[11] among other diseases. With the increase in use of bisphosphonates, the need for well-made, well-fitting removable prostheses in patients ineligible for implants will only increase with time.

Even if a patient is a candidate for implants, however, the fabrication of implant-retained overdentures must still take into account the health of the residual ridge, soft tissue, and supporting structures. Therefore, every dentist should still recognize the importance of ensuring that the structures supporting a removable prosthesis are in optimal health.

Lasers can be used as adjuncts to removable prosthetic care for many different procedures, including
- Epulis fissurata reduction
- Hyperplastic tissue reduction/vestibuloplasty
- Soft tissue tuberosity reduction
- Osseous tuberosity reduction
- Torus/exostosis reduction
- Treatment of papillary hyperplasia, nicotinic stomatitis, and other pathologic conditions associated with wearing of maxillary dentures
- Osseous adjustment of undercut and irregularly resorbed ridges
- Treatment of denture stomatitis

The general advantages of using lasers during removable prosthetic treatment planning are essentially the same as with the use of lasers in periodontal, pedodontic, cosmetic, or oral surgical treatment plans. Kesler[12] enumerated the advantages of using lasers in removable prosthetics as follows:
1. Reduced overall treatment time owing to less mechanical trauma and edema
2. Decreased bacterial contamination of the surgical site
3. Reduced swelling, scarring, and wound contraction at the surgical site
4. Excellent hemostasis, leading to superior visualization of the surgical site

Excision of Epulis Fissurata

Kruger[13] described the conventional (blade) correction of epulis: excision of the fold if small, or submucosal dissection followed by sharp submucosal excision, with suturing of the flap to the periosteum. This method frequently fails, however, because of extensive contracture of the vestibule, with loss of height. These anatomic changes will exacerbate the problem: a denture that does not properly fit in the vestibule. Lack of relapse and contracture is one advantage of using a laser over conventional techniques.

Keng and Loh[14] used a carbon dioxide (CO_2) laser to remove epulides from 20 patients, with follow-up visits at 1 day, 1 week, and 2, 3, 4, and 8 weeks postoperatively and continuously over 2 years. No patient experienced hemorrhage, infection, aspiration, or pain that could not be relieved by common oral analgesics. No sutures or packing was used, and healing was uneventful. All patients had stable results. Of interest, many patients were apprehensive about conventional (scalpel) surgery but agreed to participate in the study if a laser would be used. This major advantage of patient perception of the advantages of laser surgery over conventional surgery was supplemented by a second advantage: lack of wound contraction and relapse. Other advantages of laser surgery included lack of scarring, good reepithelialization, and precise tissue destruction. The investigators concluded that the CO_2 laser represents a significant advance for the management of epulis fissurata.[14]

The lack of wound contracture merits further discussion. Laser wounds have been shown to contain fewer myofibroblasts.[11] Fewer myofibroblasts means less wound contracture postoperatively. In a petite patient with a small vestibule, performing a vestibuloplasty with a blade versus vestibuloplasty with a laser could mean the difference between a denture that fits perfectly and a denture that no longer fits. Excessive wound shrinkage of a small vestibule will unquestionably throw off the fit of a full denture. In a larger study involving 126 patients with epulis, Barak et al.[15] concluded that the CO_2 laser is ideal for this procedure. Other investigators evaluating laser treatment

of epulis also report positive results. Gaspar and Szabo[16] reported a relapse rate after epulis reduction with conventional methods of 12.8% versus 7.9% for laser methods. They also performed a successful epulis reduction in a hemophiliac patient with no adverse effects. Komori et al.[17] performed epulis removal in seven patients using a CO_2 laser without anesthesia. All lesions were successfully removed, with no pain reported by the patients during the procedure.

No contraindications to the use of lasers for epulis treatment has been identified. Moritz[18] described the removal of an epulis in a 64-year-old diabetic patient and of an irritation fibroma interfering with a maxillary denture in an 83-year-old patient. No complications or adverse postoperative sequelae occurred in either patient. Case Study 9-1 provides a clinical scenario.

> **CLINICAL TIP**
>
> As with any excisional procedure, from a frenectomy to a biopsy to an epulis excision, tension on the redundant tissue facilitates separation from the supraperiosteal plane. There should be no movement to the periosteal tissue; if movement is observed, the dissection is not in the correct plane. Performing this step correctly will significantly reduce the need for additional corrective procedures.

The procedure is completed by excising the tissue beginning at the lateral margins, then proceeding toward the midline bilaterally, while retracting the tissue away from the alveolar ridge (see Figure 9-1B). If bleeding occurs, hemostasis can be achieved by defocusing the laser. A denture tissue conditioner material (e.g., Coe Comfort) should be placed in the existing denture for comfort; except for removal during daily cleaning, the patient should wear this while tissue is granulating. A fibrous coagulum will form during the initial phases of healing (see Figure 9-1C), which should not be confused with infection. Complete healing occurs within a few weeks, and if necessary, the old prosthesis may be relined/rebased, or discarded and a new prosthesis fabricated (see Figure 9-1D).

CASE STUDY 9-1

Typical Laser Removal of Epulis Fissurata

A 64-year-old edentulous man presented with elongated rolls of tissue in the maxillary mucolabial fold area (Figure 9-1A). He was functioning with a poorly fitting, 20-year-old complete denture with no major symptoms. The flabby tissue appeared to have a central groove from the extension of the denture flange. This condition, *epulis fissurata,* also called *denture-induced fibrous hyperplasia* (DIFH), is a common consequence of an improperly fitting denture and generally can be diagnosed on the basis of the patient's clinical history and findings. Laser excision generally is suggested; if the lesion size is relatively small, however, laser ablation will suffice. Because these lesions

may represent a squamous cell carcinoma that has proliferated around a denture flange, management for suspicious-looking tissues should consist of excision and biopsy to eradicate the disease and rule out malignancy.[19]

During this patient's initial visit, a CO_2 laser excision was performed after local anesthesia was established. A supraperiosteal excision was begun along the alveolus, perpendicular to the tissue attachment level. The growth was retracted laterally with tissue forceps for performance of a parallel ridge dissection superior to the height of the denture flange.

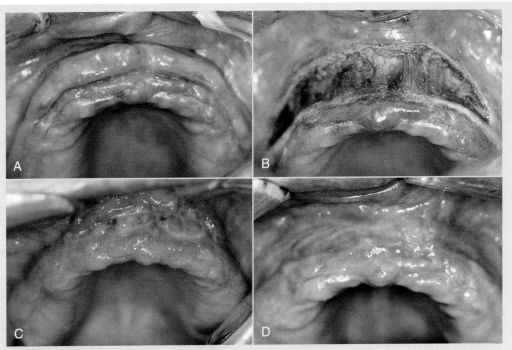

• **Figure 9-1** Epulis reduction. **A,** Large epulis fissuratum consisting of elongated mass of flabby hyperplastic tissue in mucolabial fold. **B,** Complete bilateral excision of the hyperplastic tissue along a supraperiosteal plane with excellent hemostasis. **C,** At 1-week postoperative visit, a fibrous coagulum is present and functioning as a natural protective dressing during healing. **D,** At 3-month postoperative visit, complete healing is achieved, and the area of supraperiosteal dissection has granulated with attached keratinized tissue.

Vestibuloplasty

A common condition involves alveolar bone resorption with shallow vestibular depth, resulting in the patient's inability to wear a denture with the desired comfort and function. Although traditionally this condition has been treated surgically using a scalpel, the CO_2 laser is ideal in this situation for performing a bloodless supraperiosteal vestibuloplasty, with excellent results. Neckel[20] treated 40 patients requiring vestibuloplasty with either traditional scalpel surgery or a laser procedure. Results showed equivocal gain in vestibular height between the two groups, but with less postoperative pain and discomfort in the laser group.

Beer and Beer[21] performed CO_2 laser maxillary vestibuloplasty in 10 patients in whom vestibular height ranged from 3 to 7 mm. A laser incision was performed from the second molar region of one side all the way to the second molar region of the contralateral side. After laser treatment, the patients' old prostheses were adjusted with denture material to support the new vestibular heights. At the conclusion of the study, all of the vestibules were increased a minimum of 3 to 8 mm. Many of the patients showed increases of 10 to 12 mm, with no relapse. No complications were seen at follow-up evaluation 6 to 10 months postoperatively.

Laser Technique

Figure 9-2 illustrates a technique for laser vestibuloplasty in a patient requiring excision of an epulis and a vestibuloplasty. After administration of local anesthetic, the anterior vestibule is placed under tension by pulling the lower or upper lip outward. The laser is then used to create a supraperiosteal dissection.[22] The tension maintained on the lip allows effortless establishment of an adequate plane of dissection. The tissue margin is then retained in place with sutures or a stent. If desired, an autogenous or allogeneic soft tissue graft can be used to cover the denuded area. Immobilization of the graft is key to its survival, which can be accomplished with suturing or placement of a stent.[23]

In patients not undergoing soft tissue grafting, postoperative discomfort is minimized and may be further reduced by initial continuous wear of a soft-relined denture or a tissue-conditioned denture, although this is not mandatory. In patients with significant resorption of the mandible, the genioglossus and mylohyoid muscle attachments often preclude adequate extension of the lingual flange of the denture.[24] In such cases, a floor-of-mouth lowering procedure can be performed to increase lingual vestibular height. This operation can be done with a laser as previously described, again using supraperiosteal dissection and either sutures or a stent to fix the lowered tissue in place. At least half the musculature attached to the genial tubercles should remain, to ensure adequate functioning of the tongue and oropharyngeal muscles.

Tuberosity Reduction

During treatment planning for a full or partial upper denture, significant diagnostic criteria include the size and shape

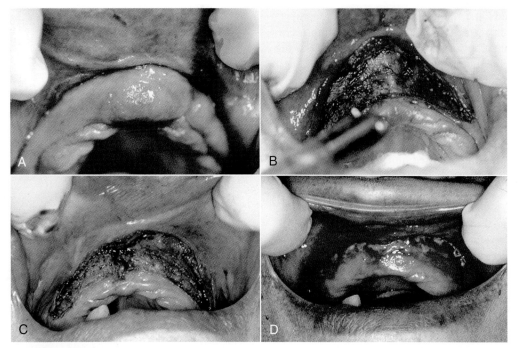

• **Figure 9-2** Vestibuloplasty with epulis excision. **A,** Preoperative view of maxillary ridge epulis fissuratum. **B,** Epulis excision with a CO_2 laser in continuous-wave mode. Note residual muscle on the periosteum. The laser is used to incise the muscle attachments, which subsequently migrate vertically. As the muscle is being dissected superiorly, tension is applied to the lip. **C,** Supraperiosteal dissection and vestibuloplasty completed. Note clean periosteum. **D,** Postoperative appearance at 10 days, with excellent vestibular depth and reepithelialization.

of the maxillary tuberosity. The tuberosity may be small and inconsequential in treatment planning. Alternatively, however, the tuberosity also may be large, flabby, and pendulous, with bilateral undercuts that would prevent fabrication of a properly fitting prosthesis. If the tuberosity is a concern, a radiographic series must be taken to evaluate the type of tissue; palpation alone will not necessarily provide the clinician with sufficient information to determine its consistency. The tuberosity may consist solely of hypertrophied soft tissue, requiring a surgical procedure to reduce the soft tissue, or it may consist of a thin layer of fibrotic tissue and mucosa overlying a thick, prominent mass of osseous tissue, requiring a hard tissue tuberosity reduction. Occasionally, the tuberosity may consist of a thin layer of fibrotic tissue and mucosa overlying a pneumatized sinus, and a sinus lift procedure may be performed (see Chapter 7).

As summarized by Terry and Hillenbrand,[25] soft tissue tuberosity reductions are performed to provide enough maxillomandibular clearance to allow sufficient space for the denture base and denture teeth. These investigators suggested a minimum of 5 mm of clearance between the tuberosity and the mandibular mucosa.

Costello et al.[26] described the procedure for a soft tissue tuberosity reduction as follows:
1. An elliptical incision is performed over the tuberosity.
2. The mucosa is undermined.
3. The fibrous tissue is removed.
4. Excessive mucosal tissue is removed.
5. Primary closure is obtained.

If the tuberosity is primarily osseous tissue, once the elliptical incision is made, the mucoperiosteum is reflected and the bone removed with a rongeur or bur. The area must be smoothed with a bone file, irrigated, and closed. Care must be taken to avoid perforating into the maxillary sinus.[26] Guernsey[27] warned that during conventional techniques, care must be taken to avoid the greater palatine artery and its branches.

Laser Tuberosity Reduction

Each step just outlined may be performed using a dental laser. Pick[28] stated that laser tuberosity reduction offers numerous advantages over conventional techniques. Common problems arise after the elliptical incision is made and the fibrous wedge of tissue removed, because the flaps of tissue need to be thinned and trimmed. The flaps often are trimmed more than once to achieve the correct size for primary closure. Occasionally, the flaps may be trimmed so that they are too short to achieve primary closure. This area is also difficult to suture.

When a laser is used for a soft tissue tuberosity reduction, the procedure is performed without an incision, so no suturing is needed. The soft tissue of the tuberosity is simply vaporized layer by layer until the correct maxillomandibular space has been achieved. This procedure may be performed both in patients currently wearing full dentures and in patients with treatment plans to receive a full or partial denture.

Convissar and Gharemani[29] described a soft tissue tuberosity reduction in a patient before making a final impression for an immediate insertion of a full upper denture. By using a laser, the treatment period was shortened by at least 3 to 6 weeks because of the accelerated healing and less traumatic technique. The final impression for the immediate-insertion prosthesis was taken only 3 weeks after the tuberosity reduction, with confidence that no further tissue shrinkage would occur, resulting in a poor fit of the prosthesis. With no incision or sutures, healing occurred quickly and uneventfully. Accidental sinus perforation is avoided because the bloodless surgical site is clearly visualized, permitting ready distinction between mucosa and periosteum and decreasing the potential for this mishap. Because lasers cauterize and coagulate, inadvertently severing a palatine artery or one of its lesser branches also is less of a risk.

Pogrel[30] described laser tuberosity reduction on four patients (average treatment time, 6 minutes). There were no reports of bleeding, swelling, or recurrence of the excess tissue. One patient underwent a bilateral tuberosity reduction: one side done with a conventional (scalpel) technique and the other with a laser; the laser-operated side felt more comfortable to the patient. The laser side healed before the scalpel side, and laser reduction took less time. Pogrel concluded that the advantages of the CO_2 laser appear to be applicable to soft tissue preprosthetic surgery.

Soft Tissue

The procedure for a soft tissue laser tuberosity reduction is relatively simple and straightforward (Figure 9-3). After diagnostic radiographs are obtained to determine the location of the sinus floor and mounted study casts to determine the amount of surgical reduction necessary, a local anesthetic of choice is administered to the tuberosity both buccally and palatally. After selection of a large spot size/fiber or handpiece, the laser of choice is used at a surgical setting to ablate the tissue of the tuberosity layer by layer until sufficient maxillomandibular space is created. The laser tip should be kept as parallel as possible to the tuberosity, to ensure maximum efficiency. The laser beam is then moved out of focus to ensure adequate hemostasis. At this time the tissue is evaluated for irregularities or tissue tags; any such tissue is ablated with the laser. The denture may then be relined with a tissue conditioner or soft reline material. The patient receives postoperative instructions (maintaining clean surgical site, stressing oral hygiene), and a follow-up appointment is scheduled.

Hard Tissue

Many options are available for hard tissue laser tuberosity reduction, depending on the wavelengths available. If only a soft tissue wavelength—CO_2, diode, or neodymium-doped yttrium-aluminum-garnet (Nd:YAG)—is available, an elliptical incision is made into the tuberosity with the laser, exposing the osseous structure. The osseous tissue is then reduced with the clinician's instrument of choice, which may be a rongeur, a round bur with copious water spray in

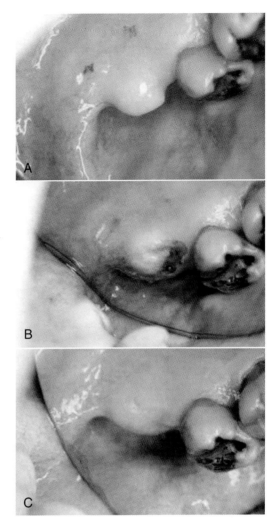

• **Figure 9-3** Tuberosity reduction. **A,** Preoperative photograph of enlarged soft tissue tuberosity. **B,** Tuberosity reduction performed using a simple ablation technique, with no incision or sutures. **C,** Postoperative view of surgical site at 17 days. Note excellent healing and reepithelialization of surgical site. Excellent contours of site have been achieved without incisions or sutures. (Courtesy Dr. Stuart Coleton, Chappaqua, New York.)

a high-speed handpiece, or a bone file. All of the advantages of using a laser over a scalpel are apparent in using this technique, including the excellent visualization resulting from superior hemostasis and a dry surgical site. The surgical site is then closed with sutures.

If a hard tissue laser is available, such as the erbium-doped yttrium-aluminum-garnet (Er:YAG) or erbium plus chromium–doped yttrium-scandium-gallium-garnet (Er,Cr:YSGG), or possibly the 9300-nm CO_2 laser, the elliptical incision into the soft tissue may be made with the laser to expose the bone. The hard tissue laser is then used to ablate the bone slowly and methodically. To ensure maximum hemostasis with the hard tissue laser with use on soft tissue, it is advised to shut off the water spray when incising the soft tissue. Once the hard tissue is ready to be removed, a copious water spray must be used on the bone. This step ensures maximum spallation (see Chapter 10) and cutting efficiency, with minimal thermal damage to the bone.

Laser Torus Reduction

Mandibular tori are present in 8% of the population, affecting men and women equally.[31] Tori occasionally can interfere with fabrication of a full or partial denture, in which case a torus reduction is indicated. The procedure for performing laser torus reduction is similar to that for hard tissue tuberosity reduction: An incision is made to expose the bone, the bone is reduced, and the incision is sutured closed.

Although risks are inherent in any surgical procedure, complications may be more serious when surgery is performed on or close to the floor of the mouth; reports include hemorrhage and infection[26] and a life-threatening swelling after a mandibular vestibuloplasty.[32] Mantzikos et al.[33] described three cases of hematoma formation on the floor of the mouth after periodontal surgery combined with extensive torus and exostosis reduction. Terry and Hillenbrand[25] also described hematoma formation as a complication of torus reduction. A literature search found no reports of hematoma formation during laser mandibular torus reduction. The superior ability of lasers to coagulate and cauterize surgical sites along with less manipulation of the tissues during a laser-assisted procedure when compared with scalpel procedures probably is responsible for this significant advantage of lasers for this procedure.

Payas[34] described a mandibular *lingual* torus reduction using a combined CO_2 plus erbium laser. An incision was made with a scalpel to expose the osseous tissue. The erbium laser was then used to cut the torus into sections. The sections were grasped and removed with a hemostat, and the surgical site was closed with multiple black silk sutures. The CO_2 laser was used for hemostasis. Healing was uneventful.

In this procedure, the soft tissue incision could have been made with any laser or with a scalpel and the osseous tissue reduced with a high-speed bur in a handpiece using copious water spray, with a rongeur, with a hard tissue laser, or with a bone file. Hemostasis could have been achieved with a laser or with digital pressure and gauze packs. There is no "best" technique.

In the "ideal" technique, the clinician maximizes use of the laser wavelength(s) available while staying within his or her comfort zone of laser use. Many practitioners embrace the use of hard tissue lasers for both torus and hard tissue tuberosity reductions; others, especially oral and maxillofacial surgeons, have not embraced the use of the erbium wavelengths because of the slowness of cutting by these lasers compared with conventional techniques. The practitioner is advised always to recognize the capabilities and limitations of the wavelengths available.

Palatal tori occur in 25% of female patients with these lesions, twice the incidence in male patients.[25] Palatal torus reduction is rarely necessary before fabrication of a maxillary prosthesis. When reduction is required, however, complications can include the following[25,26]:
- Nasal perforation
- Oronasal/oroantral fistula
- Palatal tissue necrosis
- Hematoma
- Palatal fractures

As with osseous tuberosity and mandibular torus reductions, for palatal torus reduction, an incision is made over the osseous protuberance to expose the bone. The bone usually is removed by sectioning with a bur and removal with a chisel, or by judicious use of a large, round bur with water spray. Although an erbium laser would be slower than conventional techniques, this is one clinical situation in which speed of the procedure is secondary to safety. The erbium lasers may be used safely to ablate the osseous material layer by layer, until a sufficient amount has been removed. A slow but steady ablation of bone prevents the accidental perforation of the palate or creation of a fistula. Many clinicians advocate the use of palatal stents to prevent hematoma formation. Any laser wavelength can be used to create hemostasis and decrease the risk of hematoma.

Alveolar Ridge Abnormalities

Even if the patient has no torus or tuberosity to interfere with fabrication of prostheses, the residual alveolar ridge may be unsuitable for placement of a denture. Kesler[12] identified a variety of conditions that may potentially interfere with fabrication of a prosthesis, including irregularly resorbed and irregularly undercut ridges. With an insufficiently compressed tooth socket after extraction, an irregularly shaped alveolus may result. A prominent premaxilla may manifest with significant undercuts.

Ogle[35] noted the presence of prominent mylohyoid and internal oblique ridges, ridge undercuts that interfere with proper extension of a denture flange, and sharp residual ridges. Meyer[36] identified three types of sharp ridges: sawtoothed, razorlike, and with discrete projections. All of these ridge types will affect the fit and the comfort of the denture. If the denture does not sit equally well on the entire residual ridge, the occlusal load on one part will be significantly more than on other parts of the ridge. This discrepancy will lead to discomfort and even more irregular ridge resorption, compounding the problem.

If ridge augmentation is not part of the treatment plan, all of these conditions may be addressed with laser assistance. The soft tissue may be flapped open (by laser or scalpel) to expose the ridges, followed by use of erbium lasers to reshape their contour, resulting in a ridge better able to support the prosthesis comfortably.

Soft Tissue Abnormalities

One of the more common soft tissue abnormalities diagnosed during full-denture fabrication, or during routine examination of a patient wearing a complete maxillary denture, is *papillary hyperplasia*. Regezi and Sciubba[37] reported an incidence of 10% in the population of patients wearing a full maxillary denture. Causative factors include poor hygiene, poor fit of the denture causing a localized irritation, and occasionally, a fungal infection.

The use of lasers for treatment of papillary hyperplasia is well established in the literature.[25,26,28,30,38] As reported by Terry and Hillenbrand,[25] the most common complication of conventional treatment of papillary hyperplasia is hemorrhage. The use of any soft tissue laser wavelength to perform this procedure will result in coagulation and cauterization of the site, preventing any hemorrhage. In a study of 11 patients who underwent laser treatment of papillary hyperplasia, Pogrel[30] reported no bleeding, swelling, or (in mandibular arch treatment) mental nerve damage. Advantages of using CO_2 lasers to treat papillary hyperplasia include the following[28]:

- The ability to negotiate curves and folds in the tissue easily
- No bleeding during or after the procedure
- A dry field
- Speed
- Minimal postsurgical pain
- Minimal postsurgical swelling
- Superb effectiveness in vaporization of the tissue

Papillary hyperplasia is a superficial mucosal lesion, so laser treatment does not involve an incision/excision procedure. The laser is used with a large fiber/spot size or handpiece in a defocused mode, with the aim of covering the entire lesion with laser energy. This defocused laser energy is insufficient to incise through the tissue but more than sufficient to perform a superficial vaporization of the affected tissue. Infante Cossio et al.[39] described a patient with inflammatory papillary hyperplasia initially treated with a topical antifungal gel for 1 month, which did not heal the lesion. A CO_2 laser successfully vaporized the lesion, with no recurrence at 3 years postoperatively.

Figure 9-4 shows a severe case of papillary hyperplasia. A CO_2 laser was used in a defocused mode to perform surface vaporization of the lesion. Removal of char layer revealed complete vaporization of the lesion.

> **CLINICAL TIP**
>
> Note the parallel horizontal lines of vaporization on the palate in Figure 9-4. Performing this procedure with the laser passes in parallel horizontal lines, rather than in a back-and-forth technique, prevents the clinician from retreating tissue. Laser irradiation of already-treated tissue may result in severe charring, leading to postoperative discomfort and possibly sloughing of the tissue.

Other oral mucosal lesions associated with the wearing of removable prosthetic devices include the following[40]:

- *Denture stomatitis,* which affects the palatal mucosa in up to 50% of all patients who wear a partial or full denture
- *Traumatic ulcers,* which occur in approximately 5% of all denture wearers
- *Angular cheilitis,* which affects 15% of all patients with full dentures

All of these lesions are amenable to laser treatment using defocused energy.

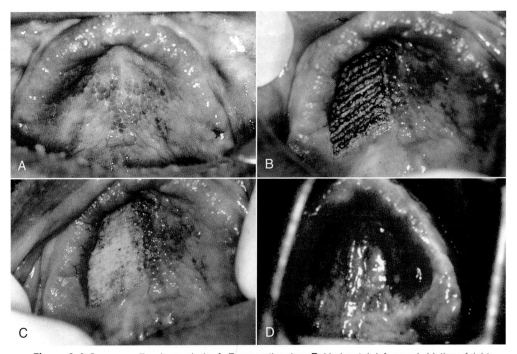

• **Figure 9-4** Severe papillary hyperplasia. **A,** Preoperative view. **B,** Horizontal defocused ablation of right side of palate. Because this is a vaporization/ablation procedure rather than an incision/excision procedure, the laser is used slightly out of focus. **C,** Wet gauze used to remove char layer, which was expected using older-model CO_2 laser unit. The newer superpulsed or ultraspeed CO_2 lasers no longer create char layers on tissue because their high peak powers are delivered in a much shorter burst, or pulse, of energy. **D,** Postoperative view at 2 weeks shows good initial healing.

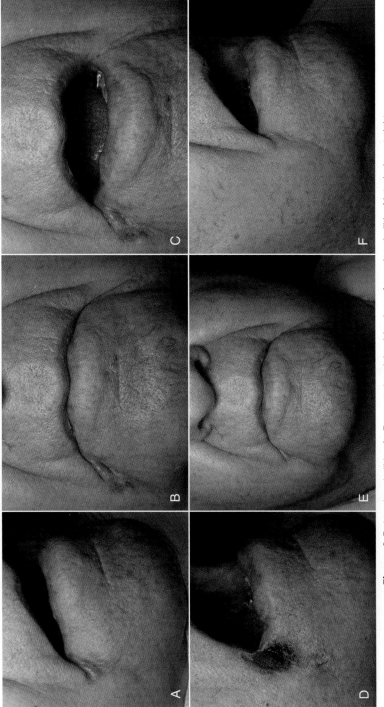

• **Figure 9-5** Angular cheilitis. **A,** Preoperative right-side view of angular cheilitis. Note lesion at right corner of the mouth. **B,** Preoperative anterior view with patient's mouth closed. Note overclosed vertical dimension, which contributes to the condition. **C,** Preoperative anterior view with patient's mouth open. **D,** Immediate postoperative view after treatment with CO_2 laser. **E,** Two-week postoperative view of treated area with patient's mouth closed. **F,** Two-week postoperative view of treated area with patient's mouth open. (Courtesy Dr. Rick Kava, Sioux City, Iowa.)

These lesions also may be treated with low-level laser therapy (LLLT). Marei et al.[41] divided 18 patients into three groups according to mode of treatment: removal of the denture for a specified period, relining the dentures with tissue-conditioning material, and low-level laser irradiation. Results showed superior healing in the LLLT group compared with the other two groups (see Chapter 15).

Figure 9-5 illustrates CO_2 laser treatment for a severe case of angular cheilitis. The laser was used with low power in a vaporization technique to remove the lesion. Note the excellent healing at 2 weeks (see Figure 9-5E, F). The patient must be advised at this point that the lesion will unquestionably recur unless a new prosthesis is made with an increased vertical dimension.

CLINICAL TIP

To speed healing of such lesions, application of vitamin E oil to the surgical site four times a day for 2 weeks, as used by the patient in Figure 9-5, may be helpful.

Conclusions

Laser dentistry is a continuously evolving discipline. As more dentists discover the superior results that laser treatment provides compared with those obtained with conventional techniques, the discipline will increase in size and scope. Although removable prosthetic reconstruction in the partially or fully edentulous patient is less common than in the past because of the increased popularity of implants, a certain percentage of the population still will require a removable prosthesis to replace missing teeth.

The advantages of laser dentistry noted throughout this book also apply to procedures involving removable prosthetic reconstruction. Unparalleled hemostasis and maintenance of a dry, sterile surgical field resulting in increased visualization of the surgical site are as important in the partially or fully edentulous patient as in the patient with a complete dentition. A decontaminated postsurgical field with much less postoperative pain will result in less need for prescription analgesics and antibiotics for the patient. The greatly reduced potential for negative drug interactions is a critically important advantage in dealing with elderly edentulous patients, who typically already take multiple medications. As part of a comprehensive treatment plan for the partially or fully edentulous patient, laser treatment benefits both the dentist and the patient.

References

1. Blanchaert RH: Implants in the medically challenged patient, *Dent Clin North Am* 42(1):35–45, 1998.
2. Holahan CM, Koka S, Kennel KA, et al.: Effect of osteoporotic status on the survival of titanium dental implants, *Int J Oral Maxillofac Implants* 23(5):905–910, 2008.
3. Mundt T, Mack F, Schwahn C, Biffar R: Private practice results of screw type tapered implants: survival and evaluation of risk factors, *Int J Oral Maxillofac Implants* 21(4):607–614, 2006.
4. Michaeli E, Weinberg I, Nahliel O: Dental implants in the diabetic patient: systemic and rehabilitative considerations, *Quintessence Int* 40(8):639–645, 2009.
5. Rasmussen JM, Hopfensperger ML: Placement and restoration of dental implants in a patient with Paget's disease in remission: literature review and clinical report, *J Prosthodont* 17(1):35–40, 2008.
6. Adami S, Baroni MC, Broggini M, et al.: Treatment of postmenopausal osteoporosis with continuous daily oral alendronate in comparison with either placebo or intranasal salmon calcitonin, *Osteoporos Int* 3(suppl 3):S21–S27, 1993.
7. Baran DT: Osteoporosis: monitoring techniques and alternate therapies. Calcitonin, fluoride, bisphosphonates, vitamin D, *Obstet Gynecol Clin North Am* 21(2):321–335, 1994.
8. Iranikhah M, Stricker S, Freeman MK: Future of bisphosphonates and denosumab for men with advanced prostate cancer, *Cancer Manag Res* 6:217–224, 2014.
9. Saag KG: Bone safety of low-dose glucocorticoids in rheumatic diseases, *Ann N Y Acad Sci* 1318(1):55–64, 2014.
10. Wang X, Yang KH, Wanyan P, Tian JH: Comparison of the efficacy and safety of denosumab versus bisphosphonates in breast cancer and bone metastases treatment: a meta-analysis of randomized controlled trials, *Oncol Lett* 7(6):1997–2002, 2014.
11. Roos FC: Kidney cancer: bisphosphonates in the era of antiangiogenic targeted therapy, *Nat Rev Urol* 11(6):315–316, 2014.
12. Kesler G: Clinical applications of lasers during removable prosthetic reconstruction, *Dent Clin North Am* 48:963–969, 2004.
13. Kruger G: *Textbook of oral and maxillofacial surgery*, St Louis, 1979, Mosby.
14. Keng SB, Loh HS: The treatment of epulis fissuratum of the oral cavity by CO_2 laser surgery, *J Clin Laser Med Surg* 10(4):303–306, 1992.
15. Barak S, Kintz S, Katz J: The role of lasers in ambulatory oral maxillofacial surgery: operative techniques, *Otolaryngol Head Neck Surg* 5(4):244–249, 1994.
16. Gaspar L, Szabo G: Removal of epulis by CO_2 laser, *J Clin Laser Med Surg* 9(4):289–294, 2001.
17. Komori T, Yokoyama K, Takako T, Matsumoto K: Case reports of epulis treated by CO_2 laser without anesthesia, *J Clin Laser Med Surg* 14(4):189–191, 1996.
18. Moritz A, editor: *Oral laser applications*, Berlin, 2006, Quintessence.
19. Marx R, Stern D: *Oral and maxillofacial pathology: a rationale for diagnosis and treatment*, Chicago, 2003, Quintessence.
20. Neckel CP: Vestibuloplasty: a retrospective study on conventional and laser operation techniques, *Lasers Dent* 3593:76–80, 1999.
21. Beer A, Beer F: Laser preparation technique in vestibuloplasty: a case report, *J Oral Laser Appl* 2:51–55, 2002.
22. Wlodawsky RN, Strauss RA: Intraoral laser surgery, *Oral Maxillofac Surg Clin North Am* 16(2):149–163, 2004.
23. Fonseca RJ, Frost DE, Hersh EV, Levin LM: *Oral and maxillofacial surgery*, vol 7, Philadelphia, 2000, Saunders.
24. Miloro M, Ghali GE, Larsen PE, Waite PD: *Peterson's principles of oral and maxillofacial surgery*, ed 2, vol 1, Hamilton, 2004, BC Decker.
25. Terry B, Hillenbrand D: Minor preprosthetic surgical procedures, *Dent Clin North Am* 38(2):193–216, 1994.
26. Costello B, Betts N, Barger HD, Fonseca R: Preprosthetic surgery for the edentulous patient, *Dent Clin North Am* 40(1):19–38, 1996.
27. Guernsey LH: Preprosthetic surgery. In Kruger GO, editor: *Textbook of oral and maxillofacial surgery*, ed 5, St Louis, 1979, Mosby.

28. Pick R: The use of laser for treatment of gingival disease, *Oral Maxillofac Surg Clin North Am* 9(1):1–19, 1997.

29. Convissar R, Gharemani E: Laser treatment as an adjunct to removable prosthetic care, *Gen Dent* 336–341, July–August 1995.

30. Pogrel MA: The carbon dioxide laser in soft tissue preprosthetic surgery, *J Prosthet Dent* 61:203–208, 1989.

31. Kolas H, Halperin V, Jeffries KR, et al.: Occurrence of torus palatinus and torus mandibularis in 2478 denture patients, *J Oral Surg* 6:1134, 1953.

32. Hull M: Life-threatening swelling after mandibular vestibuloplasty, *J Oral Surg* 35:511, 1977.

33. Mantzikos K, Segelnick S, Schoor R: Hematoma following periodontal surgery with a torus reduction: a case report, *J Contemp Dent Pract* 18(3):72–80, 2007.

34. Payas G: Clinical applications of CO_2 laser and Er:YAG laser in frenectomy, vestibuloplasty and removal of mandibular bony protuberances, *J Acad Laser Dent* 12(2):15–18, 2004.

35. Ogle R: Preprosthetic surgery, *Dent Clin North Am* 21(2):219–236, 1977.

36. Meyer RA: management of denture patients with sharp residual ridges, *J Prosthet Dent* 16:431, 1966.

37. Regezi J, Sciubba J: Connective tissue lesions. In *Oral pathology: clinical-pathologic correlation*, ed 2, Philadelphia, 1993, Saunders.

38. Strauss RA: Lasers in oral and maxillofacial surgery, *Dent Clin North Am* 44(4):851–873, 2000.

39. Infante Cossio P, Martinez-de-Fuentes R, Torres-Carranza E, Gutierrez-Perez JL: Inflammatory papillary hyperplasia of the palate: treatment with carbon dioxide laser, followed by restoration with an implant supported prosthesis, *Br J Oral Maxillofac Surg* 45:658–660, 2007.

40. Budtz-Jorgensen E: Oral mucosal lesions associated with the wearing of removable dentures, *J Oral Pathol* 10(2):65–80, 1981.

41. Marei M, Abdel-Maguid S, Mokhtar S, Rizk S: Effect of low energy laser application in the treatment of denture induced mucosal lesions, *J Prosthet Dent* 77:256–265, 1997.

10

Lasers in Restorative Dentistry

STEVEN PARKER*

Despite the advances in preventive dentistry, the primary occupation of the general dental practitioner remains the restoration of carious teeth. Together with the modification of tooth structure associated with cosmetic restorative procedures, caries restoration accounts for the dilemma of achieving diseased hard tissue removal while preserving healthy surrounding natural tooth tissue and pulp vitality. The need to cut dental hard tissue during restorative procedures presents a challenge to the ability to remove diseased carious tissue selectively and to maintain the integrity of supporting tooth tissue without structural weakening. The additional requirement of preventing further breakdown in the restoration makes the choice of instrumentation and clinical technique of primary importance. The essentially patient-driven quest for an alternative treatment mechanism to replace the conventional high-speed, fear-provoking drill has led to the development of various mechanical and chemical approaches and devices, including lasers.

Caries Removal: Background and Debate

The U.S. National Health and Nutrition Examination Survey (NHANES), in an extrapolated survey (1999 to 2002) of the noninstitutionalized civilian population, found that 41% of children 2 to 11 years of age had dental caries in their primary teeth, and that 42% of children and adolescents 6 to 19 years of age and approximately 90% of adults had dental caries in their permanent teeth.[1] Other studies reflect even greater prevalence of caries—as high as 96% among children 6 to 7 years of age in Saudi Arabia.[2] Such findings indicate a continued demand for interceptive restorative treatment.

In addition to such prevalence, a growing skepticism has emerged regarding the two classic mainstays of restorative dentistry: the cavity classification of G.V. Black (classes I to V) and the continued use of amalgam as a restorative material.[3] Black's ideology, based on the dogma "extension for prevention," often has resulted in the removal of large

areas of otherwise healthy enamel and dentin. The flaw in this approach has been exacerbated by the need to address the mechanical success of amalgam: outline form and retention form of cavity design. Studies assessing the iatrogenic damage to natural tooth tissue during restorative procedures report microfractures adjacent to cavity margins, damage to teeth adjacent to interproximal cavity design,[4] and thermal injury to the pulp caused by rotary instrumentation.[5]

Despite the gradual reduction in the number of amalgam restorations being placed (from 56 million to 52 million in the United States[6] and from 8 million to 6 million in the United Kingdom[7]), a considerable need to service existing metal restorations still exists. However, the evolution of non–metal-based composite restorations, as well as a desire for a natural-appearing result in a patient base with greater awareness and higher expectations, has led to a shift toward smaller restorations, a change in cavity design (e.g., "tunnel" restorations[8]), and a greater reliance on acid-etch microretention techniques.[9,10]

Instrumentation and Lasers

The most common procedures for removing diseased dental hard tissue during restorative procedures involve the use of excavators and burs. The accuracy of such instrumentation has been questioned,[11] with minimal objective analysis of total removal of demineralized, infected enamel and dentin, as well as the possible removal of excessive amounts of sound tissue.[12] By contrast, the use of a suitable laser wavelength may allow a much more conservative approach to the preservation of sound, mineralized tooth tissue, with preferential removal of higher-water-content caries, greater precision, and reduced bacterial contamination of the laser-prepared cavity.[13,14]

A key factor in pulpal injury is thermal conduction from the range of instrumentation chosen.[15] Studies have established that rotary instrumentation can cause conductive thermal elevation in excess of 20° C above 37.4° C.[16,17] With regard to laser irradiation of dental tissue, the explosive defragmentation resulting from water-assisted mid-infrared wavelengths allows much of the heat

---

*Dr. Lawrence Kotlow contributed information on the 9300 nm CO_2 laser.

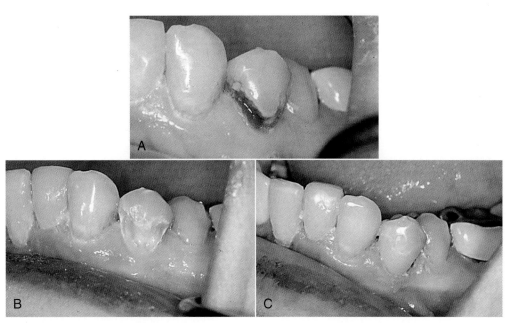

• **Figure 10-1 A,** Dental caries presents a risk to natural tooth structure and vitality of dental pulp, as well as a challenge to the clinician. In treating dental caries, it is essential to avoid precipitating further damage to the tooth. **B,** Using an Er:YAG laser, selective removal of dental caries can be achieved with maximal preservation of healthy, mineralized tooth tissue. **C,** Completed restoration achieves functional and cosmetic form.

to escape from the cavity (carried in ablated particles), resulting in pulpal thermal increase of less than 5° C.[18-20] The affinity of mid-infrared laser wavelengths for water allows the main absorption to take place in demineralized tissue richer in organic material and with a higher percentage of water, thus protecting any sound tissue overlying the pulp, with a reduced penetration of the beam (Figure 10-1). With adoption of operating parameters to standardize the normal clinical use of each instrument, evidence-based protocols now serve to provide what is best for the patient. As treatment shifts toward early diagnosis and interceptive action that is more selective in preserving healthy tissue, the choice of a laser procedure may become more common, placing the dental profession in an increasingly responsible position to deliver patient-centered restorative care.

The claimed precision of laser use in many areas of surgery would appear to complement the demands of the restorative dentist. Also, although a tooth was the first tissue to be exposed to laser light in Maiman's 1960 investigations,[21] the first laser specifically made for the general dentist did not become commercially available until 1989. The chosen wavelength of this laser, neodymium-doped yttrium-aluminum-garnet (Nd:YAG), 1064 nm, has limited therapeutic action on hard dental tissue. More recent developments include the erbium plus chromium–doped yttrium-scandium-gallium-garnet (Er,Cr:YSGG) (2780-nm) and erbium-doped YAG (Er:YAG) (2940-nm) laser wavelengths and the 9300-nm CO_2 laser for use in cavity preparation.

In addition to laser use in dental surgery, other, nonsurgical laser wavelengths have been developed for diagnostic procedures, to assist the clinician in caries detection and assessment of the effective removal of diseased tissue.

Table 10-1 summarizes the advantages of laser use in dental restorative procedures.

Laser Photonic Energy–Hard Tissue Interaction

Healthy coronal hard tissue comprises enamel and primary and secondary dentin. By volume, enamel is 85% mineral (predominantly carbonated hydroxyapatite), 12% water, and 3% organic proteins; most free water exists in the periprismatic protein matrix. Dentin has a higher water content, being 47% mineral (carbonated hydroxyapatite), 33% protein (mostly collagen), and 20% water. Water content in carious dentin may be as high as 54%.[22]

Each of these compounds represents a target *chromophore*, a tissue element or molecule capable of selective absorption of photonic laser energy. Current understanding of chromophores that offer clinically acceptable laser-tissue interaction identifies high absorption of photonic energy by water (free molecules and OH^- radical) at approximately 3.0-µm wavelength; by the phosphate (PO_4) radical of carbonated hydroxyapatite (near 7.0 µm); and by the carbonate (CO_3) radical of the tooth mineral, approximately 9.6 µm. If the incident photonic energy is assumed to be above the nominal ablation threshold of the target, the resulting conversion of photonic energy into heat can lead to structural or phase change in the target material (photothermal

TABLE 10-1	Summary of Comparable Benefits of Laser Use Over Rotary ("Air Rotor") Instrumentation in Tooth Cavity Preparation	
Restorative Procedure	**Rotary**	**Laser***
Cutting enamel/dentin	Yes	Yes
Selective removal of caries	No	Yes
Precision	Precise to >1000-2000 μm	Precise to <300 μm
Smear layer	Produced	Not produced
Thermal rise	>15° C	<5° C
Risk of iatrogenic damage	Greater	Less
Noise/vibration	>120 dB/vibration	<120 dB/no vibration
Bactericidal action	No	Surface decontamination
Speed of cutting enamel	Fast	<30% rotary speed
Speed of cutting dentin	Fast	Comparable
Contact with tooth tissue	Contact required	Noncontact possible
Pain response	High	Less/no pain

*Erbium laser family (Er:YAG, Er,Cr:YSGG).

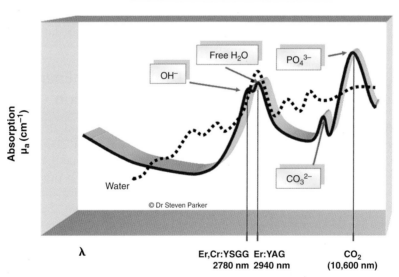

• **Figure 10-2** Graphic representation of absorption by water and carbonated hydroxyapatite (CHA) of varying mid-infrared and far-infrared laser photonic radiation energy. Coincident peaks of water and CHA between 2780 and 2940 nm represent the great affinity of these wavelengths for water. In CHA, high absorption of laser energy of approximately 10,600 nm is caused primarily by interaction with the phosphate radical of the mineral molecule.

change). With the application of laser energy in restorative dental procedures, presence of demineralized and carious hard tissue also must be considered, where the greater water and protein (pigmented) (~1.0-μm wavelength) content are chromophores.

With such a breadth of target elements, several laser wavelengths have been investigated as possible adjuncts in cutting tooth cavities and removing carious tissue. The absorption coefficients of water and mineralized dental tissue are shown in Figure 10-2.

Early investigation into the Nd:YAG laser, first marketed for soft tissue laser dentistry in the United States, was done to determine its utility for procedures involving hard tissue.[23-27] Issues included applications for ablation of

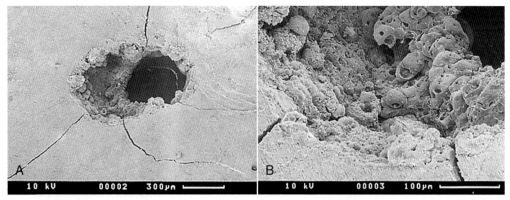

• **Figure 10-3 A,** Environmental scanning electron micrograph showing effect of incident Nd:YAG laser photonic energy on human enamel. The cracks represent thermal overload of the mineral matrix. **B,** Higher-power (×300) scanning electron micrograph of tooth tissue. Thermal damage has melted the crystalline mineral, resulting in globules of amorphous hydroxyapatite. Ironically, this re-formed mineral displays greater resistance to acid dissolution, leading to claims that such laser treatment may help prevent dental caries.

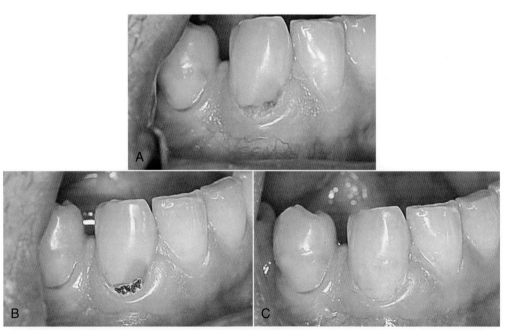

• **Figure 10-4** Preparation of buccal cavity in lower right canine tooth. **A,** The patient requested laser-assisted treatment, and the dentist erroneously assumed that the high absorption of the CO_2 laser in hydroxyapatite would allow efficient ablation. **B,** Lack of water spray and continuous-wave laser emission led to damaging carbonization to surface caries. Consequently, the cavity was prepared using hand instruments. **C,** Completed restoration. Tooth later tested positive for pulp vitality. Use of CO_2 laser in this case predated commercial availability of erbium laser wavelengths.

pigmented and diseased tissue, the antibacterial effect of this laser wavelength, and the possible effects on the vital dental pulp. Although studies established safe and effective parameters, the Nd:YAG laser's clinical significance was of only marginal benefit to the restorative dentist because of its very low absorption in sound enamel or dentin. Furthermore, several studies concluded that the Nd:YAG wavelength could cause unwanted heating effects, such as cracking and melting of mineral structures[28-30] (Figure 10-3).

Early studies on enamel ablation also focused on the other available laser wavelength of 10,600 nm, delivered by a carbon dioxide (CO_2) laser, but this laser gave poor interactions, with reports of charring, cracking, and damaging

heat buildup in tooth and bone structure.[31,32] Although examination of absorption data for this wavelength with hydroxyapatite shows an effective interaction, many currently available CO_2 lasers operate in continuous-wave (CW) emission mode with no cooling water, which results in very high energy deposition in hard tissue (Figure 10-4). The recent introduction of a CO_2 "superpulsed" laser at 9300 nm, whose chromophore is carbonated hydroxyapatite, has been shown to be safe for pulpal tissues and capable of ablating enamel, which is 93% hydroxyapatite.

In the mid-1990s, the search for a more suitable laser wavelength by Keller and Hibst[33,34] led to the development of the Er:YAG (2940-nm) wavelength laser, a free-running

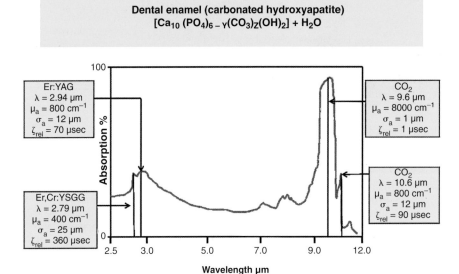

• **Figure 10-5** Comparative interaction (absorption) of four laser wavelengths (λ) with carbonated hydroxyapatite: Er:YAG (2940 nm); Er,Cr:YSGG (2780 nm); CO_2 (9600 nm); and CO_2 (10,600 nm). μ_a = absorption coefficient, σ_a = surface penetration of the beam (μm units), ζ_{rel} = thermal relaxation (μsec units). (Data from Fried D, Ragadio J, Akrivou M, et al: Dental hard tissue modification and removal using sealed transverse excited atmospheric-pressure lasers operating at λ 9.6 and 10.6 μm, *J Biomed Opt* 6(2):231-238, 2001.)

(inherently microsecond-pulsed) mid-infrared laser for effective ablation of dental hard tissues. This was followed by similar investigations into the use of another mid-infrared free-running wavelength, the Er,Cr:YSGG (2780-nm), which could effect photothermal vaporization of interstitial water and ablative disruption of target tooth mineral both safely and precisely.[35-38]

Considered in the following order, enamel, dentin, bone, cementum, and carious tissue have descending mineral density and ascending water composition.[39,40] Both Er,Cr:YSGG and Er:YAG laser wavelengths are absorbed well in water, with slightly stronger absorption for the Er:YAG than for the Er,Cr:YSGG (see Figure 10-2). This absorption is several orders of magnitude greater than seen with the Nd:YAG wavelength (Figure 10-5).

The strong absorption in water with the erbium wavelengths results from a relatively broad water band of approximately 3000 nm, together with small absorption at approximately 2800 nm by the hydroxyl group of the (carbonated) hydroxyapatite mineral of the tissues.[41-44]

When incident laser energy directed onto hard dental tissue is absorbed by the prime chromophores (either water or carbonated hydroxyapatite), one of two effects occurs. For both Er:YAG and Er,Cr:YSGG wavelengths, this energy is absorbed primarily by the water and is rapidly converted to heat, which causes superheating with a consequent phase transfer in the subsurface water, resulting in a disruptive expansion in the tissue. Through this mechanism, whole tissue fragments are ejected and a hole is cut in the tooth, with little or no alteration to the mineral itself. A common term for this effect is *spallation* (Figures 10-6 to 10-8).

Relatively high fluences (energy density or laser photonic energy per unit area) are needed at these wavelengths for spallation to occur. The emission mode of current mid-infrared lasers is defined as free-running pulsed mode. Currently available lasers emit a pulse train of 50- to 250-µsec pulses on average, which, when delivered in rates of 3 to 50 Hz (pulses per second), represent high peak-power values sufficient to ablate tooth mineral tissue. Although pulse durations are close to the thermal relaxation times of enamel and dentin, further examination of ultrashort pulse widths (and associated high peak-power values) is needed to create sufficient ablative force without inducing collateral thermal damage.[45,46]

The rate of ablation of dental hard tissue depends on the amount of incident laser energy delivered to the tissue, as well as the effects of wavelength, pulse duration, pulse shape, repetition rate, power density, thermal relaxation time of the tissue, and delivery mode.[47,48] In addition, heat buildup in the tissue (and unwanted heat conduction to the pulp) must be avoided and accumulation of products of ablation (char) prevented.

Mid-infrared ablation of dental hard tissue has led to the concept of two wavefronts of interaction: an *ablation* front and a *thermal* front. It is important that the ablation front always precedes the thermal front, to avoid the risk of a damaging heat increase through the accumulation of ablation debris within a deep cavity.[49] Accordingly, studies have examined the effects of excessive incident power and the buildup of ablation products, or their removal by means of a coaxial water spray.[50] The vital dental pulp is acutely sensitive to thermal change. The explosive defragmentation of mineralized dental tissue, induced by water-assisted erbium wavelengths, allows much of the heat to escape from the cavity, carried in the ablated particles, resulting in pulpal thermal increases of less than 5° C.[51-53]

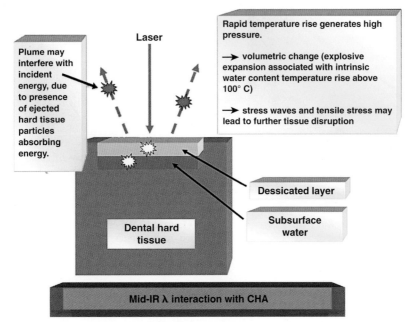

• **Figure 10-6** Graphic representation of interaction of mid-infrared laser wavelength with tooth (mineralized) tissue. Incident-pulsed laser photonic energy of mid-infrared wavelength is preferentially absorbed by water contained within the target dental tissue. Rapid heating beyond the vaporization temperature of water causes volumetric expansion and structural fragmentation of associated mineral. Such action may be accompanied by an audible "pop" and visual evidence of a microcrater formation in the tooth surface.

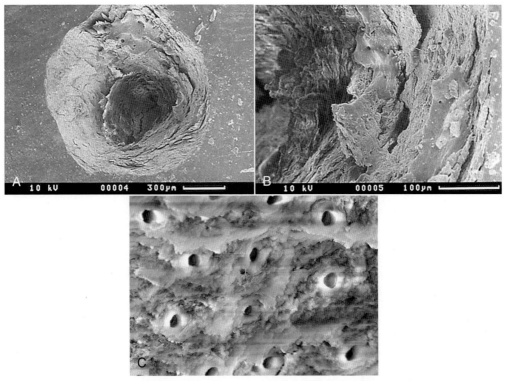

• **Figure 10-7** Scanning electron micrographs showing effects of pulsed Er:YAG (2940 nm) laser energy with water spray on human enamel and dentin. **A,** Laser-enamel interaction. Note effects of spallation and absence of signs of thermal change in mineral structure or cracking. **B,** Higher-power (×300) scanning electron micrograph of same specimen **(A)**. **C,** Laser-dentin interaction. Note absence of thermal damage, no smear layer, and open dentinal tubules.

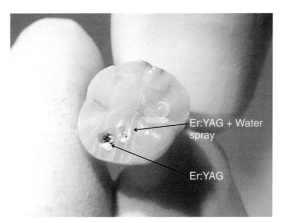

• **Figure 10-8** Handheld (sectioned) specimen (human molar) exposed to pulsed Er:YAG (2940 nm) laser energy. Use of laser energy without water spray results in carbonization of target tissue.

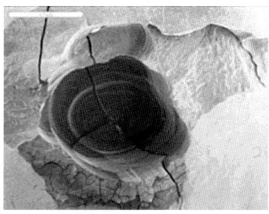

• **Figure 10-9** Scanning electron micrograph of human enamel showing cavity prepared with high-speed rotary instrumentation. Note cracking caused by vibration.

Laser Use Versus Conventional Instrumentation

To any clinician who chooses to use a laser in restorative dentistry, application of the high-speed rotary drill is seen as the "gold standard." Ease of use and speed often are accepted as plausible, despite several studies showing that high-speed drilling leads to surface and pulpal temperature rise, tissue cracking, and unnecessary removal of healthy surrounding tissue during cavity preparation[54-56] (Figure 10-9).

The precise and selective ablation of tooth tissue with the Er,Cr:YSGG and Er:YAG laser wavelengths is well documented. In general, the only drawback appears to be the lower "speed" of cutting compared with that for even a slow-speed drill,[57-59] with reports of 80% slower speed in enamel and comparable speed in dentin. Also, the desire to match laser cutting speeds with those of rotary instruments has led to power delivery greatly in excess of that postulated by Keller and Hibst, relative to the ablation threshold of enamel. Coexistent with such power levels and heat conversion, studies have shown that by reducing the pulse duration of the laser energy (pulse width), peak-power values rise, ablation is more efficient, and heat transfer is minimized,[33,60-62] to establish a clinically acceptable rate of interaction commensurate with treatment time.

Different handpiece tips have been designed to address the needs of energy delivery, efficiency of cutting, and access. Round cross-sectional tips may vary in diameter from 200 to 1300 μm. Care should be exercised in assessing the power density of the emitted beam; as the spot size (diameter) is reduced, the energy per exposed target area increases dramatically, assuming all other variables remain the same, and places a high risk of tissue overheating. Most delivery tips are made of quartz and provide efficient transmission of laser energy to the target. With the spallation effect of hard tissue ablation, impact damage from ejected ablation products may cause irregularity in both the beam configuration and the cutting dynamics. The tips should therefore be regularly inspected for damage, and the ends can be repolished using fine discs and diamond paste. Tips made of sapphire offer marginal improvements in energy delivery, as do hollow-bore tips.[63,64] Sapphire tips are more expensive and less able to be reconditioned, however, and their rigidity is associated with a greater risk of fracture during use.

> ### CLINICAL TIP
>
> Other factors, such as fluoridation of the tissue, incident angle of the delivery tip relative to the tooth, and presence of ablation products, also affect the speed of ablation. Several anecdotal reports have shown the effectiveness of orienting the delivery tip parallel to the axis of the enamel prisms, to permit access to the interprismatic, higher water-content structure. Remember that the long axis of the enamel prisms changes from the occlusal (or incisal) third to the middle third to the gingival third, necessitating a change in the incident angle of the tip onto the tissue.

Laser Use in Cavity Preparation

The use of Er:YAG and Er,Cr:YSGG lasers for almost two decades in clinical practice has resulted in emergence of protocols governing their use in restorative dentistry, from simple fissure sealing to complete cavity management and surface preparation for direct composite-resin veneers. The spallation effect of exposing the enamel surface to laser energy results in a microcavitation; although this environment is ideal for further acid etching and direct bonding, it is considered impractical to use such a surface to place indirect ceramic veneers. Nonetheless, some clinicians advocate laser use in crown and veneer preparation[65,66] despite the lack of peer-reviewed literature to validate this application (Figures 10-10 and 10-11).

Early erbium lasers had rudimentary handpieces that were comparatively heavy. In addition, the delivery of laser energy through a noncontact sapphire window proved to be inadequate for precise cutting action. Newer developments have resulted in balanced waveguides or low-OH⁻ fibers (e.g., germanium oxide), together with handpieces that are similar to turbines, use contact tips, and have coaxial illumination and water spray. This allows more precise interaction

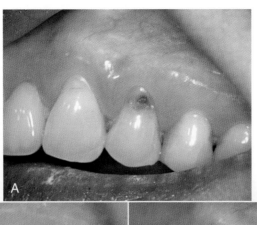

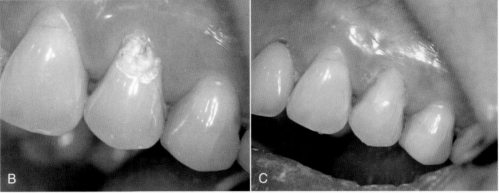

• **Figure 10-10** **A,** Buccal caries in upper left bicuspid. **B,** Cavity prepared using Er:YAG laser (2940 nm) and water spray (350 mJ/pulse, 10 Hz). Topical anesthetic was applied. **C,** Completed acid-etched composite restoration in place, before polishing.

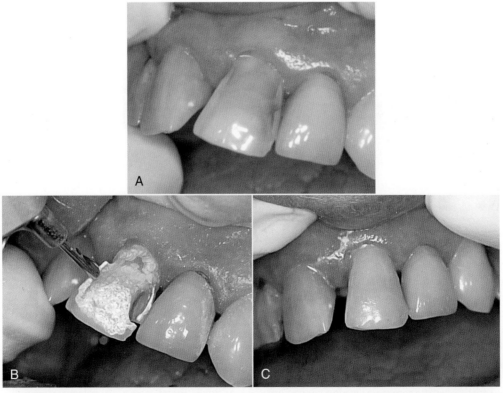

• **Figure 10-11** **A,** Upper left central incisor showing signs of labial tooth loss. Patient chose treatment to include laser use and placement of direct composite veneer. **B,** Tooth prepared using Er:YAG laser (2940 nm) and water spray (350 mJ/pulse, 10 Hz). **C,** Completed restoration.

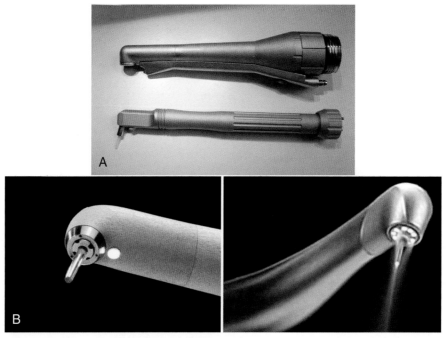

• **Figure 10-12 A,** Comparison of early handpiece for use with Er:YAG laser (2940 nm) with a later version. **B,** Modern handpiece variants of those shown in A. Note similarity to rotary ("air rotor") handpiece, coaxial water spray, and illumination (Courtesy BIOLASE, Inc., Irvine, CA.).

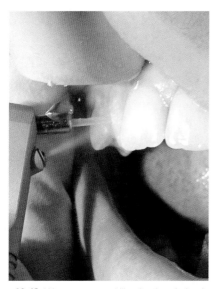

• **Figure 10-13** Water spray and illumination during laser use.

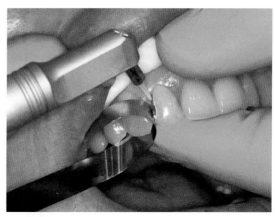

• **Figure 10-14** With significant risk of damage to adjacent nontarget tooth tissue, a suitable nonreflective material can provide protection. Here, a metal matrix band has been dulled to prevent reflection of the laser beam.

with tooth tissue, using instrumentation familiar to the dentist (Figure 10-12).

Tissue ablation results from end-on emission of laser energy from the tip. Progressive tissue removal is through surface ablation; this mode of action is at variance with that of the rotary bur, which predominantly uses a side-cutting action. Ideal laser ablation of tooth tissue is achieved by positioning the handpiece tip just out of contact with the tooth surface; during laser emission, the tip should be moved back and forth over the target to develop cavitation. Once entry into the tooth cavity has been achieved, it is important to allow adequate access for the water spray, both to provide cooling and to prevent accumulation of ablation debris. It is recommended that the laser tip be pumped in and out of the laser cavity to ensure adequate water spray (Figures 10-13 and 10-14).

No laser is capable of removing amalgam or gold restorations; intrinsically, the significant risk of beam reflection may result in nontarget exposure to laser energy. In addition, the rapid buildup of heat in the metal may cause pulpal damage and, with amalgam, result in the liberation of toxic metal fumes. Similarly, thermally fused indirect ceramic restorations are subject to rapid spot-heat buildup, leading to carbonization and crazing.

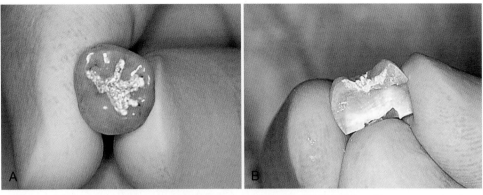

• **Figure 10-15** **A,** Occlusal surface of human molar exposed to Er:YAG (2940 nm) laser energy, showing effects of interaction after air drying. **B,** Vertical section of same tooth shows depth of penetration of the laser beam.

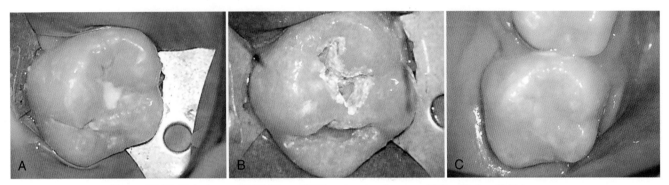

• **Figure 10-16** Clinical use of Er:YAG laser (2940 nm) and water spray (700 mJ/pulse, 10 Hz) on upper molar showing preoperative **A,** intraoperative **B,** and immediate postoperative **C,** appearance of composite restoration.

However, in an emerging world of minimal intervention and early caries management of the natural tooth, laser use may be seen as indispensable. Cavity preparation can proceed in a manner similar to that for rotary instrumentation to define the cavity and remove caries. Access form and restoration form are determined by the extent of the caries, but retention form may be viewed differently. The microexplosive ablation of mineral results in a rough surface, which, together with an acid-etch technique, permits a strong bond for composite-resin restoratives, often with reduced need for physical undercuts in the cavity margin.[67,68]

During cavity preparation, an audible "popping" can be appreciated as laser ablation occurs. This audible clue is a lower-level sound with healthy tooth tissue but becomes louder with caries ablation because more water is present. With minimal experience, this phenomenon can aid the operator in using the laser to remove diseased tissue selectively while preserving healthy enamel and dentin. In this way, laser action can benefit the clinician in establishing the success of cavity preparation as an adjunct to explorer use. At least one Er:YAG laser has a coaxial low-level laser beam to determine the fluorescence of the target tissue, corresponding to mineral content. This beam is linked electronically to the emission beam of the erbium laser, as an additional level of detection of carious tissue.

The characteristic appearance of a fresh cavity prepared with a laser may be viewed with some disdain by dentists trained in the disciplines of G.V. Black[69]; sharp cavosurface angles are absent, and the cavity outline may appear distinctly irregular. The premise of Black's cavity design drew on "extension for prevention" and the need to provide bulk strength for amalgam retention and stability. Laser-assisted cavity preparation involves a "minimalistic" approach: the advantage of removal of only diseased tissue and the choice of composite-resin restorative materials (Figures 10-15 and 10-16).

Studies on the marginal integrity of early laser-created restorations reflect poor stability, partly explained by postablation weakness in marginal enamel.[70-72] However, treating the cut surface further with conventional acid-etch techniques improves the longevity of the restoration, with enhanced bond strength.[73,74] This technique can be used as an adjunct when restorative procedures requiring facial or incisal bonding of direct composite-resin materials are required. With carious dentin, the laser beam may pass quickly through the surface layer in gross caries, leading to dehydration in deeper layers. When gross caries is present, it is advisable to use an excavator to remove bulk volume, both to prevent heat damage and to expedite cavity preparation (Figure 10-17).

Both of the erbium lasers will leave a cut surface without a smear layer, and using a proprietary bonded dentin

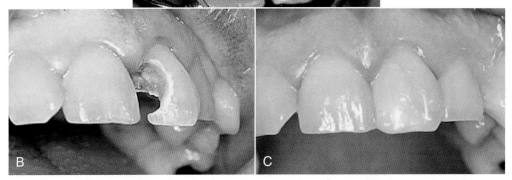

• **Figure 10-17 A,** Carious cavity Caries in upper left central incisor. **B,** Outline form was determined using Er:YAG laser (2940 nm) with water spray (450 mJ/pulse, 10 Hz). Gross caries was removed using hand excavators and the final form obtained using the laser. Laser energy levels were reduced (250 to 300 mJ/pulse, 10 Hz, water spray) to remove deeper caries and to modify the enamel margins. Tooth preparation was done with use of local anesthetic. **C,** Completed restoration.

protector, calcium hydroxide, or glass ionomer lining is recommended on open tubules exposed by the ablation process.

Establishing a "recommended" power value for laser-assisted ablation of dental hard tissue is problematic because of conflicting and anecdotal factors. The reported ablation threshold for human enamel is 12 to 20 J/cm^2, and for dentin, 8 to 14 J/cm^2, using Er:YAG and Er,Cr:YSGG laser wavelengths. For an average laser delivery spot size, using a free-running pulsed emission mode, this power value may be 150 to 250 mJ/pulse. The paramount concern is delivering sufficient laser energy, within a minimal time, to achieve clinically acceptable ablation rates without causing adjacent tissue damage. Besides studies that have determined minimal levels of power necessary, anecdotal reports abound. Certainly, the Er:YAG and Er,Cr:YSGG lasers prepare tooth cavities comparably, with similar effects on tooth tissue[75] (Figure 10-18).

Clinicians should follow the manufacturer's guidelines in establishing laser treatment protocols for a given laser, bearing in mind the differing operating parameters of air, water, spot size, delivery tip choice, and any power losses that may occur among delivery systems. Most lasers have a "power meter test" port to establish the energy levels emitted through the delivery system, which should be checked before clinical use. The test fire of the laser also will determine the patency of the energy delivery system.

The key criteria in laser ablation of dental hard tissue are (1) matching incident wavelength to target chromophores,

(2) delivering energy and interaction during a time frame that does not induce conductive thermal events, and (3) evacuating the products of ablation. The low water content of enamel may present difficulties when attempts are made to gain access to subsurface caries. This situation is seen most often in healthy, fluoridated occlusal sites, where the ablation rate is approximately 20% of that achievable with a turbine. Fluoridated enamel presents greater resistance because of a harder fluoroapatite ($Ca_{10}[PO_4]_6F_2$) mineral and replacement of the hydroxyl group by the fluoride radical. Anecdotally, this problem may be somewhat overcome through the alignment of the laser beam parallel to the prismatic boundaries, or by the use of a conservative rotary bur, such as a fissurotomy bur, to establish intraenamel access for the laser beam (Figure 10-19).

In class III, IV, and V cavity sites and where prismatic density is less (e.g., deciduous teeth), the ablation rate is comparable to that for slow-speed rotary instrumentation.[76-78]

As previously discussed, the constraints of emission modes available with existing lasers has limited the clinically significant ablation of caries and dental hard tissue to the mid-infrared wavelength erbium family of lasers. Their suitability is obtained through absorption of laser energy by water and the short micropulsing of the emission. Studies on extremely short (nanosecond and femtosecond) pulses of laser energy have shown how other wavelengths might be utilized in clinical restorative dentistry.[79] Of note is the use of the 9600-nm CO_2 wavelength, which has high absorption in hydroxyapatite.[80-82]

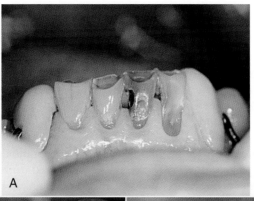

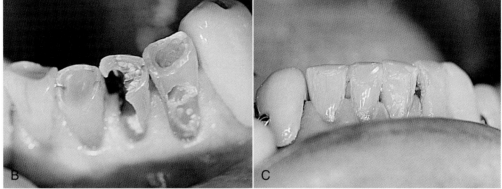

• **Figure 10-18** **A,** Multiple cavities associated with lower anterior teeth. The need for preservation of healthy tooth tissue was considered paramount. **B,** Cavity prepared using topical anesthesia. Benefits of laser use enabled precise removal of only diseased tissue. Microretention afforded by spallation of enamel and dentin reduced the need for adjunctive pins and retention pits. Microexplosive tissue ablation contributed to control of thermal rise, thereby protecting the tooth pulp. **C,** Completed direct-composite restorations.

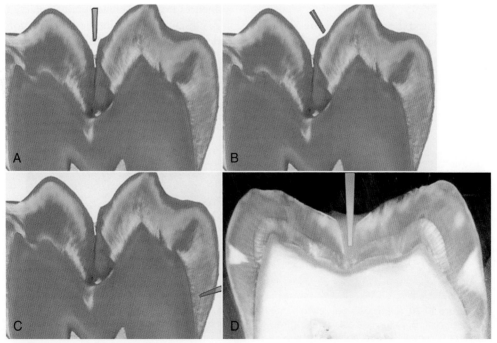

• **Figure 10-19** Ground vertical sections of human tooth. **A** to **C,** Radial arrangement of enamel prisms. Alignment of laser tip parallel to the prism axis may allow a more efficient ablation of interprismatic material and expedite cavity preparation. **D,** Fiber alignment and early fissure preparation.

The advantages of water spray during laser ablation include cooling of the target tissue and removal of ablation products. Early research on the Er:YAG laser and enamel showed that laser parameters of approximately 350 mJ per 2 to 4 pulses per second (pps) (with average power of 0.7 to 1.4 W) would initiate enamel ablation in human teeth. With the development of better coaxial coolant and shorter pulses, fast and efficient cavity preparation can be achieved with levels of 400 to 700 mJ per 10 to 20 pps (average power, 4 to 8 W), which with adequate water cooling does not cause pulpal damage. Clinical experience suggests that with "harder" occlusal enamel, the use of higher energy per pulse and lower repetition rates (pulse rates) would provide for easier ablation.

Adequate water spray must be provided during cavity preparation.[34] Successive laser pulses may interact with ablation products rather than with the cavity surface, and the need to maintain adequate water cooling may be compromised by access problems. Such concerns also apply to the use of rotary instruments in similar situations, possibly increasing the thermal assault on the pulp.[83-85]

The limitation in the end-on emission of laser energy can pose a problem in defining greater width to an already-established cavity. Any overhanging, unsupported enamel can be pared back with a suitable hand chisel; alternatively, a rotary bur can be used. Surface ablation of such overhangs also is possible. The depth of the cavity can proceed through back-and-forth sweeping movement of the beam within the cavity, ensuring proper water irrigation to prevent buildup of debris and heat. It is imperative that the laser beam be kept moving at all times. Tactile feedback is intrinsically lacking in laser use, and the clinician should visually check the progress of cavity preparation so that excessive tissue is not removed (Figure 10-20).

Laser photonic energy can be used to ablate dental hard tissue during the management of caries and cavity preparation within a clinically acceptable time frame. The use of safe power and delivery parameters allows the procedure to proceed without causing local thermal damage or pulpal injury. The prepared cavity surface can be a base for stable and retentive restorations when additional acid-etch techniques are used before composite placement.

Laser Analgesia

The noise, vibration, and perception of pain associated with the high-speed dental drill are well-recognized negatives of this technology and the bleeding, postoperative swelling/inflammation, and sutures/dressings associated with intraoral soft tissue surgical procedures interfere with all aspects of oral function for the patient during a potentially long period of healing.[86] The opportunity to address these subjective disadvantages in the patient experience and to deliver high-quality dental treatment must surely represent a new gold standard.

The avoidance of pain during restorative procedures remains a strong factor in promoting patient acceptance of treatment.[87-89] The use of the Nd:YAG laser in developing pulpal analgesia, possibly through interference with the "gate theory" of neural stimulus propagation, has been suggested; afferent nociceptive stimulation of pulpal nerve fibers undergo synapse transmission in the subnucleus chordalis, before onward transmission to the higher brain. Influence of such transmission may be affected by restimulation at a faster speed than the re-formation rate of acetylcholine at the synapse or the polarity reversal rate of the nerve fiber. The synaptic neurotransmitter refractory period is approximately 1 msec, whereas a typical pulse width of a free-running laser is 100 to 150 μsec. In addition, inhibitory influences from the higher brain, notably the periaqueduct and substantia nigra, in the form of norepinephrine and endorphins, may influence or even override the ascending

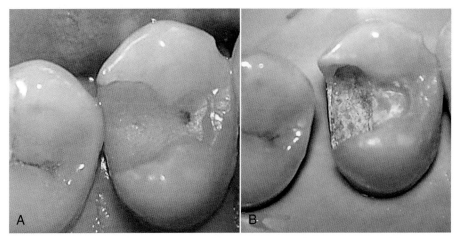

• **Figure 10-20 A,** Preoperative view of upper bicuspid tooth. Existing composite restoration requires replacement. **B,** Composite ablation using two different erbium laser wavelengths (2780 nm, 2940 nm) may be accomplished through interstitial water vaporization, vaporization of monomer component of composite, or a combination of both. Action may vary depending on type of composite. Desired depth of cavity can be attained through back-and-forth movement of the laser delivery tip. Final cavity contour may be achieved using hand chisels.

transmission of stimuli. Investigation into the subjectivity or placebo effect has rendered Er:YAG laser application inconsistent.[90,91]

Anecdotal reports claim similar gate theory effects with the 9300-nm CO_2 wavelength and both the Er:YAG and Er,Cr:YSGG lasers, each having free-running emission similar to that of the Nd:YAG laser. Use of subablative fluences during a 60-second exposure of the entire natural tooth surface appears to define an accepted protocol. The clinician needs to instill trust in the patient and should approach the success of laser-induced analgesia on a case-by-case basis. At least one study has established that when the Er:YAG laser is used to cut hard tooth structure, a positive neural response in both A and C intradental fibers is created, so there appears to be no induced change in the ionic balance of the nociceptor.[92] In my own (S. Parker) clinical practice, a 20% tetracaine topical anesthetic gel applied adjacent to the tooth often is sufficient to overcome temporary discomfort.

The following patient-centered factors may affect pain perception during cavity preparation:
- *Emotion:* fear, anxiety, stress syndrome, excitement
- *Awareness:* trust, previous experience, conditioning (e.g., hypnosis), activity subordination
- *Threshold potential:* age, infirmity, drugs, alcohol, social factors

The lack of tactile and thermal stimulation compared with rotary instrumentation is also significant in addressing claims of pain avoidance during laser-assisted tooth preparation. Other patient-centered factors include previous experience of turbine use as well as other emotional and conditioning states (Figure 10-21).

When studied with laser Doppler "vibrometric" measurement, preparation of a cavity using settings of 145 mJ at 10 Hz produced 400 times less vibration than that from a rotary bur.[93] Also, studies show that patients are disturbed more by the vibration perception with rotary use.[58] Reports indicate that use of erbium lasers in restorative dentistry is less painful.[14,94-97] Overall, anecdotal reports of delivering "pain-free" laser cavity preparation are still controversial, possibly undermining the true capability of both the Er:YAG and the Er,Cr:YSGG laser as an alternative to conventional rotary instrumentation.

The benefits of bacterial reduction associated with laser versus bur use involve less postoperative pain and reduced caries recurrence. Studies show a reduction in bacterial strains associated with caries (e.g., *Streptococcus mutans*) as well as other strains (e.g., *Escherichia coli, Enterococcus faecalis*) when the laser is used.[98,99] Although "absolute" sterilization is not possible, a decrease in bacteria (along with reduced tactile insult) may help reduce postoperative pain and decrease the possibility of recurrent decay with laser use.

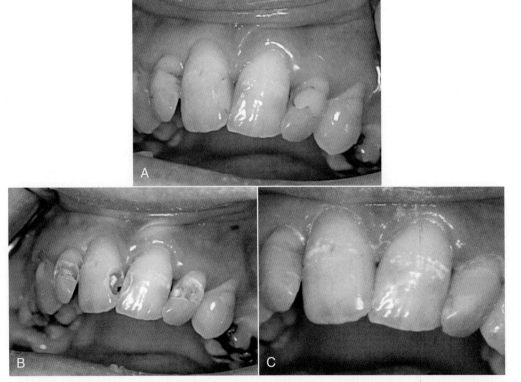

• **Figure 10-21** **A,** Replacement of worn composite restorations on upper anterior teeth. Patient had been reluctant to undergo dental treatment because of fear of rotary instrumentation and intraoral injections. **B,** Cavity preparations performed using topical anesthesia and Er:YAG laser (2940-nm wavelength) and water spray (350 mJ/pulse, 10 Hz). Multiple preparations were done at one treatment session. **C,** Completed restorations.

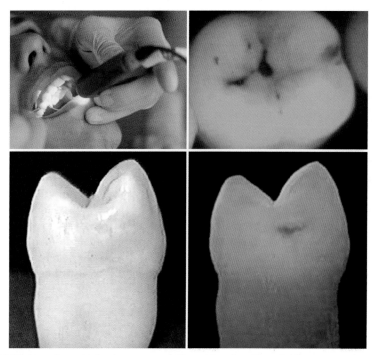

• **Figure 10-22** Use of nonablative laser energy (405 nm) to raise differential fluorescence in tooth tissue. Quantitative light-induced fluorescence (QLF) produces a green appearance in healthy tooth tissue (color shift caused by absorption phenomena and some energy loss, resulting in longer postexposure emission). Correspondingly, absorption of light by bacteria produces a discernible red shift.

Laser Use in Caries Diagnostics

The use of *fluorescence* in caries detection originally was suggested more than a century ago; current optical caries detection techniques emerged with the introduction of laser technology. In the 1980s, a clinically applicable visual detection method focusing on the natural green fluorescence of tooth tissue was developed.[100,101] The technique used a 488-nm excitation wavelength from an argon-ion laser to discriminate bright-green–fluorescing healthy tooth tissue from poorly fluorescing carious lesions. This technique was further refined in the early 1990s; the argon-ion laser was replaced by a xenon-based arc lamp, with the emission light shined through a blue-transmitting filter. This became known as *quantitative light-induced fluorescence* (QLF), using the digitization of images to quantify the observed green-fluorescence loss as an indirect measure of mineral loss.[102,103] QLF is a highly sensitive method for determining short-term changes in hard tissue lesions in the mouth[104] (Figure 10-22).

The excitation wavelength (approximately 405 nm) produced by the QLF system allows visualization and quantification of both the intrinsic green fluorescence of dental tissue and the *red fluorescence* of bacterial origin, as observed in calculus, plaque, and advanced caries.[105,106] The green fluorescence loss from demineralized enamel and natural carious lesions strongly correlates with mineral loss.[107] The red fluorescence of bacteria allows identification of leaking margins of sealants and restorations.

The phenomenon of substantial red fluorescence using laser wavelengths between 650 and 800 nm in carious lesions, much brighter than that of sound enamel or dentin,[108,109] has resulted in a handheld device to detect dental caries.[110] The first such unit was manufactured by KaVo (Biberach, Germany) in 1998, with an emission wavelength of 655 nm (Figure 10-23).

The QLF system is best incorporated as an adjunct to other diagnostic methods (tactile, visual, radiographic), to limit the possibility of false-positive results.[111,112] The unit offers reproducible analog scoring of site examination, allowing a degree of objective assay of suspect areas of caries, although the equivocal accuracy of results in primary tooth enamel is a concern, possibly a result of the reduced mineral density.[113,114] The presence of existing restorations (amalgam, gold, porcelain, composite) appears to allow detection of only marginal caries. The consistency of accurate readings has been questioned,[115,116] as has the situation with existing fissure sealants, especially when visually opaque.[117,118]

Studies comparing QLF with the diode fluorescence device suggest equal reliability, although QLF techniques appear better for determining mineral loss.[119]

Polarization-sensitive optical coherence tomography (PS-OCT) techniques have proved successful at imaging hard and soft tissue in the oral cavity, providing numerical analysis of the optical properties of the surface and subsurface enamel. At research levels, using a near-infrared beam (wavelength of 1310 nm), caries detection is possible at both surface level and under composite restorations and sealants[120,121] (see Chapter 17). Other spectroscopic devices use Raman-effect phenomena to quantify mineral loss associated with dental caries.[122-124]

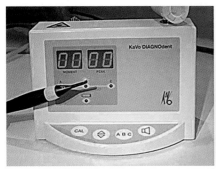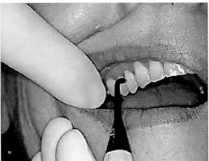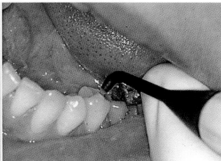

• **Figure 10-23** DiagnoDent system (KaVo, Biberach, Germany). Demineralization in tooth tissue affects fluorescence dynamics of the tooth. These changes are recorded through the handpiece tip, calibrated, and displayed through analog score and sound.

Laser Caries Prevention

Early work with the then-new Nd:YAG dental laser in 1989, ostensibly to investigate its tooth-cutting capability, revealed thermally induced changes in carbonated hydroxyapatite in enamel, from the ordered crystalline structure to the formation of amorphous mineral. These changes predominated at the margins of laser-induced cavities, suggesting the possibly beneficial action of lower emission parameters. Also, this mineral had higher resistance to acid dissolution compared with the parent crystals. These findings led to the advocacy of such laser techniques in a quasi–fissure sealant technique for erupted posterior teeth.[125-128]

During laser light generation in a CO_2 laser, the slow decay from the energized state may result in additional wavelengths produced (but not emitted) from this laser (9300, 9600, 10,300, and 10,600 nm). If a shorter wavelength other than the usual 10,600 nm is selected, the absorption coefficient of carbonated hydroxyapatite (carbonate radical) increases greatly.[129,130] Featherstone and co-workers at the University of California, San Francisco, have conducted extensive investigations into the use of an experimental ultra-pulsed 9300-nm and 9600-nm laser. In September 2013, the first CO_2 laser emitting at 9300 nm for caries removal and soft tissue surgery came to the U.S. market. The greater selectivity of these wavelengths in the targeting and removal of the carbonate group from the enamel mineral molecule results in a much more highly acid-resistant compound.[131-134] Additionally, the altered mineral has greater uptake of topically applied fluoride, with the expectation of even greater acid resistance and caries prevention (see Chapter 17).[135]

Conclusions

Restorative dentistry has evolved from the need to treat dental disease and especially dental caries. This need often is accompanied by the conditional requirements of maintaining integral strength of the teeth during function and establishing a healthy interface between the restoration and the hard/supporting soft tissue, to prevent further breakdown and allow ongoing maintenance, all within a growing patient-driven demand for pain-free and cosmetic treatment. Also, professional dental care demands more accurate diagnosis of disease, earlier interceptive treatment, and therapeutic prevention of dental disease. These factors accommodate well the potential for laser photonic energy to interact with the various target chromophores, to effect ablation or to modify structure precisely and predictably.

For the clinician providing common restorative procedures, many situations arise in which the laser can replace conventional instrumentation to achieve comparable or better results. For the patient, laser use may represent opportunities to receive less stressful and painful restorative treatment with less disruptive postoperative effects.

References

1. Beltrán-Aguilar ED, Barker LK, Canto MT, et al.: Centers for Disease Control and Prevention (CDC): surveillance for dental caries, dental sealants, tooth retention, edentulism, and enamel fluorosis—United States, 1988-1994 and 1999-2002, *MMWR Surveill Summ* 54(3):1–43, 2005.
2. Al Malik M, Rehbini Y: Prevalence of dental caries, severity, and pattern in age 6 to 7-year-old children in a selected community in Saudi Arabia, *J Contemp Dent Pract* 7(2):1–8, 2006.
3. Osborne JW, Summitt JB: Extension for prevention: is it relevant today? *Am J Dent* 11(4):189–196, 1998.
4. Qvist V, Johannessen L: Progression of approximal caries in relation to iatrogenic preparation damage, *J Dent Res* 71(7): 1370–1373, 1992.
5. Baldissara P, Catapano S: Clinical and histological evaluation of thermal injury thresholds in human teeth: a preliminary study, *J Oral Rehabil* 24(11):791–801, 1997.
6. Beazoglou T, Eklund S, Heffley D, et al.: Economic impact of regulating the use of amalgam restorations, *Public Health Rep* 122:657–663, 2007.
7. United Kingdom Government Department of Health: *Dental Practice Board report*, London, 2006, HMSO.
8. Hörsted-Bindslev P, Heyde-Petersen B, Simonsen P, Baelum V: Tunnel or saucer-shaped restorations: a survival analysis, *Clin Oral Invest* 9(4):233–238, 2005.
9. Martin FE: Adhesive bonding: some clinical considerations, *Ann R Australas Coll Dent Surg* 18:30–35, 2006.
10. Breschi L, Mazzoni A, Ruggeri A, et al.: Dental adhesion review: aging and stability of the bonded interface, *Dent Mater* 24(1):90–101, 2008.

11. Freitas PM, Navarro RS, Barros JA: de Paula Eduardo C: The use of Er:YAG laser for cavity preparation: an SEM evaluation, *Microsc Res Tech* 70(9):803–808, 2007.

12. Banerjee A, Watson TF, Kidd EA: Dentine caries excavation: a review of current techniques, *Br Dent J* 188(9):476–482, 2000.

13. Pellagalli J, Gimbel C, Hansen R, et al.: Investigational study of the use of the Er:YAG laser versus the drill for caries removal and cavity preparation: phase 1, *J Clin Laser Med Surg* 15:109, 1997.

14. Keller U, Hibst R: Effects of Er:YAG laser in caries treatment: a clinical pilot study, *Lasers Surg Med* 20:32, 1997.

15. Mjör IA, Odont D: Pulp-dentin biology in restorative dentistry. Part 2. Initial reactions to preparation of teeth for restorative procedures, *Quintessence Int* 32(7):537–551, 2001.

16. Ozturk B, Usumez A, Ozturk AN, Ozer F: In vitro assessment of temperature change in the pulp chamber during cavity preparation, *J Prosthet Dent* 91(5):436–440, 2004.

17. Vaughn RC, Peyton FA: The influence of rotational speed on temperature rise during cavity preparation, *J Dent Res* 30(5):737–744, 1951.

18. Rizoiu I, Kohanghadosh F, Kimmel AI, Eversole LR: Pulpal thermal responses to an erbium, chromium: YSGG pulsed laser hydrokinetic system, *Oral Surg Oral Med Oral Pathol Oral Radiol Endod* 86(2):220–223, 1998.

19. Paghdiwala AF, Vaidyanathan TK, Paghdiwala MF: Evaluation of erbium:YAG laser radiation of hard dental tissues: analysis of temperature changes, depth of cuts and structural effects, *Scan Microsc* 7(3):989–997, 1993.

20. Oelgiesser D, Blasbalg J, Ben-Amar A: Cavity preparation by Er-YAG laser on pulpal temperature rise, *Am J Dent* 16(2):96–98, 2003.

21. Maiman TH: Stimulated optical radiation in ruby, *Nature* 187:493–494, 1960.

22. Ito S, Saito T, et al.: Water content and apparent stiffness of non-caries versus caries-affected human dentin, *J Biomed Mater Res B Appl Biomater* 72(1):109–116, 2005.

23. Bassi G, Chawla S, Patel M: The Nd:YAG laser in caries removal, *Br Dent J* 177(7):248–250, 1994.

24. Cox CJ, Pearson GJ, Palmer G: Preliminary in vitro investigation of the effects of pulsed Nd:YAG laser radiation on enamel and dentine, *Biomaterials* 15(14):1145–1151, 1994.

25. Harris DM, White JM, Goodis H, et al.: Selective ablation of surface enamel caries with a pulsed Nd:YAG dental laser, *Lasers Surg Med* 30(5):342–350, 2002.

26. Yamada MK, Watari F: Imaging and non-contact profile analysis of Nd:YAG laser-irradiated teeth by scanning electron microscopy and confocal laser scanning microscopy, *Dent Mater J* 22(4):556–568, 2003.

27. McDonald A, Claffey N, Pearson G, et al.: The effect of Nd:YAG pulse duration on dentine crater depth, *J Dent* 29(1):43–53, 2001.

28. Goodis HE, White JM, Marshall Jr GW, et al.: Effects of Nd: and Ho:yttrium-aluminium-garnet lasers on human dentine fluid flow and dental pulp-chamber temperature in vitro, *Arch Oral Biol* 42(12):845–854, 1997.

29. Seka W, Fried D, Featherstone JD, Borzillary SF: Light deposition in dental hard tissue and simulated thermal response, *J Dent Res* 74(4):1086–1092, 1995.

30. Srimaneepong V, Palamara JE, Wilson PR: Pulpal space pressure and temperature changes from Nd:YAG laser irradiation of dentin, *J Dent* 30(7-8):291–296, 2002.

31. Lan WH, Chen KW, Jeng JH, et al.: A comparison of the morphological changes after Nd-YAG and CO_2 laser irradiation of dentin surfaces, *J Endod* 26(8):450–453, 2000.

32. Yamada MK, Uo M, Ohkawa S, et al.: Three-dimensional topographic scanning electron microscope and Raman spectroscopic analyses of the irradiation effect on teeth by Nd:YAG, Er:YAG, and CO_2 lasers, *J Biomed Mater Res B Appl Biomater* 71(1): 7–15, 2004.

33. Keller U, Raab WH, Hibst R: Pulp reactions during erbium YAG laser irradiation of hard tooth structure, *Dtsch Zahnarztl Z* 46(2):158–160, 1991.

34. Hibst R, Keller U: Mechanism of Er:YAG laser–induced ablation of dental hard substances, *Proc SPIE* 1880:156–162, 1993.

35. Fried D: IR laser ablation of dental enamel, *Proc SPIE* 3910: 136–148, 2000.

36. Walsh Jr JT, Cummings JP: Effect of the dynamic optical properties of water on mid infrared laser ablation, *Lasers Surg Med* 15:295–305, 1994.

37. Apel C, Meister J, Ioana RS, et al.: The ablation threshold of Er:YAG and Er:YSGG laser radiation in dental enamel, *Lasers Med Sci* 17:246–252, 2002.

38. Harashima T, Kinoshita J, Kimura Y, et al.: Morphological comparative study on ablation of dental hard tissues at cavity preparation by Er:YAG and Er,Cr:YSGG lasers, *Photomed Laser Surg* 23:52–55, 2005.

39. Meister J, Franzen R, Forner K, et al.: Influence of the water content in dental enamel and dentin on ablation with erbium YAG and erbium YSGG lasers, *J Biomed Opt* 11(3):340–350, 2006.

40. Wigdor H, Abt E, Ashrafi S, Walsh Jr JT: The effect of lasers on dental hard tissues, *J Am Dent Assoc* 124(2):65–70, 1993.

41. Featherstone JDB, Nelson DGA: Laser effects on dental hard tissues, *Adv Dent Res* 1:21–26, 1987.

42. Zuerlein MJ, Fried D, Featherstone JDB, Seka W: Optical properties of dental enamel in the mid-IR determined by pulsed photothermal radiometry, *J Select Top Quantum Electron* 5:1083–1089, 1999.

43. Nelson DGA, Featherstone JDB: The preparation, analysis and characterization of carbonated apatites, *Calcif Tiss Int* 34:S69–S81, 1982.

44. Featherstone JDB, Fried D: Fundamental interactions of lasers with dental hard tissues, *Med Laser Appl* 16:181–194, 2001.

45. Cozean C, Arcoria CJ, Pelagalli J, Powell GL: Dentistry for the 21st century? Erbium:YAG laser for teeth, *J Am Dent Assoc* 128(8):1080–1087, 1997.

46. Curti M, Rocca JP, Bertrand MF, Nammour S: Morpho-structural aspects of Er:YAG prepared class V cavities, *J Clin Laser Med Surg* 22(2):119–123, 2004.

47. Mercer CE, Anderson P, Davis GR: Sequential 3D X-ray microtomographic measurement of enamel and dentine ablation by an Er:YAG laser, *Br Dent J* 194(2):99–104, 2003.

48. Mehl A, Kremers L, Salzmann K, Hickel R: 3D volume-ablation rate and thermal side effects with the Er:YAG and Nd:YAG laser, *Dent Mater* 13(4):246–251, 1997.

49. Dostalova T, Jelinkova H, Krejsa O, Hamal H: Evaluation of the surface changes in enamel and dentin due to possibility of thermal overheating induced by erbium:YAG laser radiation, *Scan Microsc* 10(1):285–290, 1996.

50. Freiberg RJ, Cozean C: Pulsed erbium laser ablation of hard dental tissue: the effects of atomised water spray vs water surface film, *Proc SPIE* 4610:74–84, 2002.

51. Rizoiu I, Kohanghadosh F, Kimmel AI, Eversole LR: Pulpal thermal responses to an erbium, chromium:YSGG pulsed laser hydrokinetic system, *Oral Surg Oral Med Oral Pathol Oral Radiol Endod* 86(2):220–223, 1998.

52. Paghdiwala AF, Vaidyanathan TK, Paghdiwala MF: Evaluation of erbium:YAG laser radiation of hard dental tissues: analysis of temperature changes, depth of cuts and structural effects, *Scan Microsc* 7(3):989–997, 1993.

53. Oelgiesser D, Blasbalg J, Ben-Amar A: Cavity preparation by Er:YAG laser on pulpal temperature rise, *Am J Dent* 16(2):96–98, 2003.

54. Baldissara P, Catapano S, Scotti R: Clinical and histological evaluation of thermal injury thresholds in human teeth: a preliminary study, *J Oral Rehabil* 24(11):791–801, 1997.

55. Spierings TA, Peters MC, Plasschaert AJ: Thermal trauma to teeth, *Endod Dent Traumatol* 1(4):123–129, 1985.

56. Watson TF, Cook RJ: The influence of bur blade concentricity on high-speed tooth-cutting interactions: a video-rate confocal microscopic study, *J Dent Res* 74(11):1749–1755, 1995.

57. Aoki A, Ishikawa I, Yamada T, et al.: Comparison between Er:YAG laser and conventional technique for root caries in vitro, *J Dent Res* 77:1401–1414, 1998.

58. Evans DJ, Matthews S, Pitts N, et al.: A clinical evaluation of an erbium:YAG laser for dental cavity preparation, *Br Dent J* 188:677–679, 2000.

59. Levy G, Koubi GF, Miserendino LJ: Cutting efficiency of a mid-infrared laser on human enamel, *J Endod* 24(2):97–101, 1998.

60. Khabbaz MG, Makropoulou MI, Serafetinides AA, et al.: Q-switched versus free-running Er:YAG laser efficacy on the root canal walls of human teeth: a SEM study, *J Endod* 30(8):585–588, 2004.

61. Hibst R: Mechanical effects of erbium:YAG laser bone ablation, *Lasers Surg Med* 12(2):125–130, 1992.

62. Pozner JM, Goldberg DJ: Histologic effect of a variable pulsed Er:YAG laser, *Dermatol Surg* 26(8):733–736, 2000.

63. Polletto TJ, Ngo AK, Tchapyjnikov A, et al.: Comparison of germanium oxide fibers with silica and sapphire fiber tips for transmission of erbium:YAG laser radiation, *Lasers Surg Med* 38(8):787–791, 2006.

64. Alves PR, Aranha N, Alfredo E, et al.: Evaluation of hollow fiberoptic tips for the conduction of Er:YAG laser, *Photomed Laser Surg* 23(4):410–415, 2005.

65. Nash R, Colonna M: Crown and veneer preparation using the Er,Cr:YSGG Waterlase hard and soft tissue laser, *Contemp Esthet Restorative Pract*, October 2002.

66. Usumez A, Aykent F: Bond strengths of porcelain laminate veneers to tooth surfaces prepared with acid and Er,Cr:YSGG laser etching, *J Prosthet Dent* 90(1):24–30, 2003.

67. Borsatto MC, Corona SA, de Araújo FP, et al.: Effect of Er:YAG laser on tensile bond strength of sealants in primary teeth, *J Dent Child* 74(2):104–108, 2007.

68. Gurgan S, Kiremitci A, Cakir FY, et al.: Shear bond strength of composite bonded to erbium:yttrium-aluminum-garnet laser–prepared dentin, *Lasers Med Sci*, Dec 12, 2007.

69. Boyde A: Enamel structure and cavity margins, *Oper Dent* 1:13–28, 1976.

70. Chinelatti MA, Ramos RP, Chimello DT, et al.: Influence of the use of Er:YAG laser for cavity preparation and surface treatment in microleakage of resin-modified glass ionomer restorations, *Oper Dent* 29:430–436, 2004.

71. Corona SA, Borsatto MC, Pecora JD, et al.: Assessing microleakage of different class V restorations after Er:YAG laser and bur preparation, *J Oral Rehabil* 30:1008–1014, 2003.

72. Corona SA, Borsatto M, Dibb RG, et al.: Microleakage of class V resin composite restorations after bur, air-abrasion or Er:YAG laser preparation, *Oper Dent* 26:491–497, 2001.

73. Niu W, Eto JN, Kimura Y, et al.: A study on microleakage after resin filling of class V cavities prepared by Er:YAG laser, *J Clin Laser Med Surg* 16:227–231, 1998.

74. Gutknecht N, Apel C, Schafer C, Lampert F: Microleakage of composite fillings in Er,Cr:YSGG laser–prepared class II cavities, *Lasers Surg Med* 28:371–374, 2001.

75. Harashima T, Kinoshita J, Kimura Y, et al.: Morphological comparative study on ablation of dental hard tissues at cavity preparation by Er:YAG and Er,Cr:YSGG lasers, *Photomed Laser Surg* 23(1):52–55, 2005.

76. Stock K, Hibst R, Keller U: Comparison of Er:YAG and Er:YSGG laser ablation of dental hard tissues, *Proc SPIE* 3192:88–95, 2000.

77. Belikov AV, Erofeev AV, Shumilin VV, Tkachuk AM: Comparative study of the 3 μm laser action on different hard tissue samples using free running pulsed Er-doped YAG, YSGG, YAP and YLF lasers, *Proc SPIE* 2080:60–67, 1993.

78. Mercer C, Anderson P, Davis G: Sequential 3D x-ray microtomographic measurement of enamel and dentine ablation by an Er:YAG laser, *Br Dent J* 194:99–104, 2003.

79. Kim BM, Feit MD, Rubenchik AM, et al.: Influence of pulse duration on ultrashort laser pulse ablation of biological tissues, *J Biomed Opt* 6(3):332–338, 2001.

80. Fried D, Ragadio J, Champion A: Residual heat deposition in dental enamel during IR laser ablation at 2.79, 2.94, 9.6, and 10.6 μm, *Lasers Surg Med* 29(3):221–229, 2001.

81. Dela Rosa A, Sarma AV, Jones RS, et al.: Peripheral thermal and mechanical damage to dentin with microsecond and submicrosecond 9.6 μm, 2.79 μm, and 0.355μm laser pulses, *Lasers Surg Med* 35(3):214–228, 2004.

82. Fried D, Ragadio J, Akrivou M, et al.: Dental hard tissue modification and removal using sealed transverse excited atmospheric-pressure lasers operating at λ 9.6 and 10.6 μμm, *J Biomed Opt* 6(2):231–238, 2001.

83. Kim ME, Jeoung DJ, Kim KS: Effects of water flow on dental hard tissue ablation using Er:YAG laser, *J Clin Laser Med Surg* 21(3):139–144, 2003.

84. Fried D, Ashouri N, Breunig T, Shori R: Mechanism of water augmentation during IR laser ablation of dental enamel, *Lasers Surg Med* 31(3):186–193, 2002.

85. Hossain M, Nakamura Y, Yamada Y, et al.: Ablation depths and morphological changes in human enamel and dentin after Er:YAG laser irradiation with or without water mist, *J Clin Laser Med Surg* 17(3):105–109, 1999.

86. Malamed SF: Pain and anxiety control in dentistry, *J Calif Dent Assoc* 21:35–41, 1993.

87. Penfold CN: Pain-free oral surgery, *Dent Update* 20:421–426, 1993.

88. Maskell R: Pain-free dental treatment is changing dentistry's image, *Probe (Lond)* 33(9):36–37, 1991.

89. Delfi J: Public attitudes toward oral surgery: results of a Gallup poll, *J Oral Maxillofac Surg* 55:564–567, 1997.

90. Whitters CJ, Hall A, Creanor SL, et al.: A clinical study of pulsed Nd:YAG laser–induced pulpal analgesia, *J Dent* 23:145–150, 1995.

91. Orchardson R, Whitters CJ: Effect of HeNe and pulsed Nd:YAG laser irradiation on intradental nerve responses to mechanical stimulation of dentine, *Lasers Surg Med* 26:241–249, 2000.

92. Chaiyavej S, Yamamoto H, Takeda A, Suda H: Response of feline intradental nerve fibers to tooth cutting by Er:YAG laser, *Lasers Surg Med* 27:341–349, 2000.

93. Takamori K, Furukawa H, Morikawa Y, et al.: Basic study on vibrations during tooth preparations caused by high speed drilling and Er:YAG laser irradiation, *Lasers Surg Med* 32(1):25–31, 2003.

94. Smith TA, Thompson JA, Lee WE: Assessing patient pain during dental laser treatment, *J Am Dent Assoc* 124:90–95, 1993.

95. Kato J, Moriya K, Jayawardena JA, Wijeyeweera RL: Clinical application of Er:YAG laser for cavity preparation in children, *J Clin Laser Med Surg* 21:151–155, 2003.

96. Dostalova T, Jelinkova H, Kucerova H, et al.: Noncontact Er:YAG laser ablation: clinical evaluation, *J Clin Laser Med Surg* 16:273–282, 1998.

97. Matsumoto K, Nakamura Y, Mazeki K, Kimura Y: Clinical dental application of Er:YAG laser for class V cavity preparation, *J Clin Laser Med Surg* 14:123–127, 1996.

98. Turkun M, Turkun L, et al.: Bactericidal effect of Er,Cr:YSGG laser on *Streptococcus mutans*, *Dent Mater J* 25(1):81–86, 2006.

99. Schoop U, Kluger W, et al.: Bactericidal effect of different lasers systems in the deep layers of dentin, *Lasers Surg Med* 35(2):111–116, 2004.

100. Bjelkhagen H, Sundström F: A clinically applicable laser luminescence method for the early detection of dental caries, *IEEE J Quantum Electron* 17:266–270, 1981.

101. Bjelkhagen H, Sundström F, Angmar-Månsson B, Ryden H: Early detection of enamel caries by the luminescence excited by visible laser light, *Swed Dent J* 6:1–7, 1982.

102. Hafström-Björkman U, Sundström F, de Josselin de Jong E, et al.: Comparison of laser fluorescence and longitudinal microradiography for quantitative assessment of in vitro enamel caries, *Caries Res* 26:241–247, 1992.

103. de Josselin de Jong E, Sundström F, Westerling H, et al.: A new method for in vivo quantification of changes in initial enamel caries with laser fluorescence, *Caries Res* 29:2–7, 1995.

104. Stookey GK: Optical methods: quantitative light fluorescence, *J Dent Res* 83(suppl):C84–C88, 2004.

105. Heinrich-Weltzien R, Kühnisch J, van der Veen M, et al.: Quantitative light-induced fluorescence (QLF): a potential method for the dental practitioner, *Quintessence Int* 34:181–188, 2003.

106. van der Veen MH, Buchalla W: de Josselin de Jong E: QLF technologies: recent advances. In Stookey GK, editor: *Early detection of dental caries. III.* Proceedings of the 6th annual Indiana Conference, Indianapolis, 2003, Indiana University School of Dentistry, pp 291–304.

107. Emami Z, Al-Khateeb S, de Josselin de Jong E, et al.: Mineral loss in incipient caries lesions quantified with laser fluorescence and longitudinal microradiography: a methodologic study, *Acta Odontol Scand* 54:8–13, 1996.

108. Hibst R, Gall R: Development of a diode laser–based fluorescence detector, *Caries Res* 32:294, 1998.

109. Hibst R, Paulus R: Caries detection by red excited fluorescence: investigations on fluorophores, *Caries Res* 33:295, 1999.

110. Lussi A, Megert B, Longbottom C, et al.: Clinical performance of a laser fluorescence device for detection of occlusal caries lesions, *Eur J Oral Sci* 109:14–19, 2001.

111. Bader JD, Shugars DA: A systematic review of the performance of a laser fluorescence device for detecting caries, *J Am Dent Assoc* 135:1413–1426, 2004.

112. Huth KC, Neuhaus KW, Gygax M, et al.: Clinical performance of a new laser fluorescence device for detection of occlusal caries lesions in permanent molars, *Dentistry*, Oct 17, 2008.

113. Braga M, Nicolau J, Rodrigues CR, et al.: Laser fluorescence device does not perform well in detection of early caries lesions in primary teeth: an in vitro study, *Oral Health Prev Dent* 6(2):165–169, 2008.

114. Bengtson AL, Gomes AC, Mendes FM, et al.: Influence of examiner's clinical experience in detecting occlusal caries lesions in primary teeth, *Pediatr Dent* 27(3):238–243, 2005.

115. Bamzahim M, Aljehani A, Shi XQ: Clinical performance of DiagnoDent in the detection of secondary carious lesions, *Acta Odontol Scand* 63(1):26–30, 2005.

116. Boston DW: Initial in vitro evaluation of DiagnoDent for detecting secondary carious lesions associated with resin composite restorations, *Quintessence Int* 34(2):109–116, 2003.

117. Krause F, Braun A, Frentzen M, Jepsen S: Effects of composite fissure sealants on IR laser fluorescence measurements, *Lasers Med Sci* 23(2):133–139, 2008.

118. Gostanian HV, Shey Z, Kasinathan C, et al.: An in vitro evaluation of the effect of sealant characteristics on laser fluorescence for caries detection, *Pediatr Dent* 28(5):445–450, 2006.

119. Shi XQ, Tranaeus S, Angmar-Månsson B: Comparison of QLF and DiagnoDent for quantification of smooth surface caries, *Caries Res* 35(1):21–26, 2001.

120. Fried D, Xie J, Shafi S, et al.: Imaging caries lesions and lesion progression with polarization sensitive optical coherence tomography, *J Biomed Opt* 7:618–627, 2002.

121. Jones RS, Staninec M, Fried D: Imaging artificial caries under composite sealants and restorations, *J Biomed Opt* 9:1297–1304, 2004.

122. Ribeiro A, Rousseau C, Girkin J, et al.: A preliminary investigation of a spectroscopic technique for the diagnosis of natural caries lesions, *J Dent* 33:73–78, 2005.

123. Rousseau C, Poland S, Girkin JM, et al.: Development of fibre-optic confocal microscopy for detection and diagnosis of dental caries, *Caries Res* 41(4):245–251, 2007.

124. Ko AC, Hewko M, Sowa MG, et al.: Early dental caries detection using a fibre-optic coupled polarization-resolved Raman spectroscopic system, *Opt Express* 16(9):6274–6284, 2008.

125. Harazaki M, Hayakawa K, Fukui T, et al.: The Nd-YAG laser is useful in prevention of dental caries during orthodontic treatment, *Bull Tokyo Dent Coll* 42(2):79–86, 2001.

126. Hossain M, Nakamura Y, Kimura Y, et al.: Effect of pulsed Nd:YAG laser irradiation on acid demineralization of enamel and dentin, *J Clin Laser Med Surg* 19(2):105–108, 2001.

127. Tsai CL, Lin YT, Huang ST, Chang HW: In vitro acid resistance of CO_2 and Nd-YAG laser–treated human tooth enamel, *Caries Res* 36:423–429, 2002.

128. Kwon YH, Kwon OW, Kim HI, Kim KH: Nd:YAG laser ablation and acid resistance of enamel, *Dent Mater J* 22(3):404–411, 2003.

129. Konishi N, Fried D, Staninec M, Featherstone JD: Artificial caries removal and inhibition of artificial secondary caries by pulsed CO_2 laser irradiation, *Am J Dent* 12:213–216, 1999.

130. Mullejans R, Eyrich G, Raab WH, Frentzen M: Cavity preparation using a super-pulsed 9.6-μm CO_2 laser: a histological investigation, *Lasers Surg Med* 30:331–336, 2002.

131. Featherstone JD, Barrett-Vespone NA, Fried D, et al.: CO_2 laser inhibitor of artificial caries-like lesion progression in dental enamel, *J Dent Res* 77:1397–1403, 1998.
132. Kantorowitz Z, Featherstone JD, Fried D: Caries prevention by CO_2 laser treatment: dependency on the number of pulses used, *J Am Dent Assoc* 129:585–591, 1998.
133. Goodis HE, Fried D, Gansky S, et al.: Pulpal safety of 9.6 μm TEA CO_2 laser used for caries prevention, *Lasers Surg Med* 35:104–110, 2004.
134. McCormack SM, Fried D, Featherstone JD, et al.: Scanning electron microscope observations of CO_2 laser effects on dental enamel, *J Dent Res* 74:1702–1708, 1995.
135. Tepper SA, Zehnder M, Pajarola GF, Schmidlin PR: Increased fluoride uptake and acid resistance by CO_2 laser-irradiation through topically applied fluoride on human enamel in vitro, *J Dent* 32:635–641, 2004.

11

Lasers in Pediatric Dentistry

LAWRENCE KOTLOW

In 1960, Dr. Theodore Maiman, working on the theory of light amplification proposed by Albert Einstein, created the first laser.[1] Eighty years after Einstein's 1917 paper, the first erbium laser for hard tissue dental procedures was cleared for marketing by the U.S. Food and Drug Administration (FDA). Since that time, dentistry has undergone dramatic changes in the way both soft tissue and hard tissue disease and abnormalities are treated. In pediatric dentistry, the primary goals are the prevention and interception of oral diseases and soft tissue abnormalities without making the patient reluctant to visit the dentist. If these twin goals of prevention and interception are not attainable, restoration of diseased teeth and repair or elimination of soft tissue abnormalities become necessary.

Concerns about the dental visit usually arise from the use of needles to anesthetize the hard and soft tissues. Other noxious stimuli (e.g., sound of high-speed turbine, smell of preparing teeth with high-speed handpiece, vibrations during tooth preparation) contribute to the development of dental phobias. Lasers represent a quantum leap forward in the treatment of all patients, especially the pediatric patient.

Laser Types

Erbium Family of Lasers

The development of the erbium family of lasers—specifically, the erbium-doped yttrium-aluminum-garnet (Er:YAG) and erbium plus chromium–doped yttrium-scandium-gallium-garnet (Er,Cr:YSGG) lasers—has made the treatment of children safer and easier. The availability of laser-assisted dental techniques has changed the way dentists prepare diseased teeth, ablate bone, and treat soft tissue abnormalities and diseases. An entirely new standard of care is becoming a reality. Erbium lasers have helped create a positive treatment atmosphere, with most pediatric patients undergoing dental caries treatment without fear.[2,3]

The benefits of lasers have become well documented over the past decade. The erbium lasers provide an alternative to conventional drilling and filling, while often allowing the dentist to use the high-speed or slow-speed handpiece to complete procedures (e.g., extensive alloy preparations) without the need for local anesthesia. Erbium lasers have the unique ability to ablate hard tissues (bone, dentin, enamel) as well as perform soft tissue procedures.[4-7] The erbium family of lasers, all with similar capabilities, includes the 2940-nm Er:YAG and 2780-nm Er,Cr:YSGG lasers.

The major differences between different manufacturers' erbium lasers are in the variety of handpieces and tips and, more important, the parameters incorporated into the specific device. These parameters include the variability of settings for millijoules (mJ), hertz (Hz), and pulse duration. Other critically important differences include the delivery system (fiber versus waveguide versus articulating arm), amount and type of training offered (actual hands-on versus CD and instruction manual), and the yearly service contract (costing as much as $5000 per year) after warranty on an expensive piece of equipment (as much as $90,000). Applying knowledge of laser physics allows the dentist to adjust each parameter, reducing the need for local anesthesia and providing good control of bleeding during soft tissue surgical procedures. In addition, proper settings allow the dentist to perform minimally invasive dental care, removing only the diseased tissue and preserving healthy tooth structure.

9300-nm Carbon Dioxide Laser

Before the introduction of the 9300-nm CO_2 laser in late 2013, all available CO_2 lasers emitted at 10,600 nm, a wavelength that was used exclusively for soft tissue surgery. The 9300-nm CO_2 laser wavelength has a high absorption in carbonated hydroxapatite and water and therefore is capable of safely ablating dental hard tissues without causing dangerous elevations in pulpal temperatures.[8] Dental hard tissues are ablated using short pulse durations that heat up enamel or dentin, creating very high pressure within the mineral composition (hydroxapatite) of the tissues, resulting in turn in an ejection of molten surface tissue.[9] This wavelength also can be used to perform bloodless soft tissue procedures.

Although the 9300-nm CO_2 laser has been clinically available for only a limited period (less than a year), preliminary observations by early adopters of this technology have identified two important benefits:

- A significant increase in speed of hard tissue ablation over erbium lasers
- In many instances, elimination of the need for any local anesthesia in both hard and soft tissue procedures

Information about the mechanism of action of the 9300-nm CO_2 laser is presented in Chapter 17. As with all new advances in dental laser technology, time will tell if this new and potentially game-changing device lives up to its promise.

Soft Tissue Lasers

A variety of laser wavelengths are useful for soft tissue procedures. The primary soft tissue lasers currently used include the 10,600 nm CO_2,[10,11] neodymium-doped YAG (Nd:YAG),[12] and the diode group of lasers.[13,14] These soft tissue lasers have no capability to ablate hard tissue. Although Nd:YAG lasers have FDA clearance for ablating first-degree caries in enamel, the procedure is extremely slow and tedious and has essentially been replaced by the erbium family of lasers.

Low-Level Lasers

The third group of lasers useful in pediatric care are the *photobiostimulating* (PBS), or *low-level*, lasers.[15-17] CO_2, diode, erbium, and Nd:YAG lasers are classified by the FDA as class IV lasers because of their ability to ablate tissue. However, the FDA classifies low-level (PBS) devices as class III lasers with "no significant risk" (NSR) because they produce less than 500 mW of energy. The photobiostimulatory effects of these lasers usually are designated *low-level laser therapy* (LLLT).

The low-level (PBS) lasers do not cause temperature elevation within the target tissue, but rather produce their effects from a photobiostimulation (or modulation) effect within the target tissue. These lasers are not capable of ablating tissue. These units usually are semiconductor diode lasers consisting of indium-gallium-aluminum-phosphide (InGaAlP), with wavelengths in the range of 630 to 700 nm, or gallium-aluminum-arsenide (GaAlAs), with wavelengths in the range of 800 to 830 nm. These lasers can penetrate to depths of 2 to 3 cm, depending on the exact wavelength used and the target tissue.

Outside of dentistry, the FDA has cleared low-level laser use in medicine for treating conditions such as carpal tunnel syndrome and for pain management. Dental applications at this time should be considered *off-label* use (not cleared by FDA). Although these low-level lasers are safe, caution should be used, and contraindications include pregnancy, presence of malignancies, and use near the eye or, in some cases, over the thyroid gland[18] (see Chapter 15).

Adjuncts and Benefits

To optimize the benefits of lasers on their integration into a pediatric dental practice, concomitant use of other technologies also should be considered. Laser-assisted dental procedures constitute one part of a new approach to practicing conservative, pain-free dentistry involving fluoride, digital radiography, and visual (microscopic) enhancement. Incorporating technologies such as digital radiography allows earlier diagnosis of decay and the use of minimally invasive treatments before lesions become large. When using a hard tissue laser and the improved composite materials now available, the clinician can precisely remove only diseased dental tissue, thereby preserving more healthy tooth structure than is possible with conventional techniques.

Some degree of visual enhancement for the dentist is highly recommended when using lasers. Lasers enable the practitioner to perform microdentistry because the laser can remove minute areas of diseased hard tissue not readily visualized. In performing soft tissue procedures, it is beneficial to use magnification to view the surgical area.[19,20] Loupes are one excellent option for enhanced visualization; however, the limitation of one magnification setting makes adding a dental operating microscope the optimal investment. In my own clinical experience with use of a dental operating microscope (since 2001), children accept it without difficulty and remain quite still during dental procedures.

CLINICAL TIP

Pediatric dentists appreciate the many benefits of using rubber dams for tooth isolation. In performing laser-assisted operative dentistry, the use of local anesthetics may not be necessary for decay removal. To place a rubber dam without the need for a local anesthetic, use of a winged #3 rubber dam clamp with a small amount of topical anesthetic is recommended. This technique may allow placement of the dam without causing discomfort to the child. The additional use of a mouth prop during treatment prevents the child from closing the jaw on the rubber dam clamp or accidentally biting down and breaking the laser tip.

An excellent alternative to the rubber dam is the Isolite system of tooth isolation (Isolite Systems, Santa Barbara, California). The Isolite unit incorporates all of the benefits of a rubber dam with the addition of a self-contained light source, a mouth prop, and high-speed evacuation. The Isolite unit also prevents water from being pulled away from the tooth during caries removal, unlike with the normal high-volume evacuator. This feature prevents the tooth from dehydrating, which may lead to patient discomfort during laser dentistry.

Lasers In Pediatric Dental Practice

The erbium family of lasers initially were designed, manufactured, and cleared only for hard tissue procedures involving enamel, dentin, cementum, and bone. Only through subsequent efforts of erbium laser pioneers and manufacturer applications were many soft tissue procedures added to the list of FDA-cleared procedures for erbium lasers. Erbium lasers primarily target the water content of soft tissue and the water content (that is, OH^-) of hydroxyapatite while eliminating the smell and vibration associated with dental handpieces. Also, the need for local anesthesia is significantly reduced during removal of enamel, dentin, and dental caries. Lasers are bactericidal, thus providing an added defense against infection in soft tissue and recurrent decay in hard tissue.

Lasers have led to a reevaluation of dental cavity preparation and a fundamental change in the practice of restorative dentistry. The dental profession now needs to reevaluate and modify, as appropriate, G.V. Black's principle of "extension for prevention" with the concept of *minimally invasive microdentistry*. The use of hard tissue lasers for repair of incipient hard tissue disease provides a stress-free means of restoring teeth with minimal invasiveness and usually without the need for a local anesthetic.[21,22] Other benefits to the patient over conventional methods include reducing the number of office visits required for restorative procedures, decreasing healing time for soft tissue procedures, eliminating the need for suturing, and reducing the need for postoperative pain medication and antibiotics.

The safety and effectiveness of hard tissue lasers have been well documented in the dental literature. The Nd:YAG laser has limited usefulness in the treatment of dental caries but is cleared for removal of superficial pigmented caries.[23] By contrast, the erbium family and 9300-nm CO_2 lasers are the lasers of choice and most practical for enamel, dentin, and cementum caries removal. These lasers can be used for restoring primary and permanent teeth, again with minimal to no local anesthesia. In most cases, children do not require local anesthesia for class I, II, III, IV, or V restorative procedures using bonded restorative materials.

Using the concept of minimally invasive restorative procedures, the erbium and 9300-nm CO_2 lasers allow the operator to remove only diseased tissue, thereby preserving much more of the healthy, unaffected tooth structure. Lasers also prevent the small microfractures in enamel produced with use of conventional dental handpieces. In cases in which alloy restorations are preferred, the lasers' low-level analgesic effect may allow the dentist to create a restorative preparation using a conventional handpiece without analgesia. The erbium laser creates its ablation effect through absorption of its energy by the water within the hydroxyapatite of the tooth structure. This energy heats up the water within the mineral, creating microexplosions of the hydroxyapatite out of the tooth. Because decayed hard tissue has more water content than healthy hard tissue, erbium lasers are more specific for decay than conventional instruments. The 9300-nm CO_2 laser wavelength is highly absorbed in the water and mineral (phosphate and carbonate) content of hard tissue, so this laser is extremely effective in vaporizing enamel. Conventional instruments (handpieces, air abrasion, spoon excavators) remove whatever is in their path. Erbium and 9300-nm CO_2 lasers preferentially remove higher-water-content

(decayed) tissue, leaving the lower-water-content (healthy) tissue unaffected[24] (see Chapter 10).

Table 11-1 lists the various uses of lasers in pediatric dentistry.

Hard Tissue Procedures

Analgesia for Sealant Placement and Caries Removal

Both surgical and low-level (PBS) lasers can produce an analgesic effect on teeth. The low-level laser is placed on the occlusal and root areas of the tooth to create this analgesic effect. A similar result may be produced using surgical lasers in the defocused mode for 2 to 3 min. Lasers using extremely short pulse durations are very efficient at producing this effect. Placement of sealants, preventive resin restorations, and class I, class III, and class V caries removal may be completed using hard tissue lasers with minimal to no local anesthesia using this technique. When caries are deep, removing tooth structure with a high-speed or slow-speed dental handpiece with no local anesthetic or patient discomfort also may be performed with this modality. Low-level laser analgesia is technique-sensitive (see Chapter 15).

CO_2 and Erbium Laser Caries Removal

Class II preparations are more time-consuming when accomplished with lasers; however, use of the correct parameters will allow the procedure to be performed successfully without patient discomfort. In general, preparing the tooth for a stainless steel or other type of crown is possible but not usually practical because of the length of time needed for this procedure. Every hard tissue laser has different pulse durations, Hz/mJ settings, tip diameters (producing different spot sizes) of different materials, and different delivery rates of air and water through the handpiece. Therefore, it is impossible to include suggested settings for each procedure. The following generalities, however, apply to all laser operative dentistry procedures, based on absorption of specific wavelengths by the target tissue, the spot size (see Chapter 2), and the laser energy's preferential absorption by water and mineral content:

1. The higher the water content of a tissue, the more easily the hard tissue lasers will cut through that tissue. Therefore, extremely decayed tissue (with higher water content) will cut much more easily, with less power needed, than slightly decayed tissue.
2. Healthy enamel (with lower water content), when lasers are used, will be more difficult to cut than any other hard tissue, so the procedure will require more power than any other tissue.
3. Erbium lasers are absorbed by the water in hydroxyapatite. The 9300-nm CO_2 laser wavelength is absorbed by both the water and mineral content. In fluoridated areas, the occlusal surfaces of teeth usually are composed of *fluoroapatite*, not hydroxyapatite. Because erbium laser energies are not well absorbed by fluoroapatite, it may be difficult

TABLE 11-1   Pediatric Dental Procedures and Use of Various Lasers

Procedure	Laser Type					
	Erbium	Diode	CO₂: 10,600 nm	CO₂: 9300 nm	Nd:YAG	Low-Level*
Investment cost	$35,000+	$2500+	$20,000+	$80,000+	$20,000+	$800+
Caries removal	Yes	No	No	Yes	Extremely limited	No
Bone ablation	Yes	No	No	Yes	No	No
Hemostasis	Fair to good	Excellent	Excellent	Excellent	Very good	Limited
Analgesic effect on teeth	Yes	Limited	Very limited	Excellent	Limited	Yes
Bactericidal	Yes	Yes	Yes	Yes	Yes	No
Limited postoperative pain	Yes	Yes	Yes	Yes	Yes	Yes
Aphthous ulcer treatment	Yes	Yes	Yes		Yes	Yes
Pulpotomy	Yes	Yes	Yes	Yes	Yes	No
Maxillary frenum revision	Yes	Yes	Yes	Yes	Yes	No
Mandibular frenum revision	Yes	Yes	Yes	Yes	Yes	No
Lingual frenum revision	Yes	Yes	Yes	Yes	Yes	No
Gingival recontouring	Yes	Yes	Yes	Yes	Yes	No
Gingivectomy	Yes	Yes	Yes	Yes	Yes	No
Biopsy	Yes	Yes	Yes	Yes	Yes	No
Tissue welding	Yes	Yes	Yes	Yes	Yes	No
Primary herpes	Yes	Yes	Yes	Yes	Yes	Yes
Herpes labialis	Yes	Yes	Yes	Yes	Yes	Yes
Periodontal therapy	Yes	Yes	Yes	Yes	Yes	No
Venous lake removal	Limited use	Yes	Yes	Yes	Yes	No

*LLLT (PBS techniques).

to begin a preparation for class I or class II decay on a permanent lower molar with many pits and fissures within the fluoroapatite. For these procedures, treatment should begin with a *fissurotomy* bur, which can strip off the outer layer of fluoroapatite, leaving the hydroxyapatite exposed. Fissurotomy burs typically can be used on pits and fissures without local anesthetic, because these burs are used only on the *surface* of the enamel, which has no innervation.

4. Proceeding deeper into the cavity preparation, upon moving from ablating enamel to ablating dentin, the clinician must adjust the settings from higher energy to lower energy for two reasons:
   a. Because enamel is not innervated, but dentin is composed of dentinal tubules, which have nerve tissue, as the enamel is ablated to expose the dentinoenamel junction, the settings must be decreased. Most hard tissue lasers have preset power levels, which are lower for dentin than for enamel. As the laser ablates the decayed enamel, and the dentin becomes exposed, the

nerve tissue within the exposed dentinal tubules may be affected by the air or water from the laser, which the patient will perceive as pain. With lowering of parameters as the laser nears the dentinoenamel junction, the patient may have no sensation at all.
   b. Upon moving from a more calcified (healthy) tissue to a less calcified (higher water content) tissue, parameters must be lowered. Dentin has a higher water content than enamel, so the laser will ablate dentin more quickly than enamel, possibly cutting through the dentin too quickly and leading to excessive tooth structure removal.

5. Knowledge of spot size and power density allows selection of the proper sapphire or quartz tip for the procedure (see Chapter 2). As with selecting a #1 or a #6 round bur based on amount of decay, selection of the correct size of laser tip will affect procedural efficiency. Class V preparations generally are wide yet shallow; accordingly, a large spot size is needed for these preparations, with selection of a wide tip recommended. A small occlusal

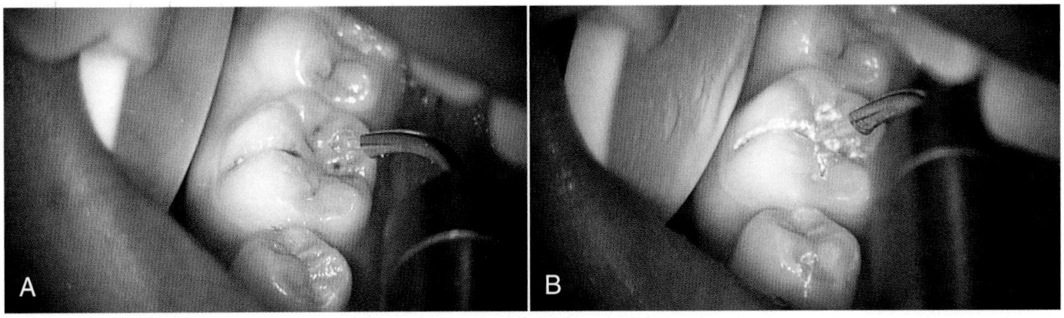

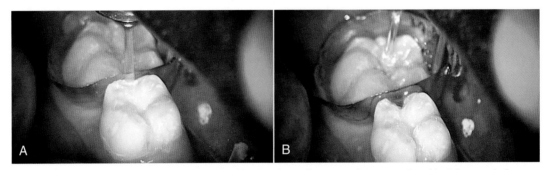

• **Figure 11-1 A,** Class I caries. **B,** Removal with erbium laser.

• **Figure 11-2 A,** Class II caries. Matrix band is placed on adjacent tooth to prevent accidental removal of its structure. **B,** Class II caries removal with erbium laser.

pit may be narrow buccolingually or mesiodistally but extend deep into the tooth. A small spot size would be more effective for this procedure, so a small-diameter laser tip would be appropriate. Other cavity preparations will require different size tips, depending on the width and depth of the decay. Because an inverse relationship exists between power density and spot size, a change in tip diameter during the procedure will require a change in laser parameters.

6. With class V preparations that extend subgingivally, it may be impossible to complete the procedure without performing an access gingivectomy. When changing from hard tissue treatment to soft tissue treatment, the water spray should be shut off. Use of the water spray during ablation of soft tissue with an erbium laser will not allow for adequate hemostasis of the soft tissue. Once the soft tissue ablation is completed, the water spray should be turned on to complete the hard tissue procedure. The power parameters also must be adjusted.

Figures 11-1 to 11-5 show erbium laser removal of class I to V caries. Figure 11-6 shows the result of conventional instrumentation for caries removal using local anesthesia in a pediatric patient.

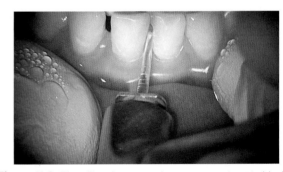

• **Figure 11-3** Class III caries removal on permanent central incisors with erbium laser.

Soft Tissue Procedures

A wide array of soft tissue procedures may be performed with lasers in the pediatric dental office.[25-31] Erbium lasers may be used to accomplish many soft tissue procedures with little or no bleeding when used at lower energy settings than for hard tissue procedures, and without water spray. In some cases, however, a diode, CO_2, or Nd:YAG laser may be better suited to the procedure. Patients with bleeding disorders (e.g., von Willebrand disease, hemophilia) or those receiving anticoagulants (e.g., aspirin, warfarin) will benefit from the superior hemostatic ability of these lasers.

Pediatric soft tissue laser procedures include the following:

• Maxillary frenum revisions
• Mandibular frenum revisions
• Lingual frenum revisions
• Treatment of pericoronal pain or infection

CLINICAL TIP

Placement of a metal matrix band on adjacent teeth is recommended with use of the laser for class II preparations, to prevent accidental etching of the noncarious adjacent tooth (see Figure 11-2A).

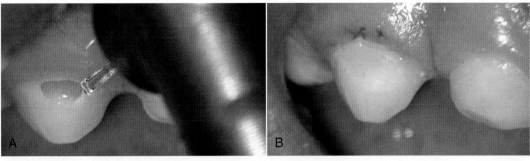

• **Figure 11-4** **A,** Class V caries removal combined with access gingivectomy. Both procedures were completed using an erbium laser. **B,** Immediate postoperative view of restoration.

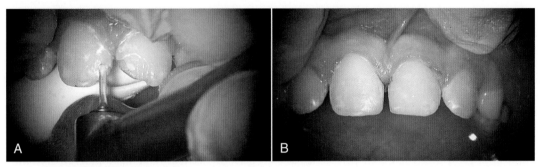

• **Figure 11-5** **A,** Class IV erbium laser preparations on maxillary central incisors fractured as a consequence of trauma. **B,** Fractures repaired and tooth structure restored.

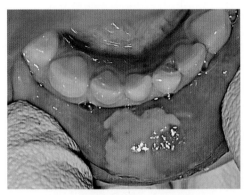

• **Figure 11-6** Lip bite in child resulting from use of local anesthetic. The ability to perform operative dentistry without injection of local anesthetic makes this a relic of twentieth-century dentistry.

- Removal of hyperplastic tissue caused by drugs or suboptimal oral care in orthodontic patients
- Biopsies
- Treatment of aphthous ulcers and herpes labialis
- Pulpotomies
- Pulp capping
- Exposure of unerupted teeth

CLINICAL TIP

Laser plume may contain benzene, formaldehyde, viral DNA, and other potential carcinogens. It is imperative that all members of the dental team use adequate plume avoidance measures; wearing 0.1-μm filtration masks is strongly suggested for *all* laser procedures.

Frenum Revisions

Indications for frenum revision in the infant, child, or adolescent patient range from an inability to nurse in newborns to speech pathology in children to orthodontic problems in preadolescent and adolescent patients. The correction of an aberrant frenum, whether by blade, electrosurgical unit, or laser, is basically the same: removal of the fibers causing the problem. For the purposes of frenectomy, the three types of frena are lingual, maxillary anterior, and mandibular anterior.

Correction of Nursing Problems

Parents have many concerns when a minor surgical treatment for infants and young children is recommended. A common scenario involves a preadmission physical examination and blood work; early-morning surgery with nothing to eat for the previous 6 h; general anesthesia in the operating room; and postoperative discomfort for a few days. The clinician may have heard the following questions and concerns regarding pediatric treatment:

- Is this an elective procedure?
- Does the child really need to be placed under general anesthesia? Is the child too young to have frenectomy performed as a general anesthetic procedure?
- Should the procedure be delayed until the child is older (and the operating room "safer")?
- Should the pediatric patient be referred to an oral surgeon, general surgeon, or ear, nose, and throat surgeon?

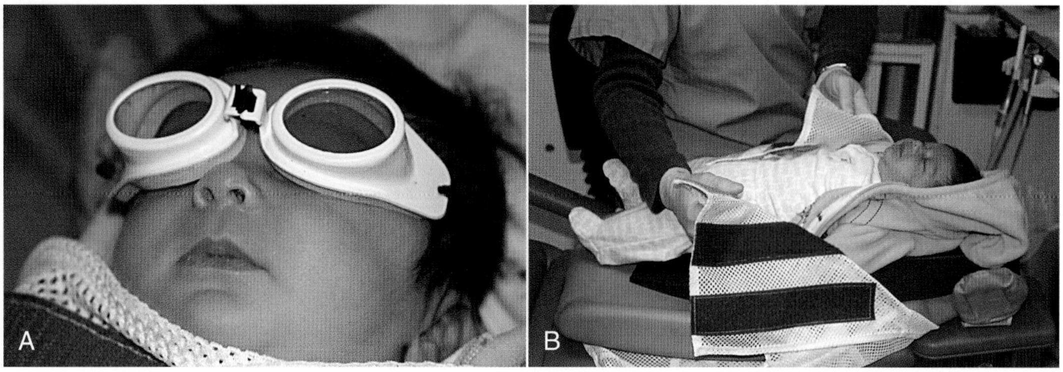

• **Figure 11-7** Preparation of a 1-day-old infant for laser surgery. This newborn required lingual frenum revision because of inability to nurse. **A,** Use of wavelength-specific protective eye goggles. **B,** The child is placed in a protective patient stabilizer.

- "Why can't we wait to see if the problem corrects itself as our child matures?"
- "I do not want to put my child through the procedure because I had horrible pain when I had it done as a child."

Although these objections may have been raised before the introduction of lasers to dentistry, their persistence as encountered in clinical practice reflects how some parents, friends, relatives, and physicians react when a child is born with a dental anomaly such as an abnormal lingual frenum or maxillary anterior frenum attachment that must be corrected. New mothers look forward to comforting and nurturing their newborn by nursing, which they view as the best way to ensure that the child receives the safest and best nourishment. When problems occur and the mother consults with a lactation specialist, the diagnosis of a short or tight lingual frenum with or without a tight maxillary frenum may be the major cause of the nursing problem.[32-37]

One of the most satisfying procedures in my own clinical practice is correcting a neonate's inability to nurse. A short lingual frenum, which occurs in approximately 3% to 4% of infants, may prevent the baby from properly latching on to the mother's nipple. This impaired function may result in failure of the infant to gain appropriate weight despite nursing every 2 h and, for the mother, painful nursing periods, followed by development of sore and flattened nipples and painful mastitis, and eventually the need to replace nursing at the breast with bottle feedings.[27,38-42]

Laser frenum correction is a safe, simple, and quick procedure that is a significantly less expensive option than conventional surgery. Any dental laser currently available (Nd:YAG, diode, CO_2, erbium) can complete this procedure literally in seconds, with no need for an operating room or general anesthesia, in a quick office visit, often with less pain than that from a local anesthetic injection, allowing the mother to begin nursing efficiently and painlessly.

The procedure is completed by placing the infant in a stabilization device or wrapping the infant in a small receiving blanket. The tongue is elevated using a grooved tongue director and a small amount of topical anesthetic placed. If the erbium wavelength is selected, no water is used. No

sutures are required. The infant is seen in 5 to 6 days for a follow-up examination (Figures 11-7 and 11-8).

Maxillary and Mandibular Frenectomy

Although all laser wavelengths can be used successfully to perform maxillary and mandibular frenectomies, in patients with bleeding disorders who require hemostasis during soft tissue surgery, diode, CO_2, or Nd:YAG lasers are the safest choice. These three lasers are much better than erbium lasers at creating excellent hemostasis immediately after frenum revision. Patients with bleeding or clotting disorders may be treated with these lasers without medical intervention, avoiding potential hospitalization to prevent or treat postsurgical bleeding complications as well as medication costs. Figure 11-9 illustrates a maxillary anterior laser frenectomy in a child with von Willebrand disease. In cases such as these involving medically compromised patients, a consultative telephone conversation with the primary care physician is always strongly recommended.

> **CLINICAL TIP**
>
> For most patients, after a small amount of topical anesthetic is applied over the area, injection of a small amount of local anesthetic will be adequate. For all maxillary frenum revisions, gently pull the lip upward while ablating the tissue. When ablating the mandibular frenum, pull the lip downward as the laser ablates the tissue. In both maxillary and mandibular frenum revisions, it is important for parents to separate the wound area twice daily by either pulling up the upper lip or pulling down the lower lip. This maneuver is effective in preventing tissue reattachment. Carefully following postoperative instructions may prevent the need for lower graft procedures (Figure 11-10).

Lingual Frenum Revisions

To assist in the diagnosis and treatment of lingual frenum abnormalities, the author created the following classification system based on the distance from the origin of the frenum at the tip of the tongue to the insertion of the frenum on the mandible: Normal frenum attachment length is more than 16 mm from tongue tip to frenum insertion.[25]

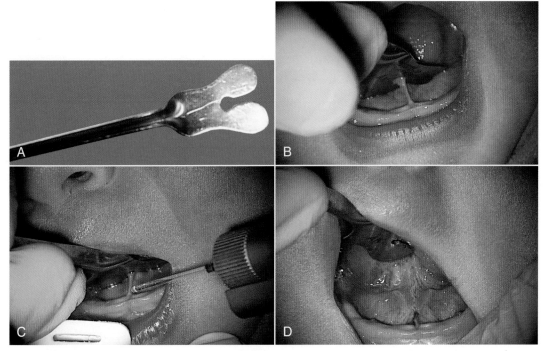

• **Figure 11-8** Lingual frenum revision procedure in the infant shown in Figure 11-7. **A,** Grooved tongue director is used to stabilize the tongue. **B,** Preoperative view of lingual frenum. **C,** Intraoperative view of lingual frenectomy. No local anesthetic was used. **D,** Immediate postoperative view.

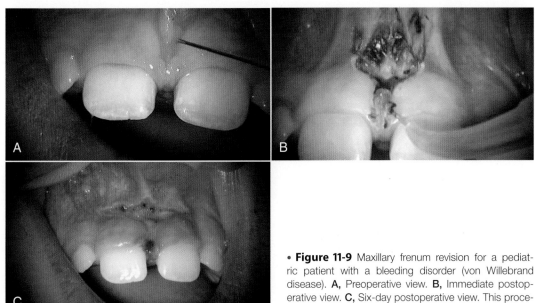

• **Figure 11-9** Maxillary frenum revision for a pediatric patient with a bleeding disorder (von Willebrand disease). **A,** Preoperative view. **B,** Immediate postoperative view. **C,** Six-day postoperative view. This procedure was performed with a 980-nm diode laser.

Class I frenum length is 12 to 16 mm; class II, 8 to 12 mm; class III, 4 to 8 mm; and class IV, 0 to 4 mm.

When the frenum insertion length is less than 8 mm, the author usually recommend a frenum revision. Whether the patient is a few days old or in the teenage years, the revision of the lingual frenum is easily completed using any laser wavelength in 15 to 30 sec. Postoperative care includes over-the-counter pain medications if discomfort occurs. To prevent reattachment, the parent is instructed to have the child exercise the tongue and to stretch the area daily. A follow-up appointment is scheduled for 6 to 7 days later (Figures 11-11 and 11-12).

CLINICAL TIP

In my experience, use of a *grooved tongue positioner* (Miltex) contributes to good surgical technique in frenum release procedures. When the frenum tissue exists as a thin fibrous attachment, local anesthesia usually is unnecessary. When the frenum tissue is thick and fibrous, local anesthesia may be required, and a single gut suture may be needed at the end of the final release point to prevent frenum reattachment. If the frenum is dense or muscular, after the frenum is anesthetized, grasp the frenum using a hemostat, placed close to the base of the tongue. The laser excision is completed on the exposed side of the hemostat, *not* on the hemostat surface touching the tongue.

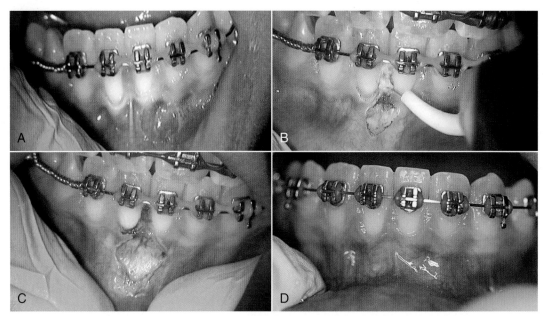

• **Figure 11-10** Anterior clefting caused by aberrant mandibular frenum in a pediatric patient. **A,** Preoperative view. **B,** Intraoperative view of mandibular frenectomy. **C,** Immediate postoperative view. **D,** Six-month postoperative view. This procedure was performed using an 810-nm diode laser.

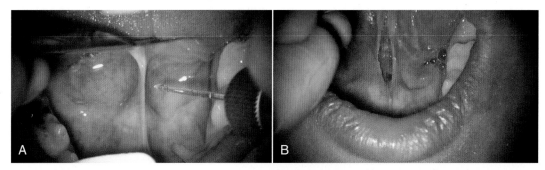

• **Figure 11-11 A,** Lingual frenum revision in 3-year-old child with use of only topical anesthetic. **B,** Immediate postoperative view. This procedure was performed using an erbium laser.

Diode and Nd:YAG laser wavelengths are absorbed by pigmented chromophores such as hemoglobin, which is abundant in vascular areas such as the floor of the mouth. CO_2 and erbium laser energies are absorbed by water, which is abundant in the mouth floor mucosa. The beginner laser clinician should place wet cotton rolls or gauze on the floor of the mouth to protect the delicate tissue from stray laser energy. Also, application of the laser significantly inferior to the lingual surface of the lower incisors should be avoided because of the proximity of the sublingual glands.

Hyperplastic Gingival Tissue

When the final result of orthodontic repositioning of the front teeth results in gingival hypertrophy, or orthodontic therapy itself causes gingival hypertrophy from poor oral hygiene, the laser can be a useful tool to increase crown length, to give the patient a more esthetic-appearing smile. Depending on the wavelength used and the amount of tissue revision needed, this procedure may be accomplished

without local anesthesia. Patients who have drug-induced hyperplastic tissue, as from phenytoin (Dilantin) administration, as well as organ transplant recipients taking cyclosporine, also can have this tissue reduced and reshaped with lasers[43,44] (Figures 11-13 to 11-15).

Lesion Removal and Biopsy

Fibrotic lesions, gingival growths, mucoceles, and other types of lesions can be quickly and safely removed using lasers. Lesion removal usually requires use of a local anesthetic (Figures 11-16 and 11-17). This topic is discussed in detail in Chapter 8.

Herpes Labialis and Aphthous Ulcer

Two of the most debilitating oral lesions that may arise in children are recurrent herpes labialis and aphthous ulcers. Dental lasers can immediately relieve the pain of aphthous ulcer lesions[45,46] and often stop or reduce

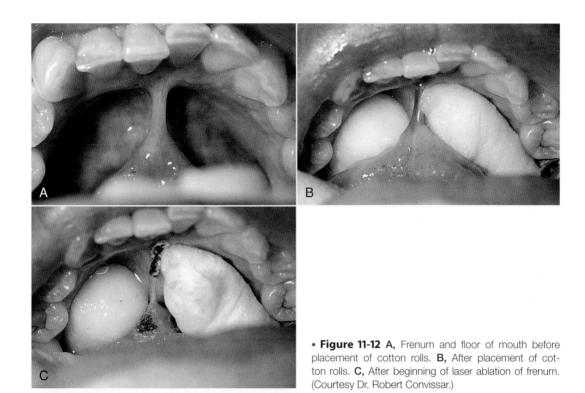

• **Figure 11-12** **A,** Frenum and floor of mouth before placement of cotton rolls. **B,** After placement of cotton rolls. **C,** After beginning of laser ablation of frenum. (Courtesy Dr. Robert Convissar.)

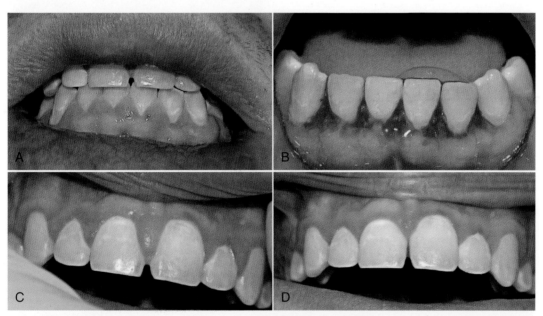

•**Figure 11-13** Phenytoin-induced gingival hyperplasia. **A,** Mandibular anterior view. **B,** Mandibular anterior view immediately after laser surgery. **C,** Maxillary anterior view. **D,** Maxillary anterior view immediately after surgery.

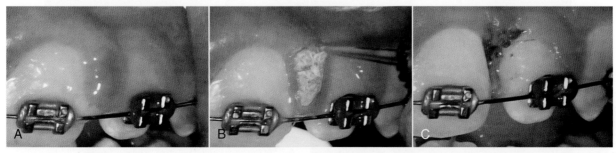

• **Figure 11-14** Laser removal of interproximal gingival hypertrophy with use of topical anesthetic. **A,** Preoperative view. **B,** Intraoperative view. **C,** Immediate postoperative view.

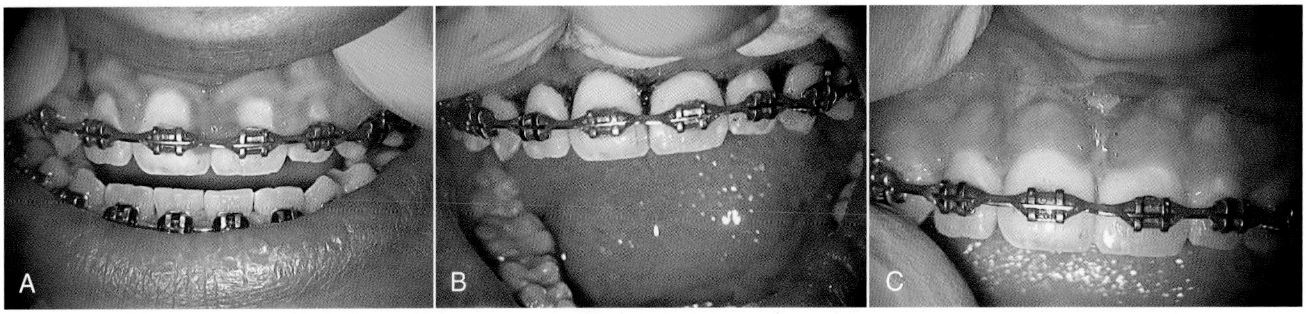

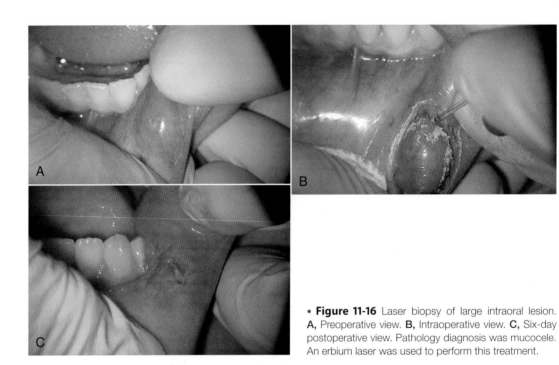

• **Figure 11-15** Orthodontically induced gingival hyperplasia removed by laser. **A,** Preoperative view. **B,** Immediate postoperative view. **C,** Postoperative view at 5 ½ days.

• **Figure 11-16** Laser biopsy of large intraoral lesion. **A,** Preoperative view. **B,** Intraoperative view. **C,** Six-day postoperative view. Pathology diagnosis was mucocele. An erbium laser was used to perform this treatment.

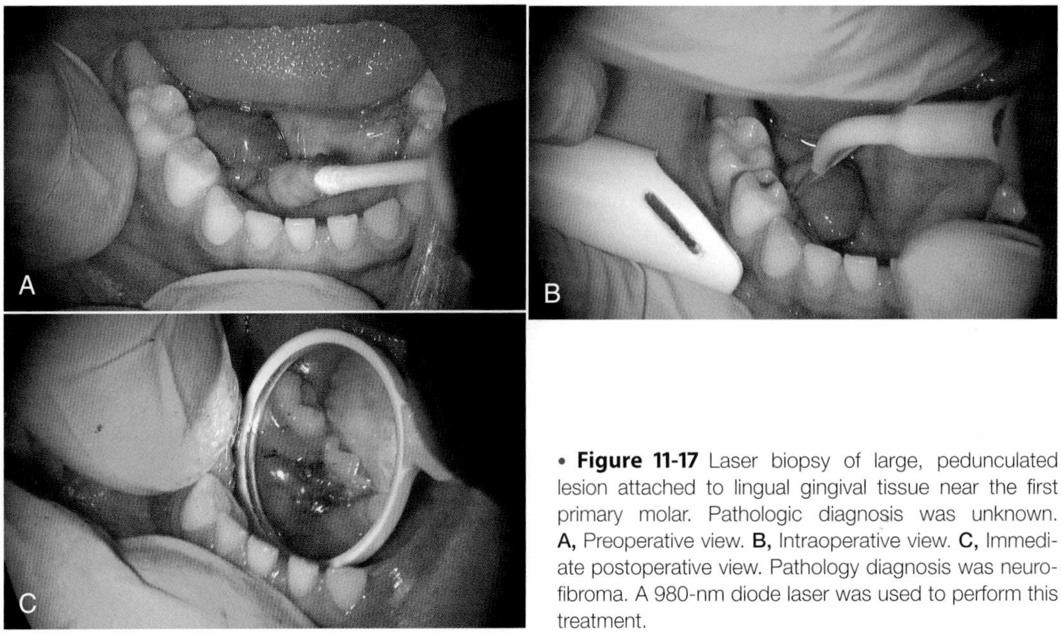

• **Figure 11-17** Laser biopsy of large, pedunculated lesion attached to lingual gingival tissue near the first primary molar. Pathologic diagnosis was unknown. **A,** Preoperative view. **B,** Intraoperative view. **C,** Immediate postoperative view. Pathology diagnosis was neurofibroma. A 980-nm diode laser was used to perform this treatment.

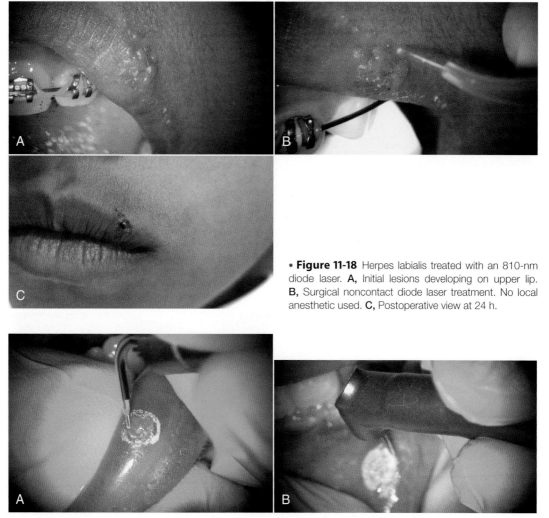

• **Figure 11-18** Herpes labialis treated with an 810-nm diode laser. **A,** Initial lesions developing on upper lip. **B,** Surgical noncontact diode laser treatment. No local anesthetic used. **C,** Postoperative view at 24 h.

• **Figure 11-19** Aphthous ulcer treatment using an erbium laser. **A,** Intraoperative view. **B,** White pock-marked lesion at completion of treatment.

pain associated with herpes labialis lesions. Treatment of these lesions usually is performed at low power settings in a defocused mode. The purpose is not to ablate the tissue but to modify the surface epithelium of the lesion (Figures 11-18 and 11-19).

Anecdotal reports indicate that the aphthous ulcer will not recur in the specific laser-treated site. The reason for this beneficial effect is unknown.

Treating herpes labialis involves passing the laser tip slowly over the entire portion of the lip that is infected, just short of observing the white change in tissue color. This procedure usually involves treating the entire one half of the lip involved. The process takes 1 to 2 min, usually without anesthesia. When herpeslike lesions are treated at the first signs of an infection, such lesions often can be eliminated permanently.

CLINICAL TIP

When treating aphthous ulcers, make certain that the treated area includes the entire lesion as well as at least 3 to 5 mm lateral to the erythematous halo marking this lesion's border. If a small area of healthy tissue around the lesion is not treated along with the entire lesion, the ulcer will recur.

Pericoronitis (Operculitis)

Pericoronal inflammation, or infection of the gingiva surrounding the crown of the tooth during the eruption of molars, may cause patient discomfort. This tissue can be removed with any wavelength of laser. If chosen, the erbium laser must not contact the enamel; otherwise, a small area of hard tissue could be ablated. The advantage of the erbium laser is that only topical anesthesia may be required. When other wavelengths are used to treat pericoronitis, injection anesthesia usually is necessary. The potential disadvantage of using the erbium laser is less hemostasis postoperatively than with the other wavelengths, and the slight risk of ablating hard tissue once the soft tissue has been removed (Figure 11-20).

Laser Tissue Welding

For children with fissures and cracks on the lips, lasers can be used for welding the tissue together.[47,48] The purpose is not to ablate tissue, so low power in defocused mode is used. The tissue appears to self-weld, improving healing. The laser's bactericidal effect also promotes healing (Figure 11-21).

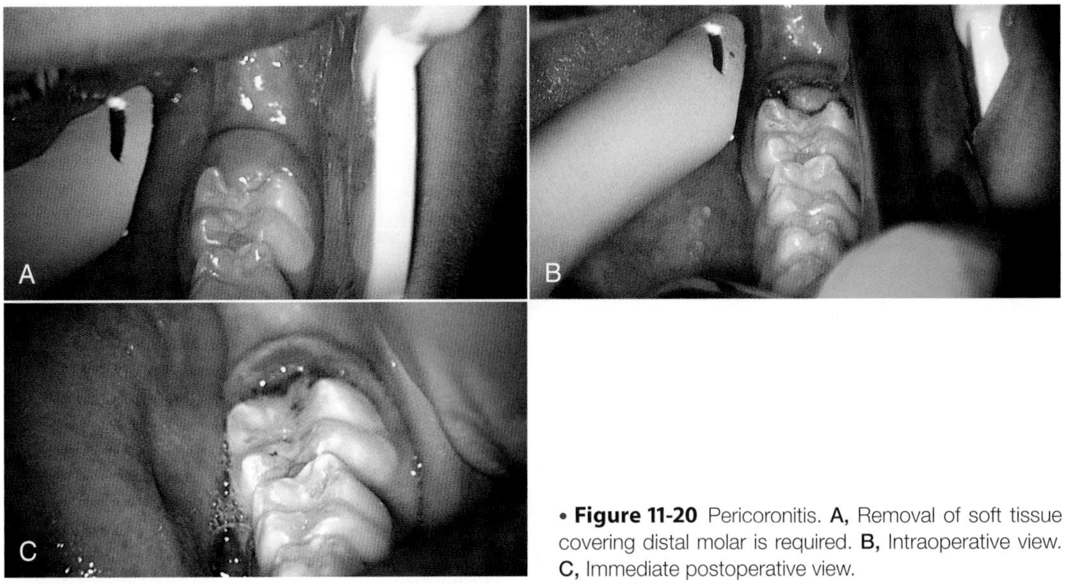

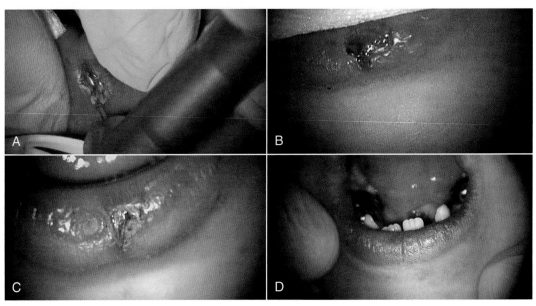

• **Figure 11-20** Pericoronitis. **A,** Removal of soft tissue covering distal molar is required. **B,** Intraoperative view. **C,** Immediate postoperative view.

• **Figure 11-21** **A,** Laser tissue welding of open fissure in lower lip. **B,** Immediate postoperative view. **C,** Postoperative view at 48 h. **D,** Tissue healed completely without reopening at 3 weeks.

Impacted Mesiodens

Lasers may be used for the surgical removal of mesiodens. The laser replaces a scalpel in cutting palatal tissue to gain access to the unerupted tooth. The area must be anesthetized. If bone is covering the tooth, or if the tooth is ankylosed and sectioning of bone or tooth is necessary, the erbium or 9300-nm CO_2 lasers may be used for the hard tissue procedure. The soft tissue is separated from the bone by means of a periosteal elevator. Laser advantages include reduced healing time, bactericidal effects at the surgical site, and greatly reduced postsurgical discomfort (Figure 11-22).

Venous Lake on Lower Lip

A venous lake, or venous pool, lesion manifests as a soft, bluish, discrete, painless nodule beneath the epithelium of the lower lip. Although such lesions usually are seen after the age of 40 years, the patient shown in Figure 11-23 presented with a venous lake lesion at the age of 8 years. A venous lake or pool often is the result of an injury to the lip. The two-step treatment involves first using the laser out of contact at low power (<1 W) for a few minutes for deep penetration into the lesion, which is rich in hemoglobin; the Nd:YAG or diode laser with an uninitiated tip would therefore be the preferred laser. After the lesion has absorbed sufficient laser energy, any laser can then be used in contact to open the tissue and remove the remaining dried blood.[49-53]

Tooth Exposure for Orthodontic Banding

Removal of soft tissue covering an unerupted permanent tooth usually requires no local anesthetic. All lasers can perform this treatment; however, caution must be used in angulating the

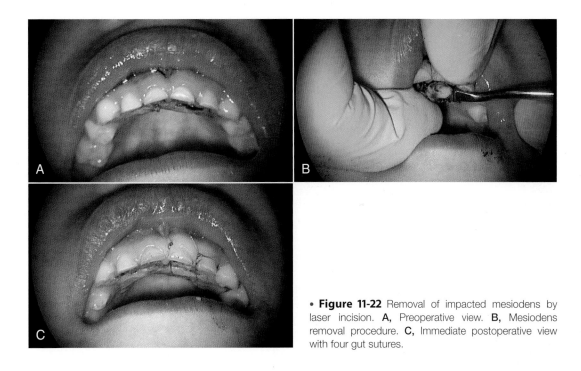

• **Figure 11-22** Removal of impacted mesiodens by laser incision. **A,** Preoperative view. **B,** Mesiodens removal procedure. **C,** Immediate postoperative view with four gut sutures.

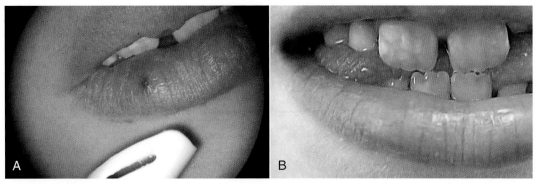

• **Figure 11-23 A,** Venous lake lesion on lip of 8-year-old girl. **B,** Six weeks after laser treatment.

laser tip toward the tissue. Direct contact of an erbium laser with the tooth could ablate tooth structure. Direct contact between a tooth and any of the other wavelengths could create charring of the enamel, which is easily polished off with a prophy cup or rubber wheel (Figure 11-24). (See Chapter 12.)

Pulpotomy and Pulpectomy

Primary teeth that have exposed pulp tissue resulting from caries, mechanical removal of carious tissue, or preventive procedures on severely abraded teeth require a pulpotomy or pulpectomy.[54,55] In a *pulpotomy*, as defined by the American Academy of Pediatric Dentistry, the coronal pulp is amputated and the remaining vital radicular pulp tissue surface is treated with a medicament (e.g., formocresol, ferric sulfate)[56] or with electrocautery to preserve the pulp's health. Mineral trioxide aggregate (MTA) also has been used as therapeutic pulp-dressing agent.[57]

A *pulpectomy* is defined as a root canal procedure for pulp tissue that is irreversibly infected or necrotic as a result of

caries or traumatic injury. The objective of both pulpectomy and pulpotomy is to maintain a tooth both functionally and painlessly without disease until the primary tooth normally exfoliates with eruption of the underlying permanent tooth, or until the tooth is adequately developed for definitive root canal therapy.

Lasers are an effective alternative for treating pulpal disease, with the additional benefit of providing pulp therapy without introducing chemicals into children's systems. Small amounts of formocresol may be absorbed and distributed throughout the child's body within minutes of its use at the pulpotomy site,[58] and parents may express concern about the effect of such medicaments.

Pulpotomy is one of the clinical indications for use of lasers.[31,59,60] Successful treatment can delay the need to extract a nonvital primary tooth until a space maintainer can be inserted. Lasers provide a safe, effective, nonchemical alternative to pulpotomy.[61,62] In the author's clinical experience, excellent results in more than 5000 laser pulpotomies, performed over more than 6 years presumably confirm the

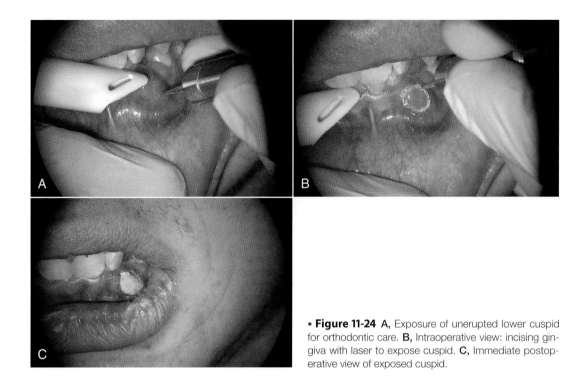

• **Figure 11-24 A,** Exposure of unerupted lower cuspid for orthodontic care. **B,** Intraoperative view: incising gingiva with laser to expose cuspid. **C,** Immediate postoperative view of exposed cuspid.

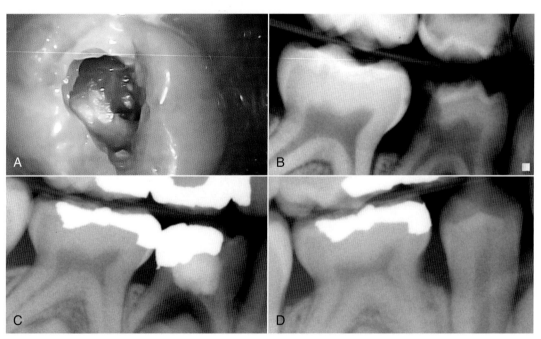

• **Figure 11-25 A,** Access for pulpotomy. **B,** Radiograph of lower first primary molar requiring pulpotomy. **C,** Radiographic view of completed pulpotomy. This successful laser-assisted treatment allowed the permanent bicuspid to erupt successfully 5 years later. **D,** Radiograph of 5-year postoperative view showing the permanent bicuspid in place.

safety and effectiveness of this technique in children without the need for chemicals or electrosurgery (Figure 11-25).

Combined Procedures

The advantage of the erbium wavelength is that it can be used for both hard tissue and soft tissue procedures, as shown in Figure 11-26.

Low-Level (Photobiostimulating) Laser Therapy

As discussed earlier, the effectiveness of low-level (PBS) lasers, also known as "cold lasers," is backed up by more than 2500 studies, although many of these are poorly controlled and do not meet the Western medical criteria (see Chapter 15).

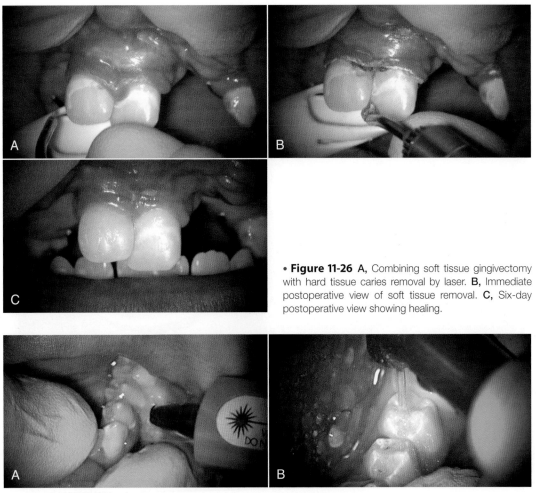

• **Figure 11-26 A,** Combining soft tissue gingivectomy with hard tissue caries removal by laser. **B,** Immediate postoperative view of soft tissue removal. **C,** Six-day postoperative view showing healing.

• **Figure 11-27** Laser analgesia. **A,** Low-level laser placed over root area of tooth for 1 minute. **B,** Erbium laser placed over occlusal surface of tooth for 2 min.

The pediatric applications described in this section are not well documented in the literature but have proved to be successful treatment modalities in the author's clinical experience, and that of many other dentists, with PBS lasers. Use of LLLT in the pediatric dental office offers another laser treatment modality for the following indications:
• Dental analgesia
• Treatment of hard tissue trauma
• Treatment of soft tissue trauma
• Treatment of primary herpes and herpes labialis
• Controlling the gag reflex

Analgesic Effect

A PBS analgesic effect can be achieved with either specific lasers limited to low-level energy [63-65] or surgical lasers used in a defocused mode, which does not cause photothermal buildup in the dental tissue. The technique involves placing the tip of the surgical laser, in defocused mode (noncontact, 1 to 3 mm off the tooth surface), over the crown of the tooth for 1 to 2 min. Tooth preparation can then be completed using a hard tissue laser. Alternatively, in preparing primary or permanent teeth, a high-speed handpiece can be used to complete

an alloy preparation without causing patient discomfort (if not previously used on the pediatric patient). Whether a composite or an alloy restoration is placed, the patient can leave the office without the need for a local anesthetic. In children, this beneficial effect eliminates the potential for traumatic injury of tissue from lip biting (Figure 11-27).

Traumatized Primary and Permanent Anterior Teeth

Children often sustain accidental injury to the maxillary or mandibular anterior primary teeth. Such injury may result in pulpal death and tooth discoloration.[66,67] These complications usually will develop within 2 to 6 weeks after trauma to the area. Infants and toddlers 7 months to 5 years of age have benefited from treatment with a 660-nm or 830-nm low-level laser placed over the root areas of the injured teeth for 1 minute. Patients with slightly mobile, partially avulsed, or displaced front teeth who received LLLT within 24 h of injury demonstrated clinically and radiographically normal teeth in color and vitality and remained asymptomatic for as long as 36 months after trauma (Figures 11-28 and 11-29).

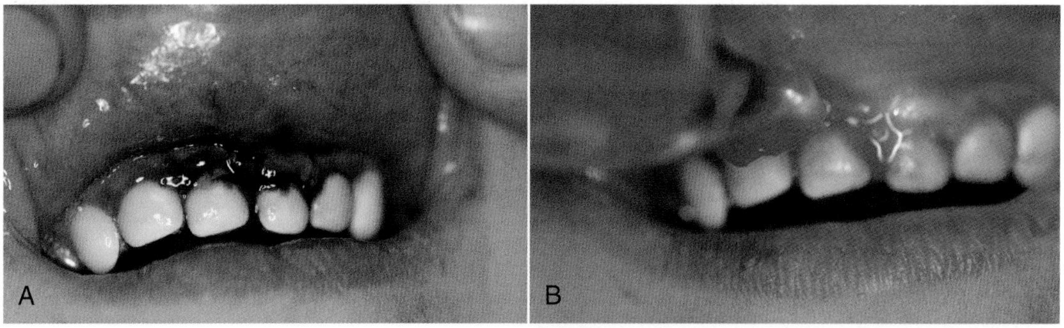

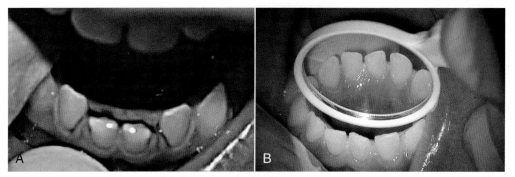

• **Figure 11-28 A,** Anterior trauma. **B,** Treatment using low-level laser for 1 minute per tooth.

• **Figure 11-29 A,** Trauma with partial avulsion of lower anterior teeth. **B,** Two years after low-level laser treatment.

CASE STUDY 11-1

An 8-year-old girl presented for emergency treatment of a partial avulsion of tooth #9. The tooth extended out of the alveolus approximately 5 mm. The tooth was gently repositioned, splinted, and treated with the 660-nm LLLT probe for 1 minute. This treatment was repeated 3 days and again 7 days later. After 23 months, the tooth remained vital and asymptomatic (Figure 11-30).

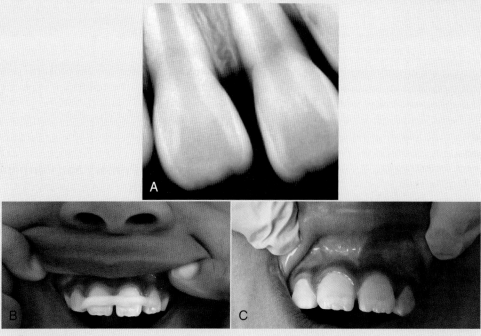

• **Figure 11-30** Partially avulsed permanent incisor. **A,** Preoperative radiograph. **B,** Tooth splinted and treated with low-level laser 1 minute over lingual and facial areas. **C,** Tooth remains vital 23 months after treatment.

CASE STUDY 11-2

An 8-year-old boy presented with multiple intraoral herpetic lesions and complained of significant discomfort. The low-level laser globe was placed extraorally for 3 min. At the follow-up appointment 4 days later, the patient had no further discomfort, with elimination of most lesions[68] (Figure 11-31).

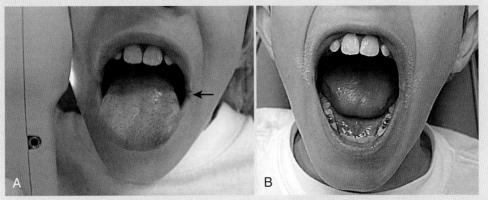

• **Figure 11-31 A,** Immediately before treatment of primary herpes using low-level (PBS) laser cluster for 3 min. **B,** Area is free of lesions 4 days after treatment.

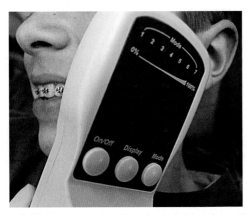

• **Figure 11-32** Treatment of patient immediately after orthodontic adjustment.

For treatment of traumatic injury to primary and permanent teeth, a radiograph is taken to ensure that the tooth has not sustained a root fracture. The low-level laser is placed over the lingual and facial areas of the root for approximately 1 minute (4 J/area). A soft diet is then instituted. Depending on the degree of injury, additional LLLT, at the same energy setting, may be performed at 3 and 5 days postoperatively (Case Study 11-1).

Intraoral Primary Herpes

See Case Study 11-2 and Figure 11-31.

Orthodontic Adjustment or Temporomandibular Joint Discomfort

Patients with discomfort caused by orthodontic adjustments or with temporomandibular joint (TMJ) discomfort may obtain relief with use of the following protocol: The laser/LED unit is held over the external facial area for 3 min, and then the 660-nm or 830-nm probe is placed into the posterior oral cavity, where trigger points for pain from TMJ

CASE STUDY 11-3

A 13-year-old boy presented with a mandibular swelling caused by an abscessed lower molar, with pain and limited ability to open the mouth. This restriction also hindered clinical examination of the oral cavity and prevented operative access to the infected tooth to allow for drainage and pain relief. Placing the diode and LED globe portion of the low-level (PBS) laser over the affected side for 3 min provided sufficient relief of muscle trismus to allow adequate mouth opening and drainage of the infected tooth (Figure 11-33).

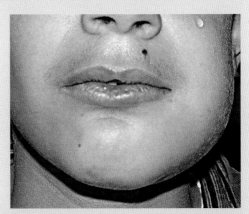

• **Figure 11-33** Patient with facial cellulitis and limited mouth opening treated with low-level laser applied for 3 min.

syndrome are present.[68-69] Repeating this treatment three to five times within 1 week for patients with TMJ pain significantly reduces or eliminates discomfort (Case Study 11-3 and Figure 11-32). The mechanism of action is outlined in Chapter 15.

Facial Injuries

Low-level laser treatment appears to stimulate the proliferation of fibroblasts within the gingival tissue.[70-74]

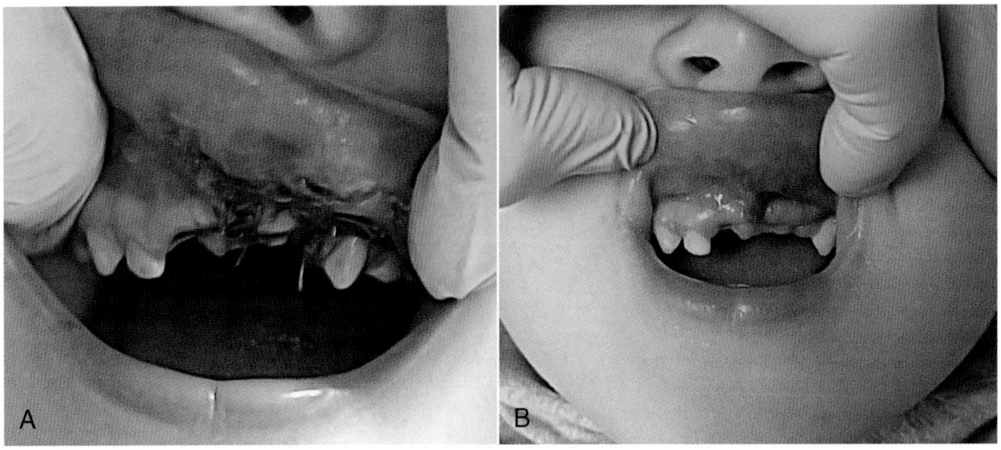

• **Figure 11-34** **A,** Facial injury treated with LLLT. **B,** Six-day postoperative view.

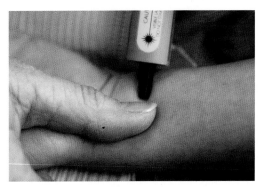

• **Figure 11-35** Control of gag reflex achieved with diode laser placed on P6 acupuncture point for 1 minute.

Pediatric surgical patients pretreated with photobiostimulation had reduced postsurgical pain and inflammation. Low-level (PBS) lasers result in enhanced healing as measured by wound contraction. Stimulation of healing in soft tissues to resolve inflammation, provide pain relief, and improve the wound's tensile strength helps the immune system resolve infection (Figure 11-34). Rochkind et al.[75] also found that the effects from irradiating one area were seen in other contemporaneous wounds, suggesting a systemic effect of LLLT. This possibility may explain why a study comparing the left and right sides in a patient will fail to show any difference between placebo effect and laser effect.

Reducing the Gag Reflex

Applying the 660-nm diode laser at approximately 4 J to the P6 acupuncture point provides relief from the gag reflex in many children. The P6 point is located on the undersurface of the wrist approximately 2.5 cm (1 inch) from the wrist crease, approximating the width of the distal thumb phalanx. In patients with gag reflexes strong enough to preclude intraoral radiography or molar evaluation, placement of the 660-nm diode laser on P6 for 1 minute resulted in good reflex control, allowing the necessary evaluation procedures[76-79] (Figure 11-35).

Conclusions

Lasers constitute an extremely versatile addition to pediatric dentistry and often can be used instead of conventional methods. Incorporating a laser into the pediatric dental practice should be viewed as an investment rather than a cost. When used with a good knowledge of laser physics and laser safety, lasers provide pediatric patients with a new standard of dental care.

References

1. Maiman T: Stimulated optical radiation in ruby, *Nature* 187: 493–494, 1960.
2. Kotlow L: The use of the erbium hard and soft tissue laser in the pediatric dental practice, *J Southeast Soc Pediatr Dent* 17:12–14, 2001.
3. Hinson P: Three, two, one, blast off! President's message, *Pediatr Dent Today Newslett* 4–5, September 2005.
4. Aoki A, Ishikawa I, Yamada T, et al.: A comparison of conventional handpiece versus erbium:YAG laser for root caries in vitro, *J Restorative Dent* 77:1404–1414, 1998.
5. Sasaki K, Aoki A, Ichinose S, et al.: Scanning electron microscopy and Fourier transformation spectroscopy analysis for bone removal using Er:YAG and CO_2 lasers, *J Periodontol* 73:643–652, 2002.
6. Hossain M, Nakamura Y, Yamada Y: Effects of Er,Cr:YSGG laser irradiation in human enamel and dentin, *J Clin Laser Med Surg* 17:105–109, 1999.
7. Hibst R, Keller U, Steiner R: The effects of pulsed Er:YAG laser irradiation on dental tissue, *Laser Med Surg* 4:163–165, 1988.
8. Goodis HE, et al.: Pulpal safety of 9.6 micron TEA CO_2 laser used for caries prevention, *Laser Surg Med* 35:104–110, 2004.
9. Seka W, Featherstoe J, Fried D, et al.: Laser ablation of dental hard tissue: from explosive ablation to plasma –mediated ablation, *Proc SPIE* 2672:144–158, 1996.
10. Frame JW: Carbon dioxide laser surgery for benign oral lesions, *Br Dent J* 158:125–128, 1985.
11. Pecaro BC, Garehime WJ: The CO_2 laser in oral and maxillofacial surgery, *J Oral Maxillofac Surg* 41:725–728, 1983.
12. White JM, Goodis HE, Rose CM: Use of the pulsed Nd:YAG for intraoral soft tissue surgery, *Lasers Surg Med* 11:455–461, 1991.

13. Moritz A, Gutknecht N, Doertbudak O: Bacterial reduction in periodontal pockets through irradiation with a diode laser, *J Clin Laser Med Surg* 15:33–37, 1997.

14. Coluzzi DJ: Lasers and soft tissue curettage: an update, *Compendium* 23:1004–1011, 2002.

15. Walsh LJ: The current status of low level laser therapy in dentistry. Part 1. Soft tissue applications, *Aust Dent J* 42(4):247–254, 1997.

16. Walsh LJ: The current status of low level laser therapy in dentistry. Part 2. Hard tissue applications, *Aust Dent J* 42(5):302–306, 1997.

17. Sun G, Tuner J: Low-level laser therapy in dentistry, *Dent Clin North Am* 48(4):1061–1076 viii, 2004.

18. Dyson M: Cellular effects of LLLT, *Laser Ther J* 2(1):14–18, 1990.

19. Van As G: Magnification and alternatives for microdentistry, *Compendium* 22(11A):108–114, 2001.

20. Nase JB: Dental operating microscopes: the next era in general dentistry, *Diamond (Maurice H. Kornberg School of Dentistry Magazine)* [Temple University] 11:12–14, 2002.

21. Coluzzi DJ: An overview of laser wavelengths used in dentistry, *Dent Clin North Am* 44:776, 2000.

22. Miserendino LJ, Pick RM: *Lasers in dentistry*, Chicago, 1995, Quintessence, pp 145–160.

23. White JM, Goodis HE, Setcos JC, et al.: Effects of pulsed Nd:YAG laser energy on human teeth: a 3-year follow-up study, *J Am Dent Assoc* 124:45–50, 1993.

24. Diaci Laser Profilometry for the characterization of craters produced in hard dental tissues by the Er:YAG and Er,Cr:YSGG lasers, *J Laser Health Acad* 2/1, 2008.

25. Rechmann P, Goldin D, Henning T: Er:YAG lasers in dentistry: an overview, *Proc SPIE* 3248:1–13, 1998.

26. Kotlow LA: Pediatric dentistry begins at birth: laser and pediatric dental care in treating soft tissue lesions in the dental office, *J Pediatr Dent Care* 13(1):12–16, 2007.

27. Kotlow LA: Oral diagnosis of abnormal frenum attachments in neonates and infants: evaluation and treatment of the maxillary and lingual frenum using the erbium:YAG laser, *J Pediatr Dent Care* 10(3):11-14, 26–28, 2004.

28. Kotlow LA: Ankyloglossia (tongue-tie): a diagnostic and treatment quandary, *Quintessence Int* 30(4):259–262, 1999.

29. Parks F, O'Toole T, Yancy J: Laser treatments of aphthous and herpetic lesions, *J Dent Res* 73:190, 1994.

30. Liu H, Yan MN, Zhao EY, et al.: Preliminary report on the effect of Nd:YAG laser irradiation on canine tooth pulps, *Chin J Dent Res* 3(4):63–65, 2000.

31. Odabas ME, Bodur H, Baris E, Demir C: Clinical, radiological, and histopathologic evaluation of Nd:YAG laser pulpotomy on human primary teeth, *J Endod* 33(4):415–421, 2007.

32. Marmet C, Shell E, Marment R: Neonatal frenotomy may be necessary to correct breastfeeding problems, *J Hum Lact* 6: 117–120, 1990.

33. Ballard J, Auer RN, et al.: Ankyloglossia: assessment, incidence and effect of frenuloplasty on the breastfeeding dyad, *Pediatrics* 110(5):e63, 2002.

34. Defabianus P: Ankyloglossia and its influence on maxillary and mandibular development: a 7-year follow-up case study, *Funct Orthod* 17(4):25–33, 2000.

35. Nostestine GE: The importance of the identification of ankyloglossia (short lingual frenum) as a cause of breastfeeding problems, *J Hum Lact* 6:113–115, 1990.

36. US Department of Health and Human Services, Office on Women's Health and the Ad Council; www.hhs.gov/news/press/ 2004pres/20040604, www.4women.gov/Breastfeeding/print-bf. cfm?page227. Accessed June 2004.

37. Ballard JL, Chantry C, Howard CR: Protocol Committee, Academy of Breastfeeding Medicine (ABM): guidelines for the evaluation and management of neonatal ankyloglossia and its complications in the breastfeeding dyad. ABM Clinical Protocol No 9, *ABM News Views* 2004.

38. Huang W: The midline diastema: a review of its etiology and treatment, *Pediatr Dent* 17(3):171–179, 1995.

39. Weissinger D: Breastfeeding difficulties as the result of tight lingual and labial frena, *J Hum Lact* 11(4):313–316, 1995.

40. American Academy of Pediatrics: *Breastfeeding: best for baby and mother* [online serial], Summer 2004.

41. Corn H: Technique for repositioning the frenum in periodontal problems, *Dent Clin North Am* 90, March 1964.

42. Oesrerle LJ: Maxillary midline diastemas: a look at the causes, the midline diastema, *J Am Dent Assoc* 130(1):85–94, 1999.

43. Barak S, Kaplan I: The CO_2 laser in the excision of gingival hyperplasia caused by nifedipine, *J Clin Periodontol* 15:633–635, 1988.

44. Pick PM, Pecaro BC, Silberman CJ: The laser gingivectomy: the use of the CO_2 laser for the removal of phenytoin hyperplasia, *J Periodontol* 56:492–494, 1985.

45. Colvard M, Kuo P: Managing aphthous ulcers: laser treatment applied, *J Am Dent Assoc* 122:51–52, 1991.

46. Convissar RA: Aphthous ulcers and lasers, *Oral Surg Oral Med Oral Pathol Oral Radiol Endod* 82(2):118, 1996.

47. Phillips AB, Ginsberg BY, Shin SJ: Laser welding for vascular anastomosis using albumin solder, *Laser Surg Med* 24:264–268, 1999.

48. Bass LS, Treat MR: Laser tissue welding: a comprehensive review of current and future clinical applications, *Laser Surg Med* 17:315–349, 1995.

49. Rice JH: Removal of venous lake using a diode laser (810 mn), *Wavelengths* 12(1):20–21, 2004.

50. Neumann RA, Knobler RM: Venous lakes (Bean-Walsh) of the lips: treatment experience with the argon laser and 18 month follow-up, *Clin Exp Dermatol* 15:115, 1990.

51. Bekhor PS: Long-pulsed Nd:YAG laser treatment of venous lakes: report of a series of 34 cases, *Dermatol Surg* 32:1151, 2006.

52. Del Pozo J, Pena C, Garcia Silva J, et al.: Venous lakes: a report of 32 cases treated by carbon dioxide laser vaporization, *Dermatol Surg* 29:308, 2003.

53. Kotlow LA: Elimination of a venous lake on the vermilion of the lower lip via 810-nm diode laser, *J Laser Dent* 15(1):20–22, 2007.

54. American Academy of Pediatric Dentistry: Guideline on pulp therapy for primary and young permanent teeth, *Pediatr Dent Ref Manual* 28(7):145, 2006-2007.

55. Farooq NS, Coll JA, Kuwabara A, Shelton P: Success rates of formocresol pulpotomy and indirect pulp therapy in the treatment of deep dentinal caries in primary teeth, *Pediatr Dent* 22(4):278–286, 2000.

56. Smith NL, Sealc NS, Nunn ME: Ferric sulfate pulpotomy in primary molars: a retrospective study, *Pediatr Dent* 22:192–199, 2000.

57. Eidelman E, Holan G, Fuks AB: Mineral trioxide aggregate vs. formocresol in pulpotomized primary molars: a preliminary report, *Pediatr Dent* 23(1):15–18, 2001.

58. Pashley EL, Myers DR, Pashley DH, Whitford GM: Systemic distribution of 14c-formaldehyde from formocresol-treated pulpotomy sites, *J Dent Res* 59(3):603–608, 1980.

59. Camp JH, Barrett EJ, Pulver F: Pediatric endodontics: endodontic treatment for the primary and young, permanent dentition. In Cohen S, Burns RC, editors: *Pathways of the pulp*, ed 8, St Louis, 2002, Mosby, pp 797–844.

60. Liu H, Yan MN, Zhao EY, et al.: Preliminary report on the effect of Nd:YAG laser irradiation on canine tooth pulps, *Chin J Dent Res* 3(4):63–65, 2000.
61. Shabholz A, Sahar-Helft S, Moshonov J: Lasers in endodontics, *Dent Clin North Am* 48(4):816, 2004.
62. Kotlow LA: Use of an Er:YAG laser for pulpotomies in vital and nonvital primary teeth, *J Laser Dent* 16(2):75–79, 2008.
63. Tsuchiya K, Kawatani M, et al.: Laser irradiation abates neuronal responses to nociceptive stimulation of rat-paw skin, *Brain Res Bull* 34:369–374, 1994.
64. Mezawa S, Iwata K, Naito K, Kamogawa H: The possible analgesic effects of soft tissue laser irradiation on heat nociceptors in the cat tongue, *Arch Oral Biol* 33:693–694, 1988.
65. Navratil L, Dylevsky I: Mechanism of the analgesic effect of therapeutic lasers, *In Vivo Laser Ther* 6:33–39, 1997.
66. Erickson F: Anterior tooth trauma in the primary dentition: incidence, classification, treatment methods, and sequelae: a review of the literature, *ASCD J Dent Child* 62(4):256–261, 1995.
67. Andreasen JO: Sequelae of trauma to primary incisors. I. Complications in the primary dentition, *Endod Dent Traum* 14(1):31–44, 1998.
68. Toida M, Watanabe F, Goto K, Shibata T: Usefulness of low-level laser for control of painful stomatitis in patients with hand-foot-and-mouth disease, *J Clin Laser Med Surg* 21(6):363–367, 2003.
69. Lim HM, Lew KK, Tay DK: A clinical investigation of the efficacy of low level laser therapy in reduction of orthodontic post adjustment pain, *Am J Orthod Dentofacial Orthop* 108(6):614–622, 1995.
70. Pourzarandian A, Watanabe H, Ruwanpura SM, et al.: Effect of low-level Er:YAG laser irradiation on cultured human gingival fibroblasts, *J Periodontol* 76(2):187–193, 2005.
71. Mendez V, Pinheiro AL, Pacheco MT, et al.: Assessment of the influence of the dose and wavelength of LLLT on the repair of cutaneous wounds, *Proc SPIE* 4950:137–143, 2003.
72. Hopkins JT: Low-level laser therapy facilitates superficial wound healing in humans: a triple-blind, sham-controlled study, *J Athlet Train* 39(3):223–229, 2004.
73. Simon A: *Low level laser therapy for wound healing: an update*, IP-22 Information Paper. Edmonton, 2004, Alberta Heritage Foundation for Medical Research.
74. Woodruff LD, Bounkeo JM, Brannon WM, et al.: The efficacy of laser therapy in wound repair: a meta-analysis of the literature, *Photomed Laser Surg* 22(3):241–247, 2004.
75. Rochkind MD, Rousso M, Nissan M, et al.: Systemic effects of low-power laser irradiation on the peripheral and central nervous system, cutaneous wounds and burns, *Lasers Surg Med* 9:174, 1989.
76. Schlager A, Offer T, Baldissera I: Laser stimulation of acupuncture point p6 reduces postoperative vomiting in children undergoing strabismus surgery, *Br J Anaesth* 81:529–532, 1998.
77. Agarwal MD, Bose N, Gaur A, et al.: Acupuncture and ondansetron for postoperative nausea and vomiting after laparoscopic cholecystectomy, *Can J Anaesth* 49(6):554–560, 2002.
78. Dundee JW, Yang J: Prolongation of the antiemetic action of P6 acupuncture by acupressure in patients having cancer chemotherapy, *J R Soc Med* 83(6):360–362, 1990.
79. Fan CF, Tanhui E, Joshi S: Acupressure treatment for prevention of vomiting and postoperative nausea and vomiting, *Anesth Analg* 84:821–825, 1997.

12

Lasers in Orthodontics

LOUIS G. CHMURA AND ROBERT A. CONVISSAR

Orthodontic patients are now looking for more than straight front teeth and a good bite. They want optimal results with minimal effort as quickly as possible. To be successful, orthodontists must not only provide the best dental and facial results possible but also deliver esthetic soft tissue results efficiently. The proper use of a laser in an orthodontic office can accelerate treatment, reduce the number and length of appointments needed, and provide superior results. Two different types of lasers may be used in orthodontic practice: soft tissue surgical lasers, which are used to incise/excise tissue; and photobiomodulating (PBM) lasers, which decrease posttreatment discomfort, favorably affect bone growth rate, and accelerate tooth movement.

Choosing a Soft Tissue Laser for Orthodontics

Dozens of soft tissue lasers are available to orthodontists, each with special features and characteristics. Choosing the "best" laser can be difficult. Because the primary concern for many orthodontists is to "avoid trouble," it may be helpful to identify features both wanted and *not* wanted in a soft tissue laser. One primary consideration important to orthodontists would be to effectively treat soft tissue while avoiding alteration of hard tissues. Additional considerations might be portability and cost.

Manufacturers claim all wavelengths are capable of performing soft tissue procedures, but some wavelengths, such as those emitted by the erbium family of lasers (Er:YAG, Er,Cr:YSGG), are also promoted as suitable for hard tissue procedures. These lasers usually require water cooling, so they tend to be bulky and relatively expensive in comparison with lasers with other wavelengths. Carbon dioxide (CO_2) laser wavelengths are well absorbed by water, and because oral mucosa is more than 90% water, CO_2 lasers are very effective soft tissue lasers. In addition, CO_2 lasers often have a "superpulse" feature, providing relatively high energy in short spurts, offering a very efficient means to ablate soft tissue. On the other hand, CO_2 lasers often are larger and more expensive than diode lasers.

Diode lasers, currently available in four distinct wavelengths (810 to 830, 940, 980, and 1064 nm), and neodymium-doped yttrium-aluminum-garnet (Nd:YAG) lasers (1064 nm) emit energies that are well absorbed by hemoglobin and melanin, so these lasers work well for ablation of pigmented and vascular tissues such as oral mucosa.[1] Diode lasers have a much shallower depth of penetration than Nd:YAG lasers and may be less likely to cause pulpal damage, making them an excellent choice in orthodontics.[2,3] In addition, diode lasers tend to be the least expensive and most portable of lasers of all wavelengths—another considerable advantage in orthodontics.

Currently available diode lasers vary in price, ranging from $3000 to $15,000, and the cost can easily be justified even without charging for procedures (to avoid offending their general dentist colleagues and other referring professionals). A $10,000 diode laser financed at 7% interest over 5 years results in a monthly payment just under $218. According to the *Journal of Clinical Orthodontics,* the value of an orthodontic appointment is between $200 and $400 (calculated by dividing the total fee collected by the number of appointments).[4] Thus, eliminating even one appointment per month justifies the cost of a laser. In reality, orthodontists who have adopted laser use "save" appointments several times each day.

Of course, the return on investment can be obtained more quickly when charges are made for some or all of these procedures. Depending on the orthodontist's personal business philosophy, the patient can be billed for the procedures or the fees can be submitted to the patient's dental or medical insurance. In submitting claims for reimbursement for any laser procedure, it is not necessary to specify that a laser was used. For example, billing for a laser gingivectomy would be submitted using the usual American Dental Association (ADA) code for a gingivectomy (D4210 or D4211, depending on the number of teeth involved). Releasing a lingual frenum (correction of "tongue-tie") may be considered a medical procedure and often is more effectively submitted to the patient's medical insurance company for reimbursement. In such cases, "Medical Insurance Claim Form" number 1500 is used (blank forms can be downloaded from the Internet or purchased from software or

TABLE 12-1	Common Codes for Medical Insurance Billing		
Procedure	ICD Diagnostic Code	Procedure Code	Description
Gingivectomy			
Chronic gingivitis	523.1	41820	
Frenotomy			
Tongue-tie	750	41115	Lingual frenum
Anomalies of accessory muscles	756.82	40819	Other frenum
Operculectomy			
Disturbance of tooth eruption	520.60	41821	
Chronic gingivitis, plaque-induced	523.10	41820	
Chronic gingivitis, non-plaque-induced	523.11	41820	

ICD, International Classification of Diseases.

office supply companies). In submitting claims for medical insurance, both a diagnosis code and a procedure code must be specified. In general, providing two or three diagnosis codes and one procedure code is optimal for each procedure (Table 12-1).

Although no "ideal" laser exists for every situation, with the use of CO_2,[5,6] diode,[7] and argon[8] lasers in orthodontic procedures reported in various studies, this chapter focuses on the use of diode lasers. The selection of the proper laser is based on individual preference. The practitioner is strongly urged to take multiple courses from instructors experienced with multiple wavelengths (see Chapter 16).

Types of Orthodontic Procedures

Many procedures can be done with a soft tissue laser, but the vast majority that orthodontists might perform fall into two categories: access gingivectomies[1] and esthetic procedures. *Access gingivectomies* involve exposing more tooth tissue for earlier or more ideal bracket or band placement. *Esthetic procedures* involve removing redundant gingival tissues to optimize gingival esthetics and improve appearance of completed orthodontic treatment. To perform these procedures most safely and efficiently, with the least discomfort for the patient, it is important to know what *not* to do. Three primary considerations should be kept in mind in performing soft tissue laser procedures: biologic width or zone, pocket depth, and keratinized tissue. For gingival esthetic procedures, several additional diagnostic considerations are of importance as well.

Diagnostic Considerations with Most Soft Tissue Procedures

Biologic Width/Biologic Zone

The concept of *biologic width,* or *biologic zone,* is important in restorative dentistry. When analyzing a series of gingivectomies, Garguilo et al.[9] found that regardless of the amount of tissue removed, tissue regrowth resulted in an average connective tissue attachment (CTA) of 1.07 mm, a junctional epithelium (JE) thickness of 0.97 mm, and a sulcus depth of 0.69 mm. These workers suggested that the distance from the height of the crestal bone to the gingival margin should be approximately 2.5 mm. Cohen[10] coined the phrase "biologic width" to refer to the combined JE and CTA: 0.97 + 1.07 = 2.04 mm.[11] Kois[12] extended this definition, adding all three—0.97 + 1.07 + 0.69 = 2.73 mm, with the result rounded to 3.0 mm—and termed this dimension the "biologic zone." Restorative dentists found that placing margins within the biologic zone resulted in chronic inflammation, and Kois has suggested that a biologic zone of 3.0 mm or more is necessary for a healthy dentogingival complex.[12] When a restoration is to be placed within the patient's biologic zone, the preferred solution would be to "sound the bone," probing through the pocket to the bone, and then exposing and removing enough bone to restore the 2.5- to 3.0-mm biologic zone.

Pocket Depth

In general, orthodontists are neither equipped for nor interested in performing hard tissue procedures such as removal of bone. In nearly all cases, removing redundant gingival tissue and leaving a pocket depth of 1 mm will be all that is needed in a typical orthodontic procedure. Although an understanding of the importance of biologic zone is essential to aid in discussions with colleagues, a much more practical approach is to simply measure pocket depth and plan to leave a 1.0-mm pocket, with the recognition that in most cases, violating the biologic zone will result in relapse to a 1.0-mm pocket. If a proposed gingival procedure will leave a pocket of *less* than 1.0 mm, laser gingivectomy may not be recommended, and referral for osseous crown lengthening is the preferred method of management (Figure 12-1).

Keratinized Tissue

Keratinized tissue is the immovable, fibrous, coral pink tissue surrounding the neck of each tooth. It extends from the free gingival margin to the mucogingival junction. Keratinized tissue is resistant to recession from toothbrushing or eating. Unattached gingiva is the movable, darker pink tissue also known as *alveolar mucosa* and is not strong enough to resist recession from normal trauma. In planning a gingival procedure, care must be taken to maintain at least 2 mm of attached gingiva. If the planned gingivectomy violates this minimum, a laser procedure may be inappropriate, and referral for surgical creation of an apically positioned flap may be more appropriate. Although special dyes can be used

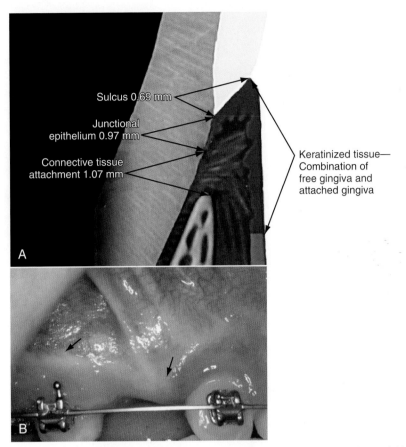

Sulcus 0.69 mm

Junctional epithelium 0.97 mm

Connective tissue attachment 1.07 mm

Keratinized tissue—Combination of free gingiva and attached gingiva

A

B

• **Figure 12-1 A,** Biologic width and area of keratinized tissue. **B,** Mucogingival junction *(arrows)*. Note the ample keratinized tissue on the upper right first bicuspid, but very little on the upper right cuspid.

to demarcate the mucogingival junction, it can easily be observed by having the patient move their lips and observing for corresponding movement of mucosa. In summary, the limiting factors to consider in planning most soft tissue procedures in an orthodontic office are to leave at least 1.0 mm of pocket depth and to preserve at least 2.0 mm of keratinized tissue.

Access Gingivectomies

Access to Partially Erupted Teeth

When a tooth is slow to emerge or a bracket is difficult to position, removing excess tissue not only enhances esthetics but also speeds treatment and reduces required appointments. Figure 12-2 shows a partially erupted maxillary cuspid. In such a case, the following options can be considered:

1. Wait for the tooth to erupt completely before bonding (6 to 12 months).
2. Bond to the exposed crown, erupt slightly, rebond and repeat, until enough crown is available to place a bracket in an ideal position.
3. Expose the tooth and bond immediately. A diode laser can be used to obtain access for near-ideal positioning of a bracket, allowing the operator to bring the cuspid into the arch and rotate it, saving months of treatment (see Figure 12-2B–D).

Access to Unerupted Teeth

When the tooth is visible just below the gingival surface but could take many months to emerge into the mouth (Figure 12-3A), the patient is often reluctant to visit the periodontist or primary care dentist for an exposure procedure, so orthodontic treatment is "on hold." If sufficient keratinized tissue is present, laser exposure with immediate bracket placement is possible, thereby saving the patient's months of waiting. In addition, the laser provides a clean, bloodless field, allowing a bracket to be bonded immediately after exposure (see Figure 12-3B, C). In the patient whose case is shown in Figure12-3, the tooth was rebonded 6 weeks later to improve bracket position and subsequently erupted to an ideal position. The initial window procedure was the only laser exposure performed. All additional tooth visibility was the result of eruption (see Figure 12-3D). The patient was thus spared months of treatment time and went on to attend school with an attractive smile and improved self-esteem.

Access for Ideal Bracket Placement

A common approach to position brackets properly involves placing brackets in the *center* of the clinical crown. To do so accurately, the practitioner must be able to visualize the clinical crown, which can be difficult when gingiva obscures tooth anatomy. A simple gingivectomy exposes the entire

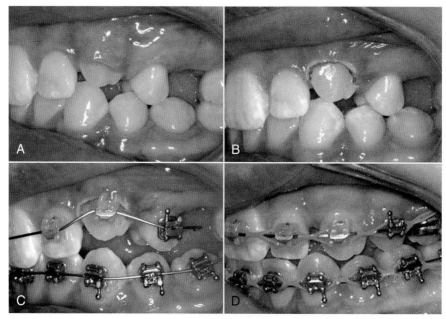

• **Figure 12-2** Gingivectomy to allow more ideal bracket placement and speed treatment. **A,** Immediately before procedure. **B,** Immediately after exposure. **C,** Bracket bonded in near-ideal position, ready for nickel-titanium wire. **D,** Six weeks later.

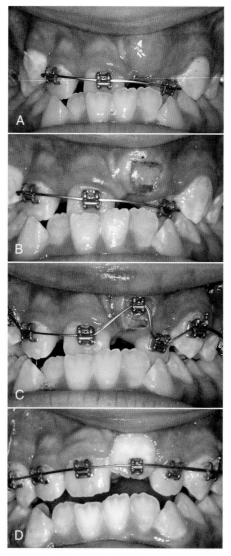

• **Figure 12-3 A,** Upper central incisors and lateral incisors not fully erupted. **B,** Simple gingivectomy exposes clinical crowns to aid ideal bracket placement. **C,** Brackets easily bonded, ideally at the same appointment in a clean field. **D,** Three weeks later, healing is complete and teeth have already aligned.

clinical crown, allows more accurate bracket placement, and speeds completion of treatment. With this procedure, not only was the patient in Figure 12-4 spared months of treatment but the exposure also afforded better access for cleaning, thereby reducing the risk of gingival hypertrophy during continued orthodontic treatment.

Access Resulting from Poor Oral Hygiene

Occasionally, a patient may have difficulty with oral hygiene, with consequent development of inflammatory gingival hyperplasia. With improved oral hygiene, the inflammation subsides, but the hypertrophy may not completely resolve. Figure 12-5 shows readiness for placement of full braces, but the gingival hypertrophy, partially erupted upper left cuspid, and unerupted upper right cuspid prevented ideal placement of brackets. A full-mouth gingivectomy was performed to remove excess tissue and expose the cuspids, allowing brackets to be placed properly and permitting the patient to maintain an improved level of hygiene during treatment.

Access Resulting from Overlying Operculum

In many patients, treatment cannot progress without banding or bonding second molars, but placement is hindered by an overlying operculum (Figure 12-6). Removing the excess tissue with immediate bonding allows treatment to progress. *Operculectomy* is one of the few procedures for which topical anesthesia may be insufficient, necessitating injection of local anesthetic.

Additional Diagnostic Considerations with Esthetic Procedures

Gingival Shape and Contour

Two important concepts of gingival architecture are gingival shape and gingival contour.[2] *Gingival shape* describes the gingival margin as seen in viewing a tooth "face on" (Figure 12-7). Several factors contribute to ideal gingival shape.[13–15] First, the gingival margins of the two central incisors should be at the same level and should form a smooth, sweeping curve; the apex of the curve should follow the contours of the cementoenamel junction (CEJ), with the height of contour inclined slightly to the distal. Second, the gingival margins of the canines should be at the same level as that of the central incisors. Third, the gingival margins of the lateral incisors should be 1.0 mm shorter than those of both the canines and the central incisors. Thus, when viewed from central incisor to cuspid, the gingival margin heights can be described as "high-low-high."

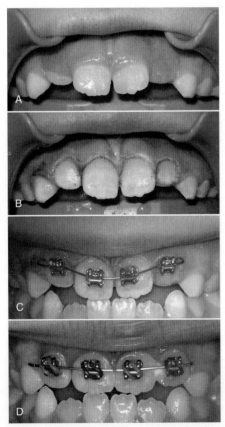

• **Figure 12-4 A,** Preoperative view of upper incisors **B,** Laser gingivectomy and exposure of upper incisors to allow bonding of brackets. **C,** Brackets bonded at the same appointment on a dry field. **D,** Four weeks later, alignment has already begun.

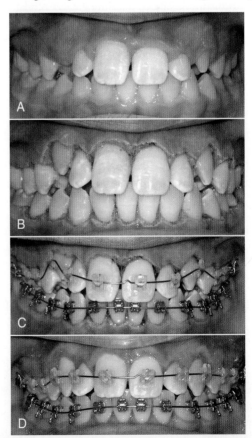

• **Figure 12-5 A,** Patient ready for treatment of gingival hypertrophy and unexposed cuspids. **B,** Immediately after gingivectomy and exposure. **C,** Teeth bonded same day. **D,** Six weeks later.

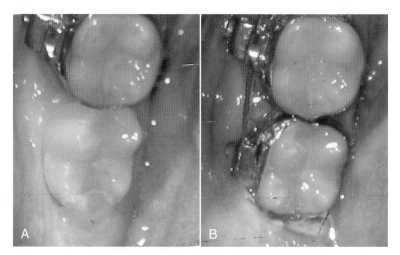

• **Figure 12-6 A,** Operculum partially covering distal of lower second molar. **B,** Operculum removed and band placed on lower second molar at same appointment, allowing immediate movement.

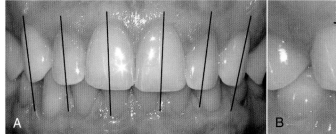
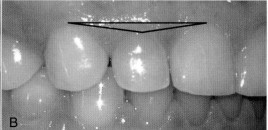

• **Figure 12-7 A,** Gingival margins define smooth curves, with the height of the gingival contour mildly distal. **B,** Gingival margins of central incisors and canines are at the same level, with the gingival margin of the lateral incisor 1.0 to 1.5 mm incisal (high-low-high from central to cuspid).

Gingival contour relates to the architecture of the gingiva parallel to the tooth surface. Healthy gingiva is relatively flat with a small, even curve just as the gingiva meets the tooth (Figure 12-8*A*). Hyperplastic gingivae are bulky and distended with a ledge at the gingival margin (see Figure 12-8*B*). If gingival shape is corrected without addressing contour, the excess bulk at the gingival margin can lead to relapse.[13]

Tooth Proportions

Widths of central incisors average from 8.4 to 9.3 mm, and lengths from 10.4 to 13.0 mm.[11–15] The ideal ratio of width to length is in the range of 75% to 80%,[12,16–20] with greater than 80% resulting in too "square" a tooth and less than 75% resulting in too long an appearance.[21] Using these ratios in concert with known dimensions of the tooth in question can help determine a more ideal treatment plan. These concepts are demonstrated in the clinical cases described in the following section.

Treatment Planning for Anterior Esthetics

Straightforward Situations

Sometimes after completion of orthodontic treatment, the teeth are aligned, but gingival contours do not conform to acceptable norms. In patients with such esthetic issues, gingival recontouring can greatly enhance the smile.

Figure 12-9 shows that the gingival architecture of the maxillary right central incisor is esthetic and harmonious relative to all other anterior teeth, except the upper left central incisor (pocket depth 2.0 mm). Removing 1.0 mm of

the left central gingiva leaves a pocket depth of 1.0 mm, with adequate keratinized tissue, and allows for harmonized gingival contours and a better result.

Figure 12-10 shows a similar discrepancy between the maxillary central incisor gingival margins in a patient ready to begin orthodontic treatment, but with no discrepancy in pocket depths and with the CEJs at different levels. Upon inspection, significant wear on the maxillary left central is evident (see Figure 12-10*B*), indicating that this tooth is hypererupted and worn. In this case, a soft tissue procedure is contraindicated. Instead, the left central incisor should be intruded to match gingival contours and then can be restored to a proper length. Diagnosing this situation at the beginning of treatment allows brackets to be placed appropriately.

Comprehensive Anterior Esthetics

In some situations, none of the anterior teeth exhibit ideal contours. Treatment planning involves evaluating the proportions of each tooth to determine ideal goals and designing the plan to ensure not only achievable goals but also sufficient time scheduled to complete the necessary procedures. First, measure the width of the central incisors. In Figure 12-11, for a patient who recently underwent debanding, the width of the central incisors is just over 9 mm (slightly wider than average). The estimated ideal width of a central usually is 80% of the length; so divide 9 by 0.8 for an estimated ideal length for the central of 11.25 mm. This becomes the initial goal for an ideal central incisor length.

Next, for each of the anterior teeth, measure the length, amount of keratinized tissue available, and depth of sulcus at the proposed gingival crest (Table 12-2). These data allow

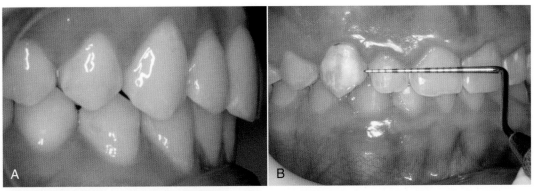

• **Figure 12-8 A,** Healthy gingiva and gingival margins, flat with a small, free-gingival groove just apical to the gingival margin. **B,** Hyperplastic gingiva, bulky at gingival margin.

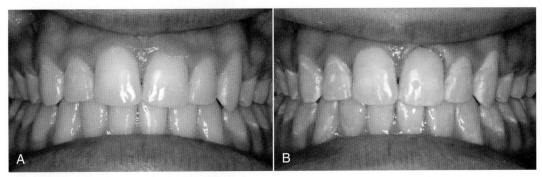

• **Figure 12-9 A,** Left central incisor with excess gingival tissue. **B,** Excess tissue is removed to match other side.

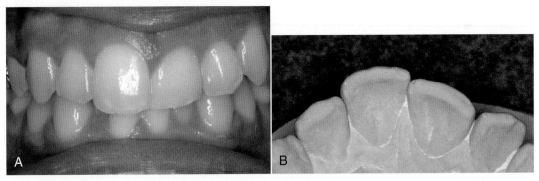

• **Figure 12-10 A,** Central incisor gingival heights do not match. **B,** Excessive wear on left central incisor suggests hypereruption.

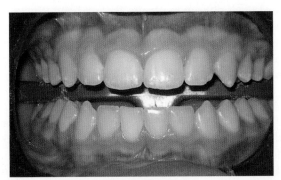

• **Figure 12-11** Improper gingival heights and contours. See Table 12-2.

TABLE 12-2	Initial Clinical Data and Treatment Goals* for the Patient in Figure 12-11					
Treatment Parameter	Anterior Tooth Measurement (mm)					
	UR3	UR2	UR1	UL1	UL2	UL3
Tooth length	9.0	8.0	9.5	9.5	9.0	8.5
Pocket depth	2.0	2.5	2.5	2.5	1.5	2.5
Keratinized tissue	3.0	5.5	5.0	5.0	5.0	4.5
Goal tooth length	10.0	9.5	11.0	11.0	9.5	10.0

UR, Upper right; *UL,* upper left.
*Calculated goal measurements based on diagnosis.

TABLE 12-3	Conditions and Results of Esthetic Recontouring for the Patient in Figure 12-12					
Timing of Evaluation	**Length of Anterior Tooth (mm)**					
	UR3	**UR2**	**UR1**	**UL1**	**UL2**	**UL3**
Preoperative	9.0	8.0	9.5	9.5	9.0	8.5
Immediately postoperative	11.0	10.0	11.5	11.5	10.0	11.0
2 weeks later	10.0	9.5	11.0	11.0	9.5	10.0

UL, Upper left; *UR*, upper right.

calculation of the limits that can be achieved with a laser in a particular case. For example, most patients will finish with approximately 1 mm of pocket depth, so by reducing the initial pocket depth by 1, the available length can be calculated for each tooth and then combined with its current length to determine the actual goal length achievable for an individual patient.

In Figure 12-11 the goal for the central incisors is 11.0 mm; for the cuspids, 10.0 mm; and for the lateral incisors, 9.5 mm. These are the maximum lengths achievable for this patient without an osseous crown-lengthening procedure, which probably is beyond the scope of many orthodontic practices. The 11.0-mm central incisor length is short of the calculated ideal (12.375 mm) by more than a millimeter. In addition, the potential lengths of central incisors and cuspids are not equal, and the differential between adjacent teeth is not ideal, so decisions must be made. At the completion of treatment, can the central incisors be left a millimeter longer than the cuspids, or should the central incisor goal be altered to match the cuspids? Because the potential lateral incisor goal is only 9.5 mm, will the discrepancy of 1.5 mm from lateral incisor to central incisor be too much? Should intrusion of the cuspids and central incisors be included in the treatment plan, to allow additional length of these teeth? These limitations were discussed with the patient and the parents, along with the option for referral for osseous crown lengthening. The decision was made to maximize the lengths of each tooth and then reevaluate for possible referral.

As shown in Table 12-3, the tooth lengths immediately after the procedure are longer than those 2 weeks later (Figure 12-12). This is an expected result; gingivae usually regrow to a level that maintains a 1-mm pocket depth. Immediately after laser exposure, tissues may appear rough and sore, albeit associated with surprisingly little tenderness. Within 2 weeks, healing is almost complete. The patient's smile is greatly improved, even with a compromised treatment plan, and both patient and parents are happy with the results.

Technique Tips

In general, it is best to address one side of the arch first, idealizing shapes (e.g., height of contours, smooth sweeping curves, mild distal tilt) before proceeding to the opposite side. When first using a laser, idealize the shape with the laser oriented perpendicular to the facial surface of the tooth (Figure 12-13).

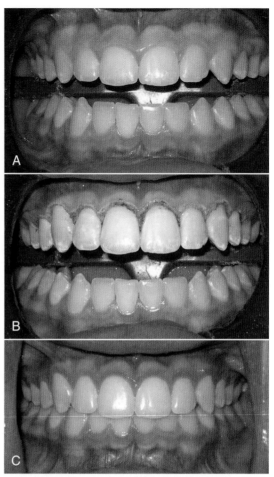

• **Figure 12-12** Esthetic gingival recontouring. **A,** Immediate preoperative view. **B,** Immediate postoperative view. **C,** Two-week postoperative view. See Table 12-3.

After the ideal shapes have been attained, the tissues are beveled at an oblique angle, usually about 45 degrees, to reduce the bulk and address contour. Once this first side is idealized, it becomes the template for completing the other side.

Once the practitioner is comfortable with the chosen laser and the diagnostic process, it is possible to bevel and to idealize shape at the same time. This more efficient approach has two distinct advantages: (1) the entire procedure will be completed in one pass and (2) laser retreatment of already-irradiated tissue that is now desiccated will be avoided. Desiccated tissues are more prone to thermal damage and charring, making the desired result difficult to obtain. For maximum efficiency, it is particularly important to learn to bevel the interproximal areas on the first pass (see Figure 12-13C). A critical point of technique is to keep the laser tip perpendicular to the lateral border of the tooth on the interproximal area, to avoid removing the papilla, leaving a "black triangular space."

A 15-mm periodontal probe with marks every 1 mm is useful in treatment planning, to measure width and length of the teeth, level of keratinized tissue, and depth of sulci. In addition, once the goal for length of each tooth is determined and gingiva anesthetized, the periodontal probe can be used to mark the goal, by producing a temporary depression in the surface of the tissues at the desired level (Figure 12-14).

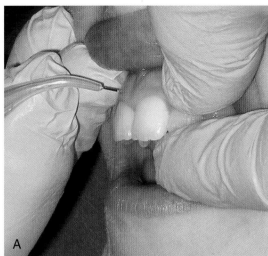

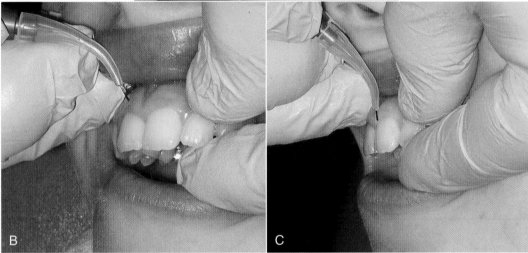

• **Figure 12-13** **A,** Laser tip perpendicular to facial surface of tooth. **B,** Laser tip at oblique angle (~45 degrees) to facial surface of tooth. **C,** Laser tip angled through interproximal area to achieve beveling without removing papilla.

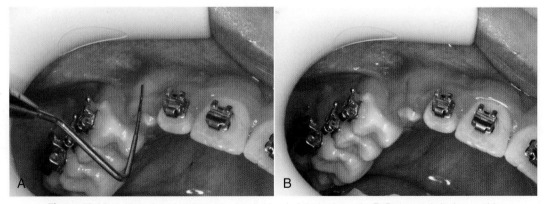

• **Figure 12-14** **A,** Periodontal probe embedded at level of desired margin. **B,** Depressed gingiva provides visual guide to goal.

Other Orthodontic Procedures

In addition to access gingivectomies and esthetic procedures, the soft tissue laser can be used to perform other valuable orthodontic services for patients.

Labial Frenum Removal

When a labial frenum extends near the free gingival margin, relieving this tension can be advantageous to the patient. Isolate, dry, and anesthetize the frenum, as with any gingivectomy procedure. When the site is ready, keep tension on

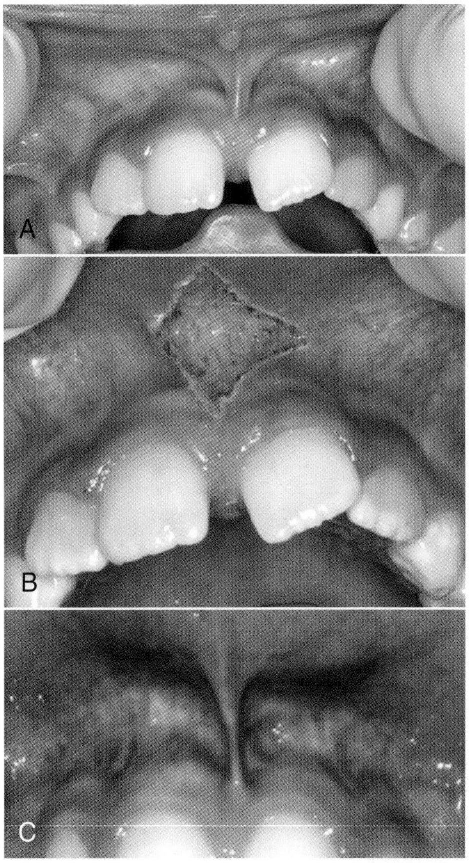

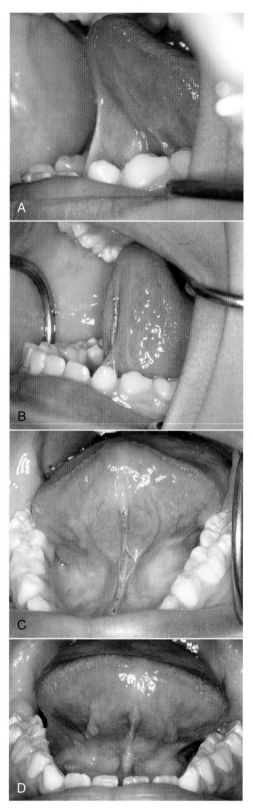

• **Figure 12-15** **A,** Labial frenum extending near diastema. **B,** Immediately after laser-assisted frenectomy (surgical time, 35 seconds). **C,** Six months later, reattachment at a higher level has been achieved.

• **Figure 12-16** **A,** Excessive lingual frenum resulting in tongue-tie. **B** and **C,** Immediately after laser procedure. **D,** Six days later.

the lip while brushing the frenum with the laser tip. Patients report no soreness with this technique, and tissues heal in approximately 1 week (Figure 12-15).

Lingual Frenum Removal

Usually an excessive lingual frenum is addressed in infancy. When early correction has not been done, however, relieving the tension from the excess attachment will not only aid in speech but also allow a more normal swallowing pattern and may improve facial growth. As with a labial frenum procedure, isolate, dry, and anesthetize. Again, tension is maintained on the tongue while the frenum is brushed with the laser tip. Postoperative soreness has not been reported, and healing occurs in approximately 1 week (Figure 12-16).

Aphthous Ulcer Pain Relief

Aphthous ulcers can be extremely painful, and laser therapy can relieve pain and speed healing (Figure 12-17). Without the need for any anesthesia, a diode laser at 0.6 W with an *uninitiated tip* is hovered over the lesion *without touching the tissue* (with the tip kept 1 to 2 mm above the tissue[22,23]). Exposing the lesion for 60 seconds will result in immediate pain relief and also accelerate healing (see also Chapter 11).

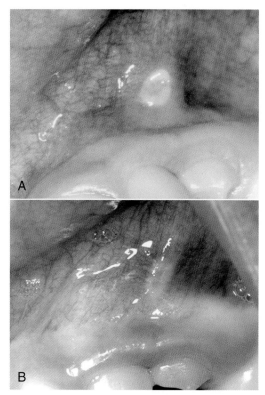

• **Figure 12-17** **A,** Aphthous ulcer. These lesions are characterized by a painful clinical course, typically 1 week to 10 days in duration. **B,** View 4 days after laser therapy.

Circumferential Fiberotomy

One way to aid postorthodontic stability for a severely rotated tooth is to perform a circumferential supracrestal fiberotomy.[24] A scalpel is inserted into the gingival sulcus to sever the epithelial attachment and transseptal fibers without removing bone. Use of a soft tissue laser seems appropriate for this procedure. The potential problem with using a diode laser for a circumferential fiberotomy is the proximity to bone. The diode laser tip emits heat, which can be absorbed to a depth of 0.8 to 4.0 mm.[25] The fiberotomy will be performed in the sulcus down to the transseptal fibers; accordingly, the diode laser heat would necessarily be delivered close to the bone. The concern is the transfer of heat to the bone resulting in necrosis.

For this reason, patients requiring circumferential fiberotomies should be referred for such treatment to the primary care dentist or periodontist. Other laser wavelengths with much smaller penetration depths, including the erbium family and CO_2 lasers, might be better alternatives than a diode laser for these procedures.

Procedural Steps

A well-trained orthodontic staff can perform most duties related to soft tissue laser procedures. Once an accurate diagnosis and treatment plan have been made, efficient delivery involves preparation of the patient and the laser, as well as providing postoperative instruction, by staff members well versed in these adjunctive aspects of treatment.

Prepare the Patient

Explain that most procedures can be performed with the use of only a topical anesthetic and that most patients experience no pain during or after the treatment. Confirm that the patient has no allergies to the anesthetic and no clotting abnormalities (e.g., hemophilia) or other medical contraindications to treatment. Discuss the pros and cons of alternative treatments.

Patients need to be informed that results cannot be guaranteed, and that relapse is a possibility. Although infection is unlikely, saltwater rinses are recommended for the first few days postoperatively. Vitamin E oil also can aid in healing and keeping the treated area moist.

The vast majority of laser procedures in an orthodontic office may be performed using topical anesthesia. Ensure that the field is isolated and dried to enhance anesthesia and improve visibility. Apply topical anesthetic liberally to the treatment area for 3 minutes, and then remove. An effective topical anesthetic for soft tissue procedures is TAC 20, a thin gel containing 20% lidocaine, 4% tetracaine, and 2% phenylephrine, with a shelf life of 3 months.

Topical anesthesia may be less effective in areas where a great deal of tissue needs to be removed, or where isolation is difficult, as in removing opercula or performing a lingual frenotomy. In such situations, the site is prepared with topical anesthetic, followed with infiltration to provide profound anesthesia. Gentle probing of the soft tissue will confirm that the patient does not feel anything sharp. The time required to achieve profound anesthesia varies with the tissue thickness and type of anesthetic.

Prepare the Laser

During the wait to obtain an appropriate depth of anesthesia, the laser is maintained in "standby" mode until the practitioner is ready to begin the procedure. Prudent laser surgeons use the minimum power necessary to accomplish a given procedure. For most tissue removal procedures, 1 to 1.4 W on a continuous wave (CW) setting is an appropriate power setting; use of a higher power is rarely necessary. Higher power settings may result in excessive energy absorption by the tissue, leading to thermal damage, tissue necrosis, sloughing, and postoperative discomfort.

Most diode lasers have two temporal emission modes: continuous wave and pulsed or "chopped" wave. Using a pulsed wave reduces the heat to surrounding tissues,[26] but continuous-wave emission is more effective if the procedure can be carried out without charring. Newer diode lasers have "superpulsed" modes, in which the laser emits a pulse of high power for a very short period. This mode results in better efficiency and less charring than with

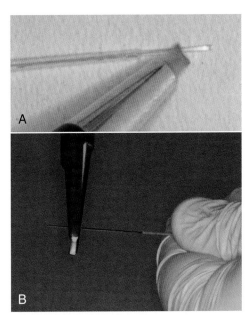

• **Figure 12-18** **A,** Cleaving fiber with scoring tool (after scoring, the remainder of the fiber is broken off). **B,** Cleaving with special scissors. Note that it is critical to keep the scissors perpendicular to the fiber. Also, the length of fiber to be discarded should be considered.

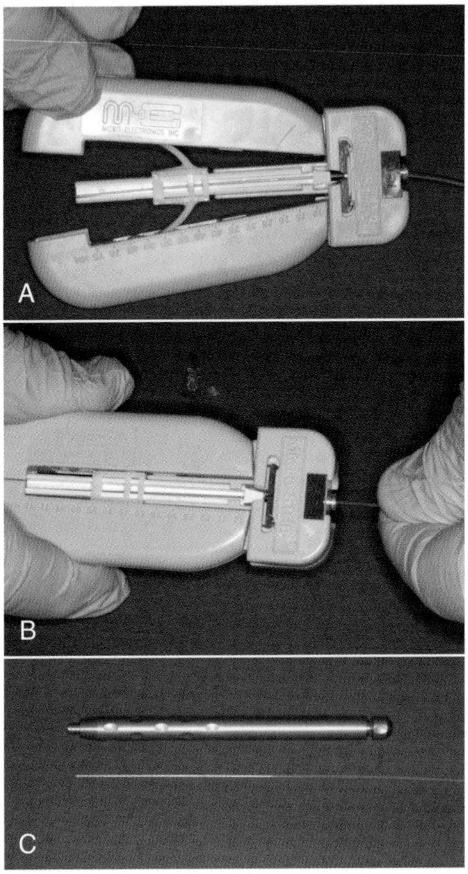

• **Figure 12-19** **A,** The protected fiber is inserted into the end of the jacket removal tool. **B,** The jacket removal tool is closed, and the fiber is firmly grasped with the other hand without bending or crimping. **C,** Removal of the protective jacket is achieved using a firm pulling motion, leaving uncovered fiberoptic cable ready to be inserted into the handpiece.

conventional continuous-wave or gated-pulse models (see Chapter 2).

It is standard protocol to cleave (cut) the quartz/glass fiberoptic cable at the end of each procedure to ensure the laser's readiness for the next procedure (Figure 12-18). After repeated use, the fiber tip can become scratched and will not emit laser energy as efficiently. Cleaving removes the scratched end of the fiber, exposing a fresh, highly polished surface capable of transmitting laser energy efficiently.

Before cleaving, it is important to ensure that sufficient cable (1 to 2 inches [2.5 to 5 cm]) extends out of the protective plastic jacket. If not enough is available, remove some of the protective jacket as suggested by the manufacturer (Figure 12-19). Next, cleave a few millimeters of the fiberoptic cable. Make sure the glass cutting scissors are perpendicular to the fiber when cleaving then confirm that the cleave left no sharp edges by shining the cable perpendicular to a flat surface, confirming that the aiming beam describes a circular pattern with no "comet tail" or oval appearance (Figure 12-20). If the beam is irregular, recleave to obtain a clean cut. Using a laser without a sharp cleave can result in bleeding as the tissues are "cut" by the irregular glass of the fiberoptic cable. With the use of a disposable-tip laser, it may sometimes be necessary to change to a fresh tip midway

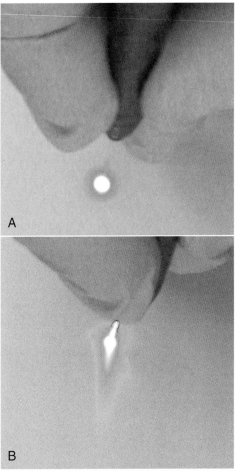

• **Figure 12-20** **A,** Appearance of aiming beam from a well-cleaved fiber. **B,** Comet-tail appearance of unevenly cleaved fiber.

through the procedure, to ensure maintenance of a sharp tip that transmits the energy efficiently.

Most lasers use a metal or plastic tube as a guide. Slip the fiberoptic cable into the handpiece and then through the guide, leaving 3 to 4 mm beyond the guide. Keep the tube straight while feeding through the fiberoptic tube until it extends 3 to 4 mm beyond the end of the metal tube. Once done, confirm fiber integrity by shining the aiming beam perpendicular to a smooth surface. If not visible, the fiber may have broken. In this case, carefully refeed the fiber through the guide without breakage. Testing the integrity of the fiberoptic cable is critical; a fracture within a metal tube would result in conversion of the laser energy to heat, with consequent burns to the patient's tissues or lips from the metal tube. Once testing is complete, carefully bend the tube to the desired angle, taking care not to kink or "overbend" it, which could fracture the fiber (Figure 12-21).

Some laser practitioners prepare the tip of the fiberoptic cable by "initiating" the tip against dark articulating film or a piece of cork. This step carbonizes the operating end of the fiberoptic cable, decreasing the depth of penetration of the laser beam and preventing deep thermal damage to the underlying tissue. A more effective method of "initiating" the laser tip is use of black ink. The fiberoptic cables are made of quartz glass. Any type of black ink that can be used on glass will work well. The ink along with thin brushes can be purchased at any art supply or hobby store. The dentist or assistant places a small amount of black ink from the bottle onto a thin brush and brushes the ink onto the tip of the fiberoptic cable. The ink dries within a matter of seconds, allowing the dentist to proceed with treatment. The ink coats the end of the fiberoptic cable much more evenly than other "initiating" methods. A more even initiation of the tip ensures that the heat emanating from the tip will be consistent throughout the surface of the tip, with no hot or cold spots. This, in turn, leads to consistent, repeatable results (see Chapter 3).

Soft tissue lasers can be hazardous to the eyes. Federal regulations mandate that all personnel in the treatment area wear safety glasses that protect against the specific wavelength used, which must be listed on the frame or the lens itself.[26] All laser units provide three sets of safety glasses: one each for the patient, the assistant, and the operator. Clip-on lenses are available for practitioners who use loupes (Figure 12-22).

With patient and laser prepared and profound anesthesia achieved, the operator turns the laser from "standby" to "on," positions the fiberoptic cable properly, and then gently passes it over the treatment site while activating the foot pedal, using a slow, brushing motion to ablate the tissues to be removed. Appropriate hand speed is critically important to the success of the procedure (see Chapter 2). The assistant holds high-speed suction as close to the tissue as possible to collect the laser "plume," reduce any odors that may arise, and cool the tissue. The assistant also holds a moist

2 × 2-inch cotton gauze to wipe ablated tissue from the fiberoptic tip. Once this step has been completed, a moistened cotton pledget may be used to clean the area; hydrogen peroxide works well. Any necessary bonding can begin immediately afterward.

The operator must guard against exposure to laser plume. Although peer-reviewed studies of laser plume generated during dental procedures are lacking, many medical plume studies document the presence of viral DNA particles and

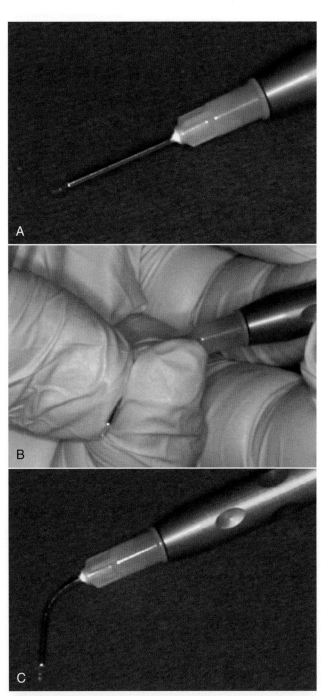

• **Figure 12-21 A,** The fiberoptic tubing is fed through the metal guide while still straight. **B,** A gentle bend is formed in the metal tubing without breaking the fiberoptic tubing. **C,** A fiberoptic cable length of 3 to 4 mm is left extending through the end of the guide.

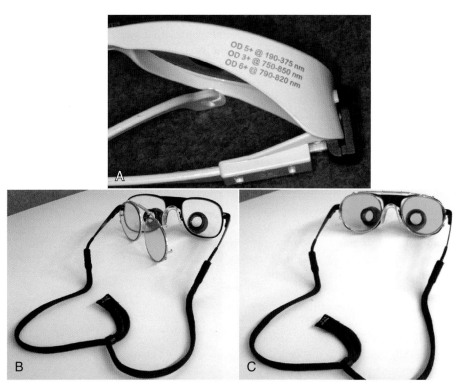

• **Figure 12-22 A,** Protective glasses designed for 810-nm lasers. **B** and **C,** Loupes with protective lens partially attached **(B)** and completely attached **(C).**

potentially carcinogenic chemicals in the plume. All personnel in the treatment area must wear a 0.1-μm filtration mask capable of filtering out laser plume; these are available in tie-on or earloop style. Tuberculosis masks, which filter out even smaller particles but are less comfortable, are also acceptable. These masks are available from most dental supply companies.

Provide Postoperative Instructions

Although varying slightly with each procedure and each patient, postoperative patient instructions include keeping the area clean, brushing softly with a soft-bristle toothbrush (or cotton swab), using warm saltwater rinses three or four times daily for several days, rubbing vitamin E gel over the healing area, and taking over-the-counter analgesics as needed. The patient should be advised that mild bleeding is normal and will resolve in a few days, but that excessive pain or bleeding is unusual.

Photobiomodulating Lasers in Orthodontics

PBM lasers by definition are nonsurgical—that is, they are incapable of cutting tissues. As their name implies, they use light (*photo*) energy to *bio*logically *modulate* cellular functions. One of the first steps in orthodontic treatment is accumulation of diagnostic data, including study

casts. Orthodontists on a daily basis encounter children who become nauseated, or even gag and vomit during the impression-making process. Orthodontists use a variety of methods to attempt to prevent this problem, including spraying topical anesthetic onto the palate and tongue, patient distraction, and other techniques. A good deal of literature is available on the use of these lasers to halt the gag reflux. A literature search of the National Library of Medicine database (PubMed) turned up many papers on the use of PBM lasers for nausea/gag control for virtually every procedure from craniotomies to general anesthesia. A Cochrane review of the literature on stimulation of the P6 acupuncture point to prevent postoperative nausea and vomiting (PONV) quite clearly concluded that "P6 acupoint stimulation prevented PONV."[27] This procedure has been successfully used in orthodontic treatment during the impression-making process. The laser is placed on the P6 (Nei guan) point in the inside of the wrist for 1 minute. Tuner and Hode[28] described placement of the laser on P6 to reduce the gag reflex, as well as in the mentolabial fold to accomplish the same effect.

Tooth movement during orthodontic therapy may cause patient discomfort both when the appliances are initially placed and when more force is placed on the appliances. PBM lasers have been successfully used to alleviate this pain.[29,30]

Turhani et al. enrolled 76 patients with edgewise-fixed appliances in a study to evaluate how effective photobiomodulation might be for treatment of orthodontic-induced discomfort.[31] One half of the patients received just one treatment of photobiomodulation for 30 seconds (group 1). The other half (group 2) received one placebo treatment (the laser was placed at the proper treatment site but was not activated). The treatment was performed immediately after placement of molar bands and ligation of the arch wires. Pain perception was evaluated at various time frames after photobiomodulation. Multiple statistical analyses of the data showed a significant difference in reporting of pain at both 6 and 30 hours after treatment. These investigators concluded that photobiomodulation clearly reduced pain prevalence immediately after multibanding and suggests that this treatment might be useful for preventing pain during orthodontic treatment.[31] Tortamano et al. performed a similar double-blind placebo study in 60 orthodontic patients ranging in age from 12 to 18 years.[32] PBM laser treatment was begun immediately after placement of the first arch wire. Analysis of the data showed that pain duration and intensity was statistically significantly less in the photobiomodulation group compared with the placebo and control groups. These researchers concluded that photobiomodulation efficiently controls pain caused by placement of the first arch wire.[32]

Another use of photobiomodulation in orthodontics is to promote bone remodeling and regeneration. Habib et al. studied changes in alveolar bone morphology in rodents during orthodontic movement.[33] Thirty rats were divided into two groups. One group of animals received PBM during orthodontic movement. The second group served as control subjects. The animals were treated every other day for a total of 3, 6, or 9 doses, and then sacrificed. The jaws were evaluated for presence of osteoblasts, osteoclasts, and collagen deposition in both pressure and tension areas. Data analysis showed a statistically significant increase in the number of osteoblasts in the photobiomodulation-treated animals, especially on the tension side. According to these authors, this newly formed bone showed better quality than non-irradiated bone. An increased amount of collagen matrix also was found on both the pressure and tension sides in the photobiomodulation-treated subjects. The investigators suggested that the greater abundance of matrix could lead to faster tooth movement and alveolar bone remodeling. Similar results and conclusions regarding faster tooth movement and bone remodeling in animal studies were found by Kawasaki and Shimizu,[34] Nicolau et al.,[35] and Silva et al.[36]

Cruz et al.[37] performed the first clinical study to evaluate the use of photobiomodulation for accelerating tooth movement. Treatment plans were formulated for 11 patients, ranging in age from 12 to 18 years, to include bilateral extraction of upper first premolars and retraction of the maxillary teeth. One side of the maxilla was irradiated with the PBM laser. The other side served as the control condition. The amount of canine movement was evaluated by measuring the distance between the distal slot of the canine and the mesial slot of the first molar brackets by means of a digital electronic caliper. Statistical analysis showed a significant increase in retraction on the treated side when compared with the nonirradiated side. Radiographs taken at the conclusion of the study showed no damage to roots or to alveolar or periodontal tissue. Cruz concluded that photobiomodulation significantly accelerates orthodontic movement with no adverse periodontal tissue effects.

Sousa et al.[38] also studied the effect of photobiomodulation on the speed of tooth movement during orthodontic therapy for canine retraction in humans. Ten patients with a mean age of 13 years undergoing first premolar extraction and canine retraction were enrolled in this study. A total of 26 canines were retracted. Half of the canines were irradiated with PBM. The other half served as control teeth. Follow-up evaluation was done at 4 months. Canine movement was evaluated by three-dimensional analysis of casts of the dentition. Periapical x-ray images of the canines also were analyzed. The study results showed a statistically significant increase in the speed of movement of the canines when compared with the non-photobiomodulation-treated canines. No statistically significant difference in bone or tooth resorption was found between the two groups. Sousa concluded that photobiomodulation increased the speed of tooth movement, which could lead to decreased orthodontic treatment time, and pointed out that this type of therapy is simple to apply and painless and has no collateral effects.

Doshi-Mehta and Bhad-Patil[39] studied the effects of photobiomodulation on both orthodontic treatment time and pain. Twenty patients 12 to 23 years of age whose treatment plan included extraction of first premolars were enrolled in this study. As with the two studies previously cited, one side was irradiated with a PBM laser and the other side was left as the untreated control region. Photobiomodulation was used on the day of coil spring placement, as well as on days 3, 7, and 14 during the first month of treatment, and subsequently every 15 days thereafter until the PBM laser-treated side was completely retracted. Casts were made for each patient three times during the study: at day 1 of canine retraction, after 3 months of canine retraction, and at the completion of canine retraction on the photobiomodulation side. A digital caliper was used to measure the distance from the first molar and the canine on each of the models. Patient questionnaires about pain were completed immediately after placement of the coil spring, again 3 days later, and then at 30 days after placement. The results showed a statistically significant difference in the rate of retraction between the photobiomodulation side and the control side. In the maxillary arch, the mean increase in the rates of tooth movement at 3 months was 54%. The mandibular arch showed a difference of 58% increased movement. The pain questionnaire visual analog scale results showed a significant decrease in pain scores on the experimental sides. This investigator concluded that photobiomodulation can safely and routinely be used to decrease treatment time with no adverse effects; and photobiomodulation is an effective method of pain relief during orthodontic therapy. Youssef et al.[40] performed a similar study in 15 patients ranging in age from 14 to 23 years. His study also showed a significant increase in the rate of tooth movement as well as a significant reduction in pain.

Rapid maxillary palatal expansion (RMPE) is a common technique in orthodontics.[41,42] A preliminary study on rats by Saito and Shimizu[43] showed that photobiomodulation affects bone regeneration after RMPE. This finding led to clinical studies: Angeletti et al.[44] evaluated the contribution of photobiomodulation in the management of 13 patients ranging in age from 18 to 33 years with a maxillary transverse deficiency greater than 7 mm. All of the patients underwent a subtotal LeFort 1 osteotomy with separation of the pterygomaxillary suture followed by activation of a Hyrax expander by 1.6 mm in the operating room. Patients then activated the screws with a turn of 0.2 mm twice a day. When the expansion was completed, the device was fixed and kept in place for 4 months. One half of the patients underwent photobiomodulation along the area of the midpalatal suture, with the other half of the patients serving as control subjects. Digital x-ray images were obtained before the surgical procedure and at 1, 2, 3, 4, and 7 months postoperatively. Optical density analysis was performed. The results showed a statistically significantly higher bone mineralization rate in the PBM group.[44]

Many more uses of these nonsurgical lasers in orthodontic therapy have been described. More information on PBM lasers can be found in Chapter 15. It must be emphasized that with *all* laser treatment, both surgical and nonsurgical, the most important criterion in deciding on the purchase of a laser is *training* received with the purchase of the device. None of the results discussed in this chapter could have been accomplished without a high level of technical expertise, achievable only with proper education and training.

Laser Education and Training

Training often is included in the purchase price of the laser but can take many forms. Some laser manufacturers provide a CD or DVD showing how to set up the laser and videos of certain procedures, but little or no discussion of diagnosis and treatment planning, no in-office or hands-on training, and most significantly, no discussion of the basics of laser physics and laser-tissue interaction. Some manufacturers include a basic course that covers general laser information and clinical applications (often including a detailed discussion about incorporating lasers into your hygiene department). Other manufacturers include a course specifically for orthodontists that reviews the clinical aspects of gingivectomies, frenectomies, exposures, and other office procedures.

To incorporate use of a laser effectively and efficiently into a busy orthodontics practice, it is critical to have all members of the office team "on board." Properly trained clinical personnel, guided by the orthodontist, can prepare the patient and parents, set up the laser, isolate the tissue areas to be treated, and apply/confirm anesthesia. Clinical team members also can assist during the procedure and provide postoperative cleanup, charting, and instructions. Office staff can document the treatment details with excellent photographs and promote laser therapy to patients and parents.

An orthodontist incorporating a laser into clinical practice also must become familiar with the appropriate periodontal literature and conferences such as the joint American Association of Orthodontists and American Academy of Periodontology meeting as resources for issues germane to orthodontics (see Chapters 1 and 2).

Many laser dentistry organizations worldwide offer training and continuing education in laser dentistry. The Academy of Laser Dentistry (ALD) (www.laserdentistry.org) provides three levels of certification: standard proficiency, advanced proficiency, and educator status. The ALD also serves as a clearinghouse for course providers and provides a list of available courses for dentists, hygienists, and office staff, including dental assistants and front desk staff. It is a nonprofit organization with no commercial associations, although many certification courses provided by ALD-certified trainers are sponsored by specific laser companies. Biolase sponsors the World Clinical Laser Institute (www.learnlasers.com) and provides its own certification pathway along with symposia and seminars, focusing on Biolase devices. Other worldwide organizations include the World Federation of Laser Dentistry and the Society for Oral Laser Applications.

In summary, proper training is critical to efficient, effective incorporation of a laser in an orthodontics office. Both orthodontist and staff should be trained, and the practitioner should consider obtaining ALD or similar certification. A list of ALD Standard Proficiency Certification Courses may be found on the ALD website (www.laserdentistry.org; click on Professionals>Education>ALD CE Calendar).

Conclusions

Use of a laser in an orthodontic office improves the quality of results, decreases treatment time and postoperative pain, and reduces the number of needed appointments. With diagnostic considerations properly addressed, these procedures can be completed quickly, painlessly, and infection-free,[45] with minimal side effects for the patient.

References

1. Hilgers JJ, Tracey SG: Clinical uses of diode lasers in orthodontics, *J Clin Orthod* 38(5):266–273, 2004.
2. Sarver DM, Yanosky M: Principles of cosmetic dentistry in orthodontics: Part 2. Soft tissue laser technology and cosmetic gingival contouring, *Am J Orthod Dentofacial Orthop* 127:85–90, 2005.
3. Dean DB: *Concepts in laser periodontal therapy using the Er,Cr:YSGG laser* [self-study course], 2005, Academy of Dental Therapeutics and Stomatology. (http://www.ineedce.com/).
4. Schulman M, McGill J: How does your orthodontic practice stand up? *J Clin Orthod* 36(5):281–283, 2002.
5. Gama S, de Araujo T, Pinheiro A: Benefits of the use of the CO_2 laser in orthodontics, *Lasers Med Sci* 23(4):459–465, 2008.
6. Gama S, de Araujo T, Pozza D, Pinhiero A: Use of the CO_2 laser on orthodontic patients suffering from gingival hyperplasia, *Photomed Laser Surg* 25(3):214–219, 2007.
7. Fornaini C, Rocca J, Bertrand M, et al.: Nd:YAG and diode laser in the surgical management of soft tissues related to orthodontic treatment, *Photomed Laser Surg* 25(5):381–392, 2007.

8. Harnick D: Use of an argon laser in the orthodontic practice, *J Gen Orthod* 5(4):11–12, 1994.

9. Garguilo AW, Wentz FM, Orban B: Dimensions and relationships of the dentogingival junction in humans, *J Periodontol* 32:261–267, 1961.

10. Cohen DW: Periodontal preparation of the mouth for restorative dentistry. In *paper presented at Walter Reed Army Medical Center*, Washington, DC, 1962.

11. Ingber JS, Rose LF, Coslet JG: The "biologic width": a concept in periodontics and restorative dentistry, *Alpha Omegan* 70(3):62–65, 1977.

12. Kois JC: New paradigms for anterior tooth preparation: rationale and technique, *Contemp Esthet Dent* 2:1–8, 1996.

13. Sarver DM: Principles of cosmetic dentistry in orthodontics. Part 1. Shape and proportionality of anterior teeth, *Am J Orthod Dentofacial Orthop* 126:749–753, 2004.

14. Rufenacht CR: *Fundamentals of esthetics*, Chicago, 1990, Quintessence.

15. Kokich VG: Excellence in finishing: modifications for the perio-restorative patient, *Semin Orthod* 9:184–203, 2003.

16. Woelful JB: *Dental anatomy: its relevance to dentistry*, ed 4, Philadelphia, 1990, Lea & Febiger.

17. Mavroskoufis F, Richie GM: Variation in size and form between left and right maxillary central teeth, *J Prosthet Dent* 43:254, 1980.

18. Gurel G: *The science and art of porcelain laminate veneers*, New Malden, UK, 2003, Quintessence.

19. Gillen RJ, Schwartz RS, Hilton TJ, Evans DB: An analysis of selective tooth proportions, *Int J Prosthodont* 7:410–417, 1994.

20. American Academy of Cosmetic Dentistry: *Diagnosis and treatment evaluation in cosmetic dentistry: a guide to accreditation criteria*, Madison, Wisc, 2001, American Academy of Cosmetic Dentistry.

21. Shillingburg Jr HT, Kaplan MJ, Grace CS: Tooth dimensions: a comparative study, *J South Calif Dent Assoc* 40:830, 1972.

22. Sarver DM, Yanosky M: Principles of cosmetic dentistry in orthodontics. Part 3. Laser treatments for tooth eruption and soft tissue problems, *Am J Orthod Dentofacial Orthop* 127:262–264, 2005.

23. Convissar RA, Massoumi-Sourey M: Recurrent aphthous ulcers: etiology and laser ablation, *Gen Dent* 40:512–515, 1992.

24. Edwards JG: A surgical procedure to eliminate rotational relapse, *Am J Orthod* 57(1):35–46, 1970.

25. *Dental applications of advanced lasers,* Burlington, Mass, 2005, JGM Associates.

26. *Safe use of lasers in health care facilities,* ANSI Z136.3, Orlando, Fla, 1996, Laser Institute of America.

27. Lee A, Fan LT: Stimulation of the wrist acupuncture point P6 for preventing postoperative nausea and vomiting, *Cochrane Database Syst Rev* (2), CD003281, 2009.

28. Tuner J, Hode L: *The new laser therapy handbook*, Grangesberg, Sweden, 2010, Prima Books.

29. Youssef M, Ashkar S, Hamade E, et al.: The effect of low-level laser therapy during orthodontic movement: a preliminary study, *Lasers Med Sci* 23(1):27–33, 2008.

30. Lim HM, Lew KK, Tay DL: A clinical investigation of the efficacy of low level laser therapy in reducing orthodontic postadjustment pain, *Am J Orthod Dentofacial Orthop* 108:614–622, 1995.

31. Turhani D, Scheriau M, Kapral D, et al.: Pain relief by single low level laser irradiation in orthodontic patients undergoing fixed appliance therapy, *Am J Orthod Dentofacial Orthop* 130:371–377, 2006.

32. Tortamano A, Calovine-Lenzi D, Soares Santos Haddad A, et al.: Low level laser therapy for pain caused by placement of the first orthodontic archwire: a randomized clinical trial, *Am J Orthod Dentofacial Orthop* 136:662–667, 2009.

33. Habib F, Gama S, Ramalho L, et al.: Laser induced alveolar bone changes during orthodontic movement: a histologic study on rodents, *Photomed Laser Surg* 28(6):823–830, 2010.

34. Kawasaki K, Shimizu N: Effects of low-energy laser irradiation on bone remodeling during experimental tooth movement in rats, *Lasers Surg Med* 26:282–291, 2000.

35. Nicolau R, Jorgetti V, Rigau J, et al.: Effect of low-power GalAlAs laser (660 nm) on bone structure and cell activity: an experimental animal study, *Lasers Med Sci* 18:89–94, 2003.

36. Silva Júnior A, Pinheiro A, Oliveira M, et al.: Computerized morphometric assessment of the effect of low-level laser therapy on bone repair: an experimental animal study, *J Clin Laser Med Surg* 20:83–87, 2002.

37. Cruz D, Kohara E, Ribiero M, et al.: Effects of low-intensity laser therapy on the orthodontic movement velocity of human teeth: a preliminary study, *Lasers Surg Med* 35:117–120, 2004.

38. Sousa M, Scanavini A, Sannomiya E, et al.: Influence of low level laser on the speed of orthodontic movement, *Photomed Laser Surg* 29(3):191–197, 2011.

39. Doshi-Mehta G, Bhad-Patil W: Efficacy of low-intensity laser therapy in reducing treatment time and orthodontic pain: a clinical investigation, *Am J Orthod Dentofacial Orthop* 141:289–297, 2012.

40. Youssef M, Ashkar S, Hamade E, et al.: The effect of low-level laser therapy during orthodontic movement: a preliminary study, *Lasers Med Sci* 23:27–33, 2008.

41. Haas AJ: Rapid expansion of the maxillary dental arch and nasal cavity by opening the midpalatal suture, *Angle Orthod* 31:73–90, 1961.

42. Haas AJ: Palatal expansion: just the beginning of dentofacial orthopedics, *Am J Orthod* 57:219–255, 1970.

43. Saito S, Shimizu N: Stimulatory effects of low power laser irradiation on bone regeneration in midpalatal suture during expansion in the rat, *Am J Orthod Dentofacial Orthop* 111:525–532, 1997.

44. Angeletti P, Pereira M, Gomes H, et al.: Effect of low-level laser therapy (GaAlAs) on bone regeneration in midpalatal anterior suture after surgically assisted rapid maxillary expansion, *Oral Surg Oral Med Oral Path Oral Radiol Endod* 109(2):e38–e46, 2012.

45. Moritz A, Gutknecht N, Doertbudak O, et al.: Bacterial reduction in periodontal pockets through irradiation with a diode laser, *J Clin Laser Med Surg* 15:33–37, 1997.

13

Lasers in Endodontics

ADAM STABHOLZ, SHARONIT SAHAR-HELFT, AND JOSHUA MOSHONOV

The rapid development of laser technology combined with better understanding of laser-tissue interaction has increased the spectrum of possible laser applications in endodontics. The development of specialized delivery systems, including thin and flexible fibers as well as new endodontic tips, allows application of this technology in the following endodontic procedures:

- Pulp diagnosis
- Pulp capping and pulpotomy
- Cleaning and disinfecting the root canal system
- Obturation of the root canal system
- Endodontic retreatment
- Apical surgery

Although interest in clinical laser systems for endodontic procedures is increasing, concerns still exist, especially regarding the lack of well-designed clinical studies that clearly demonstrate the advantage of lasers over currently used conventional methods and techniques. Selection of a suitable wavelength from among currently available laser systems requires advanced training and understanding of the different characteristics of each system. This chapter discusses the clinical applications of lasers in endodontics.

Pulp Diagnosis: Laser Doppler Flowmetry

Pulp vitality may be difficult to assess at times because current tests are poor indicators. A false diagnosis of decreased pulp vitality may lead to an unnecessary endodontic procedure. Histologic evaluation of the exact condition of the pulp tissue is not feasible because creating an opening into the pulp chamber for evaluation will necessitate removal of this tissue and subsequent root canal treatment.

Laser Doppler flowmetry (LDF) was developed to assess blood flow in microvascular systems. It can also be used as a diagnostic system for measurements of blood flow in the dental pulp.[1,2] LDF uses low-power settings (1 to 2 mW) of helium-neon (HeNe) or diode (810 nm) light sources.[3,4] This technique may represent a sensitive and accurate means for pulp vitality testing because it reflects *vascular* rather than neural responsiveness compared with other methods.[5] The laser beam must be directed through the clinical crown structure to the pulpal blood vessels, where the flow of red blood cells (RBCs) causes the Doppler shifting of the

frequency of the laser beam. Some of the light is backscattered out of the tooth and is detected by a photocell on the tooth surface. The output is proportional to the number and velocity of RBCs[6,7] (Figure 13-1).

Interest in LDF has mostly been in the field of dental traumatology. Studies have found that LDF is effective in the assessment of revascularization of replanted immature teeth in dogs,[8,9] as well as in evaluating tooth vitality in patients with avulsed permanent maxillary incisors treated with reimplantation and splinting.[4,10]

Limitations in LDF mainly derive from environmental contamination, so it may be difficult to obtain laser reflection from certain teeth.[11] The anterior teeth, in which the enamel and dentin are thin, usually do not present a problem. Molars, however, with their thicker enamel and dentin and the variability in the position of the pulp within the tooth may exhibit variations in pulpal blood flow.[1,3] In addition, differences in sensor output and inadequate calibration by the manufacturer may dictate the use of multiple probes for accurate assessment.[12] Furthermore, the probe design and bandwidth may affect the laser Doppler readings from vital and nonvital teeth.[13] It has been suggested that up to 80% of the laser Doppler blood flow signal recovered from intact human teeth without a rubber dam in place is of nonpulpal origin, and that the role of the periodontium in some pulpal blood flow recordings probably has been underestimated.[14] The use of a rubber dam in combination with a rigid splint is recommended, to enhance the validity of recordings.[15]

Frentzen et al.[16] reported the following problems with LDF:

- Scattering of signals from the surrounding tissues
- Difficulty in obtaining laser reflection in posterior teeth
- Difficulty in obtaining laser reflection in restored teeth because of insufficient transmission

In traumatized teeth, in which excitability of the pulp is reduced, LDF could provide an acceptable alternative to conventional methods of vitality testing (using thermal and electrical stimuli). Further investigations and technological improvements are still required. When equipment costs decrease and clinical application improves, this technology could be efficiently used in the management of patients who have difficulty in communicating or of young children, whose responses may not be reliable.[2]

Pulp Capping and Pulpotomy

Pulp capping, as defined by the American Association of Endodontists, is a procedure in which "a dental material is placed over an exposed or nearly exposed pulp to encourage the formation of irritation dentin at the site of injury." *Pulpotomy* entails surgical removal of a small portion of vital pulp as a means of preserving the remaining coronal and radicular pulp tissues. Pulp capping is recommended when the exposure is small (≤1.0 mm[17,18]) and the patient is young. Pulpotomy is recommended when the young pulp is already exposed to caries and the roots are not yet fully formed (open apices).

The traditional pulp-capping agent is *calcium hydroxide* [$Ca(OH)_2$].[19,20] When it is applied to pulp tissue, a necrotic layer is produced and a dentin bridge formed. The same may occur when the pulpotomy procedure is performed. A newer material, *mineral trioxide aggregate* (MTA), shows favorable results when applied to exposed pulp. It produces more dentinal bridging in a shorter time with significantly less inflammation. However, 3 to 4 hours is necessary for complete setting of the MTA.[21–23] The success rate for pulp capping, whether direct or indirect, ranges from 44% to 97%. In pulpotomy, the same agents are used until root formation has been completed. Whether full root canal treatment should then be initiated is debatable.[24,25]

Since the introduction of lasers to dentistry, several studies have examined the effect of different laser devices on dentin and pulpal tissue. Melcer et al.[26] showed that in contrast with ruby lasers, which caused pulpal damage, the carbon dioxide (CO_2) laser produced new mineralized dentin without cellular modification of pulpal tissue in beagles and primates. Shoji et al.[27] applied CO_2 laser to exposed pulps in dogs, using a focused and defocused laser mode and a wide range of energy levels (3, 10, 30, and 60 W). Charring, coagulation necrosis, and degeneration of the odontoblastic layer occurred, although no damage was detected in the radicular portion of the pulp.

Jukic et al.[28] used CO_2 and neodymium-doped yttrium-aluminum-garnet (Nd:YAG) lasers with an energy density of 4 J/cm^2 and 6.3 J/cm^2, respectively, on exposed pulp tissue. In both experimental groups, carbonization, necrosis, an inflammatory response, edema, and hemorrhage were observed in the pulp tissue. In some specimens, a dentinal bridge was formed.

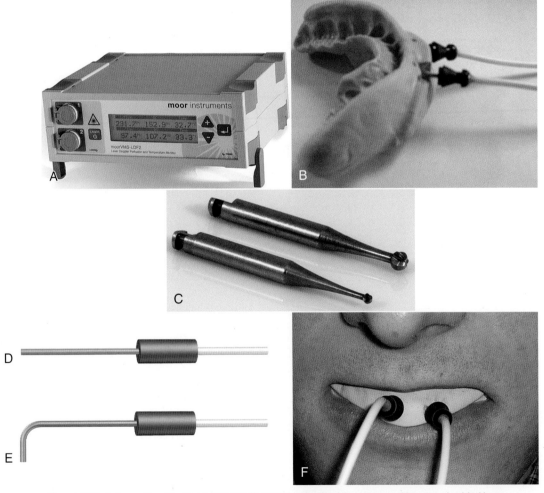

• **Figure 13-1 A,** Laser Doppler flowmeter unit. **B,** Mold made of quick-set putty with two embedded laser Doppler probes. **C,** Slow-speed round burs can be used to make holes in the putty for the placement of probes. **D** and **E,** Laser Doppler probes for assessment of blood flow in anterior teeth **(D)** and posterior teeth **(E). F,** Quick-set putty with dental probes in position in the mouth.

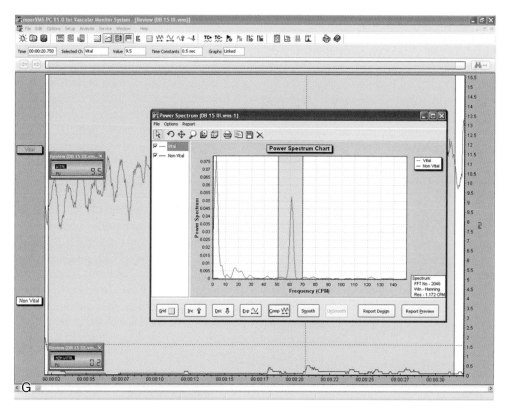

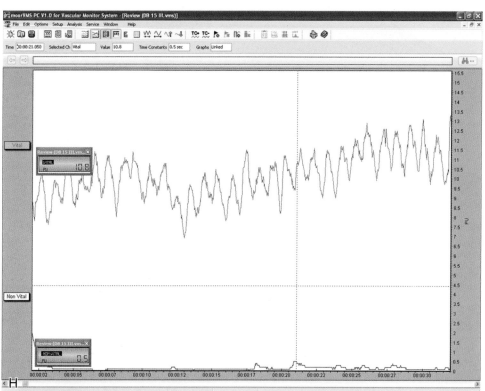

• **Figure 13-1, cont'd** **G,** Blood flow analysis readout. **H,** Fourier analysis of blood flow data. (**A, D, E, G, H,** Courtesy Moor Instruments, Ltd.)

Moritz et al.[29] used a CO_2 laser in patients requiring direct pulp-capping treatment. Laser irradiation at an energy level of 1 W with 0.1-second exposure time and a 1-second pulse interval was repeated until the exposed pulp cavities were completely sealed. The pulps were then dressed with $Ca(OH)_2$. In the control group, the pulps were capped with $Ca(OH)_2$ only. Symptom status and tooth vitality were assessed after 1 week and monthly for 1 year; 89% of patients in the experimental group had no symptoms and exhibited normal responses to vitality tests in the treated pulps versus only 68% in the control group.

With deep and hypersensitive cavities, indirect pulp capping should be considered. A reduction in the permeability of the dentin, achieved by sealing the dentinal tubules, is paramount. Nd:YAG and 9.6-μm CO_2 lasers can be used for this purpose. The 9.6-μm CO_2 laser wavelength is well absorbed by the hydroxyapatite of enamel and dentin, causing tissue ablation, melting, and resolidification.[30] The use of the 9.6-μm CO_2 laser did not cause any noticeable damage to the pulpal tissue in dogs.[31]

White et al.[32] found that use of a pulsed Nd:YAG laser with an energy level less than 1 W, with a 10-Hz repetition rate and overall 10-second exposure time, did not significantly elevate the intrapulpal temperature. According to their results, these settings may be considered safe parameters because the remaining dentinal thickness in cavity preparations cannot be measured in vivo. It is therefore recommended that clinicians choose laser parameters lower than these safety limits.

Cleaning and Disinfecting the Root Canal System

Bacterial contamination of the root canal system is considered the principal etiological factor in the development of pulpal and periapical lesions.[33–35] Creating a root canal system free of irritants is a major goal of root canal therapy, traditionally achieved through biomechanical instrumentation. Because of the complexity of the root canal system, however, complete elimination of debris resulting in a sterile root canal system is difficult.[36,37] Also, a smear layer, which covers the instrumented walls of the root canal, is formed during this treatment.[38–40]

The *smear layer* consists of two parts: a superficial layer on the surface of the root canal wall approximately 1 to 2 μm thick and a deeper layer packed into the dentinal tubules to a depth of up to 40 μm.[40] It contains inorganic and organic substances that include microorganisms and necrotic debris.[41] In addition to possible infection of the smear layer itself, it also can protect the bacteria already present deeper in the dentinal tubules by preventing intracanal disinfection agents from penetrating into the tubules.[42] Pashley[43] also has postulated that a smear layer containing bacteria or bacterial products might provide a reservoir of irritants. Thus, complete removal of the smear layer would be consistent with elimination of irritants from the root canal system.[44]

In addition, Peters et al.[45] clearly demonstrated that more than 35% of the canals' surface area remained unchanged after instrumentation of the root canal using four different nickel-titanium (NiTi) preparation techniques. Because most current intracanal medicaments have a limited antibacterial spectrum and limited ability to diffuse into the dentinal tubules, development of newer treatment strategies designed to eliminate microorganisms from the root canal system should be considered. Such strategies must include use of agents that can penetrate the dentinal tubules and destroy the microorganisms located in an area beyond the host defense mechanisms, where they cannot be reached by systemically administered antibacterial agents.[46]

Numerous studies also have documented that CO_2,[47] Nd:YAG,[47–49] argon,[47,50] Er,Cr:YSGG,[51] and Er:YAG[52,53] laser irradiation have the ability to remove debris and the smear layer from the root canal walls after biomechanical instrumentation.

However, the intracanal use of lasers has several limitations.[54] The emission of laser energy from the tip of the optical fiber or the laser tip is directed along the root canal and not necessarily laterally along the root canal walls.[55] Thus, it is almost impossible to obtain uniform 360-degree coverage of the internal aspect of the root canal system surface using a laser.[54,55] An important additional consideration, in view of the risk of thermal damage to the periapical tissues, is safety.[55] Direct emission of laser radiation from the tip of the optical fiber in the vicinity of the apical foramen of a tooth may result in transmission of the energy beyond the foramen. This in turn may adversely affect the supporting tissues of the tooth, which can be hazardous in teeth close to the mental foramen or to the mandibular nerve.[55,56]

Matsumoto[3] emphasized the possible limitations of laser use in root canal systems, suggesting that "removal of smear layer and debris by laser is possible, however it is difficult to clean all root canal walls, because the laser is emitted straight ahead, making it almost impossible to irradiate the lateral canal walls." These workers researchers strongly recommended improving laser endodontic tips to enable irradiation of all areas of the root canal walls.

Erbium lasers have gained increasing popularity among clinicians after their clearance by the U.S. Food and Drug Administration (FDA) for use on hard dental tissues.[57] Stabholz et al.[55,56] described a newer endodontic tip that can be used with an erbium laser system. The beam of the erbium laser is delivered through a hollow tube, permitting development of an endodontic tip that allows lateral emission of the laser radiation (side-firing) rather than direct emission through a single opening at the far end. This new *endodontic side-firing spiral tip* was designed to fit the shape and the volume of root canals prepared by NiTi rotary instrumentation. It emits the erbium laser radiation laterally to the walls of the root canal through spiral slits located all along the length of the tip. The tip is sealed at its far end, preventing the transmission of radiation to or through the apical foramen of the tooth. In an evaluation of the efficacy of the endodontic side-firing spiral tip in removing debris and smear layer from distal and palatal root canals of freshly extracted human molars, scanning electron microscopy (SEM) of the treated root canal walls revealed clean surfaces, free of smear layer and debris (Figures 13-2 to 13-5).[56]

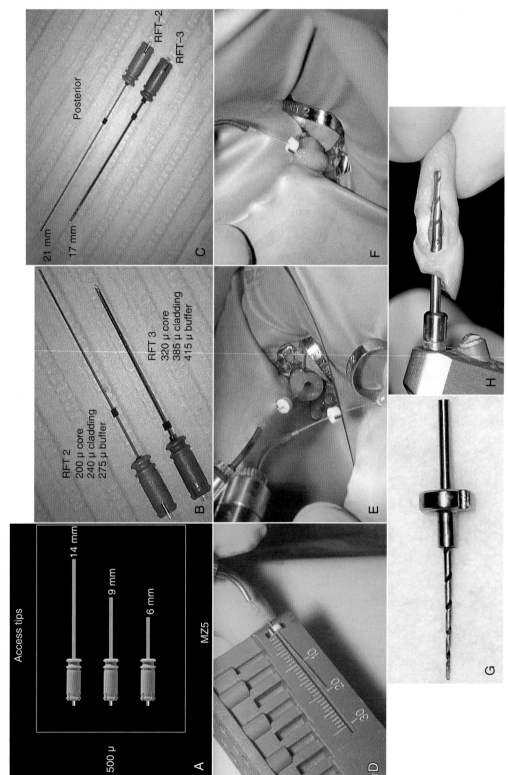

• **Figure 13-2** A to C, Er,Cr:YSGG laser tips can be used to create endodontic access openings (**A**) and for instrumentation of canals in anterior teeth (**B**) and posterior teeth (**C**). **D** to **F**, Er:YAG laser tip being fitted for a stopper for working length minus 1 mm for endodontic canal (**D**), entering the canal (**E**), and reaching measurement depth (**F**). **G**, RCLase Side-Firing Spiral Tip (Opus Dent, Tel Aviv, Israel). **H**, Prototype of RCLase Side-Firing Spiral Tip is shown in the root canal of an extracted maxillary canine in which the side wall of the root has been removed to enable visualization of the tip. (A to C courtesy Dr. David Browdy, Lynbrook, New York; D to F courtesy Dr. Donald Coluzzi, Redwood City, California.)

The palatal root of a maxillary molar tooth

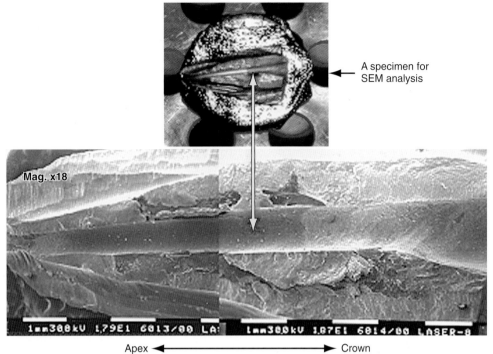

A specimen for SEM analysis

Mag. x18

Apex ◄————————► Crown

• **Figure 13-3** Longitudinally split palatal root of maxillary molar, sputter-coated by gold and ready for scanning electron microscope (SEM) evaluation. *Vertical arrow* indicates the root canal as shown on SEM photograph.

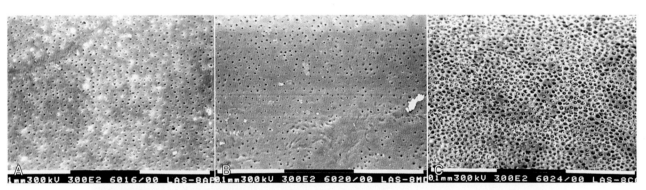

• **Figure 13-4** **A** to **C,** Scanning electron microscope photographs of laser-treated wall of root canal at its apical **(A),** middle **(B),** and coronal **(C)** portions demonstrate clean surfaces of root canal walls, free of smear layer and debris, and clean, open dentinal tubules. (Magnification ×300.)

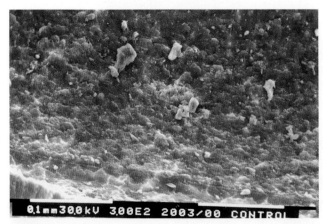

• **Figure 13-5** Scanning electron microscope photograph of a non-laser-treated wall of root canal at its middle portion demonstrates unclean surfaces of root canal walls, with smear layer and debris. Dentinal tubules cannot be seen. (Magnification ×300.)

The dentinal tubules in the root run a relatively straight course between the pulp and the periphery, in contrast to the typical S-shaped contours of the tubules in the tooth crown.[41] Studies have shown that bacteria and their byproducts, present in infected root canals, may invade the dentinal tubules. Also, the presence of bacteria in the dentinal tubules of infected teeth was noted at approximately one half the distance between the root canal walls and the cementodentinal junction.[58,59] These findings justify the rationale and need for developing effective means of removing the smear layer from root canal walls after biomechanical instrumentation. This cleansing step would allow disinfectants and laser energies to reach and destroy microorganisms within the dentinal tubules.

In various laser systems used in dentistry, the emitted energy can be delivered into the root canal system by a thin optical fiber—as in Nd:YAG, potassium titanyl phosphate (KTP)–Nd:YAG, Er:YSGG, argon, and diode lasers—or by a hollow tube—as in CO_2 and Er:YAG lasers. Thus, the potential bactericidal effect of laser irradiation can be effectively used for additional cleansing and disinfecting of the root canal system after biomechanical instrumentation. This effect was extensively studied using CO_2,[60,61] Nd:YAG,[62–65] KTP-Nd:YAG,[66] excimer,[67,68] diode,[69] and Er:YAG[70–72] lasers.

The apparent consensus is that laser irradiation performed using dental laser systems has the potential to kill microorganisms. In most cases the effect is directly related to the amount of irradiation and to its energy level. Case Study 13-1, with Figure 13-6, illustrates the use of erbium laser energy to clean and disinfect a root canal system.

CASE STUDY 13-1

An 18-year-old college student came with her mother to the endodontic clinic complaining of a bad taste in her mouth and the presence of a gum lesion in the front of the mouth. Clinical examination revealed a sinus tract opening close to the apex of the right lateral maxillary incisor. The initial radiograph showed internal resorption and a large radiolucent area in the apical third of the root. A diagnostic/length measurement radiograph showed root perforation in the apical third of the root.

The patient and her mother were advised of the poor prognosis for the tooth and the option of placing a dental implant to replace the lateral incisor. The mother asked if an attempt could be made to try to save the tooth because her daughter was leaving on a trip that could not be postponed.

The tooth was opened and the root canal cleaned and shaped using conventional methods. $Ca(OH)_2$ was placed for 3 months and then replaced with another freshly prepared mix of the same material. The sinus tract was still present after 6 months, with no signs of healing. The mother and the patient were informed that as a last resort, the tooth could be treated with a newly developed laser side-firing spiral endodontic tip (RCLase), which might provide better disinfection of the infected root canal system. The canal was then irradiated with the erbium laser energy and sealed with gutta-percha. A 2-year follow-up radiograph revealed complete healing of the periapical lesion. The sinus tract disappeared, and the patient is free of symptoms (see Figure 13-6).

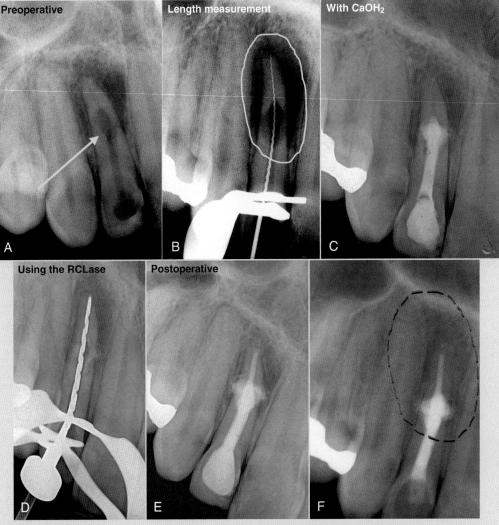

• **Figure 13-6** Laser-assisted root canal filling. **A,** Preoperative radiographs of the maxillary right incisor showing internal resorption. **B,** A root perforation is visible on the measurement radiograph. **C,** Tooth filled with calcium hydroxide. **D,** Laser tip in canal. **E,** Maxillary lateral incisor after completion of root canal filling using a hot gutta-percha technique. **F,** Two-year follow-up radiograph reveals complete healing of periapical lesion. The sinus tract has disappeared, and the patient is free of symptoms.

DeVito et al. have described a new method of removing the smear layer and disinfecting root canals using an Er:YAG laser: These researchers have patented a procedure called *Photon Induced Photoacoustic Streaming* (PIPS). According to their work, at subablative parameters, when an Er:YAG laser is activated in a root canal, the strong absorption of the wavelength in water creates a shockwave, which removes the smear layer and disinfects the canals. An in vitro study of 80 single-rooted extracted human teeth demonstrated pronounced smear layer removal with no thermal damage to the dentinal walls, and thermocouple studies have shown that the root surface temperature increases were well within an acceptable level.[73]

Lloyd et al. used 14 extracted human mandibular molars to compare single-needle irrigation of the root canal systems with photon-induced photoacoustic streaming. They concluded that the laser technique eliminated debris better than single-needle irrigation.[74] Peters et al. studied the efficacy of canal disinfection using sodium hypochlorite irrigation, sodium hypochlorite ultrasonically activated; and Er:YAG laser. These researchers concluded that all three techniques disinfected the root canal systems, with the laser treatment the most effective modality.[75] Other in vitro studies[76,77] have replicated the results of the various investigations. These in vitro studies have established proof of principle for this technique; however, longitudinal in vivo studies evaluating the long-term success rate of teeth treated endodontically with this new technique versus more conventional techniques need to be published to validate this treatment.

Obturation of the Root Canal System

Obturation of the prepared root canal space is done (1) to eliminate all avenues of leakage from the oral cavity or from the periradicular tissues into the root canal system and (2) to seal within the system any irritants that cannot be fully removed during the cleaning and shaping procedures.[78] The rationale of introducing laser technology to assist in obturating the root canal system is based on the following two assumptions about the laser's ability:

- Using the laser irradiation as a heat source for softening gutta-percha, which is employed as the obturating material
- Using the laser as a means to condition the dentinal walls before placement of an obturation bonding material

The concept of *thermoplasticized compaction* is not new and covers any technique that is based entirely on the heat softening of gutta-percha combined primarily with vertical compaction. The technique has many different names, including warm sectional technique, vertical compaction with warm gutta-percha, and the Schilder technique. Schilder[79] first described the technique to fill root canals in three dimensions more than 40 years ago. At present, some dental practitioners still use this technique, whereas others use newer, warm gutta-percha techniques such as thermomechanical compaction, thermoplasticized gutta-percha, and injection of softened gutta-percha, which have been introduced to simplify the root canal filling procedure.

The first laser-assisted root canal filling procedure used the wavelength of the 488-nm argon laser. This wavelength, which is transmitted through dentin, was used to polymerize a resin placed in the main root canal. Testing the ability of this biomaterial to penetrate into accessory root canals showed that the resin in the lateral canals was readily polymerized at low energy levels (30 mW). Further use of this wavelength became irrelevant because of its poor properties for most other dental procedures.[80]

Anic and Matsumoto[81] were the first to compare different root canal filling techniques used to fill single-rooted teeth. Lateral condensation, vertical condensation, low-temperature gutta-percha (Ultrafil), and laser-cured resin with different wavelengths (argon, CO_2, Nd:YAG) were used. The apical sealing ability achieved by the various filling techniques was compared by measuring apical dye penetration after placement of the samples in a 1% solution of methylene blue. Gutta-percha softened with an argon laser created an apical seal similar to that obtained with the lateral condensation and Ultrafil techniques.

Maden et al.[82] used the dye penetration method to measure apical leakage by comparing lateral condensation, System B technique (using thermoplasticized compaction; SybronEndo, Orange, California), and Nd:YAG-softened gutta-percha. No statistically significant differences among the different treatment groups were reported. Anic and Matsumoto[83] measured a temperature elevation on the outer root surface of 14.4° C with use of the Nd:YAG and of 12.9° C with the argon laser. Such a temperature increase may be detrimental to the tissues of the periodontal ligament and attachment apparatus of the teeth, so the implications of using such treatment methodologies remain in question.

To examine whether laser irradiation does improve the adhesion of endodontic materials to the dentinal walls of the root canal and reduce apical leakage, Park et al.[84] used different sealers and two root canal filling techniques. These investigators concluded that Nd:YAG laser irradiation at the end of the root canal preparation (at 5 W, 20 Hz) reduced the apical leakage regardless of the sealer or the technique used. Kimura et al.[85] used an Er:YAG laser (with settings of 170 to 250 mJ and 2 Hz) and showed that irradiation of the root canal did not alter the frequency of apical leakage after obturation compared with conventional methods. Also, using the Nd:YAG laser with black ink at the apical stop helped reduce apical leakage.[86]

Gekelman et al.[87] reported significant improvement in the quality of the apical sealing of root canals using the Nd:YAG laser (100 mJ/pulse, 1 W, 10 Hz). Sousa-Neto et al.[88] also demonstrated that application of Er:YAG laser (200 mJ, 4 Hz) for 60 seconds enhanced the adhesion of epoxy resin–based sealers compared with zinc oxide–eugenol (ZOE)–based root canal sealers.

The clinical evidence on laser-assisted obturation is currently insufficient. For example, it has not been determined whether the use of an optical fiber as a heat source to soften gutta-percha is safe for the surrounding structures of the tooth. Also not clear is whether the softening of gutta-percha is homogeneous in all parts of the filling, as previously suggested, when vertical condensation techniques are used.[89] However, studies show a significant role for endodontic sealers in warm gutta-percha compaction techniques.[90] It is agreed that root canal sealers affect the quality of the apical seal of vertically condensed gutta-percha, and that without a sealer, significantly more apical leakage occurs. Thus the use of sealers is recommended (e.g., ZOE-based sealers).

Currently, procedural simplification seems to be the only proven advantage of laser use. Some questions remain concerning the effectiveness of lasers for assisting in the obturation process of root canals. The clinician should determine the most suitable wavelength and ensure adequate parameters for the specific procedure to be performed.

Endodontic Retreatment

Endodontic failures can be attributed to inadequacies in cleaning, shaping, and obturation; iatrogenic events; or reinfection of the root canal system when the coronal seal is lost after completion of root canal treatment. Regardless of the initial cause, the common etiologic factor is *leakage.* The objective of nonsurgical retreatment is to eliminate the root canal space as a source of irritation to the attachment apparatus.[91]

Some failures may be successfully managed by endodontic retreatment, which can be effective in eliminating clinical and radiographic signs of pathosis. A variety of techniques have been described to remove deficient root canal filling and metallic obstructions that may lead to undesirable results.[92]

The rationale for using laser irradiation in nonsurgical retreatment arises from the need to remove foreign material from the root canal system, which is difficult to achieve using conventional methods.

Farge et al.[93] examined the efficiency of the neodymium-doped yttrium-aluminum-perovskite (Nd:YAP) laser (1340 nm) for root canal retreatment (200 mJ, frequency 10 Hz) in removing previously placed gutta-percha and ZOE-sealer root canal filling, as well as silver cones and broken instruments. These investigators concluded that laser irradiation alone could not completely remove debris and obturation materials from the root canal. Yu et al.[94] used the Nd:YAG laser at three output powers (1, 2, and 3 W) to remove gutta-percha filling (70% of samples) and broken files (55%) from the root canal space. Anjo et al.[95] reported that the time required for removing root canal obturation materials using laser ablation was significantly shorter than with conventional techniques. Some orifices of the dentinal tubules apparently were blocked with melted dentin after laser irradiation. These authors concluded that Nd:YAG laser irradiation is an effective tool for the removal of root canal obturation materials and may offer advantages over conventional methods.

The efficacy of the Er:YAG laser in removing zinc oxide sealers and phenoplastic resins from root canals also has been studied.[96] In straight root canals, laser irradiation of 250 mJ/pulse at a frequency of 10 Hz was useful to eliminate zinc oxide sealer material, in combination with hand instruments but without a specific solvent. Nevertheless, in curved root canals, the procedure had to be stopped owing to the risk of lateral perforation of the root canal wall. Under the same experimental conditions, when laser radiation was delivered to remove phenoplastic resins, ledging of the root canal occurred, and it was not possible to return to the previously established working length.

A potential clinical advantage that should be further explored is the possibility of eliminating the current use of toxic solvents in removing semisolid materials such as gutta-percha from the root canal system.

Although it was shown that filling materials can be removed from the root canal using lasers such as Nd:YAG and Er:YAG,[94–97] the decisive advantage of use of lasers for this purpose remains to be confirmed (Figure 13-7).

Apical Surgery

Surgical endodontic therapy is indicated when teeth have responded poorly to conventional treatment or when they cannot be treated appropriately by nonsurgical means. The goal of endodontic surgery is to eliminate the disease and to prevent it from recurring.[98] The surgical option should be considered only when a better result cannot be achieved by nonsurgical treatment.[99,100]

Egress of irritants from the root canal system into the periapical tissues is considered the main cause of failure after apicoectomy and retrograde filling.[101] The irritants presumably penetrate mainly through a gap between the retrograde filling and the dentin. A second possible pathway is through the dentin of the cut root surface after apicoectomy and retrograde filling. The dentin of apically resected roots is more permeable to fluids than the dentin of nonresected roots.[102]

The first attempt to use lasers in endodontic surgery was performed to seal the apical foramina of extracted teeth in which the pulp was extirpated.[103] The apices of these specimens were irradiated using a high-power CO_2 laser. Melting of the cementum and dentin was observed, with formation of a "cap" that nevertheless could be easily removed. Miserendino[104] used a CO_2 laser to irradiate the apex of a tooth during apicoectomy and described the advantages of improved hemostasis and concurrent visualization of the operative field. He also emphasized the potential sterilization effect on the contaminated root apex, as well as the reduced permeability of the root surface dentin. Recrystallization of the apical root dentin resulted in a surface that appeared smooth and suitable for placement of a retrograde filling material.

Duclos et al.[105] used a CO_2 laser to perform apicoectomies and advocated the use of a "mini" contra-angle head for efficient delivery of laser energies at a 90-degree angle, to facilitate access to the apical part of teeth in the posterior areas.

However, the unfavorable results of an in vivo study in dogs, with no improvement in success rate after apicoectomy using the CO_2 laser,[106] failed to support the rationale previously described by Miserendino.[104] A prospective

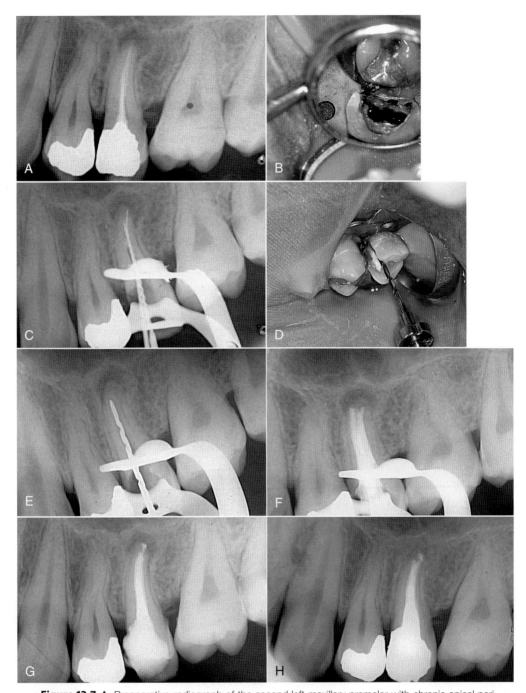

• **Figure 13-7** **A,** Preoperative radiograph of the second left maxillary premolar with chronic apical peri-odontitis. A periapical radiolucent area can clearly be seen; root canal retreatment is indicated. **B,** After access opening, previous root canal filling material was removed; occlusal view shows unclean root canals. **C,** Length-measurement radiograph shows two separate root canals. **D,** Use of Er:YAG laser irradiation for cleaning the root canal system. The RCLase Side-Firing Spiral Tip is introduced to the root canal after completion of biomechanical preparation of the canal with NiTi (ProTaper) files. **E,** RCLase tip in the root canal. **F,** Master point radiographs showing both root canals filled with gutta-percha. **G,** Completed end-odontic therapy. **H,** Six-month postoperative radiograph shows good repair.

study of two retrograde endodontic apical preparations with and without use of a CO_2 laser, in which 320 cases were evaluated, did not show that CO_2 laser irradiation improved the healing process.[107]

In vitro studies using the Nd:YAG laser have shown a reduction in the penetration of dye or bacteria through resected roots.[108–111] Stabholz et al.[109] suggested that the

reduced permeability in the lased specimens probably was the result of structural changes in the dentin after laser application. Although SEM examination showed melting, solidification, and recrystallization of the hard tissue, the structural changes were not uniform, and the melted areas appeared to be connected by areas similar to those in the nonirradiated specimens. These authors postulated that this uneven effect explained the reduced, but not completely eliminated, permeability of the dentin. Homogeneously glazed surfaces presumably would be less permeable than partially glazed surfaces.

Ebihara et al.[112] used the Er:YAG laser for retrograde cavity preparations of extracted teeth. They found no significant difference in dye penetration between the lased and ultrasonic groups. This outcome is not surprising because the Er:YAG laser neither melts nor seals the dentinal tubules; therefore, one would not expect any reduction in dentin permeability.

Gouw-Soares et al.[113] evaluated the marginal permeability in teeth after apicoectomy and apical dentin surface treatment by Er:YAG laser and by 9.6-μm transversely excited at atmospheric pressure (TEA) CO_2 laser. Both treatment groups showed a reduction in permeability to methylene blue dye.

Using the Er:YAG laser at low power in apical surgery, it is possible to cut the apices of extracted teeth, leaving smooth and clean resected surfaces devoid of charring.[114,115] Also, although the cutting speed of the Er:YAG laser is slightly slower than for conventional high-speed burs, the absence of discomfort and vibration and the reduced risk of contamination at the surgical site and trauma to adjacent tissues may compensate for the extended treatment time.[116]

In a 3-year clinical study, Gouw-Soares et al.[117] reported a new protocol to be used in apical surgery. An Er:YAG laser was applied to perform the osteotomy and root resection, whereas Nd:YAG laser irradiation was used to seal the dentinal tubules and reduce possible bacterial contamination of the surgical cavity. The improvement in healing was achieved by incorporating the use of a low-level gallium-aluminum-arsenide diode laser to the treatment protocol. The clinicoradiographic follow-up evaluation showed significant decreases in the radiolucent periapical areas, with no clinical signs and symptoms (see Chapter 15).

Studying the preparation of apical cavities by Er:YAG laser and ultrasonics, Karlovic et al.[118] found lower values of microleakage when the root end cavities were previously prepared with an Er:YAG laser, regardless of the material used to seal those cavities.

After the appropriate wavelength of melting the hard tissues of the tooth has been established, the main contribution of laser technology to surgical endodontics is to convert the apical dentin and cementum structure into a uniformly glazed area that does not allow egress of microorganisms through dentinal tubules and other openings in the apex of the tooth. Hemostasis and sterilization of the contaminated root apex are additional benefits.[119]

Conclusions

Lasers are making significant contributions to every step in the practice of endodontics, from diagnosis using Doppler flowmeter technology to preventive measures involving pulp capping and pulpotomy. Lasers may be used for cleaning, disinfecting, and obturating root canal systems. When

conventional endodontic therapy fails, laser-assisted endodontic retreatment is now a viable treatment alternative. As a last resort to prevent extraction of a tooth, lasers may be used in apical surgery to seal the root end of the tooth to prevent bacteria from entering the root canal system. As this technology matures, more uses and perhaps more wavelengths will deliver superior endodontic care.

References

1. Kimura Y, Wilder-Smith P, Matsumoto K: Lasers in endodontics: a review, *Int Endod J* 33:173–185, 2000.
2. Cohen S, Liewehr F: Diagnostic procedures. In Cohen S, Burns RC, editors: *Pathways of the pulp*, ed 8, St Louis, 2002, Mosby, pp 3–30.
3. Matsumoto K: Lasers in endodontics, *Dent Clin North Am* 44:889–906, 2000.
4. Mesaros SV, Trope M: Revascularization of traumatized teeth assessed by laser Doppler flowmetry: case report, *Endod Dent Traumatol* 13:24–30, 1997.
5. Evans D, Reid J, Strang R, Stirrups D: A comparison of laser Doppler flowmetry with other methods of assessing the vitality of traumatized anterior teeth, *Endod Dent Traumatol* 15:284–290, 1999.
6. Ebihara A, Tokita Y, Izawa T, et al.: Pulpal blood flow assessed by laser Doppler flowmetry in a tooth with a horizontal root fracture, *Oral Surg Oral Med Oral Pathol* 81:229–233, 1996.
7. Gazelius B, Olgart L, Edwall B, et al.: Non-invasive recording of blood flow in human dental pulp, *Endod Dent Traumatol* 2:219–221, 1986.
8. Yanpiset K, Vongsavan N, Sigurdsson A, Trope M: Efficacy of laser Doppler flowmetry for the diagnosis of revascularization of reimplanted immature dog teeth, *Endod Dent Traumatol* 17:63–70, 2001.
9. Ritter AL, Ritter AV, Murrah V, et al.: Pulp revascularization of replanted immature dog teeth after treatment with minocycline and doxycyline assessed by laser Doppler flowmetry, radiography, and histology, *Endod Dent Traumatol* 20:75–84, 2004.
10. Strobl H, Gojer G, Norer B, Emshoff R: Assessing revascularization of avulsed permanent maxillary incisors by laser Doppler flowmetry, *J Am Dent Assoc* 134:1597–1603, 2003.
11. Polat S, Er K, Akpinar KE, Polat NT: The sources of laser Doppler blood-flow signals recorded from vital and root canal treated teeth, *Arch Oral Biol* 49:53–57, 2004.
12. Roeykens H, Van Maele G, De Moor R, et al.: Reliability of laser Doppler flowmetry in a 2-probe assessment of pulpal blood flow, *Oral Surg Oral Med Oral Pathol* 87:742–745, 1999.
13. Odor TM, Ford TR, McDonald F: Effect of probe design and bandwidth on laser Doppler readings from vital and root-filled teeth, *Med Eng Phys* 18:359–364, 1996.
14. Soo-ampon S, Vongsavan N, Soo-ampon M, et al.: The sources of laser Doppler blood flow signals recorded from human teeth, *Arch Oral Biol* 48:353–360, 2003.
15. Hartman A, Azerad J, Boucher Y: Environmental effects of laser Doppler pulpal blood-flow measurements in man, *Arch Oral Biol* 41:333–339, 1996.
16. Frentzen M, Braun A, Koort HJ: Lasers in endodontics: an overview. In Rechmann P, Fried D, Hennig T, editors: *Lasers in dentistry VIII, SPIE Proc* 4610:1–8, 2002.
17. Isermann GT, Kaminski EJ: Pulpal response to minimal exposure in presence of bacteria and dycal, *J Endod* 5:322–327, 1979.

18. Cvek M, Cleaton-Jones PE, Austin JC, et al.: Pulp reaction to exposure after experimental crown fractures or grinding in adult monkeys, *J Endod* 8:391–397, 1982.

19. Cvek M: Endodontic treatment of traumatized teeth. In Andreasen JO, editor: *Traumatic injuries of the teeth*, ed 2, Philadelphia, 1981, WB Saunders.

20. Seltzer S, Bender IB: Pulp capping and pulpotomy. In Seltzer S, Bender IB, editors: *The dental pulp: biologic considerations in dental procedures*, ed 2, Philadelphia, 1975, JB Lippincott.

21. Torabinejad M, Chivian N: Clinical applications of mineral trioxide aggregate, *J Endod* 25:197–200, 1999.

22. Pitt-Ford TR, Torabinejad M, Abedi HR: Mineral trioxide aggregate as a pulp capping material, *J Am Dent Assoc* 127:1491, 1996.

23. Myers K, Kaminski E, Lautenschlager EP: The effect of mineral trioxide aggregate on the dog pulp, *J Endod* 22:198–202, 1996.

24. Klein H, Fuks A, Eidelman E, et al.: Partial pulpotomy following complicated crown fracture in permanent incisors: a clinical and radiographical study, *J Pedod* 9:142–147, 1985.

25. Fuks AB, Chosack A, Klein H, et al.: Partial pulpotomy as a treatment alternative for exposed pulps in crown-fractured permanent incisors, *Endod Dent Traumatol* 3:100–102, 1987.

26. Melcer J, Chaumate MT, Melcer F, et al.: Preliminary report of the effect of CO_2 laser beam on the dental pulp of the *Macaca mulatta* primate and the beagle dog, *J Endod* 11:1–5, 1985.

27. Shoji S, Nakamura M, Horiuchi H: Histopathological changes in dental pulps irradiated by CO_2 laser: a preliminary report on laser pulpotomy, *J Endod* 11:379–384, 1985.

28. Jukic S, Anic I, Koba K: The effect of pulpotomy using CO_2 and Nd:YAG lasers on dental pulp tissue, *Int Endod J* 30:175–188, 1977.

29. Moritz A, Schoop U, Goharkhay K: The CO_2 laser as an aid in direct pulp capping, *J Endod* 24:248–251, 1998.

30. Fried D, Glena RE, Featherstone JD, et al.: Permanent and transient changes in the reflectance of CO_2 laser–irradiated dental hard tissues at lambda = 9.3, 9.6, 10.3, and 10.6 microns and at fluences of 1–20 J/cm², *Lasers Surg Med* 20:22–31, 1997.

31. Wigdor HA, Walsh JT Jr: Histologic analysis of the effect on dental pulp of a 9.6-micron CO_2 laser, *Laser Surg Med* 30:261–266, 2002.

32. White JM, Fagan MC, Goodis HE: Intrapulpal temperatures during pulsed Nd:YAG laser treatment, in vitro, *J Periodontol* 65:255–259, 1994.

33. Kakehashi S, Stanley HR, Fitzgerald RJ: The effect of surgical exposures of dental pulps in germ-free and conventional laboratory rats, *Oral Surg Oral Med Oral Pathol* 20:340–349, 1965.

34. Bergenholz G: Microorganisms from necrotic pulps of traumatized teeth, *Odontologisk Revy* 25:347–358, 1974.

35. Moller AJ, Fabricius L, Dahlen G, et al.: Influence on periapical tissues of indigenous oral bacteria and necrotic pulp tissue in monkeys, *Scand J Dent Res* 89:475–484, 1981.

36. Bystrom A, Sundquist G: Bacteriologic evaluation of the efficacy of mechanical root canal instrumentation in endodontic therapy, *Scand J Dent Res* 89:321–328, 1981.

37. Sjogren U, Hagglund B, Sundquist G, et al.: Factors affecting the long-term results of endodontic treatment, *J Endod* 16:498–504, 1990.

38. McComb D, Smith DC: A preliminary scanning electron microscope study of root canals after endodontic procedures, *J Endod* 1:238–242, 1975.

39. Moodnik RM, Dorn SO, Feldman MJ, et al.: Efficacy of biomechanical instrumentation: a scanning electron microscopy study, *J Endod* 2:261–266, 1976.

40. Mader CL, Baumgartner JC, Peters DD: Scanning electron microscopic investigation of the smeared layer on root canal walls, *J Endod* 10:477–483, 1984.

41. Torabinejad M, Handysides R, Khademi AA, et al.: Clinical implications of the smear layer in endodontics: a review, *Oral Surg Oral Med Oral Pathol* 94:658–666, 2002.

42. Haapasalo M, Orstavik D: In vitro infection and disinfection of dentinal tubules, *J Dent Res* 66:1375–1379, 1986.

43. Pashley DH: Smear layer: physiological considerations, *Oper Dent Suppl* 3:13–29, 1984.

44. Drake DR, Wiemann AH, Rivera EM, et al.: Bacterial retention in canal walls in vitro: effect of smear layer, *J Endod* 20:78–82, 1994.

45. Peters OA, Schonenberger K, Laib A: Effects of four Ni-Ti preparation techniques on root canal geometry assessed by micro computed tomography, *Int Endod J* 34:221–230, 2001.

46. Oguntebi BR: Dentin tubule infection and endodontic therapy implications, *Int Endod J* 27:218–222, 1994.

47. Anic I, Tachibana H, Matsumoto K, et al.: Permeability, morphologic and temperature changes of canal dentin walls induced by Nd:YAG, CO_2 and argon lasers, *Int Endod J* 29:13–22, 1996.

48. Harashima T, Takeda FH, Kimura, et al.: Effect of Nd:YAG laser irradiation for removal of intracanal debris and smear layer in extracted human teeth, *J Clin Laser Med Surg* 15:131–135, 1997.

49. Saunders WP, Whitters CJ, Strang R, et al.: The effect of an Nd:YAG pulsed laser on the cleaning of the root canal and the formation of a fused apical plug, *Int Endod J* 28:213–220, 1995.

50. Moshonov J, Sion A, Kasirer J, et al.: Efficacy of argon laser irradiation in removing intracanal debris, *Oral Surg Oral Med Oral Pathol* 79:221–225, 1995.

51. Yamazaki R, Goya C, Yu DG, et al.: Effect of erbium, chromium:YSGG laser irradiation on root canal walls: a scanning electron microscopic and thermographic study, *J Endod* 27:9–12, 2001.

52. Takeda FH, Harashima T, Kimura Y, et al.: Efficacy of Er:YAG laser irradiation in removing debris and smear layer on root canal walls, *J Endod* 24:548–551, 1998.

53. Kimura Y, Yonaga K, Yokoyama K, et al.: Root surface temperature increase during Er:YAG laser irradiation of root canals, *J Endod* 28:76–78, 2002.

54. Goodis HE, Pashley D, Stabholz A: Pulpal effects of thermal and mechanical irritants. In Hargreaves KM, Goodis HE, editors: *Seltzer and Bender's dental pulp*, Chicago, 2002, Quintessence, pp 371–410.

55. Stabholz A, Zeltzser R, Sela M, et al.: The use of lasers in dentistry: principles of operation and clinical applications, *Compendium* 24:811–824, 2003.

56. Stabholz A: The role of laser technology in modern endodontics. In Ishikawa I, Frame JW, Aoki A, editors: *Lasers in dentistry: revolution of dental treatment in the new millennium*, Elsevier Sci BV Int Congr Series 1248:21–27, 2003.

57. Cozean C, Arcoria CJ, Pelagalli J, et al.: Dentistry for the 21st century? Erbium:YAG laser for teeth, *J Am Dent Assoc* 128:1080–1087, 1997.

58. Ando N, Hoshino E: Predominant obligate anaerobes invading the deep layers of root canal dentine, *Int Endod J* 23:20–27, 1990.

59. Armitage GC, Ryder MI, Wilcox SE: Cemental changes in teeth with heavily infected root canals, *J Endod* 9:127–130, 1983.

60. Zakariasen KL, Dederich DN, Tulip J, et al.: Bactericidal action of carbon dioxide laser radiation in experimental root canals, *Can J Microbiol* 32:942–946, 1986.

61. Le Goff A, Morazin-Dautel A, Guigand M, et al.: An evaluation of the CO₂ laser for endodontic disinfection, *J Endod* 25: 105–108, 1999.

62. Moshonov J, Orstavik D, Yamauchi S, et al.: Nd:YAG laser irradiation in root canal disinfection, *Endod Dent Traumatol* 11:220–224, 1995.

63. Fegan SE, Steiman HR: Comparative evaluation of the antibacterial effects of intracanal Nd:YAG laser irradiation: an in vitro study, *J Endod* 21:415–417, 1995.

64. Rooney J, Midda M, Leeming J: A laboratory investigation of the bactericidal effect of Nd:YAG laser, *Br Dent J* 176:61–64, 1994.

65. Gutknecht N, Moritz A, Conrads G: Bactericidal effect of the Nd:YAG laser in *in vitro* root canals, *J Clin Laser Med Surg* 14:77–80, 1996.

66. Nammour S, Kowaly K, Powell L, et al.: External temperature during KTP-Nd:YAG laser irradiation in root canals: an in vitro study, *Lasers Med Sci* 19:27–32, 2004.

67. Stabholz A, Kettering J, Neev J, et al.: Effects of XeCl excimer laser on *Streptococcus mutans*, *J Endod* 19:232–235, 1993.

68. Folwaczny M, Liesenhoff T, Lehn N, et al.: Bactericidal action of 308-nm excimer-laser radiation: an in vitro investigation, *J Endod* 24:781–785, 1998.

69. Moritz A, Gutknecht N, Goharkhay K, et al.: In vitro irradiation of infected root canals with diode laser: results of microbiologic, infrared spectrometric and stain penetration examination, *Quintessence Int* 28:205–209, 1997.

70. Mehl A, Folwaczny M, Haffner C, et al.: Bactericidal effects of 2.94-μ Er:YAG laser irradiation in dental root canals, *J Endod* 25:490–493, 1999.

71. Dostalova T, Jelinkova H, Housova D, et al.: Endodontic treatment with application of Er:YAG laser waveguide radiation disinfection, *J Clin Laser Med Surg* 20:135–139, 2002.

72. Schoop U, Moritz A, Kluger W, et al.: The Er:YAG laser in endodontics: results of an in vitro study, *Lasers Surg Med* 30: 360–364, 2002.

73. DeVito E, Peters O, Olivi G: Effectiveness of the erbium YAG laser and new design radial and stripped tips in removing the smear layer after root canal instrumentation, *Lasers Med Sci* 27:273–280, 2012.

74. Lloyd A, Uhles J, Clement D, Garcia-Godoy F: Elimination of intracanal tissue and debris through a novel laser-activated system assessed using high-resolution micro-computed tomography: a pilot study, *J Endod* 40(4):584–587, 2014.

75. Peters O, Bardsley S, Fong J, et al.: Disinfection of root canals with photon-initiated photoacoustic streaming, *J Endod* 37(7):1008–1012, 2011.

76. Devito E, Colonna M, Olivi G: The photoacoustic efficacy of an Er:YAG laser with radial and stripped tips on root canal dentin walls: an SEM Evaluation, *J Laser Dent* 19(1):156–161, 2011.

77. Jaramillo D, Aprecio R, Angelov N, et al: Efficacy of photon-induced photoacoustic streaming (PIPS) on root canals infected with *Enterococcus faecalis:* a pilot study, *Endod Pract* 5(3):28–32, 2012.

78. Gutmann JL, Whitherspoon DE: Obturation of the cleaned and shaped root canal system. In Cohen S, Burns RC, editors: *Pathways of the pulp*, ed 8, St Louis, 2002, Mosby, pp 293–364.

79. Schilder H: Filling root canals in three dimensions, *Dent Clin North Am* 11:723–729, 1967.

80. Potts TV, Petrou A: Laser photopolymerization of dental materials with potential endodontic applications, *J Endod* 16:265–268, 1990.

81. Anic I, Matsumoto K: Comparison of the sealing ability of laser-softened, laterally condensed and low-temperature thermoplasticized gutta-percha, *J Endod* 21:464–469, 1995.

82. Maden M, Gorgul G, Tinaz AC: Evaluation of apical leakage of root canals obturated with Nd:YAG laser–softened gutta-percha, System-B, and lateral condensation techniques, *Contemp Dent Pract* 15:16–26, 2002.

83. Anic I, Matsumoto K: Dentinal heat transmission induced by a laser-softened gutta-percha obturation technique, *J Endod* 21:470–474, 1995.

84. Park DS, Yoo HM, Oh TS: Effect of Nd:YAG laser irradiation on the apical leakage of obturated root canals: an electrochemical study, *Int Endod J* 4:318–321, 2001.

85. Kimura Y, Yonaga K, Yokoyama K, et al.: Apical leakage of obturated canals prepared by Er:YAG laser, *J Endod* 27:567–570, 2001.

86. Kimura Y, Yamazaki R, Goya C, et al.: A comparative study on the effects of three types of laser irradiation at the apical stop and apical leakage after obturation, *J Clin Laser Med Surg* 17: 261–266, 1999.

87. Gekelman D, Prokopowitsch I, Eduardo CP: In vitro study of the effects of Nd:YAG laser irradiation on the apical sealing of endodontic fillings performed with and without dentin plugs, *J Clin Laser Med Surg* 20:117–121, 2002.

88. Sousa-Neto MD, Marchesan MA, Pecora JD, et al.: Effect of Er:YAG laser on adhesion of root canal sealers, *J Endod* 28: 185–187, 2002.

89. Blum JY, Parahy E, Machtou P: Warm vertical compaction sequences in relation to gutta-percha temperature, *J Endod* 23:307–311, 1997.

90. Yared GM, Bou Dagher F: Sealing ability of the vertical condensation with different root canal sealers, *J Endod* 21:6–8, 1996.

91. Ruddle CJ: Nonsurgical endodontic retreatment. In Cohen S, Burns RC, editors: *Pathways of the pulp*, ed 8, St Louis, 2002, Mosby, pp 875–929.

92. Hulssman R: Methods for removing metal obstructions from the root canal, *Endod Dent Traumatol* 9:223–237, 1983.

93. Farge P, Nahas P, Bonin P: In vitro study of a Nd-YAG laser in endodontic retreatment, *J Endod* 42:359–363, 1998.

94. Yu DG, Kimura Y, Tomita Y, et al.: Study on removal effects of filling materials and broken files from root canals using pulsed Nd:YAG laser, *J Clin Laser Med Surg* 18:23–28, 2000.

95. Anjo T, Ebihara A, Takeda A, et al.: Removal of two types of root canal filling material using pulsed Nd:YAG laser irradiation, *Photomed Laser Surg* 22:470–476, 2004.

96. Warembourg P, Rocca JP, Bertrand MF: Efficacy of an Er:YAG laser to remove endodontic pastes: an in vitro study, *J Oral Laser Appl* 1:43–47, 2001.

97. Viducic D, Jukic S, Karlovic Z, et al.: Removal of gutta- percha using an Nd:YAG laser, *Int Endod J* 36:670–673, 2003.

98. Carr GB: Surgical endodontics. In Cohen S, Burns RC, editors: *Pathways of the pulp*, ed 6, St Louis, 1994, Mosby, pp 531–567.

99. Gutmann JL: Principles of endodontic surgery for the general practitioner, *Dent Clin North Am* 28:895–908, 1984.

100. Leubke RG: Surgical endodontics, *Dent Clin North Am* 18:379, 1974.

101. Stabholz A, Shani J, Friedman S, et al.: Marginal adaptation of retrograde fillings and its correlation with sealability, *J Endod* 11:218–223, 1985.

102. Ichesco E, Ellison R, Corcoran J: A spectrophotometric analysis of dentinal leakage in the resected root (abstract), *J Endod* 12:129, 1986.
103. Weichman JA, Johnson FM: Laser use in endodontics: a preliminary investigation, *Oral Surg Oral Med Oral Pathol* 31: 416–420, 1971.
104. Miserendino LL: The laser apicoectomy: endodontic application of CO_2 laser for periapical surgery, *Oral Surg Oral Med Oral Pathol* 66:615–619, 1988.
105. Duclos P, Behlert V, Lenz P: New technique of surgical treatment of periapical lesions using carbon dioxide laser, *Rev Odontostomatol* 19:143–150, 1990.
106. Friedman S, Rotstein I, Mahamid A: In vivo efficacy of various retrofills and of CO_2 laser in apical surgery, *Endod Dent Traumatol* 7:19–25, 1991.
107. Bader G, Lejeune S: Prospective study of two retrograde endodontic apical preparations with and without the use of CO_2 laser, *Endod Dent Traumatol* 14:75–78, 1998.
108. Stabholz A, Khayat A, Ravanshad SH, et al.: Effects of Nd:YAG laser on apical seal of teeth after apicoectomy and retrofill, *J Endod* 18:371–375, 1992.
109. Stabholz A, Khayat A, Weeks DA, et al.: Scanning electron microscopic study of the apical dentine surfaces lased with Nd:YAG laser following apicoectomy and retrofill, *Int Endod J* 25:288–291, 1992.
110. Arens DL, Levy GC, Rizoiu IM: A comparison of dentin permeability after bur and laser apicoectomies, *Compendium* 14:1290–1297, 1993.
111. Wong WS, Rosenberg PA, Boylan RJ, et al.: A comparison of the apical seals achieved using retrograde amalgam fillings and the Nd:YAG laser, *J Endod* 20:595–597, 1994.
112. Ebihara A, Wadachi R, Sekine Y, et al.: Application of Er:YAG laser to retrograde cavity preparation, *J Jpn Soc Laser Dent* 9: 23–31, 1998.
113. Gouw-Soares S, Stabholz A, Lage-Marques JL, et al.: Comparative study of dentine permeability after apicectomy and surface treatment with 9.6-micrometer TEA CO_2 and Er-YAG laser irradiation, *J Clin Laser Med Surg* 22:129–139, 2004.
114. Paghdiwala AF: Root resection of endodontically treated teeth by Er:YAG laser radiation, *J Endod* 19:91–94, 1993.
115. Komori T, Yokoyama K, Matsumoto Y, Matsumoto K: Er-YAG and Ho-YAG laser root resection of extracted human teeth, *J Clin Laser Med Surg* 15:9–13, 1997.
116. Komori T, Yokoyama K, Takato T, Matsumoto K: Clinical application of the Er-YAG laser for apicoectomy, *J Endod* 23:748–750, 1997.
117. Gouw-Soares S, Tanji E, Haypek P, et al.: The use of Er-YAG, Nd-YAG and Ga-AlAs lasers in periapical surgery: a three year clinical study, *J Clin Surg Med* 19:193–198, 2001.
118. Karlovic Z, Pezelj-Ribaric S, Miletic I, et al.: Er-YAG laser versus ultrasonic in preparation of root-end cavities, *J Endod* 31:821–823, 2005.
119. Stabholz A, Sahar-Helft S, Moshonov J: Lasers in endodontics, *Dent Clin North Am* 48:809–832, 2004.

14

Lasers in Major Oral and Maxillofacial Surgery

ROBERT A. STRAUSS AND MICHAEL COLEMAN

When lasers were first introduced to mainstream oral and maxillofacial surgery (OMS) in the mid-1980s, essentially the only one available to the practitioner was the carbon dioxide (CO_2) laser, primarily because of its outstanding cutting abilities. As laser technology progressed, other medical and surgical specialties introduced different wavelengths, which have been adapted for use in the oral cavity or on the face.

Greater soft tissue needs and fewer hard tissue needs differentiate OMS from other dental specialties. In addition, the use of lasers for skin procedures further complicates the choice of appropriate wavelength, technique, and postoperative care. As with any procedure, choosing the proper laser must be based on the intended target tissue and its absorption characteristics. With cosmetic procedures, the *lateral thermal effects* of a particular wavelength are important to the surgical goal, while limiting lateral damage and scarring.[1] Unlike in the oral cavity, such complications in skin are potentially devastating.

Choosing a Surgical Laser

Surprisingly, the primary laser used in major OMS and facial cosmetic surgery remains, after more than 40 years, the 10,600-nm CO_2 laser.[2] Its excellent water absorption, favorable extinction length and depth of penetration, and consistency in soft tissue make it an excellent choice for most soft tissue procedures in the mouth. In addition, when handled carefully and correctly, the CO_2 laser can be used for cosmetic facial surgery including facial resurfacing, resulting in a predictable and substantial ablation of the epithelium and dermis.

The addition of computerized scanning devices has allowed the CO_2 laser to be used in predetermined geometric and repeatable patterns, providing exceedingly uniform results. It also can be used for all major extirpative procedures, large-scale ablations, incisional cosmetic surgery (e.g., blepharoplasty), and airway procedures (e.g., laser-assisted uvulopalatopharyngoplasty [LA-UPPP]). Although new

technology now allows the CO_2 wavelength to be transmitted through new types of fiberoptic fibers, a majority of current lasers are designed with hollow-waveguide or articulated-arm delivery systems. This setup makes endoscopy in OMS procedures difficult to perform. Recently, a variation of the CO_2 laser that produces a wavelength of 9300 nm has been cleared by the U.S. Food and Drug Administration (FDA) for procedures on enamel and dentin. This wavelength makes possible the use of this laser on both hard and soft tissue with an articulated-arm delivery system. At present, little experience has accumulated with use of this wavelength in OMS procedures involving hard tissue (and although the 9300-nm CO_2 laser is not specifically cleared for bone applications, a reasonable assumption is that it will be effective on that tissue as well), but if it proves to be effective and efficient, this wavelength potentially may be very useful in many intraoral procedures including orthognathic surgery osteotomies, odontectomies, and implant surgery, as well as cosmetic surgery.

The erbium-doped yttrium-aluminum-garnet (Er:YAG) and erbium plus chromium–doped yttrium-scandium-gallium-garnet (Er,Cr:YSGG) lasers also are useful in major OMS, although they have not reached the level of popularity of the CO_2 laser. Currently, most major hard tissue procedures (e.g., osteotomies) are too time-consuming when these lasers are used. However, lesser osseous procedures (e.g., sinus lifts) are easily and quickly accomplished with these wavelengths. The Er:YAG laser also has been used for cosmetic facial resurfacing.[3,4] Because of its reduced depth of effect in skin compared with the CO_2 laser, postoperative erythema and disability are greatly decreased with the Er:YAG laser. Unfortunately, the resurfacing effect also is diminished, with a corresponding decrease in cosmetic improvement, which has resulted in less frequent adoption of erbium lasers by surgeons.

Borrowed from orthopedics and urology, the holmium-doped YAG (Ho:YAG) laser is used almost exclusively in major OMS to perform endoscopic temporomandibular joint (TMJ) surgery. This laser's wavelength has the ability to transmit through a water-filled environment such as a joint, while the soft tissue effects mimic those of a CO_2 laser (e.g., cutting, coagulating, ablating). This is done by perforating the joint with two hollow cannulas, one for endoscopic visualization and one for the Ho:YAG laser fiber. The procedure is then done under video monitoring. The small-incision surgery leads to significantly decreased recovery time and complications.[5]

The neodymium-doped YAG (Nd:YAG) laser, now cleared by the U.S. FDA for certain periodontal procedures, has found little use in major OMS other than for some vascular lesions. Its deep extinction length and penetration in soft tissue create significant lateral tissue damage, desirable for treating vascular lesions but not other pathologic conditions.

Solid-state lasers such as the diode lasers (with wavelengths of 810 to 1064 nm) have become very popular in general dentistry because of their small size, low cost, fiber-optic delivery, and ease of use for minor surgery of oral soft tissues.[6] By contrast, for major OMS procedures, these lasers are very inefficient compared with the CO_2 laser. Although hard tissue damage is a justifiable safety concern with use of CO_2 lasers, the diminished effect of the diode lasers makes them useful only for these minor oral surgical procedures.

The use of *low-level* diode lasers for noninvasive, athermal laser therapy is popular in European countries and has been studied in the United States, but this technique generally has not proved to be effective for major surgical indications. Although studies confirm that low-level lasers have beneficial physiologic effects, their specific advantages for OMS procedures remain unclear[7,8] (Figure 14-1). (See Chapter 15.)

Intense pulsed light (IPL) sources use highly concentrated light waves to perform several procedures similar to those achievable with lasers. Unlike true lasers, however, IPL sources are polychromatic and are neither collimated nor coherent (Figure 14-2). Because they generally feature deeper tissue penetration and target tissue pigments and vascularity, primary uses include treatment of dermatologic lesions and hair removal (targeting follicular pigmentation).[9]

Several lasers also are used in OMS for dermatologic applications. These wavelengths are highly specific for particular pigments or vascular tissues and include the copper vapor, gold vapor, flashlamp-pumped pulsed dye, pulsed Nd:YAG, and potassium titanyl phosphate (KTP)–YAG lasers.[10] The choice of wavelength must be based on individual patient needs, patient age, lesion color and depth, and laser availability.[11]

Safety and Anesthesia Considerations

Although the use of lasers for OMS offers many advantages, it does present certain anesthetic risks not common to traditional surgical techniques. Standard safety precautions must be observed to maintain the safety of the patient, surgeon, anesthesiologist, and other members of the surgical staff. Each laser system's user manual should be reviewed before initiation of a planned procedure. Also, discussion with the anesthesiologist regarding the type of laser and the procedure is imperative. It is important to be just as vigilant when laser surgery is performed in the outpatient office environment.

The laser beam is a high-intensity light that, if directed at a reflective surface, can change its intended path while maintaining its focal properties. When reflected in this manner, the beam can strike unintended targets with full power. Most vulnerable to injury from a misdirected beam are the eyes, the skin, and any nearby flammable objects.[12] Appropriate warning signs should be posted outside the operating suite indicating the type of laser being used, the risk class of the laser, and the required personal safety equipment[13] (Figure 14-3). Protective eyewear with eye shields must be worn at all times by the patient and personnel to avoid ophthalmic injury. For each laser, a specific type of eyewear is available that will absorb its particular wavelength.

Flammable patient drapes, including standard paper and plastic drapes used in the operating room (OR), are a source of ignition and should not be used. Instead, laser-resistant drapes or cloth drapes saturated in water should be used around the surgical field.[13] Alcohol preparation of the field

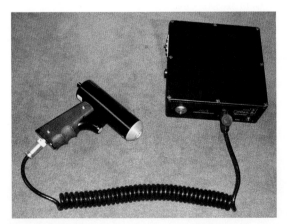

• **Figure 14-1** Low-level laser therapy using athermal diode laser.

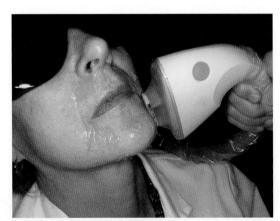

• **Figure 14-2** Intense pulsed light (IPL) source. These devices most often are used for vascular and pigmented lesion removal or hair removal. Anesthesia usually is not required for these procedures.

also should be avoided, because alcohol can serve as a potential ignition source if not allowed to vaporize completely before laser use.

Three main approaches are recognized to decrease the fire hazards associated with use of conventional endotracheal (ET) tubes during laser surgery[14]: (1) no airway, (2) protection of the surface of a conventional tube, and (3) use of a noncombustible tube. With many OMS procedures, whether done in the office or the operating suite, a total intravenous anesthesia technique may be appropriate after "chinning" the patient (i.e., applying the chin thrust maneuver as for cardiopulmonary resuscitation [CPR]) or insertion of a nasal airway. The Rousch red-rubber nasal airway has been found to be safe for laser procedures.[15]

The no-airway approach, however, is not always practical for procedures of long duration, in which case a definitive airway, with shielding from the laser beam, is necessary, such as a conventional ET tube with a protective material on its external surface. Materials available for this purpose are metallic foil wrapped around the tube and a silver anode sheet that adheres to the tube.[13] The foil often is cumbersome and vulnerable to dislodgement, so that intraoperative

manipulation can result in exposure of the tube, whereas the adherence of the silver anode sheet is less likely to lead to exposure.

Two types of noncombustible ET tubes are currently available: the metallic tube, which contains no combustible material, and the ceramic-coated tube (Xomed, Inc., Jacksonville, Florida)[13] (Figure 14-4). The metallic tube, however, cannot be used for nasal intubation and does not come with a cuff, which prevents the use of a normal anesthesia circuit.

Still other issues warrant consideration in reduction of laser-related fire hazard: Flammable gases must be avoided during laser surgery. Most inhalational anesthetics used in ORs today are not flammable and include sevoflurane, isoflurane, enflurane, and halothane. Ether and cyclopropane, which are no longer used by most anesthesiologists, are combustible and should not be used.[13]

The concentration of oxygen with inhalational agents also should be addressed. Ideally, the lowest concentration possible is used while maintaining an acceptable oxygen saturation level. To accomplish this aim, the oxygen is diluted with regular compressed air or with helium, both of which reduce flammability (Figure 14-5). Nitrous oxide mixed with oxygen, however, possesses the same flammability as that of oxygen alone and is avoided.[12]

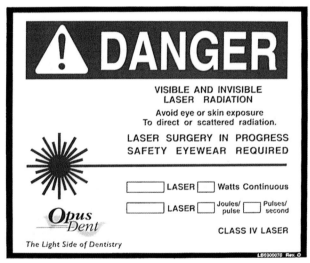

• **Figure 14-3** Warning sign posted outside operating room indicating type of laser being used, class of laser, and required personal safety equipment.

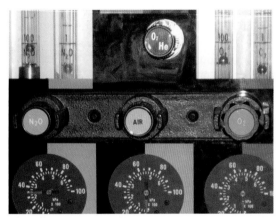

• **Figure 14-5** Standard general anesthesia machine showing compressed gases available for delivery of inhalational agent. Note availability of regular compressed air, which does not support combustion, in addition to oxygen.

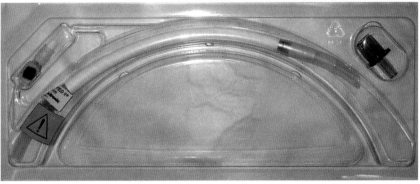

• **Figure 14-4** Example of ceramic-coated, laser-safe endotracheal tube.

Tumor-Resective Surgery: Excision versus Ablation

The laser is a versatile surgical instrument that can be used in three basic ways: excision/incision, ablation/vaporization, and hemostasis/coagulation.[16] The technique used is based on the clinical situation and three parameters controlled by the surgeon: power, spot size, and time.

Excision

When used for excisional purposes, the laser is basically a "light scalpel" producing precision cuts without the bleeding of traditional scalpel surgery. For optimal results, the *spot size* should be kept as small as possible with the particular laser used (usually 0.1 to 0.5 mm), which is accomplished by keeping the handpiece at its focal length from the tissue.[17] This is known as the *focused mode*. The *focal length* is also variable depending on the handpiece, ranging from 1 mm to 1 cm from the end of the handpiece to the tissue.

The technique for excision of a lesion remains the same regardless of the laser system used. It is recommended first to outline the intended incision line by means of the laser beam set at a lower power in an intermittent, gated, or pulsed mode. This mapping will provide superficial guide marks while avoiding deep penetration into the tissue, allowing the surgeon to adjust the location of the margins, if necessary. Of note, for performing an excisional biopsy, an additional 0.5 mm should be added circumferentially to the margin to account for the lateral zone of thermal necrosis associated with the laser.[13]

After satisfactory outlining has been performed, the laser is switched to continuous-wave mode, and the dots are connected to create the incision. Multiple passes may be required to achieve the desired depth.

Observing the effect of the laser on the tissue during the first pass will allow the surgeon to adjust the parameters of the laser during subsequent passes, if necessary, to achieve the preferred cut. For example, if the depth of the cut is too shallow, the power may be increased or the handpiece moved at slower rate to increase time of exposure. Increasing the power usually is the better option because increasing the time will allow more time for lateral conduction and subsequent lateral thermal damage. On the other hand, if the initial cut is too deep, the power may be lowered or the handpiece moved more quickly, both of which are good options.

After adequate depth of the outlining incision has been achieved, excision of the lesion can begin. This is accomplished by lightly grasping the tissue with a forceps, applying slight traction, and horizontally undermining the lesion while maintaining the laser tip at the focal length. Hemostasis at the surgical site will be excellent, and closure is rarely needed. The exception is the case in which allowing the wound to granulate would give unacceptable cosmetic results.

Ablation

Another common technique carried out with the laser is tissue ablation (also called vaporization). Ablation is used for superficial tissue removal when standard excision would lead to more extensive sectioning than necessary. The targeted lesion usually is confined to the epithelium and underlying submucosa. The advantages of this technique are less scarring, less dysfunction, and less potential for damage to important adjacent structures.

The technique for ablation begins with the same outlining procedure described for the excisional technique. Next, the laser is defocused by moving the handpiece farther from the tissue, thereby widening the laser beam and increasing the spot size. Spot sizes ranging from 1.5 to 3.0 mm typically are used. The now-defocused beam is passed over the lesion in multiple side-by-side strokes, creating multiple U patterns (Figure 14-6).

After the first pass is complete, the depth of penetration is evaluated. If the cut is too shallow, it can be deepened by increasing the power, increasing the time by moving the handpiece more slowly, or decreasing spot size. Increasing the power is the best alternative, whereas increasing time is to be avoided for reasons previously mentioned. Decreasing the spot size is a viable option but will increase the number of strokes required to cover the area.

Conversely, to decrease the depth of penetration, the surgeon can decrease the power, decrease the time by moving the handpiece more quickly, or widen the spot size. Of these, the latter two are the preferred options.

> ### CLINICAL TIP
>
> Gently wipe the char layer from the surface of the tissue with wet gauze between laser passes. This char layer contains no water for absorption of the laser wavelength, so its exposure will result in undesired excess heating and lateral thermal conduction.

Ablation alone does not allow a biopsy of the lesion to be taken; therefore, if the clinical findings are suggestive of a malignancy or premalignancy, incisional biopsy should be performed before ablation. If the lesion is histologically

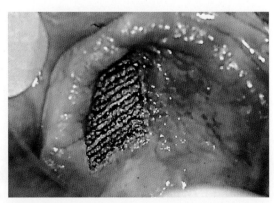

• **Figure 14-6** Ablation of papillary hyperplasia showing side-by-side U pattern.

benign, the surgeon may safely proceed with ablation. If it is malignant, however, wide laser excision is indicated.

Premalignant Lesions

Premalignant lesions may take the form of leukoplakia, erythroplakia, or a mixed form of the two known as *erythroleukoplakia.* The possibility of malignant transformation of these lesions is 36.3% to 43.0% in the presence of epithelial dysplasia, and 23.4% to 38.0% without epithelial dysplasia.[18] Also, patients with these conditions have a 50- to 60-fold greater risk of developing oral cancer than patients without the lesions. Traditional treatment has involved surgical excision with a scalpel, which has many disadvantages compared with laser excision or ablation procedures. The advantages of using a laser include better control of bleeding, less surgical time, more precise tissue removal, less morbidity and complications, and excellent healing with virtually no scarring.[19] Many surgeons also believe that the cauterization effect of the laser on blood vessels and lymphatic channels decreases the amount of hematogenous and lymphatic seeding, thereby lowering recurrence rates.[20,21]

Laser treatment of premalignant lesions is through excision or ablation. Both procedures begin with outlining the lesion, as discussed earlier, with the depth of the cut being deep to the lesion itself, usually 4 to 9 mm.[22] If excision is to be performed, the affected tissue is elevated at one end and undermined, with the laser acting as a cutting tool. If ablation is chosen (usually the treatment of choice), the laser is defocused and the tissue removed in the multiple side-by-side U pattern described earlier.

Figure 14-7 illustrates ablation of a leukoplakia on the ventrolateral surface of the tongue. Multiple passes usually are required until removal is complete. With the bloodless surgical field produced by the laser, visual confirmation of complete removal is much easier than during scalpel surgery. The area is then left to reepithelialize by secondary intention, avoiding sutures and the possible distortion and scarring.

Roodenburg et al.[18] conducted follow-up evaluations in 70 patients with 103 oral leukoplakias treated with laser ablation at a mean of 5.3 years postoperatively and found a cure rate of 90%. Similarly, Thompson and Wylie[23] reviewed the outcomes for 57 consecutive patients with laser-treated oral dysplastic lesions. After 44 months, 76% of the patients exhibited no recurrence. These results are comparable to the 80% success rate seen with conventional scalpel surgery. It is clear that ablation of premalignant lesions is somewhat controversial, although recent evidence indicates that laser ablation is an effective tool for the treatment of this disease process so long as the practitioner remains aware of the risk of recurrence and progression to malignancy.[24]

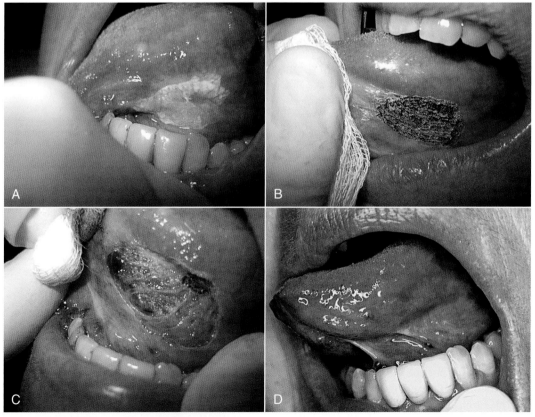

• **Figure 14-7** Laser ablation of leukoplakia. **A,** Leukoplakia of ventrolateral surface of tongue. **B,** Appearance after first pass using ablation technique. **C,** Lesion completely ablated. Note precision of tissue removal and excellent hemostasis. **D,** One-month postoperative view shows excellent healing.

Malignant Lesions and Aggressive Benign Lesions

The laser is an accepted and useful surgical tool for the treatment of malignant and aggressive benign lesions of the larynx, pharynx, oral cavity, and lips. Its use offers many advantages not seen with conventional scalpel surgery. Aside from the bloodless surgical field, shorter surgical time, and decreased patient morbidity, advantages specific to these potentially lethal conditions have been recognized. First, lasers seal lymphatic vessels at the surgical margins, which reduces seeding of malignant cells and potential metastasis.[25] Second, more nondiseased tissue adjacent to the lesion is preserved. Typical cancer margins are 1.5 to 2 cm beyond any visible or palpable tumor.[13] Better visualization, with a bloodless field, allows the surgeon to remove tissue more precisely without sacrificing unnecessary tissue.

Figure 14-8 demonstrates excision of a T1N0M0 squamous cell carcinoma of the tongue. Laser microsurgery using a surgical microscope helps the surgeon to distinguish between healthy and tumor tissue and to preserve even more normal tissue by taking narrower margins.[26] In the event of local tumor recurrence, more retreatment options are available than with conventional scalpel surgery.[27]

Verrucous carcinoma is a slow-growing, nonmetastasizing form of squamous cell carcinoma that most frequently is found in (but not limited to) the mouth.[28] Clinically, this white, cauliflower-like lesion is seen most often in elderly

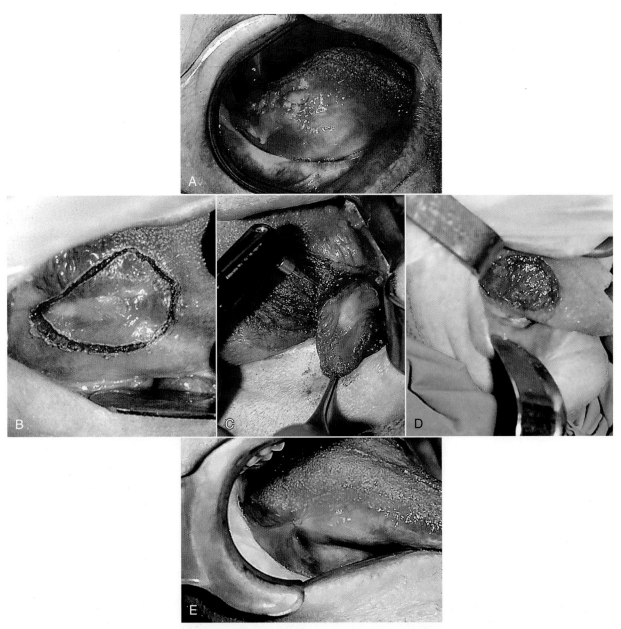

• **Figure 14-8** Laser excision of T1N0M0 squamous cell carcinoma. **A,** Malignant tumor of ventrolateral surface of tongue. **B,** Lesion outlined. **C,** Undermining the lesion. **D,** Surgical wound with the lesion excised, showing excellent hemostasis. **E,** One-month postoperative view shows excellent healing.

patients.[29] The etiology is unknown, but heavy use of tobacco (snuff, chewing tobacco, or cigarettes) may be the primary pathogenetic factor.[30,31] Some investigators postulate that human papillomavirus is associated with verrucous carcinoma, but most studies have failed to prove this correlation.[32,33] Treatment of these lesions traditionally has been with shave excision, cryosurgery, chemotherapy, or a combination, often necessitating multiple treatments that may lead to scarring.[34-36] The CO_2 laser has proved to be effective in treating verrucous carcinoma by total excision in cutting mode. Vaporization can be performed on the premalignant form, *proliferative verrucous leukoplakia*.[13]

Vascular Lesions

Vascular lesions of the head and neck region are common in patients of all ages. These lesions traditionally are classified as acquired or congenital. Common *acquired* lesions include telangiectasias, spider and cherry angiomas, pyogenic granulomas, and venous lakes. Vascular lesions are characterized by varying degrees of blood vessel dilation.[37] *Congenital* vascular lesions manifest as either hemangiomas or true vascular malformations.[37,38] Histologically, *hemangiomas* show endothelial cell hyperplasia, whereas vascular *malformations* are characterized by normal endothelial cells with vessel dilation.[39] Hemangiomas are the most common soft tissue tumors of infancy (affecting 5% to 10% of 1-year-olds).[40] Traditionally, hemangiomas spontaneously involute between ages 5 and 10 years.[41] The most common vascular malformations are *port-wine stains*, which are present at birth (in 0.3% to 0.5% of the general population[42]) and do not spontaneously involute.[37]

The ultimate goal of laser treatment of vascular lesions is selective destruction of abnormal vessels by heating of the vessel wall through the absorption of light by hemoglobin.[37] The wavelength chosen should be selectively absorbed by hemoglobin, and the pulse length should be short enough to confine heat to the blood vessels to prevent unwanted damage to adjacent tissue.[10] The most common types used for removal of vascular lesions are the KTP, Nd:YAG, and *pulsed dye laser* (PDL). In addition, IPL systems also may be used.

Telangiectasias are permanently dilated superficial vessels resulting in blue or reddish skin.[43] These common asymptomatic lesions often are a cosmetic nuisance to the affected patient. The most common devices used to treat telangiectasias are the PDL and the IPL system. The PDL emits wavelengths of 585 to 600 nm and is better suited for more focal cutaneous lesions; the IPL source emits light in the range of 500 to 1200 nm and is better suited for treatment of more diffuse telangiectasias, such as with rosacea.[37] The major drawback of the PDL versus the IPL system is the postoperative purpura, lasting 7 to 10 days.[10] The patient should be thoroughly prepared for this preoperatively, and makeup can be applied immediately after the procedure.[37]

Treatment of port-wine stains is similar to that for telangiectasias because both represent lesions of dilated superficial blood vessels. Port-wine stains typically occur in younger children and can have significant psychological effects during the child's development if left untreated. The PDL most often is used for eradication of these lesions.[40] Multiple treatments usually are required, and lesions partially resistant to the PDL may develop. Pence et al.[44] used the frequency-doubled Nd:YAG laser (with a wavelength of 532 nm) to treat 89 patients with port-wine stains of the head and neck for 1 to 12 sessions, with no treatment failures and a rate of adverse side effects (e.g., transient hyper/hypopigmentation, hypotrophic scarring) of 1% to 2%. Therefore combination therapy, with the PDL initially and then the Nd:YAG laser for deeper, more resistant lesions, is likely to produce the best results.

Superficial hemangiomas appear flat and red, whereas deeper lesions appear blue.[10] All hemangiomas eventually involute, but delaying treatment can leave lasting cosmetic and psychological scars. Laser treatment of hemangiomas on the skin is similar to that for port-wine stains. The PDL typically is used for hemangiomas with a superficial presentation, whereas the Nd:YAG laser provides the best results for deeper lesions.[45] The PDL and the Nd:YAG laser may be used in combination for hemangiomas with superficial and deep components.[40]

> **CLINICAL TIP**
>
> Hypertrophic vascular lesions are at risk for depressed scarring postoperatively, which should be discussed with the family before initiation of any laser treatment.

Although most hemangiomas have a cutaneous presentation, these lesions also can occur inside the mouth. Treatment of these intraoral forms is with vaporization or excision, depending on the size of the lesion and its proximity to important neural, vascular, and salivary structures.[46] The likelihood of damage to adjacent structures is remote if controlled vaporization is used rather than excision.[13] However, hemangiomas that manifest on the tongue, lip, or other areas isolated from important structures can be excised with the CO_2 laser. The feeding peripheral vasculature is sealed, and excision can proceed starting with outlining the margins and undermining the lesion, as described earlier.[46]

It is beyond the scope of this chapter to review all vascular lesions encountered by the oral-maxillofacial surgeon and the associated laser surgery. The interested reader is encouraged to research current trends in the dynamic field of laser surgery for the treatment of these lesions.

Snoring and Sleep Apnea

Laser-Assisted Uvulopalatopharyngoplasty

Snoring is a common social problem, affecting approximately 20% to 30% of the adult population, and has been associated with morning fatigue, restless sleep, daytime somnolence, and hypoxemia.[47] In addition to the social implications, snoring can be a risk factor for hypertension, angina pectoris, cerebral infarction, pulmonary hypertension, and congestive heart failure. A significant percentage of snorers also have associated obstructive sleep apnea syndrome (OSAS), marked by repeated episodes of apnea and hypopnea during sleep secondary to collapse of the upper airway despite respiratory effort. Serious medical consequences of OSAS include cardiac arrhythmias, myocardial infarction, systemic and pulmonary hypertension, and increased risk for involvement in motor vehicle crashes.

Although the most common treatment for patients with these sleep-disordered breathing problems has been scalpel uvulopalatopharyngoplasty (UPPP), this procedure is fraught with complications, including severe pain, hemorrhage, transient nasal regurgitation, permanent velopharyngeal insufficiency, and nasopharyngeal stenosis.[48] LA-UPPP can be performed more easily and with less morbidity than with standard scalpel UPPP. Notwithstanding the advantages and low morbidity associated with LA-UPPP, the surgeon must be thorough and systematic when evaluating patients with sleep-disordered breathing. A complete preoperative workup must encompass history and physical examination (including nasopharyngoscopy); often a polysomnogram needs to be performed before initiation of treatment. Patients with retropalatal obstruction are the best candidates for successful LA-UPPP.[49]

The basic concept of LA-UPPP is similar to that for a standard UPPP, with removal of the soft palate and uvula as well as excision of both the anterior and the posterior tonsillar pillars. In addition, some undermining into the lateral pharyngeal tissues and suturing are done to maximize the airway dilation and prevent relapse. LA-UPPP works only when the patient has previously undergone tonsillectomy or has small residual tonsils, which if present can be ablated to a depth of a few millimeters as part of the procedure. Large tonsils should be removed before the procedure, or a standard UPPP should be performed.

The LA-UPPP can be done with local anesthetic injections as used for any palatal procedure. However, because many candidates for this surgery have sleep apnea, they often will be simultaneously undergoing other surgical procedures, such as genial tubercle advancement and hyoid myotomy (GAHM) or nasal surgery. Accordingly, operative management may require use of an OR and general anesthesia. These patients may need to be admitted to the hospital for overnight observation because of the greater risk of postoperative airway compromise. In severe cases or in smaller community hospitals, a monitored intensive care unit (ICU) bed may be appropriate. The patient is prepared and positioned as for a standard LA-UPPP. Once again, the procedure is easier to do in the sitting position, although when done in the OR, the supine position may be necessary and does not pose any problem so long as the levator muscle is marked preoperatively.

After local anesthesia is obtained, the procedure begins with two vertical through-and-through incisions of the soft

palate adjacent to the uvula and extending a few millimeters short of the levator palatini muscle insertion (determined by phonation or gagging). Using a standard incisional technique, the backstop is placed behind the soft palate, and the vertical cuts are made from inferior to superior. A relatively high-power density (often 15 to 20 W with 0.1- to 0.4-mm spot size) typically is used to shorten the procedure time. Care is taken to prevent thermal conduction from the backstop to the pharyngeal wall. The laser is turned sideways, and the uvula and soft palate outlined by the vertical trenches are removed using the same incisional technique. The initial vertical trenches in the LA-UPPP are taken as far laterally as can be done comfortably within the soft palate, to include some of the anterior and posterior tonsillar pillars (Figure 14-9). Again, this maneuver can be aided by grasping the uvula with a forceps, hemostat, or suction tip and applying countertraction during the laser incisions. A horizontal incision can then be made across the top of the

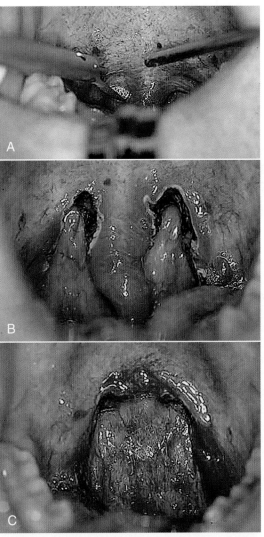

• **Figure 14-9** LA-UPPP. **A,** Laser tip is placed just lateral to the uvula for incising vertical trenches. Backstop handpiece is used to protect pharyngeal wall from damage. **B,** Bilateral vertical trenches stop just short of levator muscle insertion. **C,** Postoperative view shows significant opening of the airway.

vertical trenches to remove the uvula, soft palate, and some of the medial aspect of the tonsillar pillars. A horizontal incision is then made to connect the vertical cuts, remaining approximately 4 to 5 mm below the levator insertion. Additional ablation or excision of the pillars can be carried out until the operator is sure that the airway has been maximized. At this point, the soft palate is grasped with a long forceps and rotated anteriorly so that the long aspect of the palate is facing into the mouth, and a nonbackstop handpiece is used to remove a triangular wedge of tissue from the soft palate between the anterior and posterior aspects of the palatal mucosa, while leaving 3 to 4 mm to the levator insertion. This step essentially undermines the soft palate and allows for significant thinning.

Results of LA-UPPP should include an *anterior* mucosal flap consisting of the oral mucosa of the palate and the anterior tonsillar pillar and a *posterior* mucosal flap comprising the nasal side of the palatal mucosa and the posterior tonsillar pillar. All of the flap edges must be deepithelialized; two epithelialized surfaces will not adhere to each other. At this point, the posterior flap is stretched anteriorly and brought into apposition with the anterior flap, overlapping it for 1 to 2 mm. A series of 4-0 polyglactin or polyglycolic sutures is then used to coapt the two flaps. The resultant suture line is essentially identical to that seen with a standard UPPP.

Advantages of the laser-assisted over the standard UPPP include considerably less bleeding and slightly less postoperative discomfort. In addition, LA-UPPP is faster and, when appropriate (for snoring or mild apnea), may be performed on an outpatient basis or even in the office.

Temporomandibular Joint Surgery

Arthroscopic surgery of the TMJ has been a successful mode of treatment well accepted by patient and surgeon alike.[50,51] Lasers offer many advantages in TMJ surgery not possible with conventional arthroscopic cutting instrumentation. Eliminating the need for physical contact with the diseased tissue reduces trauma to surrounding synovial tissue and articular cartilage. Laser use also can provide rapid coagulation with minimal thermal damage, allowing better visualization of the surgical field and decreased hemarthrosis.[52] Because of the small cutting width, laser surgery is much more precise than conventional arthroscopic surgery, and the tip can be more easily manipulated in the narrow joint space.[53] Also, the risk of instrument breakage and subsequent retrieval is eliminated.[54]

The high water content of the joint space does not allow the use of a CO_2 or Er:YAG laser, because the synovial fluid would absorb the light energy before reaching the target tissue.[55] The Ho:YAG laser wavelength, however, is minimally absorbed by water, so its energy is transmitted directly to the desired tissue. The Ho:YAG laser offers the advantage of penetrating tissue to a depth of 0.5 mm or less, thereby reducing the risk of iatrogenic damage to adjacent tissues.[53] Typical settings used for Ho:YAG arthroscopic surgery are a power output of 0.8 J and a pulse rate of 10 Hz (8 W),

which will efficiently ablate the tissues without creating excessive zones of thermal damage.[17]

Arthroscopic procedures typically are performed in the OR with the patient under general anesthesia with nasotracheal intubation. A video monitor at the head of the bed receives input from a camera attached to the arthroscope. Two portals usually are used for these procedures, through which cannulas are placed to allow entry of the arthroscope, laser fiber, or other surgical instrumentation into the superior joint space (Figure 14-10). The placement of the portals can be variable (endaural, superior posterolateral, inferior posterolateral, superior anterolateral, inferior anterolateral), but ultimately a portal is placed in the posterior region of the joint and another in the anterior region. A constant flow of irrigation fluid into the joint space is essential to distend the potential space and wash away blood and debris, greatly improving visualization of the surgical field. The irrigation inflow is attached to the arthroscope, and outflow is through the second portal. Using this technique with the Ho:YAG laser, procedures such as diskectomy, diskoplasty, synovectomy, hemostasis, posterior attachment contraction, anterior release, and debridement of fibrous ankylosis can be performed on an outpatient basis.[3,17]

Koslin[56] described laser treatment for anteriorly displaced disks that are symptomatic or that limit function. The technique involves an anterior disk release procedure with or without posterior attachment contraction and repositioning. The laser is placed in the anterior cannula and the energy directed medially along the disk-synovium junction down to the lateral pterygoid muscle. Blunt probe dissection may facilitate complete release and movement of the disk posteriorly. The laser energy is then directed toward the posterior synovial tissue, where, using a lower energy, contraction of the tissue is performed. Suturing of the posterior disk-synovium junction can then be accomplished. Kaneyama et al.[52] described a similar procedure for anteriorly displaced disks and reported a 92.8% success rate.

Synovitis is a painful inflammatory TMJ condition characterized by hyperemic and hyperplastic synovium as seen

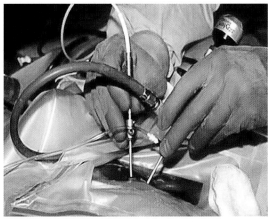

• **Figure 14-10** TMJ arthroscopy using Ho:YAG laser. Separate ports are required to provide the surgeon with visibility of the laser tip during use.

under arthroscopy.[57] When nonsurgical therapy fails, the surgery of choice is a synovectomy, traditionally done with motorized instrumentation. However, *laser synovectomy* with the Ho:YAG laser offers much greater control and precision in tissue removal.[56] The laser should be set at 0.5 J and 5 to 15 pulses per second. The laser tip is placed approximately 3 mm from the target tissue and then passed repeatedly over the surface using a paintbrush technique; the treated tissue will be seen to contract and lose its redness.[58] Normal synovium is then left to regenerate.

Mazzonetto and Spagnoli[5] reported results in 30 patients (38 joints) who underwent arthroscopic Ho:YAG laser diskectomy for the treatment of disk perforation associated with pain and restricted function. The laser excises the disk at its margins (usually in two fragments), with small alligator forceps or hemostats used to grasp and remove the tissue. With the laser then set at a lower power, the remaining fibrocartilage and redundant disk tissue are removed, and tissue peripheral to the condyle is contracted. Overall success rate was 93.3%, with a mean follow-up period of 31.7 months. Patients showed a mean increased opening of 14 mm, with decreased pain and return to a more normal diet.

Ankylosis of the TMJ can be clinically devastating, leading to difficulties with eating, speech, and other functions. Causes include traumatic injury (most common), infection, and arthritis.[59,60] Surgical treatment of TMJ ankylosis traditionally has been with arthrotomy and debridement of fibrous adhesions or bone bridges.[61] With advances in arthroscopic TMJ surgery, however, this correction can effectively be accomplished with the Ho:YAG laser. Using a dual-portal technique as previously described, bone bridges, osteophytes, and fibrous adhesions are removed layer by layer with the laser.[62] Once adequate joint mobility is obtained, final contouring of sharp bony edges can be performed with a reciprocating miniature bone file. Postoperatively, patients are instructed to resume aggressive physical therapy to prevent reankylosis and to improve function.[63]

Cosmetic Facial Surgery

In the 1970s and 1980s, *orthognathic surgery*, the manipulation of one or more facial bones to correct occlusal abnormalities and facial dysmorphisms, became both popular and well established in the OMS practice. In the early 1990s, however, it became evident that merely changing the bony skeleton and restoring occlusion without modifying the overlying soft tissues did not necessarily correct the dysmorphism. Thus began a paradigm shift in the workup and diagnosis for orthognathic patients that emphasized soft tissue appearance over bone position. To accomplish this goal, oral-maxillofacial surgeons needed to gain expertise in cosmetic facial surgery. At the same time, the use of lasers for soft tissue surgery also was becoming routine.[46]

As a consequence of their many general advantages— greater precision, improved healing, smaller incisions, and decreased suturing—and several wavelength-specific benefits, lasers inevitably found a prominent role in cosmetic

surgery procedures. Lasers not only have improved existing procedures but also have allowed new cosmetic procedures to be done safely and effectively using only specific laser wavelengths and IPL devices.[64]

Advantages specific to cosmetic procedures include the ability afforded by some lasers (depending on wavelength) to work through endoscopes and to use several very small incisions rather than one large incision. Even when the laser beam cannot be passed through an endoscope, such as with the CO_2 laser (in which the beam is absorbed by typical quartz fiberoptics), the laser beam often can be delivered through long handpiece attachments using the same small incisions. The hemostasis provided by many laser wavelengths becomes significantly more imperative for cosmetic procedures, in which the resultant scar and overall result can be greatly influenced by the associated tremendous increase in visualization in the surgical field.

The primary advantage of lasers specific to cosmetic surgery is the ability to provide superficial tissue ablation, rather than creating deep incisions. Using a laser for epidermal and dermal tissue ablation allows for the removal of very precise amounts of tissue. This technique can be used to remove facial lesions with little to no scarring or to resurface the entire face and remove wrinkles and the long-term effects of solar damage.[65] Cosmetic surgical procedures using lasers or IPL sources generally can be divided into *invasive* and *noninvasive* as well as *incisional* and *ablational* procedures, with several common procedures using each of these techniques.

Invasive Incision Procedures
Blepharoplasty

Blepharoplasty is the removal of excessive skin, muscle, and fat from the upper or lower eyelid.

In the lower eyelid, the laser (usually CO_2) is used to make an incision transconjunctivally, although it also can be used transcutaneously.[66] The laser is used in focused mode at the smallest spot size for that laser. The hemostatic nature of the laser is especially important in blepharoplasty because bleeding can be both problematic for visualization in the fornix of the eye and potentially catastrophic should the blood leak posteriorly behind the globe, causing a retrobulbar hematoma with subsequent loss of vision. Once the conjunctiva is incised, the retroorbital septal fat can be seen pseudoherniating into the septum. A small incision in the overlying fascia and lid retractors allow the fat to be delivered and incised by the laser, again in focused mode (Figure 14-11). Small residual fat pockets also can be vaporized back into the orbit using defocused mode. This is another technique unique to lasers and permits safe, precise sculpting of the fat. Once the fat is removed and hemostasis ensured, the conjunctiva can be sutured or only approximated and left unsutured.

Upper eyelid blepharoplasty is similar to the lower eyelid procedure but usually involves a transcutaneous incision. Although the laser generally is not as precise as a scalpel for making skin incisions, in the eyelids the final results appear to be identical with both modalities, and the laser has the

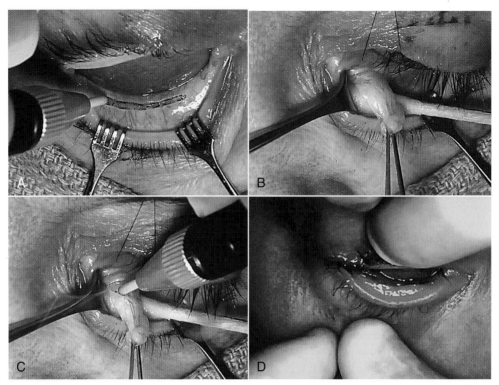

• **Figure 14-11 A,** Incision for transconjunctival lower eyelid blepharoplasty using a CO_2 laser. Note metal eye shield in place to protect the globe. **B,** Fat protruding through orbital septum. **C,** Using laser to incise fat. Laser also seals blood vessels, preventing blood from leaking behind the globe. **D,** Laser incision requires no closure, and the lid is simply inverted back into place.

advantages mentioned previously, making it the technique of choice.[64] Once the excess skin is removed, the orbicularis muscle can be partially excised. Again, the ability to do this without blood in the field is essential. Similarly, the septum is easily visualized and incised to isolate the pseudoherniated fat, which is then incised with the laser. Again, the laser also can be used to vaporize, in defocused mode, any residual pockets of fat. The skin is then closed with sutures to ensure a cosmetic scar (Figure 14-12).

Endoscopic Browlift

Although a browlift to raise sagging eyebrows can be done either endoscopically or with an open technique, the endoscopic procedure using several small incisions in the hairline best uses the many advantages of the laser. Once again, because of its excellent tissue-cutting abilities, the CO_2 laser typically is used for this procedure. Four to six 1-cm-long incisions are made with the laser in focused cutting mode, behind the hairline down to the skull. A subperiosteal pocket is made from inferior to approximately 2 cm above the orbital rims. An endoscope is then passed into the pocket and the dissection continued inferiorly to the rims, under direct vision to protect the supraorbital nerve (Figure 14-13). Using a thin laser tip 100 mm or longer (the length will vary by laser) passed through one of the incisions, an incision is made with the laser in the periosteum under direct endoscopic vision at the level of the orbital rims (arcus marginalis) (Figure 14-14). The incision is carried

just through the periosteum to release the forehead, or it can be carried through into the frontalis, corrugator, and procerus muscles to disrupt them, preventing their contraction and decreasing their wrinkle effect. The forehead tissue can then be retracted posteriorly, where it is fixed in position using sutures, screws, or tacks. The laser is used here because it provides precise incisions without bleeding.[67]

Ablation Procedures

Their predictable depth of effect allows lasers to remove successive layers of the skin to eliminate superficial lesions and sun-damaged tissue and wrinkles. The use of the laser as an ablational tool for skin conditions has allowed cosmetic surgeons to remove the surface epidermis and dermis in an unprecedented manner. Although chemical peeling and dermabrasion perform similar functions, the laser has more predictable effects and is less reliant on operator timing and interpretation than chemical peeling, and it is more predictable and less messy than dermabrasion.[68]

Cosmetic Skin Resurfacing

The basic technique for cosmetic skin resurfacing (CSR) is based on a thorough understanding of skin anatomy and wound healing. A normal full-thickness wound heals as follows: Basal cells adjacent to the wound edges cease normal vertical migration into keratinocytes and begin horizontal migration to cover the exposed connective tissues.

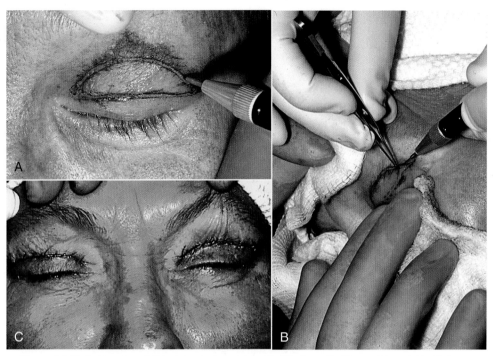

• **Figure 14-12** **A,** Upper eyelid blepharoplasty incision with CO_2 laser. **B,** After excision of skin. Note easy identification of orbicularis oculi muscle and septum (no bleeding). **C,** Unlike with the lower lid, closure of the upper lid incision is necessary for cosmetic reasons.

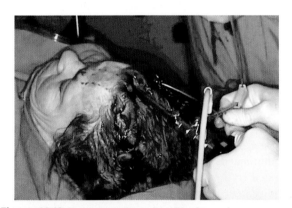

• **Figure 14-13** Endoscopic laser browlift. An endoscope camera is passed through one incision, while a 100-mm laser handpiece is passed through an adjacent incision. The laser tip is then visualized in the camera and manipulated under indirect vision.

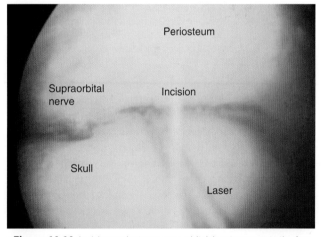

• **Figure 14-14** Incising periosteum over orbital rims to separate the forehead tissue from the orbits. Note supraorbital nerve at left of the laser tip.

At the same time, collagen builds up within the center of the wound. If the wound is large enough, the required time permits scar formation. CSR uses the laser to remove the surface epidermis and superficial papillary dermis while leaving intact the subjacent reticular dermis with its adnexal epithelial structures (hair follicles, sebaceous and sweat glands). These epithelial structures then allow for internal as well as external reepithelialization from adjacent basal cells. Many more such structures are present in facial skin than elsewhere in the body, so full epithelialization is extremely rapid and occurs before significant collagen formation.

This CSR technique is made possible by a high-energy, short-pulsed laser to maximize tissue ablation with minimal lateral thermal damage to underlying tissues. The ablation threshold of tissue is 4 to 5 J/cm^2, and the pulsewidth must be less than the thermal relaxation time for the tissue, approximately 695 μsec. Any energy application less than the ablation threshold will lead to the need for prolonged laser application, which in turn will lead to significant lateral thermal damage. Should this damage affect the adnexal structures, scarring will occur.[69]

One of the most important aspects of CSR is the preoperative preparation of the patient. Once a thorough medical history is obtained and contraindications including skin diseases, radiation therapy, connective tissue disorders, and use of isotretinoin (Accutane) (which destroys adnexal structure) within the last year have been ruled out, the patient is started on a regimen of several medications. Many surgeons begin with a retinoic acid to initiate the process of healing and repair. The use of a melanocyte-depleting agent such

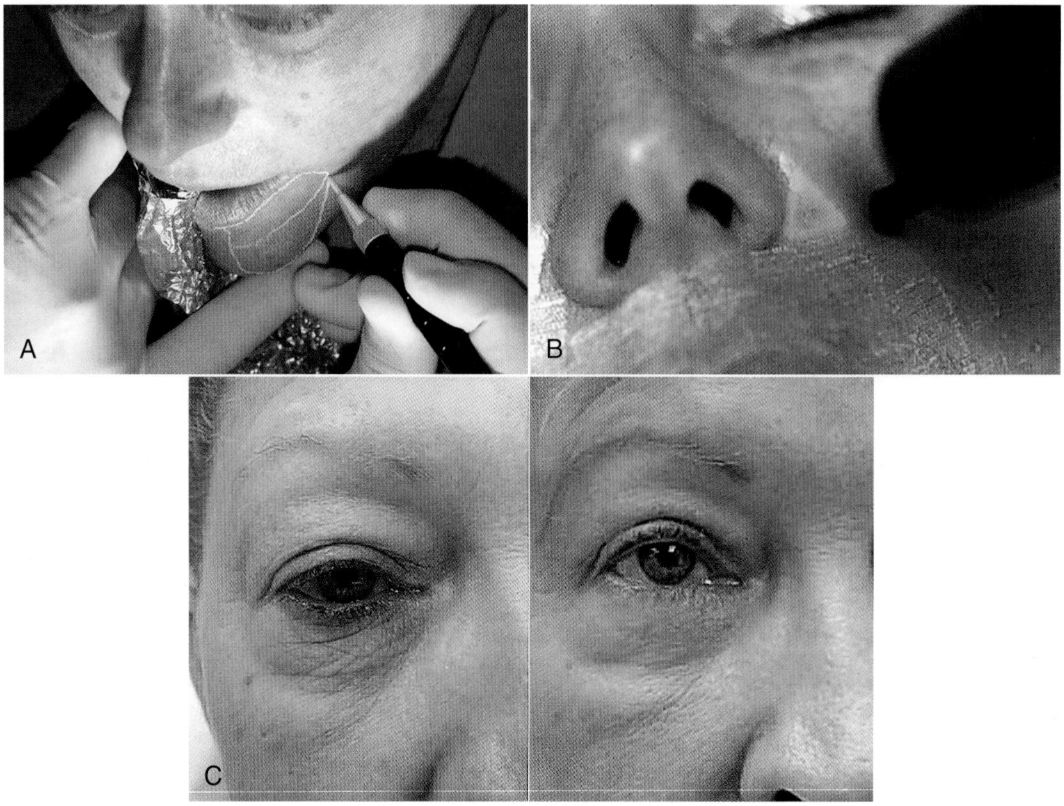

• **Figure 14-15** **A,** CO_2 laser handpiece with regular spot size. Small areas can be covered using standard 0.8-mm handpiece in an alternating-U pattern. **B,** Resurfacing of larger areas usually is done with a CPG for predictable and mechanized filling of various geometric shapes. **C,** Preoperative and postoperative views of facial rhytids.

as hydroquinone will help prevent postoperative hyperpigmentation (in addition to limiting this procedure to patients with Fitzpatrick scale skin types I to IV). Antiviral therapy prevents recurrent herpetic infection, which would have a devastating effect on denuded skin, and can be started 1 to 14 days before surgery, depending on the patient's previous herpetic history. Acyclovir, famciclovir, and valacyclovir all have been used for this purpose.[70] Finally, sunblock (with a sun-protective factor [SPF] of 30 or greater) should be used throughout the surgical and healing phases.

Choosing the correct laser and the ideal delivery is paramount for obtaining a good result with CSR. The two lasers most often used for this procedure are the CO_2 and the Er:YAG. The CO_2 laser is much more effective but is associated with long-term erythema and greater risk of scarring if exposure is done too deeply. Because the CO_2 is a continuous-wave laser, it must be pseudopulsed at high powers to obtain the short times needed to prevent significant lateral thermal damage to adjacent tissues. Greater absorption by water allows the Er:YAG laser to penetrate less deeply in tissue and ablate tissue more superficially. It also has the advantage of being a true pulsed laser, allowing for high powers with very short pulse durations. Although this leads to less postoperative erythema and decreased risk of excessive ablation, it also leads to decreased effectiveness with the Er:YAG laser.[69]

In an effort to decrease thermal damage by the laser while maximizing effect, several lasers now use various scanning devices to place the laser pulses geometrically in nonadjacent patterns, to limit the buildup of heat in proximity to each laser strike. This technology also provides uniform coverage of the face. When it is combined with high-power short-pulse laser energy, the effect is superficial ablation of skin with minimal tissue damage, allowing for rapid healing with decreased erythema and risk of scarring. Another option is fractional laser resurfacing, which creates a series of microscopic vertical columns in the skin surrounded by untreated areas. This technique results in significant improvement in the skin but with less potential tissue damage.

Topical, local, or parenteral anesthesia techniques may be used for CSR, depending on the size of the area to be resurfaced, anticipated depth of resurfacing, and patient tolerance. Once proper anesthesia has been obtained, the skin is cleansed and prepared with a non–iodine-containing antibacterial, usually chlorhexidine. Protective eye shields of metal (not plastic) should be placed over the globes and the outlying tissues protected with wet towels.[71]

If a regular handpiece is used, the laser is directed in a series of alternating-U patterns to cover the area evenly without overlapping, which would lead to charring and excessive heat buildup. With use of a computerized pattern generator (CPG), the handpiece is held stationary while the computer directs the laser in a preset geometric pattern. The pattern can be chosen to match the area to be ablated (Figure 14-15). Once the pattern is completed, the handpiece can be moved to the next area. The skin surface is then gently wiped with wet gauze to remove any dehydrated tissue, although some evidence suggests that wiping may be unnecessary.[72] It is important to complete an entire anatomic subunit of the face before wiping is performed; once the area has been cleaned, it may be difficult to distinguish treated from untreated skin, potentially leading to double striking and excess heat.

When treatment of the area to be ablated has been completed (e.g., perioral, periorbital, or entire face), it is covered with an occlusive or nonocclusive dressing. Occlusive dressings generally are left on the face for only 1 or 2 days, to prevent infection. Nonocclusive dressings (e.g., Eucerin, Aquaphor) should be used continuously for 7 to 10 days, until reepithelialization has occurred. The patient is placed on cephalosporin therapy to prevent bacterial infection and is maintained on antiviral therapy for 7 to 21 days (with the duration depending on whether the history included previous herpetic outbreaks) postoperatively, to prevent a viral infection. The patient is instructed to clean the face gently, initially with a weak vinegar solution and then with mild soap and water, several times a day, followed by careful dabbing to dry. The patient also should avoid sun exposure and must use sunscreen (with an SPF of 35 or greater) for several months. Once reepithelialization has occurred, the patient may resume wearing makeup; a green-base foundation can be recommended to counteract the significant postoperative erythema lasting for 3 to 60 days after surgery.

Complications after CSR can be devastating, so only surgeons trained to manage them should perform these procedures. Because of the denuded nature of facial skin after the procedure, with attendant loss of its natural immunity barrier, bacterial, viral, or fungal infection can occur (Figure 14-16). Treatment must be swift and powerful to prevent disastrous scarring. Postoperative erythema is expected but may be prolonged, in some cases lasting several months. Hyperpigmentation and hypopigmentation are most frequently seen in patients with Fitzpatrick skin types V and VI. Hyperpigmentation may be treated with melanocyte-depleting agents such as hydroquinone or kojic acid. Hypopigmentation is more problematic because no satisfactory treatment has been identified.[73]

Facial Lesion Removal

The laser is a very useful tool to remove benign facial lesions (e.g., epidermal and superficial dermal nevi, seborrheic keratosis), with minimal scarring in most cases (Figure 14-17). It is important to establish a benign diagnosis by visual examination and history or by histologic confirmation, because no specimen will be available after laser ablation. Alternatively, the top layer of the lesion may be removed by shaving with a scalpel (then sent for pathology examination) and the remainder by laser. This approach provides a histologic diagnosis but still allows the excellent results expected with the laser.[74]

Once local anesthesia has been obtained, the laser (in the same high-power short-pulsed mode used for CSR) is used in a spiral fashion, emanating from the center to the periphery. This aspect of technique is important because the

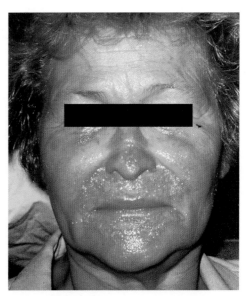

• **Figure 14-16** Bacterial infection after cosmetic laser skin resurfacing.

operator is likely to be slower when first starting the laser, which will then penetrate further at the apex of the typical dome-shaped nevus, where a deeper cut will have less effect. After each spiral pass, the area is gently wiped with wet gauze to remove any dehydrated tissue. This is continued until the laser-treated skin is at the same level as the surrounding normal epithelium. The area is then covered with an antibiotic ointment and kept moist for 7 days until reepithelialization has occurred. Cleaning techniques are the same as for CSR procedures.

Scar Revision

Because of its great precision, the laser is an excellent tool for the revision of scars. Poor cosmetic results from scarring are caused basically by color abnormalities and surface-geometry abnormalities. Using different lasers, both of these factors often can be addressed to improve the cosmetic result.

Hypervascularity is common in healing scar tissue, and the appearance of erythematous scars often can be improved by diminishing the vascularity in the tissue. Of the several lasers used to accomplish this, the 532-nm KTP-YAG and PDL devices are used most often.[75]

Surface irregularities in scars (depressed or elevated) lead to changes in light reflection. It is primarily this effect that leads the observer to focus on the scar. By elevating depressed scars or leveling elevated scars, this phenomenon can be diminished, resulting in an improved appearance to the scar. Depending on the degree of resurfacing needed, the CO_2 or Er:YAG laser may be used.[76]

For elevated scars, a uniform reduction in the scar tissue is performed, using the same CSR techniques described previously. The scar should be reduced to the level of the adjacent normal tissues. For depressed scars, the laser is used to reduce the surrounding normal tissues in an increasingly circumferential pattern, thus blending the depression into the adjacent normal tissues (Figure 14-18). However, the normal tissues must not be resurfaced deeper than the

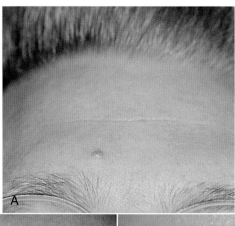

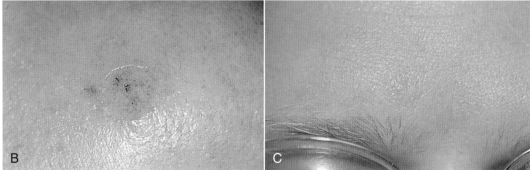

• **Figure 14-17** **A,** Cutaneous nevus. **B,** Removal down to adjacent tissue level with high-energy pseudo-pulsed CO_2 laser. **C,** Minimal to no scarring after healing.

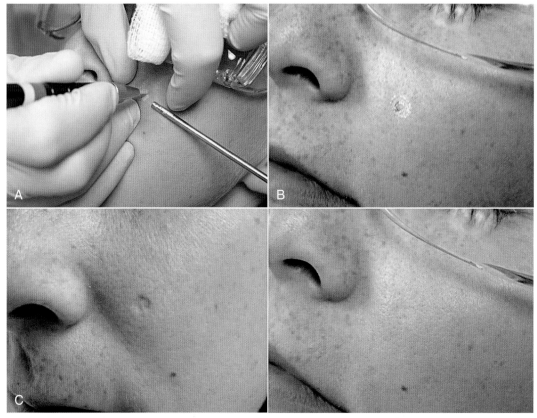

• **Figure 14-18** **A,** High-energy pseudopulsed CO_2 laser is used to blend adjacent normal tissue around a depressed scar. **B,** Area surrounding the scar is treated to soften the depression. **C,** Preoperative and postoperative views.

midreticular dermis; otherwise, scarring could occur in this region as well. If necessary, the procedure may be repeated after healing has occurred to improve the results as needed.

Conclusions

Lasers have been used in major OMS procedures for many years and will continue to provide benefits to both surgeon and patient. With clear advantages of laser use for many of these procedures, only the considerable financial cost limits its near-universal application. As with all technology, however, the hardware costs will diminish with time, allowing all surgeons access to these devices. New advances in energy delivery with less lateral thermal effects and in waveguide and fiberoptic delivery systems, as well as more specific tissue interactions based on new wavelengths, will continue to make lasers an integral part of the practice of the oral-maxillofacial surgeon.

References

1. Sanders DL, Reinisch L: Wound healing and collagen thermal damage in 7.5 microsecond pulsed CO_2 laser skin incisions, *Lasers Surg Med* 1:22–32, 2000.
2. Wheeland RG: Cosmetic use of lasers, *Dermatol Clin* 13(2):447–459, 1995.
3. Walsh JT, Deutsch TF: ER: YAG laser ablation of tissue: measurement of ablation rates, *Laser Surg Med* 9:327–337, 1989.
4. Teikemeier G, Goldberg DJ: Skin resurfacing with erbium:YAG laser, *Dermatol Surg* 23(8):685–687, 1997.
5. Mazzonetto R, Spagnoli D: Long term evaluation of arthroscopic diskectomy of the TMJ using holmium YAG laser, *J Oral Maxillofac Surg* 59(9):1018–1023, 2001.
6. Convissar R: Lasers in general dentistry, *Oral Maxillofac Surg Clin North Am* 16(2):165–179, 2004.
7. Kahraman SA: Low-level laser therapy in oral and maxillofacial surgery, *Oral Maxillofac Surg Clin North Am* 16(2):277–288, 2004.
8. Kulekcioglu S, Sivrioglu K, Ozcan O, Parlak M: Effectiveness of low-level laser therapy in temporomandibular disorder, *Scand J Rheumatol* 32(2):114–118, 2003.
9. Dierick CC: Hair removal by lasers and intense pulsed light sources, *Dermatol Clin* 20:135–146, 2003.
10. Niamtu J: Treatment of vascular and pigmented lesions in oral and maxillofacial surgery, *Oral Maxillofac Surg Clin North Am* 16(2):239–254, 2004.
11. Goldman MP, Fitzpatrick RE: Laser treatment of cutaneous vascular lesions. In Golman MP, Fitzpatrick RE, editors: *Cutaneous laser surgery*, ed 2, St Louis, 1999, Mosby.
12. De Vane GG: New technologies in anesthesia. Update for nurse anesthetists: lasers (AANA course), *J Am Assoc Nurse Anesthetists* 58(4):313–319, 1990.
13. Catone GA, Alling AC: *Laser applications in oral and maxillofacial surgery*, Philadelphia, 1997, Saunders.
14. Hermens JM, Bennett MJ, Hirshman CA: Anesthesia for laser surgery, *Anesth Analg* 62(2):218–229, 1983.
15. Ossoff RH: Laser safety in otolaryngology—head and neck surgery: anesthetic and educational considerations for laryngeal surgery, *Laryngoscope* 99(8):1–26, 1989.
16. Carruth J: Lasers in oral surgery, *J Clin Laser Med Surg* 9(5):379–380, 1991.

17. Strauss RA, Fallon SD: Lasers in contemporary oral and maxillofacial surgery, *Dent Clin North Am* 48(4):861–888, 2004.
18. Roodenburg JL, Panders AK, Vermey A: Carbon dioxide laser surgery of oral leukoplakia, *Oral Surg Med Pathol* 71(6):670–674, 1991.
19. Schoelch M, Sekandari N, Regezi J, Silverman S: Laser management of oral leukoplakias: a follow-up study of 70 patients, *Laryngoscope* 109(6):949–953, 1999.
20. Lanzafame RJ, Rogers DW, Naim JO, et al.: The effect of CO_2 laser excision on local tumor recurrence, *Lasers Surg Med* 6(2):103–105, 1986.
21. Lanzafame RJ, Rogers DW, Naim JO, et al.: Reduction of local tumor recurrence by excision with the CO_2 laser, *Lasers Surg Med* 6(5):439–441, 1986.
22. Meltzer C: Surgical management of oral and mucosal dysplasias: the case for laser excision, *J Oral Maxillofac Surg* 65(2):293–295, 2007.
23. Thompson P, Wylie J: Interventional laser surgery: an effective surgical and diagnostic tool in oral precancer management, *Int J Oral Maxillofac Surg* 31(2):145–153, 2002.
24. Ishii J, Fujita K, Komori T: Laser surgery as a treatment for oral leukoplakia, *Oral Oncol* 39(8):759–769, 2003.
25. Apfelberg DB, Master MR, Lash H, et al.: CO_2 laser resection for giant perineal condyloma and verrucous carcinoma, *Ann Plast Surg* 11(5):417–422, 1983.
26. Blanch JL, Vilaseca I, Grau JJ, et al.: Prognostic significance of surgical margins in transoral CO_2 laser microsurgery for T1-T4 pharyngo-laryngeal cancers, *Eur Arch Otorhinolaryngol* 264(9):1045–1051, 2007.
27. Eckel HE: Local recurrences following transoral laser surgery for early glottic carcinoma: frequency, management, and outcome, *Ann Otol Rhinol Laryngol* 110(1):7–15, 2001.
28. Jordan RC: Verrucous carcinoma of the mouth, *J Can Dent Assoc* 61(9):797–801, 1995.
29. Median JE, Dichtel MW, Luna MA: Verrucous-squamous carcinomas of the oral cavity: a clinicopathologic study of 104 cases, *Arch Otolaryngol* 110:437–440, 1984.
30. Kamath VV, Varma RR, Gadewar DR, et al.: Oral verrucous carcinoma: an analysis of 37 cases, *J Craniomaxillofac Surg* 17(7):309–314, 1989.
31. Rajendran R, Varghese I, Sugathan CK, et al.: Ackerman's tumor (verrucous carcinoma) of the oral cavity: a clinico-epidemiologic study of 426 cases, *Aust Dent J* 33(4):295–298, 1988.
32. Lopez-Amado M, Garcia-Caballero T, Lozano-Ramirez A, et al.: Human papillomavirus and p53 oncoprotein in verrucous carcinoma of the larynx, *J Laryngol Otol* 110(8):742–747, 1996.
33. Miller CS, Johnstone BM: Human papillomavirus as a risk factor for oral squamous cell carcinoma: a meta-analysis, 1982-1997, *Oral Surg Med Pathol Radiol Endod* 91(6):622–635, 2001.
34. Azevedo LH, Galletta VC, de Paula Eduardo C, et al.: Treatment of oral verrucous carcinoma with carbon dioxide laser, *J Oral Maxillofac Surg* 65(11):2361–2366, 2007.
35. Yeh CJ: Treatment of verrucous hyperplasia and verrucous carcinoma by shave excision and simple cryosurgery, *Int J Oral Maxillofac Surg* 32(3):280–283, 2003.
36. Schrader M, Laberke HG: Differential diagnosis of verrucous carcinoma in the oral cavity and larynx, *J Laryngol Otol* 102(8):700–703, 1988.
37. Astner S, Anderson RR: Treating vascular lesions, *Derm Ther* 18(3):267–281, 2005.
38. Mulliken JB, Glowacki J: Hemangiomas and vascular malformations in infants and children: a classification based on endothelial characteristics, *Plast Reconstr Surg* 69(3):412–422, 1982.

39. Mihm MC, North PE: Histopathological diagnosis of infantile hemangiomas and vascular malformations. In *Vascular birthmarks of the head and neck, Facial Plastic Surgery Clinics of North America*, Philadelphia, 2001, Saunders.

40. Railan D, Parlette EC, Uebelhoer NS, Rohrer TE: Laser treatment of vascular lesions, *Clin Dermatol* 24(1):8–15, 2006.

41. Fishman SJ, Mulliken JB: Hemangiomas and vascular malformations of infancy and childhood, *Pediatr Clin North Am* 40(6):1177–1200, 1992.

42. Vascular Birthmark Foundation. http://www.birthmark.org. Accessed August 2008.

43. Merlen JF: Red telangiectasias, blue telangiectasias, *Soc Franc Phlebol* 22:167–174, 1970.

44. Pence B, Aybey B, Ergenekon G: Outcomes of 532-nm frequency-doubled Nd:YAG laser in the treatment of port-wine stains, *Dermatol Surg* 31(5):509–517, 2005.

45. Ulrich H, Baumler W, Hohenleutner U, Landthaler M: Neodymium-YAG laser for hemangiomas and vascular malformations: long-term results, *J Dtsch Dermatol Ges* 3(6):436–440, 2005.

46. Wlodawsky RN, Strauss RA: Intraoral laser surgery, *Oral Maxillofac Surg Clin North Am* 16(2):149–163, 2004.

47. Seeman R, DiToppa J, Holm M, Hanson J: Does laser-assisted uvulopalatoplasty work? An objective analysis using pre- and postoperative polysomnographic studies, *J Otolaryngol* 30:212–215, 2000.

48. Maniglia AJ: Sleep apnea and snoring: an overview, *Ear Nose Throat J* 72(1):16–19, 1993.

49. Sher AE, Schechtman KB, Piccirillo JF: The efficacy of surgical modifications of the upper airway in adults with sleep apnea syndrome, *Sleep* 19(2):156–157, 1996.

50. Dijkgraaf CL, Spijkervert FK, DeBont LG: Arthroscopic findings in osteoarthritic temporomandibular joints, *J Oral Maxillofac Surg* 57:255–268, 1999.

51. Sanders B: Arthroscopic management of internal derangements of the temporomandibular joint, *Oral Maxillofac Surg Clin North Am* 6(2):259–269, 1994.

52. Kaneyama K, Segami N, Sato J, et al.: Outcomes of 152 temporomandibular joints following arthroscopic anterolateral capsular release by holmium:YAG laser or electrocautery, *Oral Surg Med Pathol* 97(5):546–552, 2004.

53. Yoshida H, Fukumura Y, Tojyo I, et al.: Operation with a single-channel thin-fibre arthroscope in patients with internal derangement of the temporomandibular joint, *Br J Oral Maxillofac Surg* 46(4):313–314, 2008.

54. Hendler B, Gateno J, Mooar P, Sherk H: Holmium:YAG laser arthroscopy of the tempooromandibular joint, *J Oral Maxillofac Surg* 50(9):931–934, 1992.

55. Israel HA: The use of arthroscopic surgery for treatment of temporomandibular joint disorders, *J Oral Maxillofac Surg* 57(5):579–582, 1999.

56. Koslin MG: Advanced arthroscopic surgery, *Oral Maxillofac Surg Clin North Am* 18(3):329–343, 2006.

57. Miloro M, Ghali GE, Larsen PE, Waite PD: *Peterson's principles of oral and maxillofacial surgery*, vol. 2, ed2. Hamilton, Ontario, 2004, BC Decker.

58. Koslin MG: Laser applications in temporomandibular joint arthroscopic surgery, *Oral Maxillofac Surg Clin North Am* 16(2):269–275, 2004.

59. Nitzan DW, Dolwick MF: Temporomandibular joint fibrous ankylosis following orthognathic surgery: report of eight cases, *Int J Adult Orthod Orthog Surg* 4(1):7–11, 1989.

60. Topazian RG: Etiology of ankylosis of the TMJ: analysis of 44 cases, *J Oral Surg Anesth Hosp Dent Serv* 22:227–233, 1964.

61. Kaban LB, Perrott DH, Fisher K: A protocol for management of TMJ ankylosis, *J Oral Maxillofac Surg* 48(11):1145–1152, 1990.

62. Moses JJ, Lee J, Arredondo A: Arthroscopic laser debridement of temporomandibular joint fibrous and bony ankylosis: case report, *J Oral Maxillofac Surg* 56(9):1104–1106, 1998.

63. Chidzonga MM: Temporomandibular joint ankylosis: review of thirty-two cases, *Br J Oral Maxillofac Surg* 37(2):123–126, 1999.

64. Niamtu J: Radiowave surgery versus CO_2 laser for upper blepharoplasty incision: which modality produces the best results? *Dermatol Surg* 34:912–921, 2008.

65. Strauss RA, McMunn W, Gregory B: Cosmetic skin resurfacing, *Sel Read Oral Maxillofac Surg* 9(3):1–27, 2001.

66. Griffin RY, Sarici A, Ozkan S: Treatment of the lower eyelid with the CO_2 laser: transconjunctival or transcutaneous approach? *Orbit* 26(1):23–28, 2007.

67. Griffin JE, Frey BS, Max DP, Epker BN: Laser-assisted endoscopic forehead lift, *J Oral Maxillofac Surg* 56(9):1040–1048, 1998.

68. Holmquist KA, Rogers GS: Treatment of perioral rhytids: a comparison of dermabrasion and superpulsed carbon dioxide laser, *Arch Dermatol* 6:725, 2000.

69. Riggs K, Keller M, Humphreys TR: Ablative laser resurfacing: high energy pulsed carbon dioxide and erbium-yttrium-aluminum-garnet, *Clin Dermatol* 25(5):462–473, 2007.

70. Gilbert S, McBurney E: Use of valacyclovir for herpes simplex virus-1 (HSV-1) prophylaxis after facial resurfacing: a randomized clinical trial of closing regimens, *Dermatol Surg* 1:50, 2000.

71. Widder RA, Severin M, Kirchhof B, et al.: Corneal injury after carbon dioxide laser skin resurfacing, *Am J Ophthalmol* 125(3):392–394, 1998.

72. Niamtu J: To debride or not to debride? That is the question: rethinking char removal in ablative CO_2 laser skin resurfacing, *Dermatol Surg*, May 2008. Epub.

73. Brandon MS, Strauss RA: Complications of CO_2 laser procedures in oral and maxillofacial surgery, *Oral Maxillofac Surg Clin North Am* 16:289–299, 2004.

74. Guttenberg SA, Emery RW: Laser dermatopathology, *Oral Maxillofac Surg Clin North Am* 16(2):189–196, 2004.

75. Alster T: Zaulyanov Laser scar revision, *Dermatol Surg* 33(2):131–140, 2007.

76. Chen MA, Davidson TM: Scar management: prevention and treatment strategies, *Curr Opin Otolaryngol Head Neck Surg* 13(4):242–247, 2005.

15

Photobiomodulation in Dentistry

JAN TUNÉR, PER HUGO BECK-KRISTENSEN, GERALD ROSS, AND ALANA ROSS

The wavelengths of surgical lasers—neodymium-doped yttrium-aluminum-garnet (Nd:YAG), carbon dioxide (CO_2), erbium, diode—effect changes in tissues not only by ablation, coagulation, and vaporization but also through stimulation of natural healing processes in the cells. Other lasers and light-emitting diodes (LEDs), applied at much lower power than that of the surgical lasers, act more as "biostimulators."

This chapter discusses the most useful dental indications for treatment with these lower-power lasers and LEDs. Such therapy was historically referred to as *low-level laser therapy* (as well as cold laser therapy, therapeutic laser therapy, and soft laser therapy), although the addition of LEDs has altered the suggested nomenclature. Currently the most accurate description is *photobiomodulation* (PBM), because this term best describes the process and encompasses the operational principles for all therapeutic light devices.

Therapeutic Lasers and Light-Emitting Diodes

Therapeutic laser and LED wavelengths typically are found in the visible red to near-visible *infrared* part of the electromagnetic spectrum, from 630 to 980 nm. Output powers typically range from 50 to 500 mW with either pulsed or continuous-wave emission, although a number of high-powered lasers are now in the marketplace. The names of these therapeutic lasers, as with surgical lasers, are derived from the active medium, such as the gallium-aluminum-arsenide (GaAlAs) and helium-neon (HeNe) lasers.

The simplest way to classify therapeutic lasers is by wavelength. Penetration depths vary; lasers in the red part of the spectrum are more superficially absorbed, whereas infrared lasers penetrate as much as 3 to 5 cm, depending on wavelength and target tissue. LED beams are noncoherent; acccordingly, the penetration of these photons is much more superficial. There is an "optical window" at approximately 820 nm, which has the greatest depth of optical penetration. Mucosa is quite *transparent* to the wavelengths (i.e., it does not absorb light well), skin and bone are moderately transparent, and muscles have the greatest absorption of light. Dosage at the target tissue must be calculated accordingly.

Another factor in depth of penetration is the distance from the target tissue, which affects the spot size (see Chapter 2). Irradiation *out of contact,* irradiation *in contact,* and irradiation with pressure on the tissue all deliver different dosages to the tissue. Laser irradiation with concomitant tissue pressure results in a slight localized ischemia, which reduces the hemoglobin concentration in the spot and allows for deeper penetration. With irradiation in out-of-contact mode, the reflection off the tissue increases, and fewer photons will be absorbed (Figures 15-1 and 15-2).

Mechanisms

The advantage of therapeutic laser light is that it stimulates natural biologic processes and mainly affects cells in a decreased oxidation–reduction (redox) reaction. A cell in a low redox state is acidic, but after laser irradiation the cell becomes more alkaline and able to perform optimally. Healthy cells cannot significantly increase their redox capability and thus will not react strongly to the laser energy, whereas cells in a low redox state will be stimulated.[1,2] The most essential effect may be the increase in adenosine triphosphate (ATP), the "fuel" of the cells, produced in the mitochondria.[3] ATP is the end product of the Krebs cycle, whereby the photon-acceptor enzyme cytochrome *c* oxidase

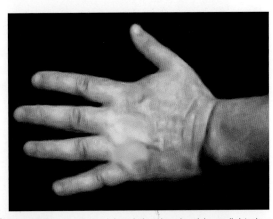

• **Figure 15-1** It is often claimed that low-level laser light does not penetrate well through skin. A 650-nm wavelength at only 30 mW shows penetration of low-level laser light through the ventral surface of the hand to the dorsum.

is inhibited by nitric oxide (NO). Laser light will dissociate the binding between NO and cytochrome c oxidase, allowing it to resume ATP production.[4] This basic mechanism initiates a cascade of cell signaling, leading to an optimization of body functions[5] (Figure 15-3).

Dosage

The most critical part of PBM is determining the optimal dosage. The tissue dosage is expressed in *fluence,* or energy density, measured in joules per square centimeter (J/cm^2). The total produced energy is determined by multiplying the output power of the laser in milliwatts by the time of

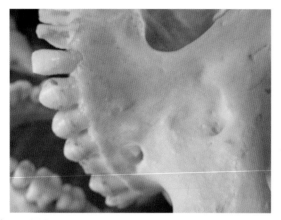

• **Figure 15-2** A 650-nm wavelength at only 30 mW shows penetration of low-level laser light through bone.

exposure in seconds; for example, 50 mW × 40 sec = 2000 millijoules (mJ), or 2.0 J.

The next factor to consider is the size of the area being irradiated. With irradiation of an area of 2 cm^2, the calculation is 2 J of energy divided by an area of 2 cm^2, or 2/2, for a fluence (energy density), or superficial tissue dose, of 1 J/cm^2. Suppose that the irradiated area was only 0.5 cm^2. An inverse relationship exists between spot size (size of irradiated area) and fluence. Decreasing the size of the irradiated area increases the fluence: 2 J divided by 0.5 cm^2 = 4. Thus the dose becomes 4 J/cm^2, because the energy was emitted over a smaller area, increasing the local intensity. Because the dose depends greatly on the spot size, a thin light probe will create high doses in J/cm^2. This probe/spot size–dose dependency does not necessarily mean that the amount of energy applied to the tissue is high—it merely determines that the *intensity* of the light energy at the emitting end of the thin probe is high.

With the difference between energy and dose now established, a more complex calculation is in order: determination of the *dose at target.* If the target is 1 cm below the surface, reflection, scattering, and absorption of the energy could occur before it arrives at the target. It is therefore necessary to consider the depth of the target area and the type of tissue between the light and the target tissue. The main absorbers of these wavelengths are pigmented *chromophores,* such as the hemoglobin in blood; acccordingly, highly vascular tissue will absorb these wavelengths well, and less vascular tissue will absorb these wavelengths poorly.

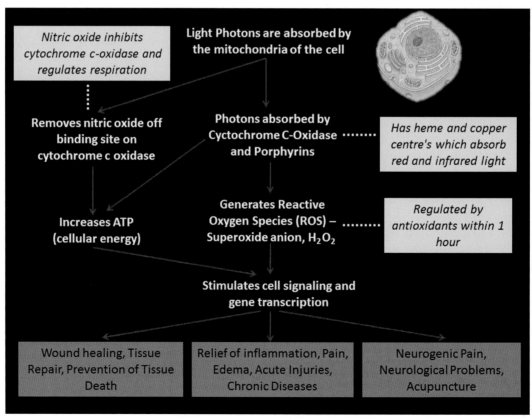

• **Figure 15-3** Summary of the primary mechanisms of PBM.

Mucosa is transparent to these low-level wavelengths; bone also is rather transparent, whereas muscle tissue, with its rich blood supply, is not. Another complicating factor is the amount of another chromophore in the target tissue, *melanin.* Because melanin is a strong absorber of these wavelengths, more light energy may be superficially absorbed rather than reaching deeper tissue, which may create local heating and even pain.

Therefore the use of J/cm^2 to describe the dose in owner's manuals can be confusing. The J/cm^2 (dose, fluence) indicates the intensity at the surface of the tissue but not the dose at the underlying target. A simpler approach is to use the term *energy per point,* calculating only the number of joules in each point. For clinical use, this is acceptable, but for scientific investigations, unacceptable.[6] A "point" often is referred to as the size of the tip of the laser probe (spot size). The relationship between spot size and power density holds true for low-level lasers as well. A small spot size creates a larger concentration of the power per square millimeter or centimeter of tissue irradiated, whereas a wider spot size dilutes the same energy over a larger area.

Stimulation/Inhibition

Low-level laser therapy follows the Arndt-Schulz law: Too small a stimulus does not trigger any effect. Increased stimulation augments the effect up to an optimal dose level. Increasing the dose even further means that the stimulation is gradually reduced, and at very high doses, stimulation is inhibited. The quest for the "optimal dose" is still not exact, but much is known about therapeutic windows for this modality. In some patients, the goal is inhibition rather than stimulation, especially for pain management. High doses of laser light will inhibit the pain signals, partly by creating transient varicosities along the neurons, impeding signal transmission.[7] Opioid-related mechanisms also have been reported,[8] as well as a reduction in the compound action potential[9] (Figures 15-4–15-6). Dosages may need to be modified throughout the course of the treatment as the desired outcome changes. Such a flexible approach is indicated during orthodontic treatments, for example. During application of the required force to the tooth, pain reduction is the primary goal, so a bioinhibitory dose is used.

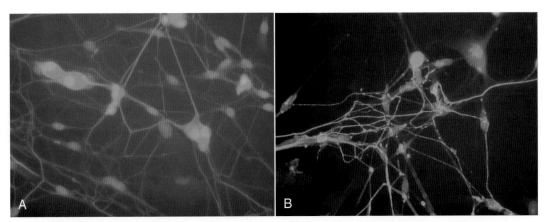

• **Figure 15-4** **A,** Neurons before low-level laser irradiation. **B,** Neurons after irradiation, using 830-nm wavelength for 120 sec. Note varicosities that formed along axons. These varicosities are transient but are thought to be obstacles in neural transmission. (Courtesy Roberta Chow, MB, Ph.D.)

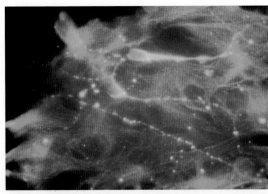

• **Figure 15-5** Varicosities formed along the axons after Nd:YAG laser irradiation. (Courtesy Ambrose Chan, BDS, MDSc.)

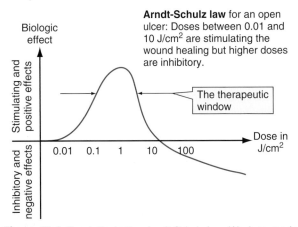

• **Figure 15-6** Graph illustrating Arndt-Schulz law. Weak to moderate stimuli activate physiologic processes. Strong stimuli (doses >10 J/cm^2) inhibit physiologic responses. Therapeutic window is therefore between 0.01 and 10 J/cm^2.

At subsequent visits, the aim is to stimulate the osteoblast-osteoclast turn over, so a lower dose is applied.[10]

Acute Versus Chronic Conditions

The general rule is to apply high doses of laser energy for acute conditions that manifest with inflammation and edema, while treating chronic conditions (e.g., wounds, paresthesias, pain) more conservatively. Initially, acute conditions often can be treated until they resolve and the pain is no longer present, whereas chronic conditions should be treated two to three times weekly.

Patients with long-standing chronic pain conditions may experience a flare of pain after PBM, which is commonly known as a treatment reaction. This reaction is transient and actually shows that the patient is responding well to the treatment. The underlying mechanism is believed to involve transformation of the chronic situation into an acute phase, allowing healing to begin. Pain levels are reduced below baseline within 24 h. *The patient should be informed about this possibility before treatment, to avoid a reduction in compliance.* Other patients undergoing treatment for chronic pain conditions may respond with deep fatigue, interpreted as an accumulated lack of rest, surfacing when the pain subsides. As with pharmaceuticals, management of the reaction and the dosage must be individualized for each patient (Figure 15-7).

As a general rule, acute pain resolves much faster than chronic. In cases of traumatic injury (as from an automobile accident), the sooner laser treatments are initiated, the faster it will resolve.

Pulsing

The importance of pulsing the light is obvious when the laser is applied to cell monolayers in the laboratory.[11–13] The pulse repetition rate (PRR) also helps in the clinical setting, although little is known about pulsing in vivo and animal/clinical studies are inconclusive. It is not yet known how to control these mechanisms through use of different PRRs. Also, the biologic effects of a "chopped" continuous-wave laser beam and a superpulsed beam are different. At present, use of a continuous beam is therefore recommended in units that have continuous-wave emission. The 904-nm gallium arsenide (GaAs) laser does not have a continuous-wave mode, so determination of the optimal PRR must rely on anecdotal evidence for selection of pulse parameters.

Moriyama et al.[14] demonstrated increased expression of the inducible nitric oxide synthase (iNOS) gene after 905-nm superpulsed laser irradiation. This finding suggests a different mechanism in activating the inflammatory pathway response in superpulsed mode compared with continuous-wave mode.

Number of Sessions

Acute conditions can be resolved with a single PBM session, but many conditions require repeated irradiation for optimal results. Dental treatments often create acute injuries, so

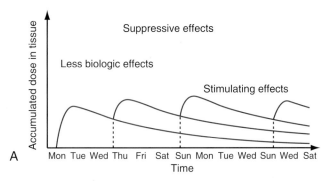

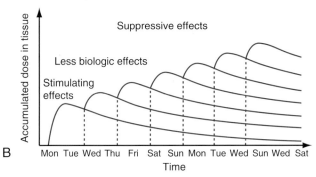

• **Figure 15-7** Cumulative effect of dosing in low-level laser therapy (i.e., PBM). **A,** With several days between doses, the total accumulated dose does not reach an inhibitory range. **B,** When doses are given too closely together, the accumulated dose reaches an inhibitory range. Such treatment inhibits rather than activates healing, according to the Arndt-Schulz law.

repeated irradiation is not necessary. As an example, in an extraction, irradiation of the site at the time of the procedure often is sufficient to reduce pain and inflammation. Other treatments, such as for facial pain or orthodontic discomfort, will require more sessions over a longer period of time. In many cases, follow-up visits requiring irradiation can be delegated to the dental assistant or the dental hygienist. Regulations vary in different areas, so clinicians should confirm local regulations before delegating. In some situations the patient can borrow, rent, or buy a simple low-power laser or LED device (even a traditional 5-mW laser pointer) for a period to optimize the treatment by applying daily doses according to the dentist's instructions (Figure 15-8).

Side Effects and Contraindications

Doses of laser energy near the therapeutic window will not cause negative effects. The worst result with PBM is that nothing happens. There are few absolute contraindications to PBM, but a few caveats follow.

Presence of known malignancies is a contraindication, because PBM stimulates cell growth (this issue is based largely on legal considerations). The literature also discusses pregnancy as a contraindication,[15] although dentists work exclusively in the oral and head-neck regions. Also, although sometimes listed as a contraindication, pacemakers are electrical and not influenced by light. Some traditional safety regulations and contraindications seem to have

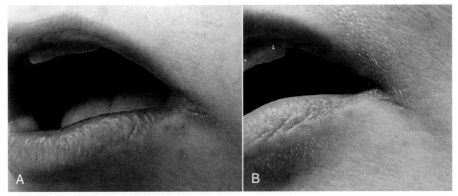

• **Figure 15-8** Patient with angular cheilitis treated with one session of PBM in the dental office (30 mW, 3 J, 650-nm wavelength) and then with once-daily self-application at home (1 J per day) for 5 days. **A,** Preoperative view. **B,** Postoperative view.

been transferred from electrosurgical and other therapies to surgical lasers.

A contraindication especially relevant to dentistry is irradiation over the thyroid gland, located within the dental treatment area. Dentists generally are not informed about possible thyroid conditions; direct irradiation over this area, therefore, should be avoided, because it could stimulate a hyperthyroid condition with a low dose or inhibit a hypothyroid condition with a high dose. However, PBM for thyroid disorders has been studied.[16]

Documentation

Because of the complex mechanisms involved in PBM, most of the literature is still not at an evidence-based level, except for a few indications. Still, research at more than 100 dental institutions worldwide is represented in the literature, comprising more than 4000 studies. Annually, approximately 250 papers on PBM appear on PubMed, many on dental issues and most reporting positive results. Reports of no effect from PBM often can be attributed to very low doses, miscalculation of the supposed dose, and ineffective treatment applications.[17] Nevertheless, some qualified negative studies underline that PBM is not a "hit and run" therapy but depends on knowledge of all relevant parameters. A correct diagnosis and sufficient dosage are key to success.

Laser Safety

Therapeutic lasers with wavelengths of less than 500 mW generally are harmless and classified as "low-risk devices" by the U.S. Food and Drug Administration (FDA).

It is prudent to use protective goggles that are wavelength-specific. Most therapeutic lasers have divergent beams, so from a distance of only a few centimeters, the intensity (and danger) is considerably reduced. PBM has even been successfully used to treat macular degeneration,[18] affirming the importance of wavelength and intensity. Some PBM lasers have a collimated lens system, producing a parallel beam. These features have no advantages in dental PBM, and when the laser is used in contact with tissue, the effect of the collimation is lost.

The regulation of laser devices varies from country to country and according to the class. LED devices generally fall in the category of Class 1 devices, for which the standards are much less stringent (Table 15-1).

All clinicians should be familiar with and follow the American National Standards Institute (ANSI) standard, which outlines all safety precautions. Almost all countries follow this standard. Clinicians should consult the appropriate local agencies and authorities to determine the regulations for use of lasers and delegation of laser procedures.

Choosing the "Right" Device

Lasers and LEDs are available with different wavelengths and also different combinations of wavelengths, powers, and probe sizes. The choice of device is therefore not "one size fits all." Any therapeutic light device can be used for many indications, but some combinations of wavelength and power are optimal for selected indications; clinicians should focus on their special interests. When choosing a device, other practical considerations include probe sterilization, education, technical service, and guarantee period.

Power and Time

During the past decade, stronger lasers have been advocated as more effective, so therapeutic lasers with output of 500 mW or more are now commercially available. For musculoskeletal conditions and pain therapy, high-output lasers may be useful, but for processes such as wound healing and bone regeneration, use of lower power over a longer time is more effective. Availability of power adjustments in a therapeutic laser, as with a surgical laser, is therefore helpful. Applying 5 J in 10 sec with a 500-mW laser is quite different from applying the same 5 J with a 50-mW laser in 100 sec. The 500-mW laser would work better for pain but might be less effective for treatment involving tissue regeneration.[19] This divergence of effect reemphasizes the importance of adequate and appropriate training in the decision-making process.

TABLE 15-1 Different Classes of Photobiomodulation Devices

Class	IEC 60825-1 (Ed-2)	U.S.: FDA/CDRH (FLPPS)	ANSI-Z136.1
Class 1	Any laser or laser system containing a laser that cannot emit laser radiation at levels that are known to cause eye or skin injury during normal operation. This does not apply to service requiring access to class 1 enclosures containing higher-class lasers.		
Class 1M	Not known to cause eye or skin damage unless collecting optics are used	N/A	Considered incapable of producing hazardous exposure unless viewed with collecting optics
Class 2A	N/A	Visible lasers that are not intended for viewing and cannot produce any known eye or skin injury during operation based on a maximum exposure time of 1000 sec	N/A
Class 2	Visible lasers considered incapable of emitting laser radiation at levels that are known to cause skin or eye injury within the time period of the human eye aversion response (0.25 sec)		
Class 2M	Not known to cause eye or skin damage within the aversion response time unless collecting optics are used	N/A	Emits in the visible portion of the spectrum and is potentially hazardous if viewed with collecting optics
Class 3a	N/A	Visible lasers less than 5 times the class 2 limit	N/A
Class 3R	Replaces class 3a and has different limits; up to 5 times the class 2 limit for visible and 5 times the class 1 limits for some invisible lasers	N/A	A laser system that is potentially hazardous under some direct and specular reflection viewing conditions if the eye is appropriately focused and stable
Class 3B	Medium-powered lasers (visible and invisible regions) that present a potential eye hazard for intrabeam (direct) viewing or for viewing specular (mirrorlike) reflections. Class 3B lasers do not present a diffuse (scatter) reflection hazard or significant skin hazard except for higher-powered class 3B lasers operating in certain wavelength regions.		
Class 4	High-powered lasers (visible or invisible) that present a potential acute hazard to the eye and skin for both direct (intrabeam) exposure and for exposure to diffuse (scatter) reflections. Class 4 lasers also present a potential hazard for fire (ignition) and byproduct emissions from target and process materials.		

ANSI, American National Standards Institute; *CDRH (FLPPS),* Center for Devices and Radiological Health (Federal Laser Product Performance Standard); *IEC,* International Electrotechnical Commission.

Hygiene

Some therapeutic lasers have a removable, sterilizable probe, similar to that of the dental curing light; if it will not affect the optics, the probe should go through a heat sterilizer and the handle should be covered with a disposable barrier. If the tip cannot be sterilized, the whole unit should be covered in a disposable barrier. Sterilizing requirements vary, so familiarity with and understanding of local regulations are imperative.

Biostimulation

Although dental lasers such as the Nd:YAG, CO_2, and erbium family are considered "hard" or "surgical" lasers, various studies indicate that they also can produce a degree of biostimulation in the areas peripheral to the focal spot, where the energy is reduced to stimulatory levels (Figure 15-9).

Some of the positive effects observed with the hard lasers may be explained by biostimulation. Pourzarandian et al.[20,21]

reported stimulation of human gingival fibroblasts by low-level Er:YAG irradiation, as well as increased prostaglandin E_2 (PGE_2) production through induction of cyclooxygenase-2 (COX-2) messenger ribonucleic acid (mRNA) in human gingival fibroblasts. Additionally, Er:YAG lasers may be used at lowest output and scanned at a slight distance (out of focus) to produce biostimulation. The problem with using these hard lasers in this manner is that no microprocessor informs the practitioner how to control the dosage, and the fibers are not specifically adapted for biostimulation.

Biostimulation is not limited to the traditional near-infrared wavelength window; such effects are even reported with use of defocused CO_2 lasers.[22-24] The CO_2 laser wavelength has extremely poor penetration through tissue because it is so well absorbed at the surface, and the biologic effects reported on deeper tissues may first appear improbable. However, the coherent light is absorbed in peripheral microvessels, and the clinical effect observed shows that PBM

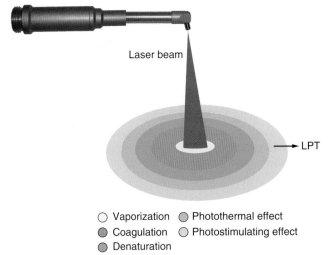

• **Figure 15-9** Various zones of effect surrounding the focal spot when using a surgical laser (CO_2, Nd:YAG, erbium, diode). At the focal spot, *vaporization* occurs. Concentric to that is a zone of *coagulation*, where the proteins in the tissue have absorbed energy and have coagulated but have not been vaporized. Concentric to that is the zone of *denaturation*, where tissue proteins have absorbed a sufficient amount of energy to be heated to the point of denaturation but have not absorbed enough energy to be coagulated. Concentric to that is the zone of *photothermal effect*, where the tissue has absorbed enough energy to be heated but is not otherwise affected. Concentric to that is the zone of *photostimulation*, where some low-level laser activity can occur.

has primary effects at the target as well as systemic effects through blood and lymph circulation. Thus, with minimal calculations in clinical practice, the owner of a "hard" laser can have a "soft" laser for free. Least complicated is the surgical diode laser, with simpler calculations and wavelengths within the traditional range of biostimulation.

Photoactivated Disinfection

There is a growing interest in the combination of different dyes with therapeutic lasers. Neither the dyes nor the therapeutic lasers used alone will have an effect on bacteria, but in combination, singlet oxygen will be produced, which has a strong bactericidal effect.

The photoactivated disinfection (PAD) method is already commercialized and recommended for use in periodontal pockets, periimplantitis, deep carious lesions, and infected root canals.[24–28] The laser must work within the absorption range of the dye used, and wavelengths generally are in the red spectrum, with a power output of 50 to 100 mW. The selected dye is applied and allowed to diffuse for a few minutes, and then laser irradiation is performed. Some transient discoloration may be seen in dentinal and mucosal areas.

Curing Light

All dentists have in their armamentarium a composite curing light, typically with a wavelength peak of approximately 470 nm. Energies delivered are within the low-level laser

therapeutic window, but studies of the photobiologic effect on the surrounding tissues are largely lacking.

In a 2009 in vitro study, Enwemeka et al.[29] demonstrated that light-emitting diode (LED) energy with a 470-nm peak successfully kills methicillin-resistant *Staphylococcus aureus* (MRSA). Irradiation produced a statistically significant, dose-dependent reduction in both the number and the aggregate area of colonies formed by each strain of cells. The higher the dose, the more bacteria were killed, but the effect was not linear, being more impressive at lower than at higher doses. Almost 30% of both strains was killed with as little as 3 J/cm^2. As much as 90.4% of the two different colonies was killed with an energy density of 55 J/cm^2. This study requires further in vivo investigation but suggests an innovative use of an available dental light source to treat MRSA infection, which carries high morbidity and mortality rates. A short wavelength such as a curing light has a very shallow penetration depth, so it will be more effective on surface lesions

Lasers Versus Light-Emitting Diodes

Laser light is coherent and is delivered as a collimated beam, whereas light from an LED light is noncoherent, without collimation. The subject of whether one is more efficacious than the other is a topic of controversy, often resulting in very heated discussion. Many research studies have investigated the effect on tissue with LEDs and lasers, with differing outcomes. A study by Nishioka et al. in 2012, however, investigated the effect of laser and LED irradiation using the same total energy deposited in tissue and found that both resulted in a significant decrease in the necrosis of the skin flap, which indicated that the light source consistency was not essential for successful results.[30]

Acupuncture

Few dentists use acupuncture, but several acupuncture points can be used in low-level laser applications by all dentists. Therapeutic lasers produce effects similar to those of acupuncture needles and are safer to use. For example, P6 (i.e., Neiguan) on the wrist is an excellent point for use in reducing nausea and vomiting.[31] The location of this point is 2.5 cm up from the wrist and 0.5 to 1.0 cm deep. The point is between two tendons. Delivery of 3 to 4 J to P6 often allows a more relaxed environment for taking impressions or working in the molar area, especially in patients with a heightened gag reflex. Another easily accessible point is the Li4 (i.e., Hegu), a pain-reducing point located in the middle of the second metacarpal bone on the radial side (Figures 15-10 and 15-11).

Functional magnetic resonance imaging (fMRI) has confirmed the similarity of needles and lasers in their effect with application on the same acupuncture point.[32] However, understanding this phenomenon becomes more difficult because a *qi* effect, the purported underlying mechanism in acupuncture, is absent with the laser. The gate control

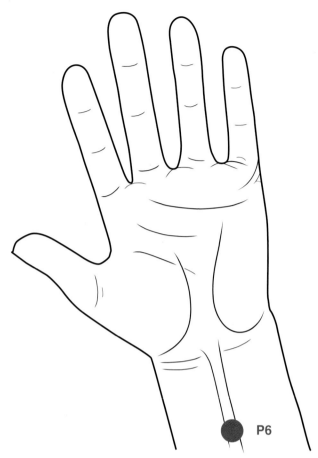

• **Figure 15-10** P6 acupuncture point can be stimulated with a low-level laser for reduction of nausea and gagging.

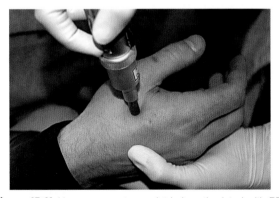

• **Figure 15-11** Hegu acupuncture point being stimulated with PBM. This point usually is used for general pain relief. Usual dose is 3 to 4 J on a superficial acupuncture point.

theory would not explain the effects because pain stimulus in the acupuncture point does not occur with use of a laser.

Dental Indications

Because PBM can influence so many pathologic conditions, the use of the therapeutic laser is not limited to the following indications. More than 30 conditions have been described in the dental literature; the most important are briefly described here. As more research is conducted, the

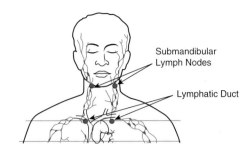

• **Figure 15-12** Diagram of subthoracic lymphatic duct and submandibular lymph nodes.

number of indications for use based on peer-reviewed literature will undoubtedly increase.

Anesthesia

Applying PBM to the mucosa, but not the hard palate, before an injection results in a slight anesthetic effect.[33] PBM applied before the injection also will improve healing, should the needle cause trauma to a vessel or nerve. PBM improves local microcirculation,[34] so the effect of the numbness can be shortened if PBM is applied to the site after completion of the dental procedure. Energy of 4 to 6 J is needed in both cases.

Aphthous Ulcers

The healing time of aphthous ulcers can be shortened and the immediate pain reduced by administering 4 to 6 J over the lesion and 4 J to the submandibular lymph nodes on the affected side[35,36] (Figure 15-12). Patients prone to development of aphthous ulcers should avoid toothpastes containing sodium lauryl sulfate, which may trigger these lesions in predisposed persons.

Edema

The lymphatic system plays an important role in the inflammatory process, and PBM applied over the involved lymph nodes decreases edema. Irradiation should start over the most distal nodes of the chain involved and proceed toward the focus of the swelling, using 4 J per node. The permeability of the lymph vessels will be reduced and lumen size increased, and repeated irradiation will stimulate growth of collaterals[37–41] (Figure 15-13). The lymphatic system also brings the lymphocytes and natural killer cells to fight infection. Meneguzzo et al.[41] reported that irradiation with an 810-nm laser reduced rat paw edema whether it was performed in the paw itself or over the inguinal lymph nodes.

Endodontics

PBM does not have a bactericidal effect, and surgical lasers are the preferred instruments to reduce bacteria in infected root canals. Few manufacturers of therapeutic lasers offer probes that could reach the root canals. However, infrared light can reach all apices, and visible red light can reach the

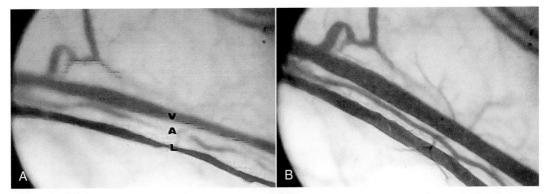

• **Figure 15-13 A,** Vein, artery, and lymphatic vessel before irradiation. Note diameter of the vessels. **B,** After low-level irradiation of vessels using a laser with 904-nm wavelength. Note dilation of vessels, which leads to increased circulation in the region they supply. (Courtesy Pierre Lievens.)

more superficial apices through the mucosa, to produce an antiinflammatory and pain-reducing effect.

Sousa et al.[42] analyzed the effect of PBM on the secretory activity of macrophages activated by interferon gamma (IFN-γ) and lipopolysaccharide (LPS) and stimulated by substances leached from an epoxy resin–based sealer (AH-Plus) and a calcium hydroxide sealer (Sealapex). The production of tumor necrosis factor alpha (TNF-α) was significantly decreased by PBM, regardless of experimental group. The level of secretion of matrix metalloproteinase-1 (MMP-1) was similar in all groups.

Laser application after overinstrumentation and overfilling is a good example of an indication for PBM in endodontics. Because PBM can stimulate bone formation, apical bone probably can heal faster after completed endodontic treatment if PBM is applied. Energy needed is related to the depth of the apex, ranging from 4 to 8 J per apex. For the same reason, intraoperative and postoperative PBM in apical surgery has potential,[43,44] but solid scientific documentation is still lacking. However, irradiation over the suture line will stimulate fibroblast proliferation and increase tensile strength.[45]

In patients with acute pulpitis, when the affected tooth or root is difficult to pinpoint, the laser can be applied over the apices in the involved area. The affected tooth may react with an increase in pain, probably because of increased microcirculatory pressure in the pulpal chamber and increased lymphatic flow. PBM also can be used as an adjunct therapy in pulp capping[46,47] and pulpotomy[48,49] (see Chapter 13). In both cases, the exposed pulp is irradiated at low intensities, applying 4 J after the exposed pulp has been cauterized but before any liners, cements, or other medicaments have been placed. The irradiation will reduce inflammation, preserve odontoblastic integrity, and stimulate cellular proliferation.

Extractions

Nontraumatic approaches and good postoperative procedures are the key to satisfactory healing after extractions. However, the occasional complication is unavoidable. Adding PBM after the extraction will reduce the inflammatory

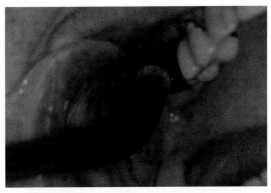

• **Figure 15-14** Application of laser probe into an extraction socket.

phase, induce pain reduction, stimulate the fibroblasts in the wound periphery, and stimulate the osteoblasts in the socket.[50–55] High doses of laser energy applied directly into the socket will reduce postoperative pain and inflammation (Figures 15-14 and 15-15).

The major goal of PBM after extractions is first to reduce pain and inflammation and then to stimulate the fibroblasts to seal the socket. In cases of post-extraction failure (dry socket), the traditional methods are used in combination with very high doses of PBM to reduce patient discomfort. The light energy is applied until the patient notices a decrease in the level of pain, and then a dressing is placed. When the dressing is changed during subsequent appointments, lower doses are given to stimulate fibroblast growth so that the epithelium can cover the exposed bone.

Herpes Simplex Virus

Patients with a herpes simplex virus type 1 (HSV-1) eruption may be reluctant to visit the dentist. However, PBM is the most efficient method of treating this infection.[36,56–58] In particular, if it is treated during the initial prodromal stage (when the patient feels the initial tingling), healing will take only a few days, or the symptoms may even disappear within hours. Of importance, in patients with recurrent HSV-1 attacks, longer intervals between the outbreaks are typical after PBM treatment.[59,60]

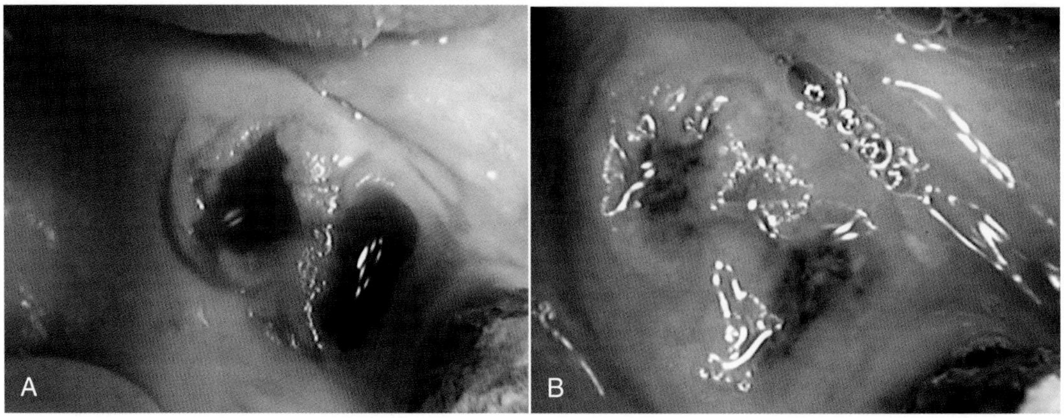

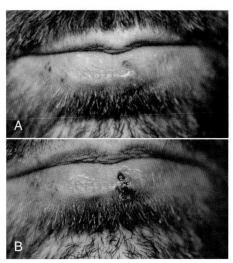

• **Figure 15-15 A,** Socket immediately after tooth extraction. **B,** Extraction socket after laser irradiation using 650-nm wavelength at 30 mW, 8 J, 1 day after extraction. (Courtesy Talat Qadri)

• **Figure 15-16** Herpes outbreak on the lower lip of a male patient. **A,** Preoperative view of. Blisters are in the vesicle stage. Outbreak started the day before the patient presented to the office. Area was treated with 808-nm laser at 500 mW, 4 J. **B,** One-day postoperative view. Lesions have crusted over, and pain has been reduced.

In the acute stage of HSV-1 infection, repeated treatment is necessary; irradiation during the prodromal stage may only be a single session of 2 to 6 J over each blister and 4 J to the submandibular lymph nodes on the affected side, in accordance with size and duration. The actual effect is not known, but research has confirmed that laser light enables the cell to resist viral attack for a longer period, presumably providing time for the immune system to react[61] (Figure 15-16).

Implants

A single high dose of irradiation after implant placement will reduce postoperative pain, inflammation, and edema. Repeated sessions at a lower dose will stimulate osseointegration by stimulating the osteoblasts. As with all healing processes, repeated irradiation is necessary; 4 to 6 J over each implant is recommended, with the laser tip in slight contact.[62–66] PBM also is a useful additional therapy in the control of periimplantitis. The effect is most prominent if PBM is applied immediately after surgery and then two or three times per week for 2 weeks.

Khadra[67] summarized five studies using the 830-nm wavelength as follows:

> PBM can promote bone healing and bone mineralization and thus may be clinically beneficial in promoting bone formation in skeletal defects. It may be also used as additional treatment for accelerating implant healing in bone. PBM can modulate the primary steps in cellular attachment and growth on titanium surfaces. Multiple doses of PBM can improve PBM efficacy, accelerate the initial attachment and alter the behavior of human gingival fibroblasts cultured on titanium surfaces. The use of PBM at the range of doses between 1.5 and 3 J/cm² may modulate the activity of cells interacting with an implant, thereby enhancing tissue healing and ultimate implant success.

Lopes et al.[64] suggested that the 830-nm wavelength can allow earlier loading of titanium implants. Kim et al.[65] found that PBM influenced the expression of osteoprotegerin (OPG), receptor activator of nuclear factor kappa B (RANK), and RANK ligand (RANKL), increasing metabolic bone activity. RANKL is a surface-bound molecule that activates osteoclast cells involved in bone resorption. Overproduction of RANKL is implicated in a variety of degenerative bone diseases, including rheumatoid arthritis and psoriatic arthritis.

Guzzardella et al.[66,68] reported similar stimulatory effects at the bone-implant surface with hydroxyapatite-coated implants using a 780-nm laser. Whether the positive effects on bone-implant integration represent a general effect or specific cell stimulation is not yet known, because several wavelengths and dosages have been used (Figure 15-17).

Inflammation

PBM will shorten the course of the inflammatory process, and it is important to recognize that acute pain reduction

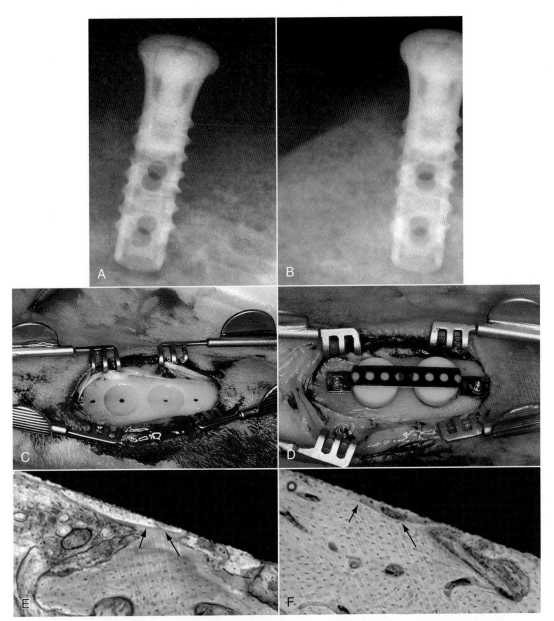

• **Figure 15-17** Low-level laser stimulation of bone healing. **A** and **B,** A failing 2-month-old implant. On the preoperative radiograph **(A),** note the radiolucent quality of bone surrounding the implant. On a post-operative radiograph **(B)** obtained 4 weeks after application of 4 J of energy twice weekly, using 30 mW with 830-nm wavelength, bone quality is greatly improved. **C** to **F,** For a study in 12 adult (8-month-old) New Zealand white rabbits, tibial bone was used as the experimental area. As seen in **C** and **D,** two coin-shaped-titanium implants were inserted into the cortical bone, covered with a polytetrafluoroethylene cap, stabilized with a titanium plate, and retained by two titanium screws. In **E** and **F,** histologic views of the implant in situ show ground section of periimplant bone with osseointegration at 8 weeks after implantation in the control group **(E)** and the irradiated group **(F).** Histomorphometric analysis showed more bone-to-implant contact in the irradiated group than in the control animals (with approximately 10% improvement). (Courtesy Maawan Khadra.)

requires high doses, whereas reduction of the inflammatory period requires less dosage. Reducing the pain may satisfy the patient but may prolong the inflammatory process. The infrared laser dose for inflammation reduction is 8 to 12 J/cm^2.

As mentioned previously, irradiation of the lymphatic system is a major aspect of PBM for antiinflammatory interventions. Lim et al.[69] concluded that 635-nm irradiation and existing COX inhibitors inhibit expression of COX and PGE$_2$ release. Unlike indomethacin and ibuprofen, 635-nm irradiation leads to a decrease in reactive oxygen species (ROS) levels and mRNA expression of cytosolic and secretory phospholipase A$_2$ (cPLA$_2$ and sPLA2). Bjordal et al.[70] also emphasized the reduction in PGE$_2$ levels.

Aimbire et al.[71] reported reduced TNF-α levels in acute inflammation after PBM. Other studies have reported antiinflammatory effects of PBM.[72,73] Steroids seem to reduce the effect of PBM,[74] possibly explaining previous studies with negative outcomes. One study compared dexamethasone (DEX) and PBM and found similar effects.[75] With the short-term and serious long-term effects of nonsteroidal antiinflammatory drugs (NSAIDs),[76] PBM seems to be a good alternative, with similar results but without the drug side effects. In a pilot study by Abiko,[77] DEX and PBM both produced antiinflammatory gene expression. More genes were expressed with DEX than with PBM, but those expressed with PBM were all favorable, whereas those expressed by DEX were those encoding a mixture of wanted and unwanted effects.

In a meta-analysis of 16 randomized controlled trials, Chow et al. demonstrated that low-level laser therapy can reduce pain immediately in cases of acute neck pain and up to 22 weeks after completion of treatment in patients with chronic neck pain. In addition, this modality compared favorably with other widely used therapies, including use of pharmaceuticals (Figures 5-18).[78]

Mucositis

Mucositis is a serious complication after radiation therapy and chemotherapy and can negatively affect quality of life; in severe cases, the patient is unable to eat. Currently, medicine has few options for successful treatment of mucositis. PBM has a cytoprotective effect[79–83] and should be used before therapy and then during the therapeutic regimen until the wounds have disappeared. PBM will reduce pain, xerostomia, and nutritional problems, thus also reducing hospitalization. Irradiation with a red laser, at 4 to 6 J/cm^2, is recommended.[84–89] Many inflammatory mucosal conditions can be treated with PBM (Figures 15-19 and 15-20).

Orthodontics

Various studies have suggested that PBM can increase orthodontic movement along with its pain-reducing effect. Low

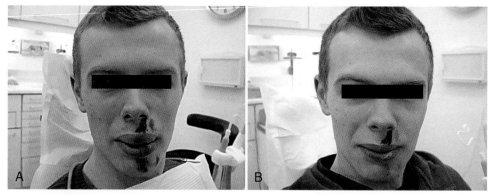

• **Figure 15-18** Low-level laser treatment of dental and soft tissue injuries incurred in a bicycle crash. **A,** Preoperative view. Note swelling and bruising on chin and upper lip. **B,** Four-day postoperative view. Note healing and greatly reduced swelling. Low-level lasers allow the dentist to treat not only injured teeth and gingival margins but traumatized soft tissues of perioral region as well. One dose of 500 mW, 4 J per zone (chin, upper lip) was applied with 808-nm wavelength.

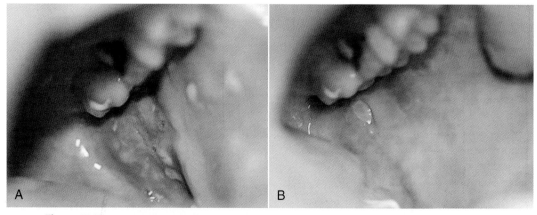

• **Figure 15-19** Low-level laser treatment of oral mucositis after chemotherapy for cancer. **A,** Preoperative view. Using a 660-nm laser at 40 mW, with 0.24 J per point, six points were irradiated. **B,** After six sessions of PBM. Healing is remarkable. (Courtesy Alyne Simões.)

doses stimulate osteoclast-osteoblast activity, whereas high doses are useful for pain control. Infrared irradiation is best owing to its superior bone penetration.

As reported in the canine study by Goulart et al.,[90] PBM may accelerate orthodontic movement at 5.25 J/cm^2, whereas a higher dosage (35 J/cm^2) may impede movement. The accelerating effect at 5 J/cm^2 has been confirmed clinically.[91,92] Youssef et al.[92] also reported a significant pain-relieving effect in the laser-treated group. Turhani et al.[93] confirmed this result, obtaining pain relief from a single exposure of PBM. Fujita et al.[94] showed that the irradiation stimulates tooth movement velocity through expression of RANK and RANKL.

The wounds created by the orthodontic appliances also can be successfully treated by PBM.[95] It may seem contradictory that PBM can stimulate osteoblastic activity on one side of the root and osteoclastic activity on the other side. However, both of these processes take place in orthodontic movement, and PBM has a general stimulatory effect. As noted earlier,[90] the specific effect is dose-dependent.

Pain

Modern dentistry need not be as painful (if at all) as traditional restorative dentistry. The pain-free side of dentistry also can be improved by incorporating the use of therapeutic lasers.[96–100] Effects include decrease in nerve conduction velocity, reduction of compound action potentials, selective inhibition of Aδ and C fibers, and suppression of noxious stimulation.

The first phase of pain reduction in acute pain is a decrease in the levels of PGE$_2$ and other inflammatory markers. Direct inhibition of peripheral afferent terminals suppresses peripheral sensitization and limits further release of neurokinins. As previously discussed, in vitro studies have confirmed formation of transient varicosities on the axons, impeding pain stimuli from reaching the brain. Reduced inflammation and a subsequent decrease in inflammatory components may be sufficient; higher doses will cause inhibition of the antiinflammatory action. However, when immediate pain reduction is the therapeutic goal, bioinhibitory doses are required to decrease neural transmission.[6]

Dosage can be correlated with patient feedback. In chronic pain, sensitization is more important than inflammation. Sensitized peripheral nociceptors may gradually be desensitized by repeated irradiation at lower energies.

Paresthesias

Several maxillofacial interventions can induce nerve damage, especially to the inferior alveolar nerve. The subsequent paresthesias may disappear shortly or within months but occasionally may be permanent. PBM has been shown to counteract the formation of paresthesias and even lessen the symptoms in long-standing aberrations. It is therefore

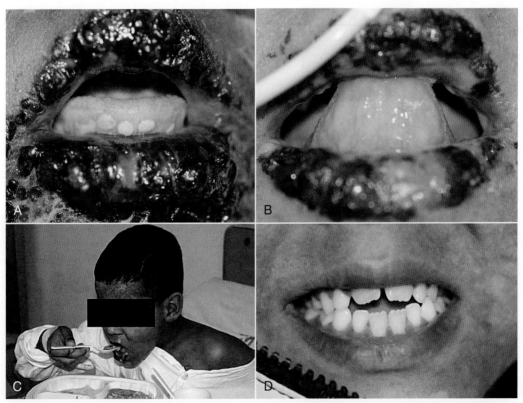

• **Figure 15-20** Erythema multiforme major in a child. **A,** Pretreatment photograph. The patient is unable to eat and is in severe pain. **B,** Fifth day of laser treatment. Note clinical improvement with relief of symptoms. **C,** Seventh day of laser treatment. The patient's appetite has returned. **D,** Complete healing of lesions at day 10. (Courtesy Alyne Simões.)

recommended to irradiate any area in which nerve damage is suspected, even intraoperatively and during follow-up. Using the infrared laser at 4 to 6 J per point along the projection of the nerve incurs a reasonable energy dosage (Figures 15-21 and 15-22).

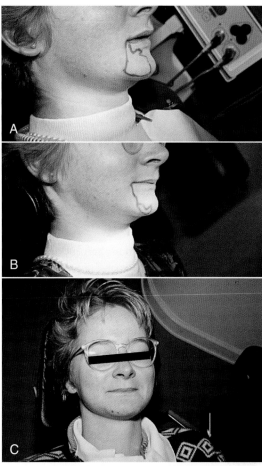

• **Figure 15-21** The patient experienced paresthesias beginning 1 year earlier, secondary to extraction of lower third molar. **A,** Affected region is outlined on the chin. **B,** Greatly reduced area of paresthesias after eight sessions of treatment at 830 nm, 33 mW. Four points along path of inferior alveolar nerve were irradiated with 2 J each. **C,** Complete resolution of paresthesias was achieved after 5 weeks and 11 sessions.

Khullar et al.[101–104] showed that paresthesias of the inferior alveolar nerve can be eliminated or decreased. The effect on motor and sensory functions will vary. Miloro and Repasky[105] confirmed these findings that PBM has a significant effect on neurosensory recovery after sagittal ramus osteotomy. Ozen et al.[106] treated four patients who still had paresthesias 1 year after third lower molar procedures, all with favorable outcomes.

Restorative Treatment

PBM can be used to stimulate analgesia in a number of situations by decreasing the conduction of nerve fibers and stimulating the production and release of endogenous opioids. Particular pediatric indications are the pain associated with tooth eruption and the need to "numb" a deciduous tooth before excavation.[107] Deciduous teeth have large pulp chambers and are easily reached by the laser energy. With open carious lesions, 8 to 16 J is applied on the affected area of the tooth. In the absence of open lesions, PBM is delivered to the buccal cementoenamel junction (CEJ), with an additional 8 to 16 J applied over the apical area (Figures 15-23 and 15-24). The technique is most effective on primary teeth but also can be used in many small to moderate-size restorations in permanent teeth and in the cementation of crowns. The main reason for success is that it affects the depolarization of the C fibers, which are nonmyelinated and thus more easily affected by the light. The release of systemic endorphins also magnifies the analgesia effect. Again, PBM also can facilitate direct and indirect pulp capping and pulpotomy.[79–81] Kurumada[49] investigated the effect of PBM on vital pulpotomy and found irradiation-induced stimulation of calcification in the wound surface, as confirmed by Thwee et al.[48] Paschaud et al.[46] used different calcium hydroxide products in combination with PBM and could show that some, but not all, products in combination with the laser stimulated dentinal bridge formation. In a canine pulp-capping study using lectin histochemistry and collagen immunohistochemistry, Utsunomiya[47] showed that concanavalin A, peanut agglutinin, wheat germ agglutinin, and collagen

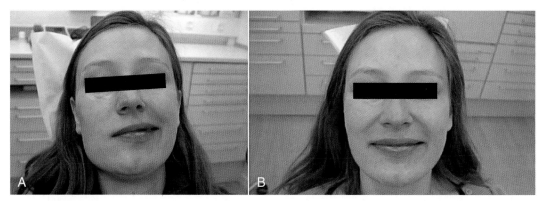

• **Figure 15-22** A female patient in whom trigeminal paresthesias developed during parturition. **A,** Appearance at 3 weeks after childbirth. In this photograph taken immediately after her first treatment, note redness from increase in the microcirculation caused by low-level laser irradiation. Treatment continued for 10 days with settings of 808 nm, 4 J, and 500 mW. **B,** Complete resolution of neuralgia was achieved at 10 days.

(types I, III, and V) were distributed in the fibrous matrix and dentin bridge. The expression of these lectins and collagens occurred earlier in the laser irradiation group than in the control group (see also Chapter 13).

Pulpal Protection

Drilling in a tooth, especially a young tooth, is traumatic for the pulp, even with modern high-speed drills with excellent cooling. Ideally, PBM should be applied after any use of the drill. Less damage to the odontoblasts and faster formation of collagen and secondary dentin have been demonstrated,[108-110] even for small and seemingly nontraumatic cavity preparations. A few joules applied to each abutment after preparation, before try-in and cementation, may prevent postoperative sensitivity and the need for future endodontic therapy. For indirect and direct pulp capping, irradiation with 2 to 4 J over the area is recommended, along with traditional methods.

Godoy et al.[109] showed the vulnerability of the dental pulp using premolars selected for extraction due to orthodontic indications. A minimal class I cavity was performed and filled with composite. One group of teeth received 2 J/cm^2 of 660-nm laser irradiation before filling; a second group received no laser treatment; and a third, no treatment at all. The histologic results are shown in Figure 15-25. These findings suggest that laser irradiation accelerates recovery of the dental structures involved in the cavity preparation at the predentin region.

Periodontics

The chronic periodontal inflammatory process leads to destruction of the periodontal ligament and subsequent loss of alveolar bone, mediated primarily by osteoclasts and triggered by PGE$_2$.[111] Studies of clinical inflammatory aspects of periodontal tissue verified that patients who underwent conventional periodontal treatment in combination with PBM enjoyed a more satisfactory prognosis.[112,113] PBM reportedly reduces gingival inflammation and MMP-8 expression when applied after scaling and root planing (SRP),[112] as well as reducing inflammatory cells in histologic preparations.[113]

Effectiveness of PBM varies, especially as related to different protocols, wavelengths, and modes used. Ozawa et al.[114] showed that PBM significantly inhibits the increase in plasminogen activator (PA) induced in human PDL cells in response to mechanical tension force. PA is capable of activating latent collagenase, the enzyme responsible for cleaving collagen fibers. PBM also was efficient in inhibiting PGE$_2$ synthesis.[115,116] In human gingival fibroblast cultures, PBM significantly inhibited PGE$_2$ production stimulated by LPS through a reduction of COX-2 gene expression in a dose-dependent manner. The decrease in PGE$_2$ levels in cultures of primary human periodontal ligament cells also was verified after mechanical stretching.[117] Garcia et al.[59] found that PBM was an effective adjuvant to conventional SRP treatment for periodontitis in rats treated with dexamethasone.

Nomura et al.[118] verified that laser periodontal therapy (LPT) significantly inhibited LPS-stimulated interleukin-1

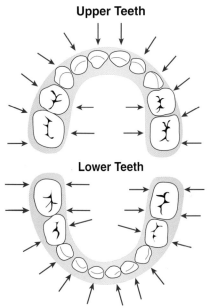

• **Figure 15-24** Irradiation chart for pediatric anesthesia. Note that deciduous molars should be irradiated toward their mesiobuccal and distobuccal aspects. All other teeth should be irradiated in the center of the buccal surface. Deciduous molars also should be irradiated on the lingual surface.

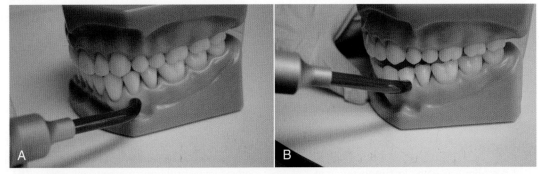

• **Figure 15-23** **A** and **B**, Irradiation sites for anesthesia of teeth. Root surfaces through the mucosa **(A)** and gingival third **(B)** are the sites of irradiation. Less successful outcomes can be expected for older teeth with more sclerotic dentin. (Courtesy Gerry Ross.)

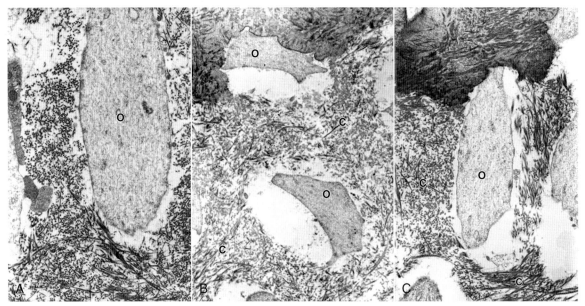

• **Figure 15-25** **A,** Scanning electron micrograph (SEM) of control tooth with no treatment. Note intact odontoblasts. **B,** Conventional preparation of tooth for minimal filling. **C,** SEM of tooth treated with PBM before filling of cavity preparation, showing intact odontoblasts. (Courtesy Martha Simões.)

beta (IL-1β) production in human gingival fibroblasts, depending on irradiation time. In an in vivo study, alterations in IL-1β concentration in periodontal pockets were not observed, although probing depth and plaque/gingival indexes were more reduced on the laser than on the placebo side.[112,119] Safavi et al.[120] evaluated the effect of LPT on gene expression of IL-1β, IFN-γ, and platelet-derived growth factor (PDGF), transforming growth factor-β (TGF-β), and basic fibroblast growth factor (bFGF) and found an inhibitory effect of PBM on IL-1β and IFN-γ production and a stimulatory effect on PDGF and TGF-β production. These alterations may be responsible for PBM's antiinflammatory effects and positive influence on wound healing.

Use of PBM after SRP will reduce postoperative discomfort[121] and reduce plaque growth.[122,123] Application of 2 to 3 J per point will incur a reasonable energy dosage. To obtain a final result exceeding that with SRP alone, three or four sessions are needed.

Ideally, PBM could be used after surgical laser interventions, to combine the bactericidal and coagulating effect of the surgical laser with the stimulating effect of the therapeutic laser. The therapeutic laser has no bactericidal effect but does trigger the immune system. Besides improved wound healing,[124–126] accelerated bone regeneration in combination with different bone graft methods can be expected.[127] PBM may be particularly useful in high-risk patients such as diabetic patients[128] and smokers[129] (Figure 15-26).

Bone Regeneration

Regeneration of new bone is of major importance in several surgical procedures and also in periodontal therapy. PBM should be used at the surgical site after suturing and

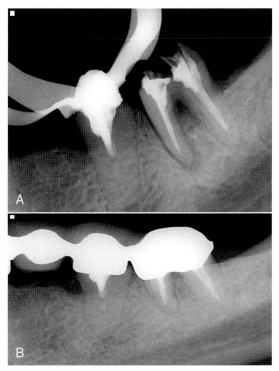

• **Figure 15-26** **A,** Mandibular molar furcation treated with Nd:YAG laser. **B,** Three-year postoperative view. Osseous growth may result from surgical use of Nd:YAG laser along with low-level effect of wavelength. (Courtesy Talat Qadri.)

then during the initial healing period, when the proliferative activity is high. Repeated irradiation, two or three times weekly for 2 weeks, is required for a pronounced effect. Many studies have confirmed the stimulatory effect of PBM on osteocytes and bone marrow cells.[130,131] PBM also can be used in combination with guided bone regeneration[132–134] and placement of different bone substitutes.[132–136]

Dentinal Hypersensitivity

Erbium, CO_2, Nd:YAG, and surgical diode lasers frequently are used to treat dentinal hypersensitivity. Studies mainly focus on obliteration of the dentinal tubules but disregard the laser's additional biostimulatory effect. PBM will not modify the dentinal tubules but will produce an effect in the odontoblastic layer, stimulate secondary dentin formation, and simultaneously reduce inflammation. In combination with traditional desensitizing agents, PBM is a valuable treatment modality (Figure 15-27).

Wakabayashi and Matsumoto[137] showed that use of a low-level diode laser was effective in 61 of 66 cases. Groth[138] showed that low-level laser treatment promoted significantly better results, establishing an irradiation protocol of three sessions with an interval of 72 h between them. Because these studies used infrared low-level lasers, Ladalardo et al.[139] studied the influence of different wavelengths on pain reduction and found that the 660-nm red diode was more effective than the 830-nm infrared diode laser. Marsílio et al.[140] observed positive clinical results with use of low-level laser wavelengths in the red spectrum, with pain reduction rates of 86.53% and 88.88% for 3 and 5 J/cm2, respectively. Corona et al.[141] compared this same wavelength with the fluoride varnish frequently used in the treatment of dentinal hypersensitivity and obtained improved results with LPT. The more sclerotic the pulp chamber, the higher the energies needed; 4 J to 10 J is used.

As with surgical lasers, patient feedback determines when dentinal sensitivity is decreased or eliminated. Kimura et al. have reviewed the application of different lasers in dentinal hypersensitivity.[142]

Sinusitis

Reduced breathing capacity through the nostrils is a clinical problem for both patient and dentist. In addition, sinus problems can refer pain to the teeth. PBM laser irradiation using a dose of 4 J first to the lymphatics and then along the base of the maxillary sinus (4 J per point) will reduce the edema and sinus pressure. The frontal and ethmoidal sinuses may be included in the irradiation therapy. In the case of a sinus infection, antibiotics will still be necessary.

Somatosensory Tinnitus

Although the etiology of tinnitus and Meniere's disease is unclear, many patients with these disorders can be treated by a dentist,[143] especially using a laser. The symptoms may emanate from muscular tension,[144] which may be caused by malocclusion, which in turn causes muscular stress.

In cases of somatosensory tinnitus, the lateral pterygoid muscles often are involved. Typically, the left muscle is tender on palpation, with premature contact on the contralateral side, whereas both left and right pterygoid muscles frequently are involved, with premature contact observed anteriorly. Premature contacts press the condyle into a

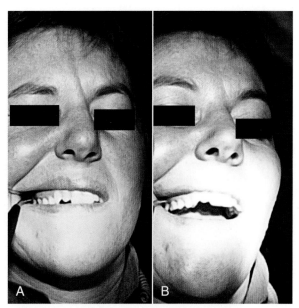

• **Figure 15-27 A,** Patient reaction to air from three-way syringe before low-level laser application. **B,** Patient reaction to same air from syringe after one low-level laser application, with 830-nm wavelength, 30 mW, and 4 J applied to gingival third of tooth.

retruded position, triggering a nociceptive reflex in the lateral pterygoid, trying to pull the condyle forward.[145] Comprehensive occlusal analysis is followed by careful removal of interferences; then the tender points in the involved muscles are irradiated to facilitate recovery. The patient should receive information about posture and stress management.

Muscles as far inferior as the trapezius are within the dental area in TMDs, and pain and tenderness in these locations are easily treatable with the laser.[146,147] Energies are chosen through patient feedback, typically 10 to 15 J per point, depending on the size of the muscle. When palpation pain is subjectively reduced, a sufficient energy has been applied. Rather than total freedom from pain, the goal is to initiate a process of muscular relaxation (Figure 15-28).

Temporomandibular Disorders

Temporomandibular joint disorder (TMD) is a term that refers to a broad spectrum of different conditions including myopathic muscle pain, joint clicking, joint locking, arthritis, and fibromyalgia. PBM is an effective tool to add to the dental arsenal for the treatment of simple and acute cases of TMDs, such as facial pain after a prolonged dental appointment, as well as chronic TMD conditions. Laser irradiation significantly reduces pain and inflammation and stimulates lymphatic flow to reduce muscle trismus.

Although low-level laser irradiation for this indication is clinically very effective, the literature reports mixed results. This confusion is due to poor study design, rather than reflecting low clinical efficacy. Frequently, research studies investigate TMDs as one condition, without due consideration of many anatomic positions and differing irradiances required, depending on the TMD condition being

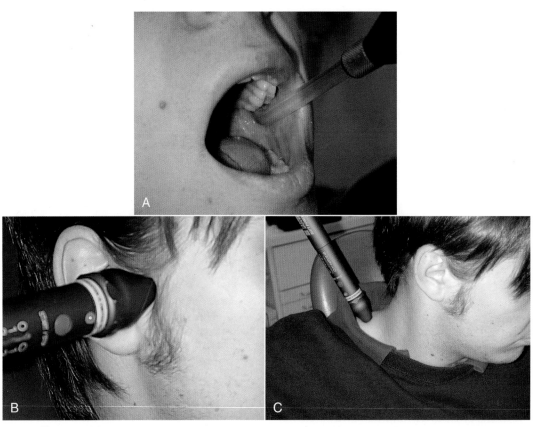

• **Figure 15-28** Low-level laser therapy for somatosensory tinnitus and TMDs. **A,** Irradiation of lateral pterygoid muscle. **B,** Irradiation of condyle. **C,** Irradiation of upper fibers of trapezius muscle. (Courtesy Marie Tullberg.)

treated. When studies investigate the individual TMD conditions, such as myopathic pain or arthritis, results are excellent.[148,149]

For treating TMD conditions, use of a combination of lasers and LED clusters generally is most effective (Figure 15-29). Lasers are ideal for treating smaller areas such as the joint or joint capsule; however, for treating larger muscles, LED clusters are indicated, because they will cover the whole muscle area, including the many trigger points. Treatments should always start with irradiation of the lymphatic system with 4 J to reduce edema, thereby normalizing the intramuscular pressure on sensory nerve endings.[150] Treating the lymphatic system with 4 J will aid in the reduction of chronic inflammation. In addition, irradiating the Li4 acupuncture point with 8 J also helps with immediate pain reduction.

Most facial pain conditions are chronic and require treatment two or three times per week for several weeks. It is critical to get feedback from the patient in regard to pain levels and associated quality of life. Treatments should always be customized in accordance with the individual patient's condition. Owing to the chronic nature of most TMD conditions, it is important to alert the patient to two potential effects before initiation of treatment. First, after the first treatment appointment, the patient may experience a feeling of malaise from the laser-induced release of inflammatory cytokines into the system. In addition, a temporary increase in pain is not uncommon; as discussed earlier, this is a positive response that indicates transition of the chronic condition into an acute

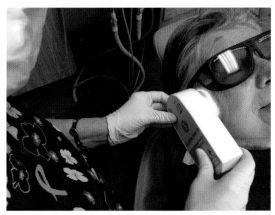

• **Figure 15-29** Application of LED cluster over maxillary muscles.

phase, which will respond well to PBM. A multidisciplinary approach to treating facial pain is ideal and should include a team of specialists who can treat problems specific to the neck, back, and other affected areas of the body.[151–157]

It is important to note that PBM treatment does not preclude the use of traditional treatments such as occlusal splints, jaw repositioning, and so on.

Wound Healing

In patients with trauma, the dentist often must manage extraoral wounds as well. With all wounds, PBM is an excellent aid in reducing edema and accelerating healing.[158–161]

Irradiation with red laser light is considered optimal for wound healing, although infrared lasers also work well within their respective therapeutic windows. Laser therapy often is used for wounds created by overextended denture margins. For the patient to be pain-free, the dentist may need to remove the overextended acrylic flanges, because the area is edematous and tender. Laser irradiation before adjustment of the denture flanges will reduce the edema and tenderness. When the patient reports reduced symptoms, the flange adjustment is complete. With excessive grinding, the symptoms will disappear quickly, but with the expectation of underextension and reduced fit of the prosthesis in the future.

Zoster and Postherpetic Neuralgia

General dentists rarely see cases of herpes zoster, but the eighth cranial nerve may be affected in this condition. Red laser is more effective in the initial phase with blisters, whereas infrared light is preferred for *postherpetic neuralgia* (PHN).[162-165] The entire dermatome should be irradiated. It is more effective to treat with high energies at spots located a few centimeters apart, rather than scanning the entire area. In the acute stage, 3 to 4 J per point should be applied daily until a distinct improvement has been noted; then treatment can be given every second or third day. Pain will soon be reduced, and treatment can stop when the vesicles have disappeared and the pain is gone. In many patients, however, the signs of zoster will disappear but the pain will remain; this PHN may linger for months or years or for life. In these patients, infrared laser irradiation is recommended, 4 to 6 J per point over the involved area. The energy dose should be related to the pain intensity and patient response. PHN is difficult to treat and has no effective pharmaceutical cure. In contrast with NSAID therapy for PHN, PBM has no side effects.

Conclusions and Outlook

Although the mechanism of action is not definitively understood for many dental applications, low-level laser therapy has shown great success. As more peer-reviewed studies are published on this topic, the use of PBM in dentistry can be expected to increase with time.

References

1. Yamamoto Y, Kono T, Kotani H, et al.: Effect of low-power laser irradiation on procollagen synthesis in human fibroblasts, *J Clin Laser Med Surg* 14(3):129–132, 1996.
2. Almeida-Lopes L, Rigau J, Zángaro R, et al.: Comparison of the low-level laser therapy effects on cultured human gingival fibroblast proliferation using different irradiance and same fluency, *Laser Surg Med* 29:179–184, 2001.
3. Amat A, Rigau J, Nicolau R, et al.: Effect of red and near-infrared laser light on adenosine triphosphate (ATP) in the luciferine-luciferase reaction, *J Photochem Photobiol A Chem* 168(1–2):59–65, 2004.
4. Hamblin MR: The role of nitric oxide in PBM, *Proc SPIE* 6846:1, 2008 (BiOS).
5. Karu T: *Ten lessons on basic science of laser phototherapy*, Grängesberg, Sweden, 2008, Prima Books.
6. Jenkins PA, Carroll JD: How to report low-level laser therapy (LLLT)/photomedicine dose and beam parameters in clinical and laboratory studies, *Photomed Laser Surg* 29(12):785–787, 2011.
7. Chow RT, David MA, Armati PJ: 830 nm laser irradiation induces varicosity formation, reduces mitochondrial membrane potential and blocks fast axonal flow in small and medium diameter rat dorsal root ganglion neurons: implications for the analgesic effects of 830 nm laser, *J Peripher Nerv Syst* 12(1):28–39, 2007.
8. Montesinos M, et al.: Experimental effects of low power laser in encephalin and endorphin synthesis, *J Eur Med Laser Assoc* 1(3):2–6, 1988.
9. Jimbo K, Noda K, Suzuki K, Yoda K: Suppressive effects of low-power laser irradiation on bradykinin evoked action potentials in cultured murine dorsal root ganglion cells, *Neurosci Lett* 240(2):93–96, 1998.
10. Huang YY, Chen AC, Carroll JD, Hamblin MR: Biphasic dose response in low level light therapy, *Dose Response* 7(4):358–383, 2009.
11. Karu TI, Ryabykh TP, Antonov SN: Different sensitivity of cells from tumor-bearing organisms to countinuous-wave and pulsed laser radiation (632.8 nm) evaluated by chemiluminescence test. I. Comparison of responses of murine splenocytes: intact mice and mice with transplanted leukemia EL-4, *Lasers Life Sci* 7:91, 1996.
12. Karu TI, Ryabykh TP, Antonov SN: Different sensitivity of cells from tumor-bearing organisms to continuous-wave and pulsed laser radiation (632.8 nm) evaluated by chemiluminescence test. II. Comparison of responses of human blood: healthy persons and patients with colon cancer, *Lasers Life Sci* 7:99, 1996.
13. Karu TI, Ryabykh TP, Letokhov VS: Different sensitivity of cells from tumor-bearing organisms to continuous-wave and pulsed laser radiation (632.8 nm) evaluated by chemiluminescence test. III. Effect of dark period between pulses, *Lasers Life Sci* 7:141, 1996.
14. Moriyama Y, Nguyen J, Akens M, et al.: In vivo effects of low-level laser therapy on inducible nitric oxide synthase, *Lasers Surg Med* 41(3):227–231, 2009.
15. Navratil L, Kymplova J: Contraindications in noninvasive laser therapy: truth and fiction, *J Clin Laser Med Surg* 20(6):341–343, 2002.
16. Azevedo LH, Correa Aranha AC, Stolf SF, et al.: Evaluation of low-level laser therapy on the thyroid gland of male mice, *Photomed Laser Surg* 23(6):567–570, 2005.
17. Tunér J, Hode L: It's all in the parameters: a critical analysis of some well-known negative studies on low-level laser therapy, *J Clin Laser Med Surg* 16(5):245–248, 1998.
18. Ivandic BT, Ivandic T: Low-level laser therapy improves vision in patients with age-related macular degeneration, *Photomed Laser Surg* 2(3):241–245, 2008.
19. Mendez TM, Pinheiro AL, Pacheco MT, et al.: Dose and wavelength of laser light have influence on the repair of cutaneous wounds, *J Clin Laser Med Surg* 22(1):19–25, 2004.
20. Pourzarandian A, Watanabe H, Ruwanpura SM, et al.: Effect of low-level Er:YAG laser irradiation on cultured human gingival fibroblasts, *J Periodontol* 76(2):187–193, 2005.

21. Pourzarandian A, Watanabe H, Ruwanpura SM, et al.: Er:YAG laser irradiation increases prostaglandin E_2 production via the induction of cyclooxygenase-2 mRNA in human gingival fibroblasts, *J Periodont Res* 40(2):182–186, 2005.

22. Lindholm A, de Mitri N, Swensson U: Clinical effect of non-focused CO_2 laser on traumatic arthritis in horses, *Lasers Med Surg Suppl* 12:51, 2000.

23. Galletti G: Low-energy density CO_2 laser as deep tissue stimulator: a comparative study, *J Clin Laser Med Surg* 9(3):179–184, 1991.

24. Morselli M, et al.: Effects of very low energy-density treatment of joint pain by CO_2 laser, *Laser Surg Med* 5(5):150–153, 1985.

25. Braun A, Dehn C, Krause F, Jepsen S: Short-term clinical effects of adjunctive antimicrobial photodynamic therapy in periodontal treatment: a randomized clinical trial, *J Clin Periodontol* 35(10):877–884, 2008.

26. Meire MA, De Prijck K, Coenye T, et al.: Effectiveness of different laser systems to kill *Enterococcus faecalis* in aqueous suspension and in an infected tooth model, *Int Endod J* 42(4):351–359, 2009.

27. Bonsor SJ, Pearson GJ: Current clinical applications of photo-activated disinfection in restorative dentistry, *Dent Update* 33(3):143–144, 147–150, 153, 2006.

28. Williams JA, Pearson GJ, Colles MJ, Wilson M: The photo-activated antibacterial action of toluidine blue O in a collagen matrix and in carious dentine, *Caries Res* 38(6):530–536, 2004.

29. Enwemeka CS, Williams D, Enwemeka SK, et al.: Blue 470-nm light kills methicillin-resistant *Staphylococcus aureus* (MRSA) in vitro, *Photomed Laser Surg* 27(2):221–226, 2009.

30. Nishioka MA, Pinfildi CE, Sheliga TR, et al.: LED (660 nm) and laser (670 nm) use on skin flap viability: angiogenesis and mast cells on transition line, *Lasers Med Sci* 27:1045–1050, 2012.

31. Schlager A, Offer T, Baldissera I: Laser stimulation of acupuncture point P6 reduces postoperative vomiting in children undergoing strabismus surgery, *Br J Anaesth* 81(4):529–532, 1998.

32. Siedentopf CM, Golaszewski SM, Mottaghy FM, et al.: Functional magnetic resonance imaging detects activation of the visual association cortex during laser acupuncture of the foot in humans, *Neurosci Lett* 327(1):53–56, 2002.

33. Xu M, Deng T, Mo F, et al.: Low-intensity pulsed laser irradiation affects RANKL and OPG mRNA expression in rat calvarial cells, *Photomed Laser Surg* 27(2):309–315, 2009.

34. Núñez SC, Nogueira GE, Ribeiro MS, et al.: He-Ne laser effects on blood microcirculation during wound healing: a method of in vivo study through laser Doppler flowmetry, *Lasers Surg Med* 35(5):363–368, 2004.

35. Von Ahlften U: [Experiences with the treatment of aphthous and herpetiform oral mucosal diseases with an infrared laser], *Quintessenz* 5(38):927–933, 1987.

36. Guerra A, Munoz P, Esquivel T, et al: *The effect of 670-nm laser therapy on herpes simplex and aphthae* [Abstract 003], paper presented at the 5th Congress of World Association for Laser Therapy, 2004, São Paulo, p 90 [*Photomed Laser Surg* 23(1), 2005].

37. Lievens PC: The effect of a combined HeNe and IR laser treatment on the regeneration of the lymphatic system during the process of wound healing, *Lasers Med Sci* 6:193–199, 1991.

38. Giuliani A, Fernandez M, Farinelli M, et al.: Very low level laser therapy attenuates edema and pain in experimental models, *Int J Tissue React* 26(1–2):29–37, 2004.

39. Albertini R, Aimbire FS, Correa FI, et al.: Effects of different protocol doses of low power gallium-aluminum-arsenate (Ga-Al-As) laser radiation (650 nm) on carrageenan induced rat paw oedema, *J Photochem Photobiol B Biol* 74(2–3):101–107, 2004.

40. Markovic A, Todorovic LJ: Effectiveness of dexamethasone and low-power laser in minimizing oedema after third molar surgery: a clinical trial, *J Oral Maxillofac Surg* 36:226–229, 2007.

41. Meneguzzo DT, Pallotta R, Ramos L, et al: Near infrared laser therapy (810 nm) on lymph nodes: effects on acute inflammatory process. *Proceedings of 7th International Congress of World Association for Laser Therapy*, 2008, Sun City, South Africa, p 157 [*Photomed Laser Surg* 27(1), 2009].

42. Sousa LR, Cavalcanti BN, Marques MM: Effect of laser phototherapy on the release of TNF-alpha and MMP-1 by endodontic sealer–stimulated macrophages, *Photomed Laser Surg* 27(1):37–42, 2009.

43. Kreisler MB, Haj HA, Noroozi N, Willershausen B: Efficacy of low-level laser therapy in reducing postoperative pain after endodontic surgery: a randomized double-blind clinical study, *Int J Oral Maxillofac Surg* 33(1):38–41, 2004.

44. Liu Q, et al: The effectiveness of semiconductor laser in the treatment of post-endodontic filling pain [Abstract 28]. *Proceedings of 7th International Congress of Lasers in Dentistry*, 2000, Brussels.

45. Stadler I, Lanzafame RJ, Evans R, et al.: 830 nm irradiation increases the wound tensile strength in a diabetic murine model, *Lasers Surg Med* 28(3):220–226, 2001.

46. Paschoud Y, et al.: [The effect of soft-laser on the neo-formation of a dentinal bridge after direct pulp capping on human teeth using calcium hydroxide], *Rev Mens Suisse Odont-Stomatol* 98(4):345–349, 1988.

47. Utsunomiya T: A histopathological study of the effects of low-power laser irradiation on wound healing of exposed dental pulp tissues in dogs, with special reference to lectins and collagens, *J Endod* 24(3):187–193, 1998.

48. Thwee T, Kato J, Hashimoto M, et al.: Pulp reaction after pulpotomy with He-Ne laser irradiation. In *Abstract handbook*, vol. 4. International Society for Lasers in Dentistry, Hong Kong, 1994, Denics Pacific.

49. Kurumada F: A study on the application of Ga-As semiconductor laser to endodontics: the effects of laser irradiation on the activation of inflammatory cells and the vital pulpotomy, *Ohu Daigaku Shigakushi* 17(3):233–244, 1990.

50. Grzesiak-Janas G, Kobos J: Influence of laser radiation on acceleration of postextraction wound healing, *Laser Technol V Appl Med Ecol* 3188:142–146, 1997.

51. Kim KS, et al.: Effects of low-level laser irradiation with 904 nm pulsed diode laser on the extraction wound, *J Korean Acad Oral Med* 23:301–307, 1998.

52. Takeda Y: Irradiation effect of low-energy laser on alveolar bone after tooth extraction: experimental study in rats, *Int J Oral Maxillofac Surg* 17:388–391, 1988.

53. Tay EJ, Lee LI, Yee S, Loh HS: Laser-induced reduction of postoperative pain following third molar surgery, *Laser Surg Med Suppl* 13:17, 2001.

54. Bjordal JM, Tunér J, Iversen VV, et al.: *A systematic review of postoperative pain relief by low-level laser therapy (PBM) after third molar extraction* [abstract], paper presented at the Congress of European Division of World Federation for Laser Dentistry, Nice, 2007.

55. Aras MH, Güngörmüş M: The effect of low-level laser therapy on trismus and facial swelling following surgical extraction of a lower third molar, *Photomed Laser Surg* 27(1):21–24, 2009.

56. Vélez-González M, Camarasa JM, Trelles MA: Treatment of relapse in herpes simplex on labial and facial areas and of primary herpes simplex on genital areas and "area pudenda" with low power laser (HeNe) or acyclovir administered orally, *Proc SPIE* 2630:43–50, 1995.

57. Rallis TR: Low-intensity laser therapy for recurrent herpes labialis, *J Invest Dermatol* 115(1):131–132, 2000.

58. Perrin D, Jolivald JR, Triki H, et al.: Effect of laser irradiation on latency of herpes simplex virus in a mouse model, *Pathol Biol* (Paris). 45(1):24–27, 1997.

59. Muñoz Sanchez PJ, Capote Femenías JL, Díaz Tejeda A, Tunér J: The effect of 670-nm low laser therapy on herpes simplex type 1, *Photomed Laser Surg* 30(1):37–40, 2012.

60. Schindl A, Neuman R: Low-intensity laser therapy is an effective treatment for recurrent herpes simplex infection: results from a randomized double-blind placebo-controlled study, *J Invest Dermatol* 113(2):221–223, 1999.

61. Eduardo FP, Mehnert DU, Monezi AM, et al.: In vitro effect of phototherapy with low intensity laser on HSV-1 and epithelial cells, Mechanisms for low-light therapy II, *Proc SPIE* 6428:642805, 2007.

62. Khadra M, Ronold HJ, Lyngstadaas SP, et al.: Low-level laser therapy stimulates bone-implant interaction: an experimental study in rabbits, *Clin Oral Implants Res* 15(3):325–332, 2004.

63. Khadra M, Kasem N, Lyngstadaas SP, et al.: Laser therapy accelerates initial attachment and subsequent behaviour of human oral fibroblasts cultured on titanium implant material: a scanning electron microscopic and histomorphometric analysis, *Clin Oral Implants Res* 16(2):168–175, 2005.

64. Lopes CB, Pinheiro AL, Sathaiah S, et al.: Infrared laser light reduces loading time of dental implants: a Raman spectroscopic study, *Photomed Laser Surg* 23(1):27–31, 2005.

65. Kim YD, Kim SS, Hwang DS, et al.: Effect of low-level laser treatment after installation of dental titanium implant: immunohistochemical study of RANKL, RANK, OPG—an experimental study in rats, *Lasers Surg Med* 39(5):441–450, 2007.

66. Guzzardella GA, Torricelli P, Nicoli-Aldini N, et al.: Laser technology in orthopedics: preliminary study on low-power laser therapy to improve the bone-biomaterial interface, *Int J Artif Organs* 24(12):898–902, 2001.

67. Khadra M: The effect of low level laser irradiation on implant-tissue interaction: in vivo and in vitro studies, *Swed Dent J Suppl* 172:1–63, 2005.

68. Guzzardella GA, Torricelli P, Nicolo-Aldini N, et al.: Osseo-integration of endosseous ceramic implants after postoperative low-power laser stimulation: an in vivo comparative study, *Clin Oral Implants Res* 14(2):226–232, 2003.

69. Lim W, Lee S, Kim I, et al.: The anti-inflammatory mechanism of 635 nm light-emitting-diode irradiation compared with existing COX inhibitors, *Lasers Surg Med* 39:614–621, 2007.

70. Bjordal JM, Lopes-Martins RA, Iversen VV: A randomised, placebo-controlled trial of low-level laser therapy for activated Achilles tendinitis with microdialysis measurement of peritendinous prostaglandin E$_2$ concentrations, *Br J Sports Med* 40(1):76–80, 2006.

71. Aimbire F, Albertini R, Leonardo P, et al.: Low-level laser therapy induces dose-dependent reduction of TNF-alpha levels in acute inflammation, *Photomed Laser Surg* 24(1):33–37, 2006.

72. Aimbire F, Albertini R, de Magalhães RG, et al.: Effect of PBM Ga-Al-As (685 nm) on LPS-induced inflammation of the airway and lung in the rat, *Lasers Med Sci* 20(1):11–20, 2005.

73. Bortone F, Santos HA, Albertini R, et al.: Low level laser therapy modulates kinin receptors mRNA expression in the subplantar muscle of rat paw subjected to carrageenan-induced inflammation, *Int Immunopharmacol* 8(2):206–210, 2008.

74. Lopes-Martins RA, Albertini R, Lopes-Martins PS, et al.: Steroids receptor antagonist Mifepristone inhibits the anti-inflammatory effects of photoradiation, *Photomed Laser Surg* 24(2):197–201, 2006.

75. Reis SR, Medrado AP, Marchionni AM, et al.: Effect of 670-nm laser therapy and dexamethasone on tissue repair: a histological and ultrastructural study, *Photomed Laser Surg* 26(4):307–313, 2008.

76. Bjordal JM, Ljunggren AE, Klovning A, Slordal L: NSAIDs, including coxibs, probably do more harm than good, and paracetamol is ineffective for hip OA, *Ann Rheum Dis* 64(4):655–656, 2005.

77. Abiko Y: *Functional genomic study on anti-inflammatory effects by low-level laser irradiation* [abstract], paper presented at the 8th Congress of World Federation for Laser Dentistry, 2008, Hong Kong.

78. Chow RT, Johnson MI, Lopes-Martins RA, Bjordal JM: Efficacy of low-level laser therapy in the management of neck pain: a systematic review and meta-analysis of randomised placebo or active-treatment controlled trials, *Lancet* 374:1897–1908, 2009.

79. Kurnar SP, Prasad K, Shenoy K, et al.: High-level evidence exists for low-level laser therapy on chemoradiotherapy-induced oral mucositis in cancer survivors, *Indian J Palliat Care* 19(3):195–196, 2013.

80. Bjordal JM, Bensadoun R, Tuner J, et al.: A systematic review with meta-analysis of the effect of low-level laser therapy (LLLT) in cancer therapy-induced oral mucositis, *Support Care Cancer* 19:1069–1077, 2011.

81. Iijima K, Shimoyama N, Shimoyama M, Mizuguchi T: Red and green low-powered HeNe lasers protect human erythrocytes from hypotonic hemolysis, *J Clin Laser Med Surg* 9(5):385–389, 1991.

82. Itoh T, et al.: The protective effect of low power HeNe laser against erythrocytic damage caused by artificial heart-lung machines, *Hiroshima J Med Sci* 45(1):15–22, 1996.

83. Da Cunha SS, Sarmento V, Ramalho LM, et al.: Effect of laser therapy on bone tissue submitted to radiotherapy: experimental study in rats, *Photomed Laser Surg* 25(3):197–204, 2007.

84. Bensadoun RJ, Franqiun JC, Ciais C, et al.: Low-energy He/Ne laser in the prevention of radiation-induced mucositis: a multicenter Phase III randomized study in patients with head and neck cancer, *Support Care Cancer* 7(4):244–252, 1999.

85. Abramoff MM, Lopes NN, Lopes LA, et al.: Low-level laser therapy in the prevention and treatment of chemotherapy-induced oral mucositis in young patients, *Photomed Laser Surg* 26(4):393–400, 2008.

86. Jaguar GC, Prado JD, Nishimoto IN, et al.: Low-energy laser therapy for prevention of oral mucositis in hematopoietic stem cell transplantation, *Oral Dis* 13(6):538–543, 2007.

87. Cruz LB, Ribeiro AS, Rech A, et al.: Influence of low-energy laser in the prevention of oral mucositis in children with cancer receiving chemotherapy, *Pediatr Blood Cancer* 48(4):435–440, 2007.

88. Genot MT, Klastersky J: Low-level laser for prevention and therapy of oral mucositis induced by chemotherapy or radiotherapy, *Curr Opin Oncol* 17(3):236–240, 2005.

89. França CM, Núñez SC, Prates RA, et al.: Low-intensity red laser on the prevention and treatment of induced-oral mucositis in hamsters, *J Photochem Photobiol B Biol* 94(1):25–31, 2009.

90. Goulart CS, Nouer PR, Mouramartins L, et al.: Photoradiation and orthodontic movement: experimental study with canines, *Photomed Laser Surg* 24(2):192–196, 2006.

91. Cruz DR, Kohara EK, Ribeiro MS, Wetter NU: Effects of low-intensity laser therapy on the orthodontic movement velocity of human teeth: a preliminary study, *Lasers Surg Med* 35(2):117–120, 2004.

92. Youssef M, Ashkar S, Hamade E, et al.: The effect of low-level laser therapy during orthodontic movement: a preliminary study, *Lasers Med Sci* 23(1):27–33, 2008.

93. Turhani D, Scheriau M, Kapral D, et al.: Pain relief by single low-level laser irradiation in orthodontic patients undergoing fixed appliance therapy, *Am J Orthod Dentofacial Orthop* 130(3):371–377, 2006.

94. Fujita S, Yamaguchi M, Utsunomiya T, et al.: Low-energy laser stimulates tooth movement velocity via expression of RANK and RANKL, *Orthod Craniofac Res* 11(3):143–155, 2008.

95. Rodrigues MT, Ribeiro MS, Groth EB, et al.: Evaluation of effects of laser therapy (wavelength = 830 nm) on oral ulceration induced by fixed orthodontic appliances, *Lasers Med Surg* [abstract issue]: 15, 2002.

96. Toida M, Watanabe F, Kazumi Goto K, Shibata T: Usefulness of low-level laser for control of painful stomatitis in patients with hand-foot-and-mouth disease, *J Clin Laser Med Surg* 21(6):363–367, 2003.

97. Ferreira DM, Zangaro RA, Villaverde AB, et al.: Analgesic effect of He-Ne (632.8 nm) low-level laser therapy on acute inflammatory pain, *Photomed Laser Surg* 23(2):177–181, 2005.

98. Nakaji S, Shiroto C, Yodono M, et al.: Retrospective study of adjunctive diode laser therapy for pain attenuation in 662 patients: detailed analysis by questionnaire, *Photomed Laser Surg* 23(1):60–65, 2005.

99. Bjordal JM, Johnson MI, Iversen V, et al.: Photoradiation in acute pain: a systematic review of possible mechanisms of action and clinical effects in randomized placebo-controlled trials, *Photomed Laser Surg* 24(2):158–168, 2006.

100. Shirani AM, Gutknecht N, Taghizadeh M, Mir M: Low-level laser therapy and myofascial pain dysfunction syndrome: a randomized controlled clinical trial, *Lasers Med Sci* 24(5):715–720, 2009.

101. Khullar SM, Brodin P, Messelt EB, Haanaes HR: The effects of low-level laser treatment on recovery of nerve conduction and motor function after compression injury in the rat sciatic nerve, *Eur J Oral Sci* 103:299–305, 1995.

102. Khullar SM, Brodin P, Barkvoll P, et al.: Preliminary study of low-level laser for treatment of long-standing sensory aberrations in the inferior alveolar nerve, *J Oral Maxillofac Surg* 54(2):2–7, 1996.

103. Khullar SM, Emami B, Westermark A, et al.: Effect of low-level laser treatment on neurosensory deficits subsequent to sagittal split ramus osteotomy, *Oral Surg Med Pathol Radiol Endod* 82(2):132–138, 1996.

104. Khullar SM, Brodin P, Fristad I, Kvinnsland IH: Enhanced sensory reinnervation of dental target tissues in rats following low-level laser (LLL) irradiation, *Lasers Med Sci* 14(3):177–184, 1999.

105. Miloro M, Repasky M: Low-level laser effect on neurosensory recovery after sagittal ramus osteotomy, *Oral Surg Med Pathol Radiol Endod* 89(1):12–18, 2000.

106. Ozen T, Orhan K, Gorur I, Ozturk A: Efficacy of low level laser therapy on neurosensory recovery after injury to the inferior alveolar nerve, *Head Face Med* 15(2):3, 2006.

107. Ross G, Ross A: Low-level lasers in dentistry, *Gen Dent* 56(7):629–634, 2008.

108. Ferreira ANS, Silveira LB, Genovese WJ, et al.: Effect of GaAlAs laser on reactional dentinogenesis induction in human teeth, *Photomed Laser Surg* 24(3):358–365, 2006.

109. Godoy BM, Arana-Chavez VE, Nunez SC, Ribeiro MS: Effects of low-power red laser on dentine-pulp interface after cavity preparation: an ultrastructural study, *Arch Oral Biol* 52(9):899–903, 2007.

110. Prezotto Villa GE, Catirse AB, Lizarelli RF: Evaluation of secondary dentin formation applying two fluences of low-level laser [Abstract 024], 5th Congress of World Association for Laser Therapy, São Paulo, 2004, p 95 [*Photomed Laser Surg* 23(1) p95, 2005].

111. Choi BK, Moon SY, Cha JH, et al.: Prostaglandin E_2 is a main mediator in receptor activator of nuclear factor-kappaB ligand–dependent osteoclastogenesis induced by *Porphyromonas gingivalis*, *Treponema denticola*, and *Treponema socranskii*, *J Periodontol* 76:813–820, 2005.

112. Qadri T, Bohdanecka P, Tunér J, et al.: The importance of coherence length in laser phototherapy of gingival inflammation: a pilot study, *Lasers Med Sci* 22:245–251, 2007.

113. Pejcic A, Zivkvic V: Histological examination of gingival treated with low-level laser in periodontal therapy, *J Oral Laser Appl* 71:37–43, 2007.

114. Ozawa Y, Shimizu N, Abiko Y: Low-energy diode laser irradiation reduced plasminogen activator activity in human periodontal ligament cells, *Lasers Surg Med* 21:456–463, 1997.

115. Amorim JC, de Sousa GR, de Barros Silveira L, et al.: Clinical study of the gingiva healing after gingivectomy and low-level laser therapy, *Photomed Laser Surg* 24:588–594, 2006.

116. Shimizu N, Yamaguchi M, Goseki T, et al.: Inhibition of prostaglandin E_2 and interleukin 1-beta production by low-power laser irradiation in stretched human periodontal ligament cells, *J Dent Res* 74:1382–1388, 1995.

117. Sakurai Y, Yamaguchi M, Abiko Y: Inhibitory effect of low-level laser irradiation on LPS-stimulated prostaglandin E_2 production and cyclooxygenase-2 in human gingival fibroblasts, *Eur J Oral Sci* 108:29–34, 2000.

118. Nomura K, Yamaguchi M, Abiko Y: Inhibition of interleukin-1beta production and gene expression in human gingival fibroblasts by low-energy laser irradiation, *Lasers Med Sci* 16(3):218–223, 2001.

119. Qadri T, Bohdanecka P, Miranda L, et al.: The importance of coherence length in laser phototherapy of gingival inflammation: a pilot study, *Lasers Med Sci* 22(4):245–251, 2007.

120. Safavi SM, Kazemi B, Esmaeili M, et al.: Effects of low-level He-Ne laser irradiation on the gene expression of IL-1beta, TNF-alpha, IFN-gamma, TGF-beta, bFGF, and PDGF in rat's gingiva, *Lasers Med Sci* 23:331–335, 2008.

121. Ribeiro IW, Sbrana MC, Esper LA, Almeida AL: Evaluation of the effect of the GaAlAs laser on subgingival scaling and root planing, *Photomed Laser Surg* 26:387–391, 2008.

122. Silveira LB, Prates RA, Novelli MD, et al.: Investigation of mast cells in human gingiva following low-intensity laser irradiation, *Photomed Laser Surg* 26(4):315–321, 2008.

123. Iwase T, Saito T, Nara Y, Morioka T: Inhibitory effect of HeNe laser on dental plaque deposition in hamsters, *J Periodont Res* 24:282–283, 1989.

124. Kiernicka M, Owczarek B, Galkowska E, Wysokinska-Miszczuk J: Comparison of the effectiveness of the conservative treatment of the periodontal pockets with or without the use of laser biostimulation, *Ann Univ Mariae Curie Sklodowska Med* 59(1): 488–494, 2004.

125. Kreisler M, Christoffers AB, Willershausen B, et al.: Effect of low-level GaAlAs laser irradiation on the proliferation rate of human periodontal ligament fibroblasts: an in vitro study, *J Clin Periodontol* 30(4):353–358, 2003.

126. Ozcelik O, Cenk Haytac M, Kunin A, Seydaoglu G: Improved wound healing by low-level laser irradiation after gingivectomy operations: a controlled clinical pilot study, *J Clin Periodontol* 35(3):250–254, 2008.

127. Ozcelik O, Cenk Haytac M, Seydaoglu G: Enamel matrix derivative and low-level laser therapy in the treatment of intra-bony defects: a randomized placebo-controlled clinical trial, *Clin Periodontol* 35(2):147–156, 2008.

128. Maiya GA, Kumar P, Rao L: Effect of low-intensity helium-neon (He-Ne) laser irradiation on diabetic wound healing dynamics, *Photomed Laser Surg* 23(2):187–190, 2005.

129. Fujimaki Y, Shimoyama T, Liu Q, et al.: Low-level laser irradiation attenuates production of reactive oxygen species by human neutrophils, *J Clin Laser Med Surg* 21(3):165–170, 2003.

130. Pires Oliveira DA, de Oliveira RF, et al.: Evaluation of low-level laser therapy of osteoblastic cells, *Photomed Laser Surg* 26(4):401–404, 2008.

131. Dortbudak O, Haas R, Mallath-Pokorny G: Biostimulation of bone marrow cells with a diode soft laser, *Clin Oral Implants Res* 11(6):540–545, 2000.

132. Pinheiro ALB, Gerbi MEM, Ponzi EAC, et al.: Infrared laser light further improves bone healing when associated with bone morphogenetic proteins and guided bone regeneration: an in vivo study in a rodent model, *Photomed Laser Surg* 26(2):167–174, 2008.

133. Torres CS, dos Santos JN, Monteiro JS, et al.: Does the use of laser photobiomodulation, bone morphogenetic proteins, and guided bone regeneration improve the outcome of autologous bone grafts? An in vivo study in a rodent model, *Photomed Laser Surg* 26(4):371–377, 2008.

134. Gerbi ME, Marques AM, Ramalho LM, et al.: Infrared laser light further improves bone healing when associated with bone morphogenic proteins: an in vivo study in a rodent model, *Photomed Laser Surg* 26(1):55–60, 2008.

135. Aboelsaad NS, Soory M, Gadalla LM, et al.: Effect of soft laser and bioactive glass on bone regeneration in the treatment of bone defects (an experimental study), *Lasers Med Sci* 24(4):527–533, 2009.

136. Aboelsaad NS, Soory M, Gadalla LM, et al.: Effect of soft laser and bioactive glass on bone regeneration in the treatment of infra-bony defects (a clinical study), *Lasers Med Sci* 24(3):387–395, 2009.

137. Wakabayashi H, Matsumoto K: Treatment of dentin hypersensitivity by GaAlAs laser irradiation [abstract], *J Dent Res* 67:182, 1988.

138. Groth EB: Treatment of dentin hypersensitivity with low-power laser of GaAlAs [abstract], *J Dent Res* 74:794, 1995.

139. Ladalardo TC, Pinheiro A, Campos RA, et al.: Laser therapy in the treatment of dentine hypersensitivity, *Braz Dent J* 15:144–150, 2004.

140. Marsilio AL, Rodrigues JR, Borges AB: Effect of the clinical application of the GaAlAs laser in the treatment of dentine hypersensitivity, *J Clin Laser Med Surg* 21:291–296, 2003.

141. Corona SA, Nascimento TN, Catirse AB, et al.: Clinical evaluation of low-level laser therapy and fluoride varnish for treating cervical dentinal hypersensitivity, *J Oral Rehabil* 30:1183–1189, 2003.

142. Kimura Y, Wilder-Smith P, Yonaga K, Matsumoto K: Treatment of dentine hypersensitivity by laser: a review, *J Clin Periodontol* 27:715–721, 2000.

143. Bjorne A, Agerberg G: Symptom relief after treatment of temporomandibular and cervical spine disorders in patients with Ménière's disease: a 3-year follow-up, *J Craniomandib Pract* 21(1):50–60, 2003.

144. Shore SE, Vass Z, Wyss NL, Altschuler RA: Trigeminal ganglion innervates the auditory brainstem: *J Compar Neurol* 419:271–285, 2000.

145. Tullberg M, Ernberg M: Long-term effect on tinnitus by treatment of temporomandibular disorders: a two-year follow-up by questionnaire, *Acta Odont Scand* 64(2):89–96, 2006.

146. Chow RT, Heller GZ, Barnsley L: The effect of 300 mW, 830 nm laser on chronic neck pain: a double-blind, randomized, placebo-controlled study, *Pain* 124(1–2):201–210, 2006.

147. Gür A, Sarac AJ, Cevik R, et al.: Efficacy of 904-nm gallium arsenide low-level laser therapy in the management of chronic myofascial pain in the neck: a double-blind and randomized controlled trial, *Laser Surg Med* 35(3):229–235, 2004.

148. Ahrari F, Madani AS, Ghafouri ZS, Tuner J: The efficacy of low-level laser therapy for the treatment of myogenous temporomandibular joint disorder, *Lasers Med Sci* 29(2):551–557, 2014.

149. Fikackova H, Dostalova T, Vosicka R, et al.: Arthralgia of the temporomandibular joint and low-level laser therapy, *Photomed Laser Surg* 24(4):522–527, 2006.

150. Öz S, Gökçen-Röhlig B, Saruhanoglu A, Tuncer EB: Management of myofascial pain: low-level laser therapy versus occlusal splints, *J Craniofac Surg* 21(6):1722–1728, 2010.

151. De Medeiros JS, Vieira GF, Nishimura PY: Laser application effects on the bite strength of the masseter muscle, as an orofacial pain treatment, *Photomed Laser Surg* 23(4):373–376, 2005.

152. Venancio RA, Camparis CM, Lizarelli RF: Low-intensity laser therapy in the treatment of temporomandibular disorders: a double-blind study, *J Oral Rehabil* 32(11):800–807, 2005.

153. Cetiner S, Kahraman SA, Yucetas S: Evaluation of low-level laser therapy in the treatment of temporomandibular disorders, *Photomed Laser Surg* 24(5):637–641, 2006.

154. Nuñez SC, Garcez AS, Suzuki SS, Ribeiro MS: Management of mouth opening in patients with temporomandibular disorders through low-level laser therapy and transcutaneous electrical neural stimulation, *Photomed Laser Surg* 24(1):45–49, 2006.

155. Fikackova H, Dostalova T, Navratil L, Klaschka J: Effectiveness of low-level laser therapy in temporomandibular joint disorders: a placebo-controlled study, *Photomed Laser Surg* 25(4):297–303, 2007.

156. Emshoff R, Bösch R, Pümpel E, et al.: Low-level laser therapy for treatment of temporomandibular joint pain: a double-blind and placebo-controlled trial, *Oral Surg Med Pathol Radiol Endod* 105(4):452–456, 2008.

157. Carrasco TG, Mazzetto MO, Mazzetto RG, Mestriner W Jr: Low-intensity laser therapy in temporomandibular disorder: a Phase II double-blind study, *J Craniomandib Pract* 26(4):274–281, 2008.

158. Al-Watban FA, Zhang XY, Andres BL: Low-level laser therapy enhances wound healing in diabetic rats: a comparison of different lasers, *Photomed Laser Surg* 25(2):72–77, 2007.

159. Byrnes KR, Barna L, Chenault VM, et al.: Photobiomodulation improves cutaneous wound healing in an animal model of type II diabetes, *Photomed Laser Surg* 22(4):281–290, 2004.

160. Hopkins JT, McLoda TA, Seegmiller JG, Baxter GD: Low-level laser therapy facilitates superficial wound healing in humans: a triple-blind, sham-controlled study, *J Athlet Train* 39(3): 223–229, 2004.

161. Silveira PCL, Streck EL, Pinho RA: Evaluation of mitochondrial respiratory chain activity in wound healing by low-level laser therapy, *J Photochem Photobiol B Biol* 86(3):279–282, 2007.

162. Moore K, Hira N, Kumar O: Double-blind crossover trial of low-level laser therapy in the treatment of postherpetic neuralgia, *Laser Ther* 1(pilot issue):7–10, 1988.

163. Otsuka H, Numasawa R, Okubo K, et al.: Effects of helium-neon laser therapy on herpes zoster pain, *Laser Ther* 7(1):27–32, 1995.

164. Iijima K, Shimoyama N, Shimoyama M, Mizuguchi T: Evaluation of analgesic effect of low power HeNe laser on postherpetic neuralgia using VAS and modified McGill Pain Questionnaire, *J Clin Laser Med Surg* 9(2):121–126, 1991.

165. Foyaca-Sibat H, Ibañez-Valdés L: Laser therapy in zoster neuropathy, HIV related. In *Proceedings of 7th International Congress of World Association for Laser Therapy*, 2008, Sun City, South Africa, p 100 [*Photomed Laser Surg* 27(1) p100, 2009].

16

Introducing Lasers into the Dental Practice

DAVID M. ROSHKIND AND ROBERT A. CONVISSAR

Dental practitioners who incorporate lasers into their clinical armamentarium can expect to expand the spectrum of their routine procedures with several additional unique techniques, although a primary concern will remain the basics of dental practice management. Laser use in dentistry requires the practitioner to balance the science of lasers, the artistry of dentistry, and the business of practice management. Dental practices in which laser procedures are integrated into the array of treatment options typically are considered "cutting edge," with up-to-date clinical facilities, and have a unique psychological and promotional advantage over those that do not offer such services. For the laser-equipped practice, increased credibility leads to promotion of patient confidence, readier conversion of clinical needs into "wants," and a deeper level of trust, translating in turn to referrals from satisfied patients.

As recommended by Catone and Alling,[1] surgeons should possess at least a "fundamental understanding of qualitative laser physics and essential operation" of the lasers most useful in the clinical practice setting. Proper understanding of the science of lasers in dental practice is imperative for delivery of optimal treatment to patients. Many laser procedures are technique-sensitive; accordingly, knowing the scientific basis of the treatment will enable the practitioner to improve and refine the techniques associated with the clinical practice and artistry of dentistry.

Team Approach

The introduction of lasers into the dental practice should proceed in an orderly, calculated manner. Proper planning will help ensure successful integration of the new laser and associated procedural changes into daily operations. For a smooth transition and the most productive outcome, the entire dental team, including both clinical and administrative personnel, must be involved. Everyone on the team should be educated on the uses and capabilities of the specific laser. It is strongly suggested that the entire staff attend a laser introductory course together so that each person can raise questions specific to his or her function as a member of the dental team. The interaction of the team members can produce new ideas to accelerate the acceptance of the laser by both staff and patients.

An introductory course on laser dentistry is designed to be an informative overview of the capabilities of the various lasers currently available. It should include a hands-on segment in which the participant uses lasers of several different wavelengths on a pig jaw. The entire team should be encouraged to experience the hands-on portion, even members who are not dentists or hygienists, to help them take ownership of the promotion of laser dentistry to their patients.

This type of participatory introduction to laser dentistry allows all members of the staff to see firsthand the effects and capabilities of the type of laser that may be purchased for their office. The practitioner can begin to formulate potential uses for a laser in the practice while considering the other parameters pertinent to the purchase decision.

General Practice

A variety of laser wavelengths are available for use in the general dentistry practice. For a practice focused on cosmetic procedures, a diode laser, neodymium-doped yttrium-aluminum-garnet (Nd:YAG) laser, or carbon dioxide (CO_2) laser would be sufficient. These lasers also are appropriate if gingival recontouring or tissue retraction would be the primary laser procedure used.

If the practice is oriented to family and pediatric dental care, for which performing surgical procedures on virgin teeth is a priority, an erbium laser or a 9.3-μm CO_2 laser must be considered. However, the large size, weight, air/water requirements, and multiple components of these lasers mean that their use often is restricted to a specific treatment room; erbium and 9.3-μm CO_2 laser-specific procedures must then be scheduled according to this room's availability, to maximize laser use. This requirement may reduce the number of procedures using the laser, thereby affecting the return on investment (ROI) of the purchase.

By contrast, a small diode laser, although not useful for hard tissue procedures, may easily be moved from treatment room to treatment room for almost constant use by both dentists and hygienists (in states in which hygienists are permitted to use lasers).

Once lasers are introduced into the practice, clinician demand may increase to the point that a second laser is eventually purchased. This device may be of a different type or wavelength, depending on needs identified in clinical practice.

Specialty Practice

Dental professionals in various specialties typically approach laser use according to the number and types of procedures they can perform in their practice. For example, oral-maxillofacial surgeons may want an extremely precise yet fast-cutting laser for soft tissue use. Virtually every surgeon who has a laser in the dental office, or who has access to a laser in a hospital, uses a CO_2 laser because of its ability to incise, excise, and ablate tissue quickly. Except for a few specific procedures (e.g., temporomandibular joint [TMJ] arthroscopy, performed with a holmium laser), the CO_2 is the laser of choice for oral and maxillofacial surgery (OMS). Although surgeons in this specialty also work on bone, they have not embraced the erbium wavelength for osseous procedures because of its rather slow speed in cutting any significant amount of osseous tissue. Erbium lasers, however, are becoming popular in some OMS practices in states in which these surgeons are permitted to perform facial cosmetic surgery, such as skin resurfacing.

An orthodontist may want a laser that is useful for frenectomies, crestal fiberotomies, tooth exposure, and orthodontically induced gingival hyperplasia. An inexpensive diode laser may be sufficient for orthodontic use. Pediatric dentists may find the greatest use for both hard and soft tissue lasers, so an erbium laser, a combined erbium–soft tissue laser, or a 9.3-μm CO_2 laser may be best suited to their needs. Some manufacturers market combined erbium–soft tissue lasers specifically for the dentist who wants both a hard tissue laser and a dedicated soft tissue laser. Similarly, endodontic, periodontic, and prosthodontic practices must weigh the types and number of different procedures planned for the laser in deciding which device best suits their needs.

The proper selection of a laser for specific practice needs is not the focus of this chapter. The dental practitioner is strongly encouraged to attend a laser course in which at least two different laser types (such as a CO_2 and a diode) are available for hands-on training and the lecturer owns multiple wavelengths. Attending a lecture at which the speaker owns just one wavelength is likely to be skewed toward the purchase of that specific wavelength.

Cost of Acquiring a Laser

Cost is always one of the first considerations in the acquisition of a laser. The term *cost* can be viewed in several ways: "the amount or equivalent paid or charged for something: price; the outlay or expenditure (as of effort or sacrifice) made to achieve an object; [or] loss or penalty incurred esp. in gaining something."[2]

Opportunity cost, also referred to as *economic cost,* is the cost of "passing up the next best choice"[2] in making a decision. Opportunity cost is "the added cost of using resources (as for production or speculative investment) that is the difference between the actual value resulting from such use and that of an alternative (as another use of the same resources or an investment of equal risk but greater return)."[2] Opportunity cost analysis is an important part of financial decision-making processes but is not treated as an actual cost in any financial statement.[3] Opportunity cost is an important concept because it implies a choice between desirable but mutually exclusive results. Just as the acquisition of a laser has its cost, the choice *not* to purchase a laser also has associated costs. Among these opportunity costs are the loss of income that would have been produced by the new procedures that otherwise are referred out of the practice or not done at all, as well as the loss of referrals to the practice for those procedures that could be performed with a laser that were not previously done. Because of the "high-tech cutting edge" image projected by the use of lasers in the office, the loss of referrals is an additional opportunity cost lost to the practice resulting from the decision not to use lasers.

The first definition of cost mentioned is the *price.*[2] The current price of a laser is approximately $4000 to $85,000 or more, depending on the type of laser and the manufacturer. The use of a laser can be paid for in any of four ways: purchase, finance, lease, or rent. The outright *purchase* of a laser may have distinct advantages if the cash flow of the practice or the assets of the owners allow for this option. Favorable tax laws may make the actual price significantly lower than the invoice price.

The option of *financing* a purchase usually is available from several sources. Often the manufacturer's relationship with a finance company can facilitate the transaction, although the fees, rates, and terms should be compared with those for other sources of financing. The practice's banking or loan institution is another good source of information and perhaps financing. Additionally, finance companies that specialize in acquisition of capital equipment may be consulted. These same points apply to *leasing* if this is considered in the acquisition of a laser. Other finance methods, such as purchase by a family trust, pension plan, or limited partnership, are viable options but are beyond the scope of this discussion. Tax consequences will differ depending on the method of acquisition. The practitioner should discuss all of the options with a trusted financial advisor.

A fourth way to acquire a laser for use in the dental practice is to *rent* the laser. This arrangement could be on an "as-needed" or a scheduled basis. Although the rental approach is common in the medical field, it is rare in dentistry because of the "cottage industry" nature of dental practices, as well as the relatively low prices of dental lasers compared with medical lasers. The vast majority of dental practices are either solo or small groups of five or less clinicians. This smaller number of potential operators in a dental practice, compared with the hospital setting, where many surgeons would have access to expensive capital equipment and could generate a large number of procedures, makes the cost–benefit ratio unfavorable for a company to rent equipment on a per-diem or per-procedure basis to smaller dental offices.

Many other considerations go into the cost of acquiring a laser, including ergonomics. In urban areas in which office space is at a premium, most dental treatment rooms are small. In considering a small, tabletop diode laser, size and plumbing requirements are not a factor. With the larger "footprint" of an erbium or a CO_2 laser, however, the following questions must be considered:

- Will the laser fit comfortably into the treatment room?
- Will the treatment room need to be remodeled to allow for easy access to the laser?
- Will a "water quick connect" be needed? An "air quick connect"?
- Will plumbing or carpentry costs be incurred from placing the laser in the treatment room?
- Will a refillable easy-access water bottle be needed and available?

Disposables are another factor associated with laser use. Laser procedures require many disposable items for which prices should be compared. Specific considerations include:

- How many laser tips are included with the device at purchase? (e.g., Manufacturer A may supply 20 sapphire tips, whereas manufacturer B may include 10 sapphire tips and 10 quartz tips.)
- What is the replacement cost of the sapphire tips? The quartz tips?
- How many uses can be expected from the tips?
- How should fees for operative dentistry be adjusted now that procedures include use of a laser, with a cost per "bur" sapphire or quartz tip of $10 to $85, rather than 99¢ for a carbide bur?
- What is the replacement cost of the fiber? Does the fiber have a full warranty (if so, for how long?)?, or is the fiber warranty prorated depending on length of service?
- What does a service contract cost?
- If the laser breaks down, how fast will a loaner or service call be provided?

All of these questions must be answered before the true cost of the laser over time can be fully determined.

Laser as Profit Center

There are many ways to evaluate the viability of a laser as a profit center in the dental office. Time is money, and all practices must achieve a certain level of gross income per hour to flourish, so the ability to perform many procedures more quickly and efficiently means additional income. Procedures that can be performed much more quickly and efficiently with lasers include (but are not limited to) the following:

- Laser tissue retraction for impressions
- Implant recovery and impression immediately after uncovering

- Gingivectomy to improve access for operative dentistry, especially class V lesions and root caries in geriatric patients
- Multiple-quadrant operative dentistry
- Soft tissue and hard (osseous) tissue crown lengthening
- Smile lift procedures
- Apicoectomy
- Exposure of unerupted teeth
- Frenectomy
- Implant placement/sinus lift/periimplantitis treatment
- Vestibuloplasty before full-denture fabrication

Procedures not previously done that enhance the results of routine procedures include the following:

- Ovate pontic site preparations
- Periodontal pocket disinfection
- Graft donor site palliation
- Graft bed site preparation
- Esthetic remodeling of bulky graft sites
- Esthetic crown lengthening/gingivoplasty
- Melanin depigmentation
- Laser tooth whitening
- Tooth desensitization

Certain formerly referred procedures can now stay in the practice, as follows:

- Tuberosity/torus reduction
- Biopsy
- Orthodontic and drug-induced tissue hypertrophy
- Osseous periodontal surgery/deepithelialization
- Lingual frenum removal
- Oral medicine procedures, such as treatment of aphthous ulcers, herpetic gingivostomatitis, and lichen planus

Return on Investment

Once the laser has been purchased, good business principles dictate that there should be a fair ROI. Just to break even, the income generated by the laser must include covering the price of the laser, maintenance, and supplies, as well as an additional amount to cover the income lost from the money used to purchase the equipment and not otherwise generating its own income. The profit exceeding the break-even point is the actual ROI.

Some of the items that should be included in this ROI determination would include profits from the following:

1. New procedures performed with the laser
2. Certain procedures no longer referred because of the availability of a laser
3. Referrals to the practice resulting from acquisition of a laser

On the basis of such considerations, a laser could be considered a profit center.

Table 16-1 demonstrates the significant positive financial impact a laser can have on the dental practice's net profit. It also illustrates possible income derived from the use of a laser for just a few procedures per month with very low fees (even without using the laser to full potential). If the laser's price is $50,000, the income generated

TABLE 16-1	Return on Investment Chart for Dental Laser Purchase		
Data Category	No. of Procedures per Month	Billable Amount per Procedure	Monthly Total
Treatment			
Gingival cosmetic recontouring	10	$75	$750
Ovate pontic site formation			
Gingival hyperplasia treatment			
(All procedures: per tooth)			
Melanin depigmentation/amalgam tattoo	1	$250	$250
Lingual frenectomy	1	$450	$450
Biopsy	1	$350	$350
Operculum release or tooth exposure	1	$225	$225
Venous lake removal	1	$275	$275
Aphthous ulcer	2	$75	$150
Sulcular debridement/quadrant	8	$200	$1600
Cervical sensitivity	2	$75	$150
Tuberosity/torus reduction	1	$300	$300
Total			$4500
Other Data			
Monthly lease			($1000)
Monthly profit			$3500
Annual profit			$42,000

over this price in the first year approaches $40,000, so the laser would almost pay for itself in 1 year.

Table 16-1 can be used as a worksheet to evaluate the potential profit a laser can bring to the practice. To begin, the number of procedures that could be performed with the laser for 1 week is recorded. The appropriate fees are then inserted for the necessary calculations. Of note, this rough estimate does *not* include the amount of hours per week gained by using the laser for procedures that save time compared with conventional techniques (e.g., gingival retraction, implant recovery, gingivectomy), which will allow the practitioner to see more patients per week, thereby generating even more income. This estimate also does not take into account the reduced time per week spent tending to postoperative visits for discomfort after surgical procedures, which are greatly reduced when lasers are used. Strauss[4] has emphasized that "one of the

main advantages of using the laser is the lack of postoperative problems and the minimal need for wound care."

Tracking

To evaluate the financial return of introducing a laser into the dental practice, the income derived from the laser must be known over time. Current computerized practice management systems simplify tracking the factors used to determine the performance of the office profit centers, using key performance indicators (KPIs). The tracking of desired KPIs starts by listing the factors used in evaluating the success of the profit center, as follows:
- Procedures performed with a laser
- Patients referred to the practice by other patients for laser procedures
- Patients referred to the practice for laser procedures by other professionals (dentists, physicians)
- Patients who come to the practice because they know a laser is available

Unique Selling Proposition

The introduction of a laser into the dental practice brings an entirely new area of marketing to highlight in counseling patients regarding treatment: the unique selling point, or unique selling proposition (USP). Lasers are still not available in a majority of practices, whereas other USPs are common to many practices, such as tooth bleaching or veneers. The relative newness of laser technology provides the opportunity to capitalize on its availability.

The USP is a marketing concept first proposed as a theory to explain a pattern among successful advertising campaigns of the early 1940s, making unique propositions to the customer that convinced them to switch brands. The USP is the "factor or consideration presented by a seller as the reason that one product or service is different from and better than that of the competition."[5] The USP of laser availability can be highlighted by emphasizing the following advantages of laser dentistry:
- Nonsurgical periodontal treatment
- Less need for antibiotics and analgesics
- Easier healing
- Less bleeding
- Less postoperative discomfort
- Less chair time
- No scalpels, no blades, no cutting

Dental practices with lasers that perform both hard and soft tissue procedures can highlight the following:
- Reduced anxiety and elimination of fear of the drill
- Reduced noise—no more "whine" of the high-speed handpiece
- Anesthesia-free operative dentistry
- Restorative dentistry without the side effect of numb lips
- Multiquadrant operative dentistry, with faster completion of the treatment plan

Advantages and Influence

Laser techniques are considered the standard of care in ophthalmology, dermatology, plastic surgery, and many other disciplines. Most patients have a friend or relative who has had laser treatment for diabetic retinopathy, a dermatologic disorder, vascular surgery, or plastic surgery procedure. The term *laser* evokes a positive attitude and response in consumers of medical services, who associate it with the latest medical advances. The perception is that laser treatments are better, faster, and less painful, with higher success rates.[6] Dental practices that offer laser treatment generally are viewed with more confidence and as more patient-oriented offices that provide better treatment and services. Wigdor[7] surveyed 100 patients on their perception of lasers and found that 69% thought that lasers would make their visit to the dentist easier.

Setting Fees

An initial question on incorporating a laser into the practice is how to charge for laser procedures. Several philosophies may be used to set fees for laser dental procedures. At one extreme, the fees are set based on an hourly rate plus a charge for materials. The other extreme allows for the dental insurance company to set the fees, regardless of the real costs. Most practices, however, use what they have developed as a *standard fee schedule,* or what the insurance industry might refer to as the office's *usual, customary, and reasonable* (UCR) fee schedule.

The approach for many offices that incorporate lasers into their practice is to leave the fees as they are and simply benefit from the increased productivity, as follows:

1. Efficiency and time savings with laser use
2. Addition of new procedures that can now be performed in the office
3. Enhancement of procedures being performed
4. Attraction of new patients

Another approach is to add a surcharge for any procedure using the laser. A third option is either to increase all fees across the board by a certain percentage to help cover the added expenses or to increase all fees simply because adding a laser provides a good reason, possibly long overdue, to update the office fee schedule.

Dental UCR Fee Reports

One way of gauging the fee level compared with that for the rest of the dental community is to use a "fee subscription service." Determining the correct fee schedule is an important annual decision. Two types of fee reports are available to dentistry: those based on "surveys," whereby offices from each area voluntarily submit fee information, and those based on insurance company data from actual claims. These reports allow clinicians to determine where they want to set fees with respect to percentiles of the fees charged in the community. Fees charged by a dentist who offers laser services should be in at least the top 50th percentile for the community, and probably much higher. These services allow fees to be compared with the 40th, 50th, 60th, 70th, 80th, 90th, and 95th percentile fees and provide "geographic multipliers" for all U.S. three-digit zip code prefixes.[8,9] Fees differ significantly relative to the cost of living in different locations.

It is difficult and time-consuming to determine a fair fee for dental services and still remain competitive. Knowing what value the marketplace and third-party payers place on dental procedures performed in the community allows dentists to set fees at a level that will best achieve their practice goals. These reports are excellent sources of information for reviewing or updating the office's fee schedule. Knowing what third-party payers may allow will help prevent pricing oneself out of the marketplace.

Preparing the Staff

After it has been decided to add laser-assisted dental services to the practice and an appropriate laser has been chosen, the next step is delivery of those services in accordance with the community's "standard of care." This standard of care begins with proper training for all staff members involved with delivery of dental services (dentists, assistants, hygienists, administrative staff) and successful completion of a comprehensive overview of laser dentistry. The Academy of Laser Dentistry (ALD) Standard Proficiency Certification Course meets the Curriculum Guidelines and Standards for Dental Laser Education developed at the University of California–San Francisco College of Dentistry,[10] which are recognized by many organizations, states, government agencies, and universities. In December 2005, the Board of Dental Examiners of Nevada passed language in Chapter 631 of the Nevada Administrative Code (NAC) that requires educational criteria for these guidelines, as interpreted by the ALD. Dentists and dental hygienists in that state must comply with the new regulations presented in sections NAC 631.033 and NAC 631.035, as follows:

> Each licensee who uses or wishes to use laser [ir]radiation in his practice of dentistry or dental hygiene must include with his application for renewal of his license:
>
> 1. A statement certifying that each laser used by the licensee in his practice of dentistry or dental hygiene has been cleared by the Food and Drug Administration for use in dentistry; and
> 2. Proof that he has successfully completed a course in laser proficiency that:
>   (a) Is at least 6 hours in length; and
>   (b) Is based on the *Curriculum Guidelines and Standards for Dental Laser Education,* adopted by reference pursuant to NAC 631.035.

A standard proficiency certification course includes the curriculum for basic education in laser use and specific device instruction with demonstrated proficiency in didactic and hands-on knowledge. Hands-on exercises include demonstration and clinical simulation with appropriate oral tissues (e.g., cow or pig jaws) and must meet participation course guidelines. Practitioners must demonstrate competency in the safety aspects of laser use. *This is the level of education that defines the standard of care.* Dental auxiliaries also are encouraged to demonstrate competency in the safety aspects of laser use.

These courses are available through the ALD's "recognized course providers," as well as several major dental meetings, dental school continuing education (CE) programs, and state and local dental societies. At least one laser manufacturer mandates that each laser customer participates in this type of course as a condition of purchase. Many "professional liability" insurance carriers now require proof of proper training for policyholders engaged in laser procedures (e.g., AIG's Dentist's Advantage Professional Liability Insurance). Additionally, from a medical-legal perspective, proper laser training is indispensable.

Preparing the Patient

Dentists can introduce lasers to their patients in several ways. The most subtle approach is to wait until an appropriate use of the laser arises and then inform the patient that a laser will be used to accomplish a specific procedure, pointing out the benefits of laser treatment for this indication over other, conventional methods. This approach is the basis of informed consent and is the minimal introduction used to inform patients about laser use in the practice. From that level, it is then appropriate to implement marketing (internal and external) and promotional options now available to the dental profession.

Internal Marketing and Patient Education

Internal marketing is one of the simplest and most productive business promotional activities that can be used to enhance patient relations. Internal marketing educates the employees about the practice's new services and alerts existing patients to new options through in-office promotional devices.

Prerecorded Educational Videos and Computer Simulations

An effective outreach approach is to show an educational video that describes the new laser and the enhanced procedures in the reception room for all visitors to see. Commercially available video programs such as Guru and Casey feature sections on laser dentistry that can be adapted to a specific dental practice, with news or promotional clips made for the office or featured on local or national news. An informed patient is much more likely to be a satisfied patient, with fewer surprises encountered during treatment and postoperatively. The resulting positive opinion formed by such a patient will now be communicated to family members, co-workers, and acquaintances, creating another source of patient referrals.

Posters

The strategic placement of posters (such as in the waiting room) can spark questions or discussion about the laser treatments depicted. Before-and-after pictures showing laser use in "patient-friendly" procedures such as cosmetic recontouring of a gummy smile before veneer placement, bleaching, and tooth-colored fillings prepared with a laser without use of an anesthetic can be displayed. Such posters tell the patient that not only does the practice offer laser procedures, but that other patients are satisfied with the results. Office staff can check with the laser manufacturer or distributor about poster availability.

Patient Information Brochures

Brochures about lasers are available from several sources, including laser manufacturers, dental supply companies, and the ALD. Brochures often can be personalized, or customized brochures can be produced in-house or professionally (Figure 16-1).

Photographs

Photographs are one of the best means of communication available. The practitioner should take photos of the various laser procedures performed in the office, or secure photos from the laser distributor and then make a book of laser procedures that can be used to show patients their recommended treatment. Also, a clinical atlas with preoperative and postoperative photos of most laser procedures is useful in explaining procedures to patients.[11]

Before taking photographs of patients, the practitioner must be sure to obtain proper releases to use the photos. Such photos should be restricted to preoperative and fully healed postoperative views. Intraoperative photos or those

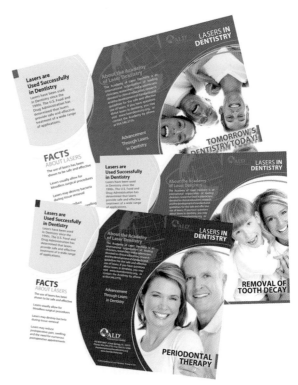

• **Figure 16-1** Laser brochure typical of those available from the ALD, Smart Practice, and other sources (Courtesy of Academy of Laser Dentistry).

that show a bloody or healing surgical site are off-putting or unappealing to most people.

Staff's Role

All administrative staff members have a role in internal marketing to the current and prospective patients. This component of the dental team includes all "front desk" personnel: the receptionist, financial coordinator, insurance coordinator, and patient care coordinator. If they themselves have experienced laser dental procedures, they can speak with firsthand knowledge, experience, and enthusiasm. This kind of communication affords special opportunities to influence the patient as a consumer. The attitude and involvement of the office team are critical to successful integration of a dental laser into the practice. The clinician should make educational opportunities available to all personnel, who also may be treated with laser procedures so that they are well qualified to deliver personal testimonies. The practitioner should consider allowing employees to offer selected new laser services at a discount to appropriate patients. Employees who become advocates for the practice's services become the practitioner's best referral source for new patients. Nothing is better than word-of-mouth advertising.

Front Desk

The receptionist has unique opportunities to promote the practice when greeting patients and answering the telephone. This person should have a clear understanding and working knowledge of the use of the practice's laser, to provide effective answers to basic questions. All front desk personnel should be able to communicate to patients the advantages, and thus the value, of laser use. Gaining the patient's confidence for future treatments is a major goal. If the practice uses a "message on hold" telephone answering system, laser use should figure prominently in the message.

Patient Care Coordinator

The patient care coordinator has several opportunities to promote the practice when interacting with patients and reviewing treatment proposals. This person too should have a clear understanding and working knowledge of the use of the office's lasers so that he or she can answer basic questions. The care coordinator should be able to relate to the patients the advantages of laser use, such as greater comfort, quicker healing, less postoperative discomfort, little to no bleeding, greater precision, and less need for anesthetic or antibiotics, reinforcing its value to the patient. The care coordinator also may be the person to discuss informed consent with the patient, both oral and written, requiring confirmatory signatures of the patient, the person reviewing the information, and the dentist. The patient must be given the opportunity to discuss any questions with the dentist before the procedure is performed (see later discussion on informed consent).

Financial Coordinator

The financial coordinator should be familiar with the fee structure and how charges are made for laser procedures. If there is a special fee for laser use, this person must be able to convince the patient that the extra fees are well worth the added expense. The financial coordinator should be able to discuss any payment and billing options offered to make the choice as easy as possible.

Insurance Coordinator

The insurance coordinator must be familiar with how to code any of the procedures for which a laser is used. The general rule is that the procedures are coded as they would normally be, and the appropriate fees charged. The use of a laser is not indicated on any insurance forms. A laser is an instrument that is used to perform or assist in performing a procedure—it is not a procedure in itself. One exception exists to this rule: the American Dental Association (ADA) code "D7465 destruction of lesion(s) by physical or chemical method, by report. (Examples include using cryo, laser or electro surgery.)."[12] In this very limited procedure, the entire lesion is ablated (vaporized), and no histopathologic tests are done, such as in treating an aphthous ulcer or hepetic lesion. Other than in these specific situations, use of this code is not recommended, because any lesion removed must be biopsied to obtain the correct pathologic diagnosis.

For many procedures, laser dentists may provide narratives with the claim form to help the insurance company properly process the claim. General codes can be used along with the narratives; for example, the D3999, D4999, D7999, and D9999 codes are, respectively, unspecified endodontic, periodontal, oral surgery, and adjunctive procedures, "by report," whereby narratives can be used to describe those procedures performed that do not otherwise fit the available ADA code descriptions. These should be used judiciously with proper documentation. These may be labeled "Laser-Assisted Procedure." It is important to recognize that insurance companies probably will not pay for such procedures as coded, but the use of this code on insurance forms may show the patient that the dental office is doing everything possible to maximize insurance reimbursement (Box 16-1).

Stationery

The dental office stationery should reflect that the practitioner is now a laser dentist. Business cards, appointment cards,

---

BOX 16-1 Example of Descriptive Coding for Insurance Documentation of Laser Procedure

Laser treatment provided to decrease the bioburden microbiologic flora in the tooth pocket after periodontal therapy—minimizing further infection and enhancing tissue reattachment.
ADA Code D4999

recall cards, and any other printed matter with the practice's name should include the international logo of lasers and the phrase "laser dentistry" (Figures 16-2 and 16-3).

External Marketing

External marketing, promoting the dental practice to potential prospects, is still a relatively new phenomenon. Some dentists still have difficulty with the acceptability of "advertising." As stated by Willis,[13] however, "educating potential patients to the procedures you offer actually provides a service. There are many individuals looking for a dental home or a specific service you may be offering that they need."

External marketing can become expensive for the dental practice. A well-designed and carefully planned marketing plan is recommended if anything more than the simplest methods of advertising are used. Also, if the plan is properly chosen, the results and savings from experts in dental marketing can be well worth their cost.

Signage

Perhaps one of the least understood forms of external marketing is the on-street sign. It is the practitioner's calling card to the community, and it can affect public perception of the dental practice. The type of sign and the information the sign is intended to convey, on both conscious and subconscious levels (Figure 16-4), should be carefully considered. Specific issues have been identified by Du Molin[14]:

> The issues are much more complex than just what to say on your dental office sign. You have to take into consideration the position of the signs relative to the building and the flow of traffic. And, of course, observe the all-important signage zoning codes. The economics of good dental signage are too important to just wing it. A well-designed set of signs—you'll notice I used the plural, meaning more than one—can easily put $1,000,000 extra into your pension fund for retirement.

Direct Mail

According to the ADA Intelligent Dental Marketing (ADAIDM)[15]:

> When executed properly, direct mail can yield more new patients per dollar spent than any other type of advertising available to dentists. New patients can be targeted by zip code, carrier route and even income or age. Dentists from all over the country have successfully created new patient flow quickly and painlessly by using . . . direct mail.

Targeted direct-mail postcards are easily custom-designed and can be eye-catching and cost-efficient. Postcards can offer a creative and effective way to reach the practice's target audience. Postcards can be used to introduce new treatments or services in laser dentistry and to make special offers to attract new patients.

Another direct-mail piece for both internal and external marketing is the newsletter. These mailings can be designed in-house or professionally. A "special issue" that highlights the introduction of a laser into the practice could be sent to existing patients, and extras could be used as a direct-mail item sent to designated demographic populations.

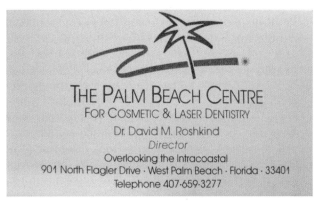

• **Figure 16-2** Sample appointment/business card showing a stylized version of the international symbol of lasers.

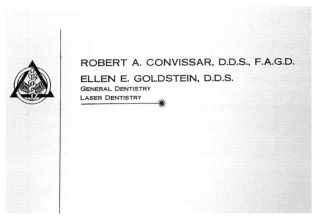

• **Figure 16-3** Sample letterhead displaying international symbol of lasers.

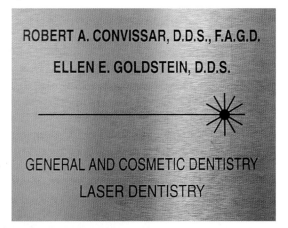

• **Figure 16-4** Sample office sign displaying international symbol of lasers.

Yellow Pages

Probably the most common method of external marketing of dental services has been a listing in the Yellow Pages or a similar telephone directory. The listing can be as simple as a name and telephone number or may be an elaborate color package with advertising, in-column ads, boldface listings, and other combinations. Often such packages include coordination with other media, such as yellowpages.com and associated online search engines. The USP of laser use should be strongly emphasized in an advertisement—or may even be the focus of the ad. The producers of these publications will assist in all phases of design, development, and production. They may be highly knowledgeable about their markets; however, it often is wise to seek the assistance of a marketing expert with experience in the dental field.

Newspapers and Magazine

Advertising and marketing programs in newspapers are now commonplace in the dental field. As with phone directory advertising, a well-planned and coordinated program will save much in terms of time and expense while yielding the best returns. Some programs are designed to run multiple small ads, whereas others run one or two larger positions. Lasers often make a good focal point for the dental practice's ad and can be a significant USP in the community.

Both the readership of newspapers and the use of telephone directories continue to decline, as a direct result of Internet use. This development might allow for better rates for advertising programs once considered too expensive.

Website

The Internet is becoming the source of choice as the demographics of the U.S. population change. The generation of people who grew up with Internet accessibility and cell phones as the norm has become dependent on electronic media as their primary source of information. Any dental practice interested in attracting new patients must have a website as well as a mobile website. More important, an office positioning itself as a cutting-edge, high-tech practice must have a website to match that image. Many website designers have experience with dental offices, making a professional, customized website easily available. Search engine optimization (SEO) has become essential in designing websites; companies can provide assistance in optimizing your place in a given online search. A website is now another part of the dental office's overall marketing plan that requires careful planning, coordinating, and budgeting.

Social Media

In addition to maintenance of a website and mobile website, the use of social media such as Facebook, Twitter, LinkedIn, and others is a necessity in today's ubiquitous digital environment. These public sites can be an excellent forum by which the practitioner can communicate with patients about the various uses of lasers in the practice, as well as many other topics. Social media also can provide a way for patients to follow specific practitioners and office staff in their pursuits of CE, special events, or lectures, or to convey any promotions offered by the practice. In addition, educational and "infomercial" tidbits can be posted for patients on topics that the practitioner wishes to highlight or promote.

Other Forms of Mass Marketing

Billboards, mass-transit marketing, and broadcast media (radio, television) are becoming more frequently used by dental practices. In some markets, these media can be affordable and demographically targeted as part of an overall marketing plan, whereas in larger markets, the costs can be prohibitive. Again, all of these external marketing options must be carefully planned, coordinated, and budgeted for the best ROI.

Marketing to Other Professionals

When lasers are introduced into the dental practice, often-overlooked sources of referrals are other local professionals. Potential contacts include physicians, pharmacists, physical therapists, speech pathologists, and chiropractors, as well as other dental professionals, both general and specialty.

Other general dentists in the area often are thankful to know about a referral source available for handling difficult situations that might best be managed with laser therapy (Case Study 16-1, with Figure 16-5), or if the dental practice is in an area where specialists are too distant for easy access. A simple, professionally written personal letter on the office letterhead that introduces the practitioner and the practice and describes what services are offered to help their patients often is welcome information (Figure 16-6). The letter could suggest contacting the laser dental practice for more information or extend an invitation to see the office and the laser equipment and to further discuss potential advantages for patients. It is always good policy to have a competent referral source. All of the reasons discussed earlier for specialty referral apply here. A specific protocol for management of referral patients should be established, because they will be returning to the referring general practice for their primary care.

CASE STUDY 16-1

A 72-year-old patient whose medical history included placement of a pacemaker many years earlier and a current regimen of warfarin (Coumadin) needed periodontal surgery in all four quadrants, which he refused. To restore the patient's upper left lateral incisor, his general dentist determined that a soft tissue crown-lengthening procedure was needed. The general dentist, however, felt uncomfortable performing the procedure with a blade because of the warfarin and could not use his electrosurgical unit because of the possible interaction with the pacemaker. The patient was referred to a laser dentist for laser crown lengthening (Figure 16-5).

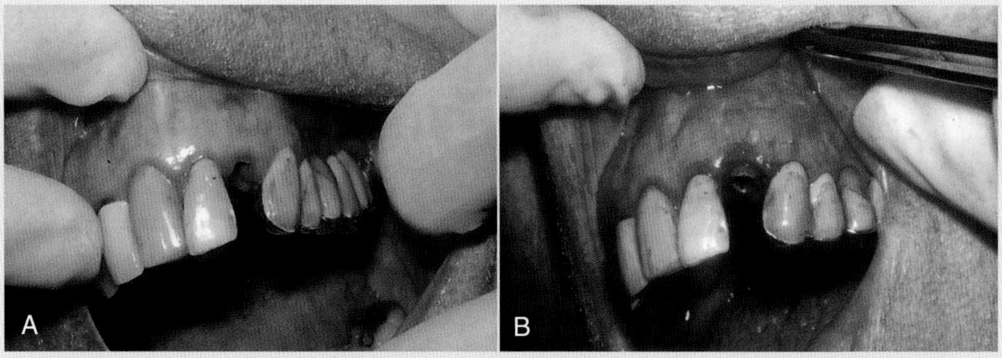

• **Figure 16-5** The patient, who has a pacemaker and takes warfarin (Coumadin), was in need of laser soft tissue crown lengthening. **A,** Preoperative view. **B,** Postoperative view.

GAINESVILLE DENTAL ASSOCIATES
DAVID M. ROSHKIND, DMD
Family, Cosmetic, and Laser Dentistry

January 15, 20XX

Dear Dr. Smith,

I am pleased to be able to write this letter to you introducing new services that we have now made available to patients throughout the community. You may on occasion have a need for dental laser treatment that is most appropriate for your patient's needs but is not available in your office. There are many reasons why you may wish to refer patients to our practice for a procedure that could best be treated with a laser. One of the most significant reasons is the minimal bleeding that accompanies laser surgery. We are making that service available to your patients on a case-by-case referral basis. These patients will be treated in consultation with your assessment of their needs, treated for only those issues, and then quickly returned to you for their continued care. Some of the procedures that we can assist you with are:

- drug-induced hyperplasia with little bleeding
- desensitization of sensitive teeth
- implant recovery (for patients on blood thinners)
- recurrent aphthous ulcers
- herpetic lesions
- Venus lake/hemangioma removal
- frenum pulls
- frenum release for spacing
- orthodontically induced gingival hyperplasia
- exposure of teeth due to delayed eruption
- frenum release in infants for suckling and speech
- periodontal graft that needs some recontouring or debulking
- lesion removal for patients on blood thinners that can be treated without going off medication
- ridge formation of an ovate pontic form for improved cosmetics

To my fellow general dentists, it is often good to know that there is a referral source when you have a difficult situation that might best be handled with laser therapy or if specialists are too far away to be easily accessed. Any of the above reasons for specialty referral could apply in those situations.

Thank you for your confidence and referrals. Please be assured that these referrals will be treated in a very special manner so that the patient is returned quickly to your practice.

Sincerely,

David M. Roshkind, DMD, MBA, FAGD, MALD

• **Figure 16-6** Sample letter introducing dentists in the community to laser dentistry, to obtain referrals.

Dental Specialists

The dental specialists in the practice's referral area are prime candidates for referrals. Many reasons for referring patients for procedures best treated with a laser have been recognized (Table 16-2).

TABLE 16-2	Common Dental Specialist Referrals for Laser Treatment	
Specialist	**Procedures for Which Referral for Laser Treatment May Be Appropriate**	
Orthodontist	Treatment for orthodontically induced gingival hyperplasia; Frenum pull correction; Exposure of tooth caused by delayed eruption; Laser fiberotomy before rotation of teeth	
Periodontist	Recontouring or debulking of periodontal grafts; Laser desensitization; Surgical procedures in patients taking warfarin (Coumadin) or other blood thinners in whom international normalized ratio (INR) is poorly controlled	
Prosthodontist	Formation of ovate pontic site for improved cosmesis; Crown-lengthening procedures; Preprosthetic procedures, such as tuberosity/torus reduction	
Oral surgeon	Treatment for recurrent aphthous ulcers; Treatment for herpetic lesions	
Pediatric dentist	Frenum release	

Physicians

Physicians potentially constitute an excellent source of referrals. Many patients must be maintained on blood thinners and are urged by their physicians to keep taking their medications during dental treatment. This management approach is made possible with laser surgery, which is associated with minimal bleeding. In addition, cyclosporine, phenytoin (Dilantin), and calcium channel blockers also may cause gingival hypertrophy, which is most easily treated using a laser. This proven application is the rationale for contact of various physicians by the laser dentist, to obtain referrals (Table 16-3, with Figure 16-7).

Besides sending letters, one of the best ways to alert physician specialists in the area to availability of the dental office's laser services is through a hospital "Grand Rounds" lecture. Hospitals often recruit speakers to discuss innovative methods of patient treatment for such lectures. The practitioner can contact the local hospital and ask to do a presentation on "laser treatment of phenytoin (Dilantin)-induced gingival hyperplasia," for example.

Chairside Considerations

With laser-assisted dental treatment performed in the office, several additional considerations must be addressed: informed consent, record-keeping, laser maintenance, operatory organization, and others, as discussed in this section.

An important point in this context is that laser treatment should not be performed only for the sake of using the laser. As medical professionals, dental practitioners carry the ethical and moral responsibility that any treatment performed with a laser should have an outcome at least as good as if the laser were not used.

TABLE 16-3	Common Physician Specialist Referrals for Laser Treatment
Specialist(s)	**Potential Reason for Referral**
Transplant surgeon	*Transplant surgeons* prescribe cyclosporine to prevent organ rejection and could refer patients for treatment of cyclosporine-induced gingival hyperplasia. Among the transplant procedures that require patients to take cyclosporine are those involving the liver, lung, kidney, and heart (Figure 16-7).
Cardiologist, hepatologist, pulmonologist	*Cardiologists, hepatologists, pulmonologists,* and *nephrologists* see posttransplantation patients regularly and usually are their primary care physicians. They may refer patients for treatment of cyclosporine-induced gingival hyperplasia.
Rheumatologist	*Rheumatologists* may treat patients with severe rheumatoid arthritis that does not respond to conventional therapies and requires the use of cyclosporine.
Dermatologist	*Dermatologists* may prescribe cyclosporine for patients with severe psoriasis that does not respond to other therapies.
Neurologist, neurosurgeon, pediatrician, primary care physician	*Neurologists, neurosurgeons,* and possibly *pediatricians* and *primary care physicians* regularly see patients taking phenytoin (Dilantin) for treatment of seizure disorders, which also may be prescribed for prevention of seizures after neurosurgery.
Primary care physician, cardiologist	Both *primary care physicians* and *cardiologists* prescribe calcium channel blockers to treat hypertension.

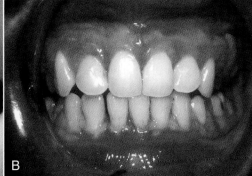

• **Figure 16-7** The patient, a 27-year-old kidney transplant recipient on both warfarin (Coumadin) and a calcium channel blocker, received CO_2 laser treatment for cyclosporine-induced gingival hyperplasia. **A,** Preoperative view. **B,** Two-week postoperative view.

Informed Consent

Obtaining proper informed consent is necessary before initiation of any dental procedure (Figure 16-8). The rationale for this step has been detailed in an online seminar on dental office risk management (sponsored by an insurance company well versed in the issues)[16]:

Informed consent represents the intersection of communication and documentation at critical junctures in patient care. . . . Informed consent is a *process*, not a piece of paper. In our experience, informed consent is still widely underutilized in dentistry. In many instances where consent forms *are* used, the consent is just a signature at the bottom of a form full of clinical jargon. It's unfortunate there is so much resistance to informed consent, since it pays dividends far in excess of the time it takes to do it right. Most dentists will have occasion to use informed consent procedures and forms at one time or another, so it's worth a few moments' consideration about how to get the most benefit out of the informed consent process with your patients. Informed consent offers the dentist an opportunity to enhance rapport with patients, as well as to create reasonable patient expectations about the desired outcome of a procedure or course of treatment. How best to take advantage of this opportunity? Keep in mind that while you know the issues at hand very well, the same is not true for patients. Most patients don't go through the informed consent process very often, so treat each informed consent discussion as though it is the first for your patient. Don't rush your verbal presentation of information, and try to avoid situations where the patient is expected to read (and understand!) a consent form while you are simultaneously speaking to them. Informed consent is not just about getting a form signed: it involves a process of advising the patient and obtaining voluntary, knowledgeable consent for a procedure. When the process is executed properly, there should be clear documentation of a patient's voluntary consent to treatment. This process can be successfully completed without a form, but using a standard form accomplishes several goals. Several parts of the patient record can and should be used during the informed consent process as they summarize the foundation for the patient's knowledgeable, voluntary decision to accept or refuse care, along with commonly known risks and benefits associated with the patient's choice of treatment.

Some practitioners do not include written informed consent in preparation for laser procedures, believing that laser treatment is currently the standard of care—and that use of a written informed consent form conveys the idea that laser treatment is somehow "different" and potentially more dangerous. Other laser dentists insist on written informed consent forms specifically to highlight that laser surgery *is* "different" and, by implication, superior. Some practitioners use standard informed consent forms, whereas other practices use specific laser dentistry informed consent forms. How to approach informed consent is the choice of each practitioner.

Record-keeping

Record-keeping is essential in any dental practice. Whether a paper chart or an electronic record is used, all details of treatment should be recorded. Such documentation can be invaluable for retrospective studies, practice analysis, management of adverse outcomes, and legal purposes.

All of the pertinent laser parameters should be recorded in a legible manner, including the following, along with any other relevant information or statistics:

• Laser name
• Wavelength
• Power or energy setting in watts (W) or millijoules (mJ)
• Temporal emission mode: hertz (Hz) and duty cycle or continuous wave (CW)
• Approximate time in contact with tissue
• Protective glasses/masks used
• Tip or fiber size

Case Study 16-2 provides an example of a chart entry for a laser treatment procedure.

Operatory Organization

For efficient use of a laser device and to maximize ROI, the dental treatment room must be well organized and ergonomically designed. A well-planned system allows proper attention to the many necessary details of readying the instrument and the treatment room between

CONSENT FORM

Patient's Name:_____ Date:_____

Address:_____ DOB: _____

1. I consent (give my permission) and request the performing, on myself (or my child _____), of the dental or oral surgical procedure known as:

    _____

    With ( ) local anesthesia ( ) analgesia

2. The doctor has explained this procedure to me in terms that I understand, and has answered any questions I have asked to my satisfaction. Alternative procedures have been offered and discussed and I have chosen to undertake this procedure.

3. I have been informed of the possible risks and complications of treatment including but not limited to:
    - ❏ Pain, swelling, bleeding
    - ❏ Infection or prolonged healing
    - ❏ Numbness, tingling, burning, or altered sensation (feeling) which may be temporary, prolonged, or permanent of the lip, chin, tongue, gums or teeth.
    - ❏ Sinus problems resulting from entering into (or displacement of teeth or roots into) the sinus, with possible sinus infection or remaining communication (opening) from the mouth into the sinuses
    - ❏ Damage to adjacent teeth, filling, or caps
    - ❏ Fracture of bone or roots
    - ❏ Muscle soreness or pain in the temporomandibular joint (TMJ)
    - ❏ Further procedures that may be necessary to treat any complications
    - ❏ Other: _____

I understand that drug reactions or reactions to anesthetics (local and general) may occur and that veins may become inflamed (phlebitis).

I understand that dental medicine and surgery are not exact sciences, and my dentist has explained to me that he cannot guarantee the precise outcome of this procedure nor can he guarantee that a perfect result will be achieved.

Instructions for postoperative care and any necessary prescriptions have been given to me with directions for use.

Signed: _____ Signed: _____
      Patient or Legal Guardian   Doctor

Witness: _____

If you have any questions or comments concerning your understanding of this form and its contents, please write them below. If not, please write "No questions."

• **Figure 16-8** Sample informed consent form.

CASE STUDY 16-2

Patient presents for removal of fibroma of the right buccal mucosa using a 1064-nm diode laser. Alternative treatments, risks, and benefits were discussed with the patient, and informed consent was obtained. Laser safety glasses were placed on the patient, and one carpule (1.8 mL) of 2% lidocaine with 1:100,000 epinephrine was administered by infiltration for local anesthesia. A 300-μm fiber was attached, cleaved, and test-fired. The settings used were 2.0 W and 50% duty cycle at 20-msec duration. Light contact with the base of the growth, with gentle traction from tissue forceps, was repeated until the entire lesion was removed, for a total surgical time of approximately 30 seconds. The open surface of the wound site was then irradiated with the laser in defocused mode. The patient was given postoperative instructions and scheduled to return for a postoperative checkup in 1 week.

procedures, while maximizing turnover. The dental assistant or the laser safety officer (LSO) can be assigned to perform these tasks and will become proficient in a short time. Steps that need to be done in minimal time to ensure efficient turnover for the laser operatory include the following:

- Laser shutdown/standby protocol followed
- Laser protective glasses cleaned
- Fiber/tip removed and wiped, bagged, and sterilized or disposed of in sharps container
- Handpieces and cannula wiped, bagged, and sterilized or disposed of in sharps container
- Laser unit wiped
- Protective coversheets changed
- New fiber/tip placed and ready to use

Laser Maintenance

The laser user should be familiar with any laser maintenance requirements. Most dental lasers are low maintenance. All lasers need to be calibrated periodically, and mirror alignment should be checked according to the manufacturer's recommendations or when energy output decreases. Some lasers have self-calibration modes or are furnished with calibration devices; others need to be professionally serviced by a laser technician, preferably from the manufacturer. If no manufacturer service is available, laser technicians at hospitals may be a good source of service.

Laser Safety Officer

The LSO is the person given the authority to monitor and enforce the control of laser hazards. For U.S. health care facilities, the American National Standards Institute (ANSI) defines the position of LSO and its responsibilities in both ANSI Z136.1 and ANSI Z136.3, laser safety standards. This person should be able to knowledgeably evaluate laser hazards in the facility and propose controls to mitigate them. The LSO's duties are as follows:

- Serves as "keeper of the keys"
- Sets up standard operating procedures
- Understands the operational characteristics of the laser
- Knows output limitations of the device
- Supervises staff education and training
- Ensures laser maintenance, beam alignment, and calibration
- Posts warning signs
- Oversees personal protective wear
- Supervises medical surveillance and incident reporting
- Is familiar with the biologic and other potential hazards of the laser
- Knows all regulations of appropriate agencies
- Determines the potential hazard zone and the nonhazard zone

Adverse Reporting Mechanisms

If any adverse effects are noted during or after laser use, either to the patient or to a staff member, a protocol to follow for proper reporting has been established: The practitioner is obligated first to address the immediate problem and then, as time allows, report the adverse effect to the manufacturer and any necessary regulatory authorities. Which authorities are notified depends on the severity of the problem; the local, state, and federal regulations; and the setting in which the procedure was performed.

If a facility has information that reasonably suggests that a device has or may have caused or contributed to a patient's *serious injury,* this information must be reported to the device manufacturer. If the manufacturer is not known, the report should be sent to the U.S. Food and Drug Administration (FDA). Each specific report of death or serious injury must be submitted on Form FDA 3500A within *10 work days* from the time at which any medical personnel of the facility becomes aware of a reportable event.

Laser Registration

Many practice owners may not be aware that some states (e.g., Florida, Texas) as well as other government jurisdictions require laser devices to be registered, often with the same state agency that registers other radiation devices. Usually, a small fee is levied for each device on the premises. The responsibility of registration could fall under the duties of the LSO or the office manager.

Continuing Education

All professionals also must be perpetual students who embrace CE to further their knowledge and skills. This aim can be accomplished by attending high-quality CE courses. Excellent sources of CE in laser dentistry are available through the ALD, the World Federation of Laser Dentistry, and the Society of Oral Laser Applications, as well as through several laser manufacturers. The many excellent laser journals include *Lasers in Medical Science, PhotoMedicine and Laser Surgery,* and *Lasers in Medicine and Surgery,* covering both medicine and dentistry.

Conclusions

It is well established that dental offices in which lasers are incorporated into treatment plans are considered "cutting edge" and have a unique psychological and promotional advantage over those that do not offer such services. Increased and immediate credibility for the practice is established as an up-to-date facility, where patient confidence is more easily attained, where needs are more readily turned into wants, and where trust is more easily established and turned into referrals. However, laser dentistry practices must still follow the basic tenets of sound dental practice management.

It is important for the clinician to reward and recognize the people who let patients know about new services, whether financially or with a simple "thank you." Laser use in dentistry has expanded and improved treatment options. The practitioner must receive proper training, maintain an adequate level of clinical experience, and proceed within the scope of the practice.

References

1. Catone GA, Alling III CC: *Laser applications in oral and maxillofacial surgery,* Philadelphia, 1997, WB Saunders.
2. *Merriam-Webster online dictionary;* http://www.merriam-webster.com/dictionary/cost/opportunitycost. Accessed May 11, 2014.
3. McConnell C: *Microeconomics: principles, problems, and policies,* Columbus, Ohio, 2005, McGraw-Hill.
4. Strauss R: Laser management of discrete lesions. In Catone GA, Alling CC III , editors: *Laser applications in oral and maxillofacial surgery,* Philadelphia, 1997, WB Saunders.

5. Reeves R: *Reality in advertising*, New York, 1961, Alfred A Knopf.

6. Cankat K: Evaluation of patient perceptions of frenectomy: a comparison of Nd:YAG laser and conventional techniques, *Photomed Laser Surg* 26(2):147–152, 2008.

7. Wigdor H: Patients' perception of lasers in dentistry, *Lasers Surg Med* 20:47–50, 1997.

8. Wasserman Y: *National Dental Advisory Service comprehensive fee report*, Milwaukee, Ill, 2009, Wasserman Medical Publishers.

9. Renaissance Systems and Services dental software; support@rss-llc.com. Also available from Renaissance Systems & Services, LLC, 1502 W Edgewood, Suite A, Indianapolis, IN 46217 (866-712-9584; 866-712-9585).

10. White JM, Barr R, Goldstein A, et al.: Curriculum guidelines and standards for dental laser education, *Lasers in Dentistry V, SPIE Int Soc Optical Eng* 3593:110–122, 1999.

11. Coluzzi DJ, Convissar RA: *Atlas of laser applications in dentistry*, Hanover Park, Ill, 2007, Quintessence.

12. American Dental Association: *Code on dental procedures and nomenclature*, 2008. Effective for Jan 1, 2009, through Dec 31, 2010; www.ada.org/goto/dentalcode.

13. Willis R: Promote your practice; www.promoteyourpractice.com. Accessed March 2009. Also available from 10020-C S Mingo Road, Tulsa, OK 74133.

14. Du Molin J: *The wealthy dentist's $1,000,000 sign!*; http://www.thewealthydentist.com/DentalSigns.htm. Accessed May 15, 2014. Also available from The Wealthy Dentist, PO Box 1220, Tiburon, CA 94920 (712-585-3606).

15. American Dental Association: *Intelligent dental marketing: harness the power of direct mail*; www.adaidm.com [no longer available]. Accessed March 2009. Now available from ADA Intelligent Dental Marketing, 10542 South Jordan Gateway, Suite 375, South Jordan, UT 84095 (888-290-0763).

16. Beckett TJ: Fortress dental risk management on-line seminar, 2007-2009; https://www.dds4dds.com/fortress/pages/RiskManagement_eLearningCenter.aspx. Also available from Fortress Insurance Company, 6133 North River Road, Suite 650, Rosemont, IL 60018–5173.

17

Laser Dentistry Research

CARLOS de PAULA EDUARDO, ANA CECILIA CORRÊA ARANHA,
KAREN MULLER RAMALHO, MARINA STELLA BELLO-SILVA, PATRICIA MOREIRA
de FREITAS, AND JOHN D.B. FEATHERSTONE

New developments and technologies have redefined dentistry in recent years. The field of *biophotonics* has grown rapidly and become an area of great interest. Research on light emission related to dental applications has been supported and performed by different groups worldwide, focusing specifically on laser research. New lasers with a wide range of characteristics, such as the erbium family of lasers, and many different diode wavelengths are now being used in the various fields of dentistry. Of note, most studies focus on minimally invasive treatments.

This chapter presents an overview of new laser technologies for clinical applications in dentistry and updates the use of different types of lasers in surgery, diagnostic testing, and microbiology. Discussions include the accuracy and reproducibility of optical coherence tomography in diagnosis, use of photodynamic therapy in disinfection and microbial reduction, and the introduction of new carbon dioxide (CO_2) lasers for surgical applications.

Optical Coherence Tomography

The history of dental imaging began in the late 1800s with the development of the x-ray image. In 1973, computed tomography (CT) created images by combining x-ray and computer technology to capture thin slices of tissue.[1] After that, magnetic resonance imaging (MRI) allowed soft tissue analysis.

Periapical and cephalometric radiographs have been the most important tools in dental radiology for detecting primary and secondary caries, analyzing specific anatomic characteristics and structures, planning surgical procedures in implantology, diagnosing possible alterations in the bone, and supervising patient progress. However, disadvantages include the interposition of anatomic parts, with suboptimal detail on images, as well as the potential detrimental effects on biologic tissues produced by the ionizing radiation.[2]

Recent developments in the field of optical engineering offer new optical techniques for biomedical imaging applications.[2] In addition to the increased availability of compact, modular diode light sources, highly sensitive detectors make it possible to distinguish very small numbers of photons after they interact with the tissue.

The term *tomography* was first used to describe a sectional radiographic technique in which the x-ray tube moved along in the same plane as that of the film, but in the opposite direction. The image of a selected anatomic plane remains stationary on the moving film while the shadows of all other planes are blurred out of view. The resultant tomographic image is a slice or cross section of the structure. Tomographic images created by CT and panoramic radiography result from the interaction of biologic tissues with x-ray photons and represent a selected "layer" or "slice" of the structure obtained using the images recorded.[2]

Optical coherence tomography (OCT) is a well-established diagnostic imaging technique that has many potential dental applications. OCT is safe, versatile, inexpensive, noninvasive, and readily adapted to the dental office (Figure 17-1). Based on the principles of interferometry, OCT uses light from the nonionizing part of the electromagnetic spectrum along with biomedical optics to generate cross-sectional images of tissue up to 3 mm in depth. OCT displays microstructural details that cannot be obtained with other current imaging modalities[1,3] (Figure 17-2). This concept of using light and optics for imaging biologic tissues was first proposed by Duguay in 1971. After its first biologic application, by Huang et al.[4] in 1991, OCT initially was applied to tomographic imaging of transparent tissue in the eye for diagnosing retinal macular disease.[5-7]

Otis et al.[2] presented one of the earliest intraoral OCT prototypes for dentistry in 2000. Their system created cross-sectional images by quantifying the reflections of infrared light from dental structures interferometrically. It consisted of a computer, compact diode light source, photodetector with associated electronics, and handpiece that scanned a fiberoptic cable over the oral tissues. In OCT images, the structures appear without the superimposition of other anatomic structures. The final OCT image consists of many axial signal arrays, producing a two-dimensional representation

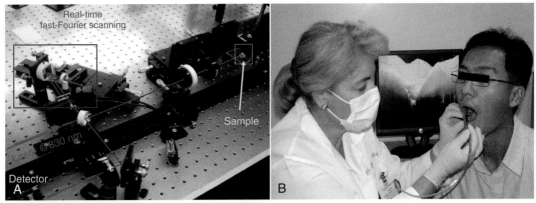

• **Figure 17-1** **A,** Real-time OCT imaging prototype. **B,** Real-time OCT imaging with the handpiece probe. (**A** Courtesy Professor Anderson Zanardi de Freitas; **B** courtesy Dr. Petra Wilder-Smith.)

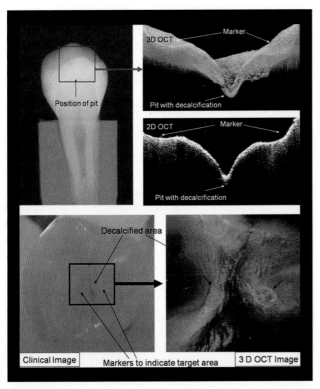

• **Figure 17-2** Two-dimensional (2D) and three-dimensional (3D) OCT images with clinical intraoral photographs and x-ray images for comparison. (Courtesy Dr. Petra Wilder-Smith.)

of the tissue reflections. Images can be viewed in real time and stored digitally.[2,3]

Although OCT is not yet widely clinically available in dentistry, the technique promises fast technological development.[8] Applying OCT to other clinically relevant biologic structures has been complicated because of optical scattering problems. Within the oral cavity, relevant biologic tissues typically are close to the surface, so OCT is a promising technique for obtaining images of human dental tissue in vivo and of carious lesions in particular.

Despite the significant gains in reducing its incidence, dental caries remains the principal cause of tooth loss worldwide. New treatment approaches emphasize early detection followed by minimal intervention. The most common approach to dental caries detection consists of dental radiography in conjunction with visual and tactile exploration.[7] At present, however, these routine procedures are not precise enough to detect early lesions, especially in occlusal surfaces, or gaps at the tooth-restoration interface, which potentially lead to secondary caries.[8] The early detection of restoration failures in the tooth-restoration interface could be the first step in preventing secondary caries formation and progression, as well as hypersensitivity of restored teeth, development of pulpal pathology, marginal staining, and the ultimate breakdown of a restoration.

Also, intraoral radiographs are highly sensitive and specific for the detection of primary caries but are less reliable for identifying recurrent caries around existing restorations.[2] OCT offers a potentially more sensitive method for detecting recurrent caries. In 2005, de Araujo et al.[8] showed the potential usefulness of OCT in clinical diagnosis compared with x-ray films. The 10-μm longitudinal resolution of the OCT system identified "induced" gaps. Conventional radiographs did not show the failure gaps. According to these authors, OCT has the advantage of showing the restored region as well as the gap, precisely localizing its position.

Amaechi et al.[9] quantitatively assessed the mineral changes in a carious lesion based on the effectiveness of preventive measures to remineralize the lesion at an incipient stage. These researchers monitored the changes over time in the mineral status of the caries by using OCT with a system that could collect A-scans (depicting depth versus reflectivity curve), B-scans (longitudinal images), and C-scans (transverse images at constant depth). Bovine teeth were subjected to demineralization in acidic buffer solution for 3 days, with images obtained before demineralization and again after 3 days of demineralization. Whereas the B-scans and C-scans qualitatively described the lesion, the A-scans showed the depth (in mm)–resolved reflectivity (in dB) of the tooth tissue and were used for the quantitative analysis. The results showed that R (dB/mm) decreased with increasing demineralization time, and that the percentage reflectivity loss ($R\%$) in demineralized tissue (amount of mineral loss) increased with increasing demineralization time, showing that OCT could quantitatively monitor the mineral changes in a carious lesion over the long term.

Fried and co-workers have spent more than 12 years studying and refining OCT, based on use of 1310-nm light for the detection of carious lesions in enamel, including the very problematic occlusal surfaces.[10-13] Their early work showed the advantage of using polarization-sensitive OCT (PS-OCT) over nonpolarized OCT.[10] PS-OCT gave much better resolution and imaging of early lesions in enamel and produced quantitative imaging as well as qualitative imaging of artificial and natural carious lesions.[12,14] Numerous experiments were conducted in vitro that demonstrated quantitative assessment of demineralization and remineralization of enamel carious lesions using PS-OCT.[12,15,16] The technique also can be applied to lesions in dentin and tooth roots for the assessment of demineralization and remineralization.[17-21] Secondary caries can be imaged with PS-OCT.[22] Of importance, quantitative assessment of carious lesions in vivo has recently been reported by this group of investigators, demonstrating that this methodology is very close to widespread use in clinical dentistry.[23] At the same time, further refinements of the technique have been achieved, leading to the development of cross-polarization OCT (CP-OCT).[24-28] CP-OCT has now been shown to be capable of monitoring carious lesion progress in human mouths.[13,29]

Prosthetic materials (e.g., metal, composites, ceramic fillings/crowns) also have been imaged with OCT, showing its potential advantage over conventional methods by visualizing structural and marginal restoration defects *before* significant leakage occurred, thereby minimizing tooth loss and decreasing the need for replacement restorations.[2,7] Although accessibility of the probe tip to the area of interest is likely to be the limiting factor in this application, OCT also easily identifies marginal adaptation of the metal coping to the cavosurface margin and visualizes the internal aspects and marginal adaptation of porcelain and composite restorations.

In periodontics, because of visualization of the microstructural detail of the periodontal soft tissues, OCT offers the potential for identifying active periodontal disease before significant alveolar bone loss occurs. Visual recordings of periodontal tissue contour, sulcular depth, and connective tissue attachment are possible. OCT is a powerful method for generating high-resolution, cross-sectional images of oral structures, with in vivo imaging studies showing much more structural detail of dental tissues than obtainable with previous measurements.[2,7]

In endodontics, the OCT probe can be used to obtain a detailed microscopic image through the surrounding root canal circumferential wall to the outside cementum layer of the root.[30] The probe also can image the anatomy and assess the cleanliness of the canal walls and measure the exact thickness of the dentinal wall, which helps prevent canal overpreparation and perforation of the canal walls.

OCT also could prove extremely useful in the diagnosis of vertical fractures.[31]

OCT has potential applications in dentistry as a noninvasive method for imaging dental microstructure. The cross-sectional images exhibit microstructural details that cannot be obtained with other current imaging modalities. Using this new technology, visual recordings of the detection of very early demineralization and remineralization processes, tooth defects and restorative failures, periodontal disease, soft tissue dysplasias, precancerous lesions, and root canal anatomy can be obtained. OCT is a diagnostic aid that could meet the dental challenges of prevention and early intervention.

Widespread availability of OCT for clinical use can be anticipated in the near future. This technique tracks carious lesion progress or remineralization using infrared light and no ionizing radiation, meaning that high-caries patients could be monitored frequently as therapeutic interventions are carried out, without any concerns regarding excess radiation exposure.

Photoactivated Disinfection and Microbial Reduction

Reduction in levels of microorganisms is the main goal of various procedures in daily dental practice, especially in the treatment of root canal and periodontal tissue. Protocols that provide significant microbial reduction have established this modality as a coadjutant to the treatment of dental infections, especially in patients with resistant microorganisms and anatomic complications.

The temperature increase resulting from high-intensity laser irradiation can cause protein denaturation and can destroy microorganisms, with high decontamination indexes.[32] Low-level laser therapy (LLLT) is not capable of increasing tissue temperature,[33] so the same antimicrobial effects of the high-intensity laser cannot be expected when LLLT is used as the sole clinical modality.[34] Despite this limitation, low-intensity lasers have been studied and introduced clinically for microbial reduction. Their antimicrobial effect is achieved using the combination of low-power lasers with extrinsic photosensitizers, which results in highly reactive oxygen species (ROS).[35] These cause damage to cell membranes, mitochondria, and DNA,[36-38] and microbial destruction is inevitable. This process is called *photoactivated disinfection* (PAD), also called photodynamic therapy (PDT), photochemotherapy, and lethal photosensitization (see also Chapter 15).

The antimicrobial capacity of PAD has been used to improve microbial reduction during conventional therapy in periodontics, endodontics, restorative dentistry, and implantology.[39-42] Viral inactivation and successful treatment in herpes simplex virus type 1 (HSV-1) infection also have been reported.[43]

Photoactivated disinfection presents various advantages over traditional antimicrobial agents. PAD promotes faster microbial killing, without the need to maintain higher concentrations of photosensitizer in the infected area, as with antiseptics and antibiotics.[44] The main advantage is attributed to its local action; PAD affects microorganisms at the site of photosensitizer deposition exclusively, whereas systemic drugs exert their actions throughout the body.[45] Moreover, PAD does not damage or alter adjacent structures, such as periodontal and periapical tissue, even when higher concentrations of photosensitizer and higher energy densities are used.[46]

For the effective treatment of bacterial infections, it is paramount to have an adequate light source and a photosensitizer capable of binding to the target pathogen, so that photosensitization may occur in either subgingival or superficial oral tissues. The most frequently used light source for photosensitization in dentistry is the low-power laser because it (1) presents a narrow spectral band that enables a more specific interaction with photosensitizers, (2) can be coupled to optical fibers, and (3) does not cause increased tissue temperatures, as observed with polychromatic light sources.[47,48] The use of light-emitting diodes (LEDs) for this application also has been reported.[49]

Several photosensitizers are available for PAD; however, disinfection of oral pathogens generally necessitates use of cationic-charged photosensitizers, such as toluidine blue, methylene blue, and poly-L-lysine-chlorin-(e6) conjugates.[50,51] Interaction between photosensitizers and microorganisms occurs within a few minutes, and this period (incubation or preirradiation time) must be respected before laser irradiation begins.[35,51]

Disadvantages of PAD include lack of standardization and absence of an established protocol. Researchers have only started to evaluate the antimicrobial action of PAD; therefore much remains to be elucidated regarding the ideal light source, the most adequate photosensitizer for each type of bacteria and target tissue, and the proper energy density and power settings. Nevertheless, protocols adopted from in vitro and in vivo studies have presented safe and favorable scientific results that already enable the clinical application of PAD.

Recent studies by Feuerstein and co-workers have reported effects of blue light on biofilm formation. Two major conclusions have come from this laboratory work, and the results are yet to be confirmed in vivo. First, exposure of *Streptococccus mutans* in biofilm to blue light affected the re-formation of a new biofilm, showing an increase in the amount of dead bacteria.[52] This phenomenon suggests that blue light has a delayed antibacterial effect, although it does not interfere with bacterial capability to re-form an initial biofilm. Second, earlier work showed that blue light coupled with hydrogen peroxide has a major antibacterial effect on biofilm.[53,54] An antibacterial synergic effect between blue light and hydrogen peroxide was observed. The mechanism of the phototoxic effect on *S. mutans* was basically a photochemical process involving ROS. Application of such light in combination with hydrogen peroxide to an infected tooth could be an alternative to or serve as an additional minimally invasive antibacterial treatment.

Influence of Pulse Duration on High-Intensity Laser Application

High-intensity lasers frequently are used in the daily practice of dentistry. The variety of wavelengths and their interaction with the different chromophores allow their application for many purposes, in either oral soft or hard tissues. The results depend on numerous parameters, including wavelength, pulse energy, fluence (joules per square centimeter), pulse duration, and repetition rate. Laser ablation of hard tissue and selective removal of dental caries have attracted attention because these are considered safe procedures[55] that reduce pain,[56,57] without the noise and vibrations of a conventional drill.[58]

Laser interaction with dental hard tissue may result in efficient and safe removal of compromised dental structure. Achieving this aim will require full awareness of those factors and technical skills involved in limiting lateral thermal and mechanical damage and in optimizing final surface characteristics.

Recent study has focused on the influence of pulse duration on the ablation process. The development of high-technology laser devices now allows the selection of pulse duration in the range of microseconds (1 μsec = one millionth [0.000001] of a second), nanoseconds (1 nsec = one billionth [10^{-9}] of a second), and lately, picoseconds (1 psec = one trillionth [10^{-12}] of a second) and femtoseconds (1 fsec = one quadrillionth [10^{-15}] of a second). The equipment includes different wavelengths in ultraviolet, visible, and infrared regions of the electromagnetic spectrum, such as 2940 nm (erbium-doped yttrium-aluminum-garnet [Er:YAG] laser in free-running and Q-switched modes), 9300 nm (TEA [transverse excited atmospheric] flowing gas CO_2 laser), 9600 nm (CO_2 and TEA CO_2 lasers), 10,600 nm (CO_2 laser), 308 nm (xenon monochloride [XeCl] laser), 2780 nm (erbium plus chromium–doped yttrium-scandium-gallium-garnet [Er,Cr:YSGG] laser), 1064 nm (neodymium-doped yttrium-aluminum-garnet [Nd:YAG] laser with regenerative amplifier [RGA] system), and 425 nm (low-power visible femtosecond laser).[59-63]

Considering that the increase in temperature and the peripheral thermal damage may provoke fracture, cracking, structural breakdown, or melting in dental hard tissue[64-67] and healing inhibition and necrosis in bone, it is assumed that high-power pulses, with pulse durations shorter than the thermal relaxation time, are necessary to avoid thermal denaturation of the tissues adjacent to the irradiated surfaces.[61,68] Longer pulse durations are thought to be responsible for inducing damage and thermomechanical stress to tissue, because they allow thermal energy to accumulate and penetrate deeply.[69]

Studies on pulse duration in the ablation process indicate that not only does the threshold energy for ablation decrease,[69] but that the morphologic shapes of the crater are altered when ultrashort pulses are used.[70-72] Although lasers with ultrashort (fsec) pulse duration are being developed, pulses in the microsecond range are already considered to be extremely short.[73] The tissue relaxation time for enamel is 100 μsec, and supershort pulse (SSP) durations (50 μsec) are already sufficient for precise ablation.[59] Pulses with 100-μsec duration (very short pulses [VSPs]) are considered the standard for routine work, as well as short pulses (SPs), of 300 μsec. Pulse durations of 700 μsec (long pulses) and 1000 μsec (very long pulses) are indicated for soft tissues because the residual thermal energy provides coagulation. Consequent to the reduction in pulse duration to picoseconds and nanoseconds, studies are now using wavelengths not previously used for dental tissue ablation (e.g., Nd:YAG lasers).[74-77]

Use of shorter pulse duration and higher energy intensity accelerates the ablation process.[78] This acceleration results from the quicker vaporization of the water present in the irradiated tissue, which causes the rapid microexplosion of the water molecules and removal of hard tissue structures.[79,80] In this case, ablation efficacy is improved; reduced residual thermal damage is induced because of the minimization of heat diffusion; enamel acid resistance to caries is increased[81,82]; and less vibration is provoked. The result is a reduction in painful stimulus to the pulp and greater patient comfort and treatment acceptance.[83]

Carbon Dioxide Lasers

Overview

With all CO_2 lasers, the active laser medium is a gas mixture that contains CO_2, helium (He), nitrogen (N_2), and possibly some hydrogen (H_2), water vapor, and xenon (Xe). Such lasers are electrically pumped by gas discharge. N_2 molecules are excited by the discharge into a metastable vibrational level and transfer their excitation energy to the CO_2 molecules when they collide. Helium serves to depopulate the lower laser level and to remove the heat. Hydrogen and water vapor can help to reoxidize carbon monoxide (CO) formed in the discharge to CO_2. These lasers typically emit at a wavelength of 10.6 μm (10,600 nm), but they also can emit as several wavelengths in the region of 9 to 11 μm—specifically, 9.3, 9.6, 10.3, and 10.6 μm.

Laser systems such as the CO_2 permit very-high-energy radiation to be focused on a tiny spot and have found applications in many dental specialties. For dental applications, all CO_2 lasers are used in a noncontact technique and can be operated in continuous-wave or pulsed-beam mode.[84]

Laser Types and Applications in Dentistry

The three main CO_2 laser wavelengths that have been researched and/or used in dental procedures are 9.3, 9.6, and 10.6 μm (9300, 9600, and 10,600 nm). Even with such similar wavelengths, the absorption by biologic tissues is different, so the clinical applications may vary. Dental mineral tissues (enamel and dentin) have weak absorption in the visible (400 to 700 nm) and near-infrared (1064 nm) spectrum.[85,86] CO_2 lasers are well absorbed by biologic tissues because of their strong affinity for water and, in the case of the 9.3- and 9.6-μm wavelengths, interact strongly with apatite absorption bands, mainly with phosphate and carbonate groups. Therefore the 9.3- and 9.6-μm CO_2 laser wavelengths can be used for procedures involving both hard and soft tissues. The absorption coefficients in dental enamel for 9.3, 9.6, and 10.6 μm are 5500, 8000 and 825 cm⁻¹, respectively,[87] compared with the Nd:YAG wavelength (1.06 μm), which has an absorption coefficient in enamel of approximately 1 cm⁻¹. These data mean that the 9.3- and 9.6-μm wavelengths are extremely well absorbed in dental mineral, causing very efficient localized heating[88] as compared with the conventional 10.6-μm laser that is absorbed at one tenth of the efficiency.

9.3- and 9.6-μm Carbon Dioxide Lasers

Results of using the 9.3-μm and 9.6-μm CO_2 laser wavelengths on hard tissues (enamel and dentin) show promising clinical applications for this wavelength.[89,90]

Many studies have been published over the past 20 years or so, and only some are highlighted here. Studying the effects of CO_2 lasers on dental enamel morphology, McCormack et al.[89] demonstrated that surface changes can be produced at low fluences if the hard tissues efficiently absorb the wavelengths used. Exposure included an extensive range of CO_2 laser wavelengths (9.3, 9.6, 10.3, and 10.6 μsec), with 5, 25, or 100 pulses at absorbed fluences of 2, 5, 10, or 20 J/cm² and pulse widths of 50, 100, 200, or 500 μsec. Longer pulses at constant fluence conditions decreased the extent of surface melting and crystal fusion, and the total number of laser pulses delivered to the tissue did not significantly affect surface changes so long as at least 5 to 10 pulses were used. Within the wavelengths of the CO_2 laser, differences in the observed surface changes of the enamel were dramatic. On dentin, the effects of CO_2 laser at 9.3 μm showed no craters or cracks but included many small, molten and rehardened particles on the surface, suggesting that laser irradiation affected only the dentin surface (<20 μm) and would be less harmful to dental pulp for dentin ablation.[91]

Both 9.3-μm and 9.6-μm CO_2 lasers have been extensively studied for caries prevention. Several studies in the past three decades have demonstrated the potential of laser pretreatment of enamel or tooth roots to inhibit subsequent acid-induced dissolution or artificial caries-like challenges in vitro.[92-94] The overall objective is to determine the optimum parameters for CO_2 laser irradiation that will effectively inhibit dental caries (primary and secondary) in enamel and dentin. Featherstone et al.[92] reported that the rate of CO_2 laser inhibition of artificial caries-like lesions in dental enamel ranged from 40% to 85% for all laser conditions tested, comparable to inhibition with daily fluoride dentifrice treatments, with minimal subsurface temperature elevation (<1° C at 2-mm depth).

Use of CO_2 lasers in cavity preparation can result in caries-preventive effects on the prepared tooth structure, decreasing the demineralization process after restorative procedures (prevention of secondary caries).[81,93,95] Fried et al.[81]

conducted dissolution studies of bovine dental surfaces modified by high-speed scanning ablation with the 9.3-µm TEA CO_2 laser. TEA CO_2 lasers tuned to the strong mineral absorption of hydroxyapatite near 9 -µm are well suited to the efficient ablation of dental hard tissues if the laser pulse is stretched to greater than 5 to 10 µsec, to avoid plasma shielding phenomena, and also to match the thermal relaxation time. Moreover, such CO_2 lasers can be operated at very high repetition rates and are inherently less expensive and more versatile than erbium lasers. An enamel surface with enhanced resistance to acid dissolution is produced after CO_2 laser ablation if sufficiently high scanning rates are used, with or without a water spray. The 9.3-µm CO_2 laser may even have greater potential for caries prevention than topical fluoride.[95]

Wilder-Smith et al.[96] investigated the surgical and "collateral damage" effects of the 9.3-µm CO_2 laser on soft tissue, specifically the incision width and depth as well as effectiveness. Incision depths correlated positively with average power; higher powers produced deeper incisions. These authors also verified that collateral damage to adjacent tissues was related to the laser pulse-emitting mode. Multiple factors were found to influence the outcomes with laser irradiation at 9.3 µm A wide range of surgical and collateral effects can be achieved with one specific laser device, depending on the parameters or configuration selected.

Although caries-preventive studies have used different CO_2 laser wavelengths, 9.3 µm and 9.6 µm are the wavelengths of choice for the reasons noted. To produce similar caries-inhibitory effects using a 9.6-µm laser and a 10.6-µm laser, a 14-fold increase in the energy density is necessary when the 10.6-µm (10,600-nm) wavelength is used.[97] Pulsed lasers provide a method of increasing the peak power density while keeping the pulse energy density at low levels (hundreds of mJ/cm^2), thereby minimizing the cumulative energy deposition.[85,98] This means that changes such as fusion, melting, carbonate loss, and recrystallization of enamel crystals can be confined to a thin surface region without affecting the underlying dentin or pulp.[97]

Viscovini et al.[99] reported another alternative for caries prevention not previously investigated—the use of waveguide CO_2 lasers, operating at high repetition rates (kHz), with pulses in the 100-msec duration and low peak powers (100 W). The advantage would be the simplification of the technology and low cost of this system compared with the TEA CO_2 laser system.

Observations of CO_2 laser effects on dental enamel morphology revealed evidence of melting, crystal fusion, and exfoliation in a wavelength-dependent manner.[89] Crystal fusion occurred at absorbed fluences as low as 5 J/cm^2 per pulse at 9.3-µm and 9.6-µm wavelengths, in contrast with no crystal fusion at 10.6-µm with the same fluence conditions. Longer pulses at constant fluence conditions decreased the extent of surface melting and crystal fusion.

Slutzky-Goldberg et al.[100] examined the effect of 9.6-µm CO_2 laser energy on the microhardness of human dental hard tissues (enamel and dentin) compared with that of high-speed drill cavity preparation, to determine the applicability of this laser in clinical treatment. These investigators concluded that the clinical use of 9.6-µm CO_2 laser energy for cavity preparation on dentin requires further analysis. Also, the effect of CO_2 lasers on dentin permeability was shown to be promising for therapy in the clinical setting.[100]

Studying the thermal effects of the 9.6-µm wavelength during hard tissue (dentin) removal, Nair et al.[101] investigated the short-term and long-term pulpal effects of cavity preparations in healthy human teeth. Although these preliminary histologic results suggest that the laser induced only minimal response of the dentin-pulp complex when used as a hard tissue drilling tool (with specific energy settings, pulse duration within thermal relaxation time), larger clinical trials involving various types of teeth are necessary to reach definitive conclusions regarding broad application of this laser for clinical procedures.

For the laser to be accepted, effects on dental pulp tissues must be similar to or less noxious than those caused by the high-speed drill. A histologic analysis using a 9.6-µm CO_2 laser confirmed these results. This animal study also showed that lasers produced no noticeable damage to the pulp and appeared to be a safe method for removing dental hard tissues.[102]

Investigations on laser-induced thermal decomposition of dental enamel have demonstrated a reduction in the rate of acid dissolution, size of artificial caries-like lesions, and acid reactivity.[92,98,103] Additionally, researchers have correlated the loss of carbonate from dental enamel with a reduction in acid dissolution. Dental mineral consists of hydroxyapatite with many substitutions, primarily carbonate (3% to 5% by weight), which greatly affects acid reactivity. Zuerlein et al.[104] determined the precise depth of modification (i.e., thermally induced decomposition) of dental enamel (carbonate loss) at the predicted optimum laser irradiation parameters. The depth of modification is consistent with the model that incorporates the absorption depth and thermal relaxation time/pulse duration. However, repeated irradiation is required for complete removal of carbonate.

CO_2 laser applications in oral surgery and implant dentistry also have been reported. For some indications, laser treatment has become the state of the art, replacing conventional techniques. A review of the literature reports that a major development was the introduction of the 9.6-µm CO_2 laser.[105] This laser can preserve tissue with almost no adverse effects and has been used to treat premalignant lesions, for intraoperative PDA, and for periimplant care, with reportedly better results than with conventional methods. However, further studies are needed to assess standard protocols.

For application in endodontics, a comparative study of dentin permeability after apicoectomy and surface treatment with 9.6-µm TEA CO_2 and Er:YAG laser irradiation showed a reduction in permeability to methylene blue dye for both wavelengths.[106] This clinical application is important because the failure of apicoectomies generally is attributed to dentin surface permeability, as well as the lack of an adequate marginal sealing of the retrofilling material, which allows the percolation of microorganisms and their products from the root canal system to the periodontal region, compromising periapical healing. Application of pulsed CO_2 laser radiation on root canals with AgCl fibers can open dentin tubules and fuse hydroxyapatite; however, further development in fiber technology is necessary to achieve predictable results.[107]

10.6-μm Carbon Dioxide Laser

Unlike the other CO_2 wavelengths, the 10.6-μm CO_2 laser has been studied not only in vitro but also in vivo, because the system is more commercially available for clinical use.

In the field of caries prevention, many studies have been conducted, and these have verified the potential effect of 10.6-μm CO_2 laser irradiation on the reduction in enamel solubility[108-112] without compromise of pulp vitality.[110] Much higher energy levels, however, were needed compared with those in studies using the 9.3- or 9.6-μm laser.

The 10.6-μm CO_2 laser has been extensively used in dentistry for management of soft tissue problems (diseases of periodontal tissue or oral mucosa). The effects on oral soft tissue disease showed some advantages for the CO_2 laser, such as a greatly reduced operating time, simpler procedure, decreased postsurgical infection, and decreased or eliminated wound contracture and wound scarring (in soft tissue preprosthetic surgery).[113]

Many authors have referred to the 10.6-μm CO_2 laser as an important tool in the treatment of oral lesions, such as carcinomas, carcinomas,[114] premalignant lesions,[114-118] and hemangiomas.[116,119] The CO_2 laser allows precise excision of the lesion and involved mucosa and provides an excellent specimen for histologic verification of the margins.[115,120] The same would apply to 9.3- and 9.6-μm lasers if either were readily commercially available with appropriate settings for the desired surgery.

Evaluating the effects of the CO_2 laser on underlying bone tissue irradiated during biopsy procedures, Krause et al.[121] verified that all specimens, regardless of tissue composition, energy density, or number of beam passes, exhibited a distinct layer of residual carbonized tissue, a zone of thermal necrosis characterized by tissue coagulation, and a zone of tissue exhibiting thermal damage. On the other hand, Frentzen et al.[122] showed that histologically, an osteotomy using 80-μsec CO_2 laser pulses resulted in only minimal damage to bone ablated at the specified parameters, and that this laser procedure might have advantages over mechanical instruments. Prevention of significant peripheral damage is possible if the thermal relaxation times are matched with the pulse duration of the laser.

Pinheiro et al.[123] investigated a possible means of reducing the thermal damage during CO_2 laser surgery of the oral mucosa. Tissue damage was evaluated by studying changes in mast cells and in the activity of lactate and succinate dehydrogenase. Results revealed a significant association with greater levels of immediate mast cell degranulation for uncooled laser wounds, but not precooled laser wounds, over those seen in scalpel wounds.

Lin et al.[124] reported on the effect of the 10.6-μm CO_2 wavelength on tooth permeability, using a CW laser and a newly developed DP-bioactive glass paste (DPGP) to fuse or bridge tooth cracks or fracture lines. Both the DPGP and tooth enamel have relatively strong absorption bands at 10.6-μm Therefore, under CO_2 laser irradiation, DPGP and enamel should both achieve an effective absorption and melt together. Morphologic analysis revealed that the melted masses and the platelike crystals formed a tight chemical bond between the enamel and the DPGP. This technique of DPGP application associated with laser irradiation is expected to be a successful alternative to the treatment of tooth cracks or fractures, but further studies are required to confirm this hypothesis.

Clinical Studies on 9.3- and 9.6-μm Carbon Dioxide Lasers

Recent pulpal safety studies on each of the 9.3- and 9.6-μm wavelengths with conditions suitable for enamel ablation and caries prevention treatments showed no signs of pulpal damage whatsoever.[125,126] The studies were done on vital teeth that were scheduled for extraction, and detailed histologic analysis was done on the extracted teeth.

Results of clinical studies on caries prevention in humans, using a 9.6-μm laser with appropriate pulse and energy characteristics, were recently reported. The first study was done on smooth surfaces adjacent to orthodontic brackets on teeth scheduled for extraction.[127] After laser treatment, teeth were left in the mouth for 4 weeks or 12 weeks. Extracted teeth were sectioned and assessed quantitatively for mineral loss. The laser-treated group of teeth demonstrated an 87% reduction in mineral loss compared with the non–laser-treated control teeth. The patients all used a fluoridated toothpaste daily. A subsequent study was done using a specially designed handpiece and the same 9.6-μm laser on occlusal surfaces of children's teeth.[128] The teeth were treated with fluoride varnish and the laser, with the control group receiving fluoride varnish only. Caries was assessed at baseline and over time using the International Caries Detection and Assessment System (ICDAS). Caries progressed on average over a period of 1 year in the teeth treated only with fluoride, showing an increase in mean ICDAS score of approximately 60%. In the laser plus fluoride group lesions, the mean ICDAS score decreased by approximately 25%. These clinical studies have confirmed the ability of 9.3- or 9.6-μm laser irradiation with appropriate pulse and energy conditions to inhibit caries progression in human mouths.

In 2013 a U.S. company launched a new 9.3-μm carbon dioxide laser with pulse characteristics, energy levels, and all other parameters developed on the basis of the foregoing laboratory and clinical studies. Of importance, the pulse durations and wavelength are optimal for ablation as well as for caries prevention. The delivery system is designed so that the dentist can readily ablate carious or sound enamel or dentin and, by switching modes, carry out soft tissue surgery equally efficiently. This laser is cleared by the FDA for both hard and soft tissue uses.

Conclusions

Current laser research focuses on OCT in dental diagnosis and on photoactivated disinfection in daily practice. CO_2 lasers also have been shown to be effective in many fields of dentistry, with advantages such as less bleeding, selective removal of tissue, shorter operating time, and reduced postoperative pain. A more recently marketed 9.3-μm carbon dioxide laser shows great promise for ablation of hard tissue, soft tissue surgery, and potentially caries-preventive treatments. Further studies are needed to demonstrate how well this new laser, or others like it, will perform these tasks. Other wavelengths, such as those for the erbium lasers, also have been widely investigated but are not the subject of this chapter.

References

1. Gimbel C: Optical coherence tomography diagnostic imaging, *Gen Dent* 56:750–757, 2008.
2. Otis LL, Everett MJ, Sathyam US, Colston BW Jr: Optical coherence tomography: a new imaging technology for dentistry, *J Am Dent Assoc* 131:511–514, 2000.
3. Colston BW Jr, Everett MJ, Da Silva LB, et al.: Imaging of hard- and soft-tissue structure in the oral cavity by optical coherence tomography, *Appl Opt* 37:3582–3585, 1998.
4. Huang D, Swanson EA, Lin CP, et al.: Optical coherence tomography, *Science* 254:1178–1181, 1991.
5. Hee MR, Puliafito CA, Wong C, et al.: Quantitative assessment of macular edema with optical coherence tomography, *Arch Ophthalmol* 113:1019–1029, 1995.
6. Coker JG, Duker JS: Macular disease and optical coherence tomography, *Curr Opin Ophthalmol* 7:33–38, 1996.
7. Everett MJ, Colston BW, Da Silva LB, Otis LL: *Fiber optic based optical coherence tomography (OCT) for dental applications*, paper presented at the Fourth Pacific Northwest Fiber Optic Sensor Workshop, 1998, Portland, Ore.
8. de Araujo RE, de Melo LSA, Freitas AZ, et al.: Applying optical coherence tomography in dental restoration, *IEEE Xplore*, [serial online] 2005. http://ieeexplore.ieee.org.
9. Amaechi BT, Higham SM, Podoleanu AG, et al.: Use of optical coherence tomography for assessment of dental caries: quantitative procedure, *J Oral Rehabil* 28:1092–1093, 2001.
10. Fried D, Xie J, Shafi S, et al.: Imaging caries lesions and lesion progression with polarization sensitive optical coherence tomography, *J Biomed Opt* 7(4):618–627, 2002.
11. Lee C, Hsu DJ, Le MH, et al.: Non-destructive measurement of demineralization and remineralization in the occlusal pits and fissures of extracted 3 molars with PS-OCT, *Proc Soc Photo Opt Instrum Eng* 7162(1): pii: 71620V, Mar 6, 2009.
12. Jones RS, Darling CL, Featherstone JD, Fried D: Remineralization of in vitro dental caries assessed with polarization-sensitive optical coherence tomography, *J Biomed Opt* 11(1):014016, 2006.
13. Nee A, Chan K, Kang H, et al.: Longitudinal monitoring of demineralization peripheral to orthodontic brackets using cross polarization optical coherence tomography, *J Dent* 42:547–555, 2014.
14. Ngaotheppitak P, Darling CL, Fried D: Measurement of the severity of natural smooth surface (interproximal) caries lesions with polarization sensitive optical coherence tomography, *Lasers Surg Med* 37:78–88, 2005.
15. Chong SL, Darling CL, Fried D: Nondestructive measurement of the inhibition of demineralization on smooth surfaces using polarization-sensitive optical coherence tomography, *Lasers Surg Med* 39:422–427, 2007.
16. Can AM, Darling CL, Fried D: High-resolution PS-OCT of enamel remineralization, *Proc Soc Photo Opt Instrum Eng* 6843:68430T1–68430T7, 2008.
17. Manesh SK, Darling CL, Fried D: Polarization-sensitive optical coherence tomography for the nondestructive assessment of the remineralization of dentin, *J Biomed Opt* 14(4):044002, 2009.
18. Manesh SK, Darling CL, Fried D: Nondestructive assessment of dentin demineralization using polarization-sensitive optical coherence tomography after exposure to fluoride and laser irradiation, *J Biomed Mater Res B Appl Biomater* 90(2):802–812, 2009.
19. Manesh SK, Darling CL, Fried D: Assessment of dentin remineralization with PS-OCT, *Proc Soc Photo Opt Instrum Eng* 7162: pii: 71620W, Jan 1, 2009.
20. Manesh SK, Darling CL, Fried D: Imaging natural and artificial demineralization on dentin surfaces with polarization sensitive optical coherence tomography, *Proc Soc Photo Opt Instrum Eng* 6843: pii: 68430M, Jan 1, 2008.
21. Le MH, Darling CL, Fried D: Methods for calculating the severity of demineralization on tooth surfaces from PS-OCT scans, *Proc Soc Photo Opt Instrum Eng* 7162(1):71620U, Feb 18, 2009.
22. Stahl J, Kang H, Fried D: Imaging simulated secondary caries lesions with cross polarization OCT, *Proc Soc Photo Opt Instrum Eng* 7549:754905, Mar 5, 2010.
23. Louie T, Lee C, Hsu D, et al.: Clinical assessment of early tooth demineralization using polarization sensitive optical coherence tomography, *Lasers Surg Med* 42:738–745, 2010.
24. Kang H, Darling CL, Fried D: Repair of artificial lesions using an acidic remineralization model monitored with cross-polarization optical coherence tomography, *Proc Soc Photo Opt Instrum Eng* 7884(78840Q):78840B_1, Jan 23, 2011.
25. Darling CL, Staninec M, Chan KH, et al.: Remineralization of root caries monitored using cross-polarization optical coherence tomography, *Proc Soc Photo Opt Instrum Eng* 8208, Feb 9, 2012. http://dx.doi.org/10.1117/12.914633.
26. Kang H, Darling CL, Fried D: Nondestructive monitoring of the repair of natural occlusal lesions using cross-polarization optical coherence tomography, *Proc Soc Photo Opt Instrum Eng* 8208:82080X, Feb 9, 2012.
27. Kang H, Chan K, Darling CL, Fried D: Monitoring the remineralization of early simulated lesions using a pH cycling model with CP-OCT, *Proc Soc Photo Opt Instrum Eng* 8566, Mar 25, 2013. http://dx.doi.org/10.1117/12.2011016.
28. Chan KH, Chan AC, Fried WA, et al.: Use of 2D images of depth and integrated reflectivity to represent the severity of demineralization in crosspolarization optical coherence tomography, *J Biophotonics*, 2013 Dec 5. http://dx.doi.org/10.1002/jbio.201300137 [Epub ahead of print.].
29. Fried D, Staninec M, Darling CL, et al.: Clinical monitoring of early caries lesions using cross polarization optical coherence tomography, *Proc Soc Photo Opt Instrum Eng* 8566, Mar 25, 2013, http://dx.doi.org/10.1117/12.2011014.

30. Shemesh H, van Soest G, Wu MK, et al.: The ability of optical coherence tomography to characterize the root canal walls, *J Endod* 33:1369–1373, 2007.

31. Shemesh H, van Soest G, Wu MK, Wesselink PR: Diagnosis of vertical root fractures with optical coherence tomography, *J Endod* 34:739–742, 2008.

32. Schoop U, Kluger W, Moritz A, et al.: Bactericidal effect of different laser systems in the deep layers of dentin, *Lasers Surg Med* 35:111–116, 2004.

33. Dickers B, Lamard L, Peremans A, et al.: Temperature rise during photo-activated disinfection of root canals, *Lasers Med Sci* 24:81–85, 2009.

34. Ishikawa I, Aoki A, Takasaki AA: Potential applications of erbium:YAG laser in periodontics, *J Periodont Res* 39:275–285, 2004.

35. Wainwright M: Photodynamic antimicrobial chemotherapy (PACT), *J Antimicrob Chemother* 42:13–28, 1998.

36. Bhatti M, MacRobert A, Meghji S, et al.: A study of the uptake of toluidine blue O by *Porphyromonas gingivalis* and the mechanism of lethal photosensitization,, *Photochem Photobiol* 68:370–376, 1998.

37. Bhatti M, Nair SP, Macrobert AJ, et al.: Identification of photolabile outer membrane proteins of, *Porphyromonas gingivalis, Curr Microbiol* 43:96–99, 2001.

38. Harris F, Chatfield LK, Phoenix DA: Phenothiazinium based photosensitisers—photodynamic agents with a multiplicity of cellular targets and clinical applications, *Curr Drug Targets* 6:615–627, 2005.

39. Christodoulides N, Nikolidakis D, Chondros P, et al.: Photodynamic therapy as an adjunct to non-surgical periodontal treatment: a randomized, controlled clinical trial, *J Periodontol* 79:1638–1644, 2008.

40. Garcez AS, Nunez SC, Hamblin MR, Ribeiro MS: Antimicrobial effects of photodynamic therapy on patients with necrotic pulps and periapical lesion, *J Endod* 34:138–142, 2008.

41. Giusti JS, Santos-Pinto L, Pizzolito AC, et al.: Antimicrobial photodynamic action on dentin using a light-emitting diode light source, *Photomed Laser Surg* 26:281–287, 2008.

42. Hayek RR, Araujo NS, Gioso MA, et al.: Comparative study between the effects of photodynamic therapy and conventional therapy on microbial reduction in ligature-induced peri-implantitis in dogs, *J Periodontol* 76:1275–1281, 2005.

43. Smetana Z, Ben-Hur E, Mendelson E, et al.: Herpes simplex virus proteins are damaged following photodynamic inactivation with phthalocyanines, *J Photochem Photobiol B* 44:77–83, 1998.

44. Malik Z, Hanania J, Nitzan Y: Bactericidal effects of photoactivated porphyrins: an alternative approach to antimicrobial drugs, *J Photochem Photobiol B* 5:281–293, 1990.

45. Chan Y, Lai CH: Bactericidal effects of different laser wavelengths on periodontopathic germs in photodynamic therapy, *Lasers Med Sci* 18:51–55, 2003.

46. Komerik N, Nakanishi H, MacRobert AJ, et al.: In vivo killing of *Porphyromonas gingivalis* by toluidine blue–mediated photosensitization in an animal model, *Antimicrob Agents Chemother* 47:932–940, 2003.

47. Bevilacqua IM, Nicolau RA, Khouri S, et al.: The impact of photodynamic therapy on the viability of *Streptococcus mutans* in a planktonic culture,, *Photomed Laser Surg* 25:513–518, 2007.

48. Prates RA, Yamada AM Jr, Suzuki LC, et al.: Bactericidal effect of malachite green and red laser on, *Actinobacillus actinomycetemcomitans, J Photochem Photobiol B* 86:70–76, 2007.

49. Wood S, Nattress B, Kirkham J, et al.: An in vitro study of the use of photodynamic therapy for the treatment of natural oral plaque biofilms formed in vivo, *J Photochem Photobiol B* 50:1–7, 1999.

50. Soukos NS, Hamblin MR, Hasan T: The effect of charge on cellular uptake and phototoxicity of polylysine chlorin(e6) conjugates, *Photochem Photobiol* 65:723–729, 1997.

51. Jori G, Fabris C, Soncin M, et al.: Photodynamic therapy in the treatment of microbial infections: basic principles and perspective applications, *Lasers Surg Med* 38:468–481, 2006.

52. Chebath-Taub D, Steinberg D, Featherstone JD, Feuerstein O: Influence of blue light on Streptococcus mutans re-organization in biofilm, *J Photochem Photobiol B* 116:75–78, 2012.

53. Feuerstein O, Moreinos D, Steinberg D: Synergic antibacterial effect between visible light and hydrogen peroxide on, *Streptococcus mutans, J Antimicrob Chemother* 57(5):872–876, 2006.

54. Feuerstein O: Light therapy: complementary antibacterial treatment of oral biofilm, *Adv Dent Res* 24(2):103–107, 2012.

55. Dostalova T, Jelinkova H, Krejsa O, et al.: Dentin and pulp response to erbium:YAG laser ablation: a preliminary evaluation of human teeth, *J Clin Laser Med Surg* 15:117–121, 1997.

56. Keller U, Hibst R: Experimental studies of the application of the Er:YAG laser on dental hard substances. II. Light microscopic and SEM investigations, *Lasers Surg Med* 9:345–351, 1989.

57. Dostalova T, Jelinkova H, Kucerova H: Er:YAG laser ablation: evaluation after two-years-long clinical treatment, *Proc SPIE* 3248:23–32, 1998.

58. Komori T, Yokoyama K, Takato T, Matsumoto K: Clinical application of the erbium:YAG laser for apicoectomy, *J Endod* 23:748–750, 1997.

59. Dayem RN: [Withdrawn] Evaluation of the ablation efficacy and morphology of some hard tissues irradiated with different types and modes of laser, *Lasers Med Sci*, 2007 Oct 19 [Epub ahead of print.]

60. Tsen KT, Tsen SW, Chang CL, et al.: Inactivation of viruses by coherent excitations with a low power visible femtosecond laser, *Virol J* 4:50, 2007.

61. Dela Rosa A, Sarma AV, Le CQ, et al.: Peripheral thermal and mechanical damage to dentin with microsecond and submicrosecond 9.6 μm, 2.79 μm, and 0.355 μm laser pulses, *Lasers Surg Med* 35:214–228, 2004.

62. Koort HJ, Frentzen M: *The effect of TEA-CO2-laser on dentine*, paper presented at the Third International Congress on Lasers in Dentistry, 1992, Salt Lake City.

63. Sheth KK, Staninec M, Sarma AV, Fried D: Selective targeting of protein, water, and mineral in dentin using UV and IR pulse lasers: the effect on the bond strength to composite restorative materials, *Lasers Surg Med* 35:245–253, 2004.

64. Zach L, Cohen G: Pulp response to externally applied heat, *Oral Surg Oral Med Oral Pathol* 19:515–530, 1965.

65. Boehm R, Rich J, Webster J, Janke S: Thermal stress effects and surface cracking associated with laser use on human teeth, *J Biomech Eng* 77:189–194, 1977.

66. Sandford MA, Walsh LJ: Differential thermal effects of pulsed vs. continuous CO2 laser radiation on human molar teeth, *J Clin Laser Med Surg* 12:139–142, 1994.

67. Shariati S, Pogrel MA, Marshall GW Jr, White JM: Structural changes in dentin induced by high energy, continuous wave carbon dioxide laser, *Lasers Surg Med* 13:543–547, 1993.

68. Van Gemert MJ, Welch AJ: Time constants in thermal laser medicine, *Lasers Surg Med* 9:405–421, 1989.

69. Kimura Y, Wilder-Smith P, Arrastia-Jitosho AM, et al.: Effects of nanosecond pulsed Nd:YAG laser irradiation on dentin resistance to artificial caries-like lesions, *Lasers Surg Med* 20:15–21, 1997.

70. Grad L, Mozina J: Laser pulse shape influence on optically induced dynamic processes, *Appl Surf Sci* 127–129, 1998.

71. Papadopoulos DN, Papagiakoumou E, Khabbaz MG, et al.: *Experimental study of Er:YAG laser ablation of hard dental tissue at various lasing parameters*, paper presented at the 7th International Conference on Laser Ablation, 2003, Crete.

72. Nishimoto Y, Otsuki M, Yamauti M, et al.: Effect of pulse duration of Er:YAG laser on dentin ablation, *Dent Mater J* 27:433–439, 2008.

73. Lukač M, Marinček M, Grad L: Dental laser drilling: achieving optimum ablation with the latest generation Fidelis laser system, *J Laser Health Acad* 2, 2007.

74. Lizarelli RF, Kurachi C, Misoguti L, Bagnato VS: A comparative study of nanosecond and picosecond laser ablation in enamel: morphological aspects, *J Clin Laser Med Surg* 18:151–157, 2000.

75. Lizarelli RF, Kurachi C, Misoguti L, Bagnato VS: Characterization of enamel and dentin response to Nd:YAG picosecond laser ablation, *J Clin Laser Med Surg* 17:127–131, 1999.

76. Lizarelli RF, Moriyama LT, Bagnato VS: Temperature response in the pulpal chamber of primary human teeth exposed to Nd:YAG laser using a picosecond pulsed regime, *Photomed Laser Surg* 24:610–615, 2006.

77. McDonald A, Claffey N, Pearson G, et al.: The effect of Nd:YAG pulse duration on dentine crater depth,, *J Dent* 29:43–53, 2001.

78. Melcer J, Farcy JC, Hellas Gand Badiane M: *Preparation of cavities using a TEA CO2 laser*, paper presented at the Third International Congress on Lasers in Dentistry, 1992, Salt Lake City, Utah.

79. Lukač M, Marinček M, Grad L: Super VSP Er:YAG pulses for fast and precise cavity preparation, *J Oral Laser Appl* 4, 2004.

80. Delfino CS, Souza-Zaroni WC, Corona SA, et al.: Effect of Er:YAG laser energy on the morphology of enamel/adhesive system interface, *Appl Surf Sci* 252, 2006.

81. Fried D, Featherstone JD, Le CQ, Fan K: Dissolution studies of bovine dental enamel surfaces modified by high-speed scanning ablation with a lambda = 9.3-μm TEA CO2 laser, *Lasers Surg Med* 38:837–845, 2006.

82. Wheeler CR, Fried D, Featherstone JD, et al.: Irradiation of dental enamel with Q-switched lambda = 355-nm laser pulses: surface morphology, fluoride adsorption, and adhesion to composite resin, *Lasers Surg Med* 32:310–317, 2003.

83. Anic I, Miletic I, Krmek SJ, et al.: Vibrations produced during erbium:yttrium-aluminum-garnet laser irradiation, *Lasers Med Sci* 24:697–701, 2009.

84. Gonzalez CD, Zakariasen KL, Dederich DN, Pruhs RJ: Potential preventive and therapeutic hard-tissue applications of CO2, Nd:YAG and argon lasers in dentistry: a review, *ASDC J Dent Child* 63:196–207, 1996.

85. Wigdor HA, Walsh JT Jr, Featherstone JD, et al.: Lasers in dentistry, *Lasers Surg Med* 16:103–133, 1995.

86. Frentzen M, Koort HJ: Lasers in dentistry: new possibilities with advancing laser technology? *Int Dent J* 40:323–332, 1990.

87. Zuerlein MJ, Fried D, Featherstone JD: Modeling the modification depth of carbon dioxide laser-treated dental enamel, *Lasers Surg Med* 25:335–347, 1999.

88. McCormack SM, Fried D, Featherstone JD, et al.: Scanning electron microscope observations of CO2 laser effects on dental enamel, *J Dent Res* 74:1702–1708, 1995.

89. McCormack SM, Fried D, Featherstone JD, et al.: Scanning electron microscope observations of CO2 laser effects on dental enamel, *J Dent Res* 74:1702–1708, 1995.

90. Darling CL, Fried D: Real-time near IR (1310 nm) imaging of CO2 laser ablation of enamel, *Opt Express* 16:2685–2693, 2008.

91. Kimura Y, Takahashi-Sakai K, Wilder-Smith P, et al.: Morphological study of the effects of CO2 laser emitted at 9.3 μm on human dentin, *J Clin Laser Med Surg* 18:197–202, 2000.

92. Featherstone JD, Barrett-Vespone NA, Fried D, et al.: CO2 laser inhibitor of artificial caries-like lesion progression in dental enamel, *J Dent Res* 77:1397–1403, 1998.

93. Takahashi K, Kimura Y, Matsumoto K: Morphological and atomic analytical changes after CO2 laser irradiation emitted at 9.3 microns on human dental hard tissues, *J Clin Laser Med Surg* 16:167–173, 1998.

94. Konishi N, Fried D, Staninec M, Featherstone JD: Artificial caries removal and inhibition of artificial secondary caries by pulsed CO2 laser irradiation, *Am J Dent* 12:213–216, 1999.

95. Can AM, Darling CL, Ho C, Fried D: Non-destructive assessment of inhibition of demineralization in dental enamel irradiated by a lambda = 9.3-micron CO2 laser at ablative irradiation intensities with PS-OCT, *Lasers Surg Med* 40:342–349, 2008.

96. Wilder-Smith P, Dang J, Kurosaki T, Neev J: The influence of laser parameter configurations at 9.3 microns on incisional and collateral effects in soft tissue, *Oral Surg Med Pathol Radiol Endod* 84:22–27, 1997.

97. Rodrigues LK, Nobre-dos-Santos M, Pereira D, et al.: Carbon dioxide laser in dental caries prevention, *J Dent* 32:531–540, 2004.

98. Kantorowitz Z, Featherstone JD, Fried D: Caries prevention by CO2 laser treatment: dependency on the number of pulses used, *J Am Dent Assoc* 129:585–591, 1998.

99. Viscovini RC, Cruz FC, Telles EM, et al.: Frequency stabilization of waveguide CO2 laser by a digital technique, *Int J Infrared Millimeter Waves* 22:757–772, 2001.

100. Slutzky-Goldberg I, Peleg O, Liberman R, et al.: The effect of CO2 laser on the microhardness of human dental hard tissues compared with that of the high-speed drill, *Photomed Laser Surg* 26:65–68, 2008.

101. Nair PN, Baltensperger M, Luder HU, Eyrich GK: Observations on pulpal response to carbon dioxide laser drilling of dentine in healthy human third molars, *Lasers Med Sci* 19:240–247, 2005.

102. Wigdor HA, Walsh JT Jr: Histologic analysis of the effect on dental pulp of a 9.6-μm CO2 laser, *Lasers Surg Med* 30:261–266, 2002.

103. Rodrigues LK, Nobre-dos-Santos M, Featherstone JD: In situ mineral loss inhibition by CO2 laser and fluoride, *J Dent Res* 85:617–621, 2006.

104. Zuerlein MJ, Fried D, Featherstone JD: Modeling the modification depth of carbon dioxide laser-treated dental enamel, *Lasers Surg Med* 25:335–347, 1999.

105. Deppe H, Horch HH: Laser applications in oral surgery and implant dentistry, *Lasers Med Sci* 22:217–221, 2007.

106. Gouw-Soares S, Stabholz A, Lage-Marques JL, et al.: Comparative study of dentine permeability after apicectomy and surface treatment with 9.6 micron TEA CO2 and Er:YAG laser irradiation, *J Clin Laser Med Surg* 22:129–139, 2004.

107. Onal B, Ertl T, Siebert G, Muller G: Preliminary report on the application of pulsed CO2 laser radiation on root canals with AgCl fibers: a scanning and transmission electron microscopic study, *J Endod* 19:272–276, 1993.

108. Lakshmi A, Shobha D, Lakshminarayanan L: Prevention of caries by pulsed CO2 laser pre-treatment of enamel: an in vitro study, *J Indian Soc Pedod Prev Dent* 19:152–156, 2001.

109. Klein AL, Rodrigues LK, Eduardo CP, et al.: Caries inhibition around composite restorations by pulsed carbon dioxide laser application, *Eur J Oral Sci* 113:239–244, 2005.

110. Steiner-Oliveira C, Rodrigues LK, Soares LE, et al.: Chemical, morphological and thermal effects of 10.6-μm CO_2 laser on the inhibition of enamel demineralization, *Dent Mater J* 25: 455–462, 2006.

111. Tagliaferro EP, Rodrigues LK, Nobre-dos-Santos M, et al.: Combined effects of carbon dioxide laser and fluoride on demineralized primary enamel: an in vitro study, *Caries Res* 41:74–76, 2007.

112. Steiner-Oliveira C, Rodrigues LK, Lima EB, Nobre-dos-Santos M: Effect of the CO_2 laser combined with fluoridated products on the inhibition of enamel demineralization, *J Contemp Dent Pract* 9:113–121, 2008.

113. Kato J, Wijeyeweera RL: The effect of CO_2 laser irradiation on oral soft tissue problems in children in Sri Lanka, *Photomed Laser Surg* 25:264–268, 2007.

114. Flynn MB, White M, Tabah RJ: Use of carbon dioxide laser for the treatment of premalignant lesions of the oral mucosa, *J Surg Oncol* 37:232–234, 1988.

115. Strong MS, Vaughan CW, Healy GB, et al.: Transoral management of localized carcinoma of the oral cavity using the CO_2 laser, *Laryngoscope* 89:897–905, 1979.

116. Luomanen M: Experience with a carbon dioxide laser for removal of benign oral soft-tissue lesions, *Proc Finn Dent Soc* 88:49–55, 1992.

117. Van der Hem PS, Egges M, van der Wal JE, Roodenburg JL: CO_2 laser evaporation of oral lichen planus, *Int J Oral Maxillofac Surg* 37:630–633, 2008.

118. Pinheiro AL, Frame JW: Surgical management of premalignant lesions of the oral cavity with the CO_2 laser, *Braz Dent J* 7: 103–108, 1996.

119. Apfelberg DB, Maser MR, Lash H, White DN: Benefits of the CO_2 laser in oral hemangioma excision, *Plast Reconstr Surg* 75:46–50, 1985.

120. Bornstein MM, Winzap-Kalin C, Cochran DL, Buser D: The CO_2 laser for excisional biopsies of oral lesions: a case series study, *Int J Periodont Restorative Dent* 25:221–229, 2005.

121. Krause LS, Cobb CM, Rapley JW, et al.: Laser irradiation of bone. I. An in vitro study concerning the effects of the CO_2 laser on oral mucosa and subjacent bone, *J Periodontol* 68:872–880, 1997.

122. Frentzen M, Gotz W, Ivanenko M, et al.: Osteotomy with 80-μs CO_2 laser pulses: histological results, *Lasers Med Sci* 18: 119–124, 2003.

123. Pinheiro AL, Browne RM, Frame JW, Matthews JB: Assessment of thermal damage in precooled CO_2 laser wounds using biological markers, *Br J Oral Maxillofac Surg* 31:239–243, 1993.

124. Lin CP, Tseng YC, Lin FH, et al.: Treatment of tooth fracture by medium-energy CO_2 laser and DP-bioactive glass paste: the interaction of enamel and DP-bioactive glass paste during irradiation by CO_2 laser, *Biomaterials* 22:489–496, 2001.

125. Goodis HE, Fried D, Gansky S, et al.: Pulpal safety of 9.6 microm TEA CO_2 laser used for caries prevention, *Lasers Surg Med* 35:104–110, 2004.

126. Staninec M, Darling CL, Goodis HE, et al.: Pulpal effects of enamel ablation with a microsecond pulsed lambda = 9.3-micron CO_2 laser, *Lasers Surg Med* 41:256–263, 2009.

127. Rechmann P, Fried D, Le CQ, et al.: Caries inhibition in vital teeth using 9.6-μm CO_2-laser irradiation, *J Biomed Opt* 16(7):071405, 2011.

128. Rechmann P, Charland DA, Rechmann BM, et al.: In-vivo occlusal caries prevention by pulsed CO_2 laser and fluoride varnish treatment—a clinical pilot study, *Lasers Surg Med* 45:302–310, 2013.

Glossary

DONALD J. COLUZZI

A

Ablation Removal of tissue using thermal energy. Also called *vaporization,* although not technically correct.

absorption Transfer of radiant energy into the target tissue, resulting in a change in that tissue.

absorption coefficient Measurement of the amount of absorption of laser energy, expressed as a relative number per square centimeter (cm^2).

active medium Material within the optical cavity that, when stimulated and amplified into a population inversion, will emit laser energy. This medium, which can be a solid, liquid, gas, or combination of gases, may be incorporated as an ion, molecule, crystal, or semiconductor wafer. Also called *lasant.*

aiming beam Beam of visible light delivered coaxially along the delivery system so that the invisible laser radiation can be detected.

amplification Process that occurs within the optical resonator whereby stimulated emission produces a population inversion.

articulated arm Laser delivery system that uses segments of a hollow tube coupled with right-angle mirrors and allows propagation of the laser beam along its length.

attenuation Observed decline in energy as a beam passes through an absorbing or scattering medium.

average power Expression of the average of the peak power and the laser "off" time.

B

beam Any collection of radiant electromagnetic waves, which may be divergent, convergent, or collimated.

C

carbon dioxide (CO_2) laser Laser with active medium composed of helium, CO_2, nitrogen, and small amounts of hydrogen. The active medium is excited by a pumping mechanism (usually an electrical discharge), and the emission is caused by the population inversion of CO_2 molecules in the range of 9300 to 10,600 nm, in the far-infrared thermal portion of the electromagnetic spectrum.

chopped-pulse mode See **gated-pulse mode.**

chromophore Light-absorbing compound or molecule normally occurring in tissues that is an attractor of specific wavelengths of laser energy.

cladding Thin coating that surrounds the core of glass in a fiberoptic delivery system. The cladding maintains the propagation of the laser beam along the glass and is surrounded by a thicker jacket to aid in flexibility.

coagulation Observed denaturation of soft tissue proteins that occurs at 60° C. At this temperature, hemostasis can occur.

coherence State in which all of the radiant waves in a light beam are traveling in phase, both temporally and spatially.

collimation State in which all electromagnetic waves are parallel, with virtually no divergence.

contact mode Direct touching of the laser delivery system to the target tissue. The opposite is *noncontact mode.*

continuous mode A manner of applying laser energy in which beam power density remains constant over time. Also called *continuous-wave (CW) mode.*

D

delivery system Manner in which laser energy is transferred to the target tissue. Dental lasers have fiberoptic, hollow-waveguide, and articulated-arm systems. Some of these systems include additional laser tips.

diode laser Laser with active medium composed of an array of semiconductor wafers, pumped with electrical current; individual beams are collected and focused into a single beam. The emission wavelengths can range from the visible into the near-infrared thermal portion of the electromagnetic spectrum.

divergence Observed degree of spread of the laser beam as it increases its distance from the emission aperture or focal point. The opposite of *collimation.*

doping Addition of an element to the laser crystal, resulting in a specific wavelength of energy emitted—for example, doping an yttrium-aluminum-garnet (YAG) crystal with the rare earth element erbium (Er).

duty cycle See **emission cycle.**

E

electromagnetic spectrum Graphic representation of all forms of radiant energy, from gamma rays to radio waves, usually depicted with increasing wavelength and/or decreasing frequency.

emission cycle The ratio, usually expressed as a percentage, of the individual pulse duration to the total time of that pulse plus the interval between it and the next pulse. For example, if the laser is operated at 10 Hz with a pulse duration of 0.01 second, there is a 0.09-second interval, for a total time of 0.1 second. The emission cycle would thus be 10%. Also known as *duty cycle.*

energy Ability to perform work, expressed in joules (J).

energy density Measurement of energy per unit area, usually expressed as joules per square centimeter (J/cm^2). Also called *fluence.*

erbium (Er) Rare earth element that is used to dope a crystal of yttrium-aluminum-garnet (YAG) or yttrium-scandium-gallium-garnet (YSGG).

excited state Atom or molecule with electron orbit(s) in an energized or higher level than the resting state. The pumping mechanism is responsible for exciting the electrons into the higher level.

external power source Energy system outside the laser's optical resonator that provides for the excitation and stimulation of the active medium. Also called *pumping mechanism.*

extinction length Thickness of a substance in which 98% of the incident laser energy is fully absorbed.

F

fiberoptic Delivery system composed of a glass fiber used to propagate the laser beam along its length. The glass is surrounded by cladding and a jacket or layers of jackets.

fluence See **energy density.**

focal length Distance between the focusing lens and the focal point, which is the place where the laser beam's power and energy are delivered at maximum value. It usually is measured in millimeters (mm). With bare, fiberoptically delivered laser beams, the focal length is essentially zero, because the greatest emission is at the end of the fiber, used in contact with the tissue. In other delivery systems, such as an articulated arm, the focal point usually is one to several millimeters from the end of the delivery system.

free-running pulsed mode Laser operating mode in which the emission is truly pulsed and not gated. A flashlamp is used as the external energy source so that very short pulse durations and peak powers of thousands of watts are possible. A laser operating in this mode cannot be operated in continuous-wave mode.

frequency Number of oscillations or cycles of a wave, usually expressed per second.

G

gated-pulse mode Laser operating mode in which the emission is a repetitive "on and off" cycle. The laser beam is actually emitted continuously, but a mechanical shutter or electronic controls "chop" the laser beam into pulses. Also called *chopped-pulse mode.*

H

handpiece Instrument attached to the distal portion of the delivery system that contains the focusing lens system. In some cases, an additional tip is attached to the handpiece to complete the assembly.

hertz (Hz) For lasers, the number of pulses per second, or *pulse rate,* also known as *repetition rate.* Frequency also can be expressed in hertz, but this unit is not used in laser science.

hollow waveguide Delivery system that uses a flexible hollow tube with a mirrored inner surface to propagate the laser beam along its length.

I

intensity See **power density.**

irradiance See **power density.**

J

jacket Thick, flexible coating surrounding the glass core of a fiberoptic that protects the core and adds to the flexibility of the delivery system.

joule (J) A unit of expression of energy.

L

lasant See **active medium.**

laser Device that generates a highly concentrated light beam, with various medical and other uses, through light amplification by stimulated emission of radiation. The basic components of a laser instrument are the active medium, an external energy source or pumping mechanism, the optical resonator, and the focusing and delivery systems.

laser cavity See **optical resonator.**

M

meter (m) Unit of measurement; used to describe the wavelength of electromagnetic waves. For dental laser wavelengths, *micrometer* (μm) and *nanometer* (nm) units are used. 1 μm = one millionth of a meter (formerly micron [μ]); 1 nm = one billionth of a meter.

monochromatic Characteristic of a laser beam composed of only one wavelength.

N

neodymium (Nd) Rare earth element, used to dope a crystal of yttrium-aluminum-garnet. The emission produced has a wavelength of 1064 nm, in the near-infrared thermal portion of the electromagnetic spectrum.

noncontact mode Delivery system in which there is no contact between the fiber or handpiece or tip and the target tissue. This is the opposite of *contact mode.*

O

optical resonator (optical cavity) Component of a laser containing the active medium in which the population inversion occurs. At each end of the resonator is a reflective surface or mirror that produces amplification and coherence. The distal mirror is partially transmissive; when there is sufficient energy, the beam can exit through that mirror. Also called *laser cavity.*

P

peak power Measurement of power in each pulse.

photon A unit or quantum of radiant energy.

plume Essentially the "smoke" from aerosolization of byproducts caused by the laser-tissue interaction. It is composed of particulate matter, cellular debris, carbonaceous and inorganic materials, and potentially biohazardous products.

population inversion State within the laser cavity in which the quantity of excited species of the active medium exceeds that of the unexcited species (those in the resting, stable state).

power Amount of work performed per unit time, expressed in watts (W).

power density Measurement of power per unit area, usually expressed as watts per square centimeter (W/cm^2); also known as *intensity, irradiance,* and *radiance.*

pulse duration Measurement of the total amount of time that the pulse is emitted. Also called *pulsewidth.*

pulse rate See **hertz (Hz).**

pulsewidth See **pulse duration.**

pumping Process of applying energy to the active medium from an external energy source.

pumping mechanism See **external energy source.**

R

radiant energy Energy transferred by an electromagnetic wave; also called *radiation.*

reflection The returning of electromagnetic radiation by surfaces on which it is incident. The two general types are *specular* reflection, which is generated from a smooth, polished surface, and *diffuse* reflection, which emanates from a rough surface.

refraction The bending of a light ray as the light passes through a medium. Also called *diffraction.*

repetition rate See **hertz (Hz).**

S

scattering Change in direction of the photons as they propagate through tissue, which could lead to increased absorption. This is the dominant effect of near-infrared laser irradiation in soft tissue. Sometimes incorrectly used to indicate *divergence.*

selective photothermolysis Precise laser tissue interaction in which the radiation is well absorbed and the pulse duration is shorter than the thermal relaxation time, which minimizes tissue damage.

Spallation A term commonly used to describe the process by which erbium lasers ablate hard tissue.

spontaneous emission Release of energy (a photon) as the previously excited particle returns to its resting, stable state.

spot size Diameter of the laser beam, which can vary with the focal distance.

stimulated emission Release of energy (a photon) from an already-excited particle by interaction with a particle of identical energy, producing two coherent particles. This process was theorized by Einstein and is the basis for laser operation.

superpulsed mode Variant of gated-pulse mode in which the pulse durations are very short, producing high peak power. Also called *very-short-pulsed mode.*

T

thermal effect For lasers, the absorption of the radiant energy by tissue, producing an increase in temperature.

thermal relaxation time Amount of time required for temperature of the tissue that was raised by absorbed laser radiation to decrease, with cooling, to one half of that value immediately after the laser pulse.

transmission Passage of electromagnetic radiation through any medium without causing a therapeutic effect.

V

vaporization Physical process of converting a solid or liquid into a gas. For dental procedures, it describes conversion of liquid water into steam.

W

watt (W) A unit of power.

wavelength Distance between any two similar points on a wave, for example, from peak to peak; measured in meters.

Y

YAG Acronym describing a solid crystal of yttrium, aluminum, and garnet that can be doped with various rare earth elements (e.g., Nd) and is used as an active medium for some lasers.

YSGG Acronym describing a solid crystal of yttrium, scandium, gallium, and garnet that can be doped with various rare earth elements (e.g., Er) and is used as an active medium for some lasers.

Index

Note: Page numbers followed by "b", "f" and "t" indicate boxes, figures and tables respectively.